Health Informatics
(formerly Computers in Health Care)

Kathryn J. Hannah   Marion J. Ball
Series Editors

Health Informatics Series
(formerly Computers in Health Care)

Series Editors
Kathryn J. Hannah   Marion J. Ball

(continued after index)

Patrick W. O'Carroll   William A. Yasnoff
M. Elizabeth Ward   Laura H. Ripp
Ernest L. Martin
Editors

Public Health Informatics and Information Systems

With a Foreword by David A. Ross, Sc.D.,
Alan R. Hinman, M.D., M.P.H., Kristin Saarlas,
M.P.H., and William H. Foege, M.D., M.P.H.

With 69 Figures

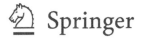 Springer

Patrick W. O'Carroll, M.D., M.P.H.,
F.A.C.P.M.
Centers for Disease Control and
Prevention
Northwest Center for Public Health
Practice
University of Washington School
of Public Health
Seattle, WA 98105, USA
e-mail: ocarroll@u.washington.edu

William A. Yasnoff, M.D., Ph.D.,
F.A.C.M.I.
Public Health Informatics
Institute
Decatur, GA 30030, USA
e-mail: wyasnoff@taskforce.org

M. Elizabeth Ward, R.N., M.N.
Community Health Information
Technology Alliance
Foundation for Health
Care Quality
Seattle, WA 98104, USA

Laura H. Ripp, R.N., M.B.A.,
M.P.H.
Crystal Insights
Government Division of
Metatomix, Inc.
Waltham, MA, 02451 USA

Ernest L. Martin Ph.D., M.B.A.,
F.L.M.I.
Electronic Data Systems
Roswell, GA 30075, USA
and
Truett-McConnell College
Watkinsville, GA 30677, USA

Series Editors:

Kathryn J. Hannah, Ph.D., R.N.
Adjunct Professor, Department
of Community Health Sciences
Faculty of Medicine
The University of Calgary
Calgary, Alberta, T3B 4Z8 Canada

Marion J. Ball, Ed.D.
Vice President, Clinical Solutions
Healthlink, Inc.
2 Hamill Road
Quadrangle 359 West
and
Adjunct Professor
The Johns Hopkins University
School of Nursing
Baltimore, MD 21210, USA

Library of Congress Cataloging-in-Publication Data
Public health informatics and information systems / editors, Patrick W. O'Carroll ... [et al.].
     p. ; cm.— (Health informatics)
  Includes bibliographical references and index.

  1. Public health—Information services.   2. Medical informatics.   I. O'Carroll, Patrick W.
II. Series.
R858 .P83 2002
025.0661—dc21   2002020946

ISBN 978-1-4419-3018-7   e-ISBN 978-0-387-22745-0

The following chapters were produced in whole or in part by officers or employees of the United States Government as part of their official duties, and as such, the text is in the public domain: Chapters 1, 5, 7, 8, 10, 16, 23, 32, and 34.

Printed in the United States of America.

9 8 7 6 5 4 3 2 1

www.springer-ny.com

Springer-Verlag New York Berlin Heidelberg
A member of BertelsmannSpringer Science+Business Media GmbH

Foreword

Let us not go over the old ground, let us rather prepare for what is to come.

—*Marcus Tullius Cicero*

Improvements in the health status of communities depend on effective public health and healthcare infrastructures. These infrastructures are increasingly electronic and tied to the Internet. Incorporating emerging technologies into the service of the community has become a required task for every public health leader.

The revolution in information technology challenges every sector of the health enterprise. Individuals, care providers, and public health agencies can all benefit as we reshape public health through the adoption of new information systems, use of electronic methods for disease surveillance, and reformation of outmoded processes. However, realizing the benefits will be neither easy nor inexpensive.

Technological innovation brings the promise of new ways of improving health. Individuals have become more involved in knowing about, and managing and improving, their own health through Internet access. Similarly, healthcare providers are transforming the ways in which they assess, treat, and document patient care through their use of new technologies. For example, point-of-care and palm-type devices will soon be capable of uniquely identifying patients, supporting patient care, and documenting treatment simply and efficiently.

Although technology offers great hope and promise for innovation in health care and public health, it is by no means certain that every investment in innovative technologies will yield improved health outcomes. Exciting technologies will not be enough by themselves. They must be understood and managed by those committed to improving community health status. Public health officials will have to understand basic principles of information resource management in order to make the appropriate technology choices that will guide the future of their organizations. Basing technology deployment decisions on well-informed assessments of value and cost must become a standard of practice for public health managers.

Experience shows us that developing and implementing new information systems is a risky business. This was true for the introduction of the telegraph (the "Victorian Internet") and is true today. New system development efforts frequently fail because they are poorly conceived and managed, underfunded, or simply take too long to deploy. Organizations often fail to conceptualize or state explicitly the characteristics they need in the system and also do not quantify the benefits they seek to realize from their investment. Insufficient attention is given to preparing personnel to adopt and use new systems.

Public health now confronts an unprecedented era of accountability. The Internet has provided every citizen with a means of gathering information (and misinformation) on a vast spectrum of diseases, treatments, and threats to health. The communications superhighway provides new means for monitoring governmental programs, understanding policies and laws, and influencing cultural practices.

The US Department of Health and Human Services (DHHS) has articulated the importance of the Internet and interactive technologies for health improvements, and the rationale for quality standards for Web sites in *Wired for Health and Well-Being*, the final report of the Science Panel for Interactive Communication and Health. The commitment of DHHS to improving the quality of health Web sites is reflected in a national "Healthy People 2010" objective calling for an increase in the number of health Web sites that disclose quality standards information. Information to be disclosed to users includes the identity of the Web site developers and sponsors; how to contact the owners/developers of the site; potential conflicts of interest or biases; explicit purpose of the site, including commercial purposes and advertising; original sources of content; how the privacy and confidentiality of personal information is protected; how the site is evaluated; and how content on the site is updated. The goal is to promote the development of a consistent, comprehensive approach to identifying high-quality sites that consumers will find reliable and easy to use.

This book marks the first systematic effort to provide informatics principles and examples of practice in a public health context. In doing so, it clarifies the ways in which newer information technologies will improve individual and community health status. Public health executives, program managers, and technology experts will find this book of great use. We commend the authors for their contributions and the editors for their drive in bringing this important work to completion. We think this text is essential reading for managers and innovators throughout the diverse disciplines of public health.

David A. Ross, Sc.D.
Director, All Kids Count
Decatur, Georgia
Alan R. Hinman, M.D, M.P.H.

Principal Investigator, All Kids Count
Task Force for Child Survival and Development
Decatur, Georgia

Kristin Saarlas, M.P.H.
Deputy Director, All Kids Count
Decatur, Georgia

William H. Foege, M.D, M.P.H.
Senior Advisor to the Bill and Melinda Gates Foundation
Presidential Distinguished Professor
Rollins School of Public Health
Emory University
Atlanta, Georgia

Series Preface

This series is directed to healthcare professionals who are leading the transformation of health care by using information and knowledge. Launched in 1988 as Computers in Health Care, the series offers a broad range of titles: some addressed to specific professions such as nursing, medicine, and health administration; others to special areas of practice such as trauma and radiology. Still other books in the series focus on interdisciplinary issues, such as the computer-based patient record, electronic health records, and networked healthcare systems.

Renamed Health Informatics in 1998 to reflect the rapid evolution in the discipline now known as health informatics, the series will continue to add titles that contribute to the evolution of the field. In the series, eminent experts, serving as editors or authors, offer their accounts of innovations in health informatics. Increasingly, these accounts go beyond hardware and software to address the role of information in influencing the transformation of healthcare delivery systems around the world. The series also increasingly focuses on "peopleware" and the organizational, behavioral, and societal changes that accompany the diffusion of information technology in health services environments.

These changes will shape health services in this new millennium. By making full and creative use of the technology to tame data and to transform information, health informatics will foster the development of the knowledge age in health care. As coeditors, we pledge to support our professional colleagues and the series readers as they share advances in the emerging and exciting field of health informatics.

Kathryn J. Hannah
Marion J. Ball

Preface

In 1995, the US Centers for Disease Control and Prevention (CDC) partnered with the University of Washington (UW) School of Public Health and Community Medicine to develop a training resource for a new and (at that time) practically unknown field: *public health informatics*. That the field of informatics was new to public health is not to say that computers, networks, databases, and so forth were unknown to public health—far from it. Computers had been used by public health scientists for generations; by 1995, personal computers were being enthusiastically adopted by public health scientists all over the world. But with the advent of large-scale *networked* computing (from local-area networks to the global Internet), traditional seat-of-the-pants methods for developing public health information systems were proving untenable. A much more systematic, experience-based, and research-grounded approach to systems development was demanded by the complex, multiuser nature of applications such as national electronic surveillance systems and immunization registries. Indeed, the CDC-UW public health informatics training course was originally developed to support public health managers responsible for the development of statewide immunization registries.

The development of that training course was the beginning of the development of this textbook. Defining the scope and nature of that first public health informatics curriculum required us to define the scope and nature of public health informatics itself. That definition has changed over time, and many others (including many who have contributed to this volume) have enormously broadened and deepened the field of public health informatics since then. But the goal and the essential nature of public health informatics remains unchanged. Its goal is to harness the power of computers, networks, and other information technologies to improve the public's health. Its essential nature is a set of time- and research-proven principles and practices that maximize one's chances of success when developing new public health information systems or technologies.

Here at the outset of the 21st century, few public health professionals have received any formal training in informatics. Indeed, most are still unfamiliar with the nature and purpose of informatics as a discipline and are only partly aware of the potential that information technology has to improve and even to transform public health practice. The goal of this textbook is to help address this important knowledge gap. This book is intended to provide both students of public health and working public health professionals with an introduction to the new and rapidly growing field of public health informatics. The reader will become familiar with the principles and practices of informatics, gain an understanding of the sciences underlying this new discipline, recognize key informatics challenges facing public health professionals, and explore emerging information systems currently in development. The reader will also be introduced to the major public health information systems that form the scientific underpinnings of public health assessment and research and that inform the development of public health policy.

One of the challenges of teaching informatics is that its scientific and practical bases are drawn from multiple disciplines and domains. Thus, informatics-relevant material is to be found in textbooks and journals on information science, computer science, technology, management, psychology, and a dozen other domains. A primary purpose of this book is to consolidate key information currently scattered over many media and locations or else residing only in the minds of a few experts. By pulling this information together into a textbook on public health informatics, we hope to provide a coherent and readable resource for use by faculty and students in schools of public health across the United States. We also hope that this resource will be of use to the practicing public health professional. Many public health leaders and managers have found themselves making critical information technology decisions or managing complex information technology projects—tasks for which few of us ever received formal informatics training heretofore.

Nature and Organization of This Book

This book is not intended to be a review of cutting-edge information technology. After all, such a book would be doomed to obsolescence before the first printing was shipped. In fact, the term *Internet years* was coined to refer to a time span of a few months to a few weeks, an apt reflection of the dizzying pace at which information technology evolves.

Instead, this book is intended to promote a strategic approach to information systems use and development. Such a strategic approach is based on well-established informatics principles and practices that will remain valid long after today's technologies are supplanted by those of tomorrow. To use an analogy, in the practice of medicine, disease treatment regimens change constantly, but the principles and practices of medicine are stable and time-tested. The principles and practices of informatics are similarly time-tested and do not change dramatically from year to year.

The material in this book is presented in five parts:

- Part I, *The Context for Public Health Informatics,* provides important background and context for the rest of the book. After an introductory chapter, this section reviews a variety of recent social, legislative, and technical developments that, taken together, create both an imperative and a historic opportunity to apply information technology to the improvement of the public's health effectively and systematically. This section summarizes the history and significance of the development of computerized information systems in public health and provides a snapshot of the governmental and legislative context of public health informatics.

- Part II is titled *The Science of Public Health Informatics.* As noted, today's public health students and practitioners generally have never had formal training in the scientific underpinnings and principles of public health informatics. This section reviews the key scientific and technical elements of this new and developing discipline and clarifies the need for and the nature of the role of an "informatician" (sometimes called an "informaticist") in the public health enterprise. It also explores organizational and management issues related to information systems development and addresses the ethics of information use.

- Part III, *Key Public Health Information Systems*, reviews key information systems relevant to public health research and practice. These systems include vital statistics systems, morbidity data systems, risk factor data systems, and environmental data systems. The review of numerous data systems is complemented by an exploration of knowledge-based information systems for public health, as exemplified by peer-reviewed journal articles, meta-analyses, prevention guidelines, and a plethora of other information resources that are increasingly available on-line on the World Wide Web.

- Part IV is *New Challenges, Emerging Systems.* In view of the evident promise of information technology, the public health community has embraced certain systems development challenges that are apparently straightforward (e.g., immunization registries) but are in fact enormously challenging. This section describes several important areas of opportunity afforded by modern information technology, such as new means of data collection and new means of increasing data accessibility. This section also addresses key information technology challenges with which the public health community is currently grappling, including geographic information systems, expert systems for public health, and the use of information technology to promote the delivery of preventive medicine in primary care.

- Part V is *Case Studies: Applications of Information Systems Development.* The promise of information technology is widely appreciated, but the true value of information technology lies in bringing that promise to fulfillment. This section presents a variety of real-world case studies, each of which is designed either to exemplify a particular kind of value derived from the deployment of actual information systems (e.g., the value of using scientific data to drive policy) or to illustrate critical issues associated with the development of new information systems (e.g., dealing with the policy and privacy issues raised by electronic disease surveillance). This section is intended to illustrate the value of applying informatics principles and practices as well as cutting-edge information technologies to both new and traditional public health information applications. These case studies illustrate and amplify the meaning and importance of informatics and effective information systems to modern public health practice.

At the end of each chapter is a section titled "Questions for Review." These questions focus on many of the most important concepts discussed in a chapter. In many instances, they are based on a short case that demonstrates and requires a student to recognize and apply the concepts in action.

In order to aid public health instructors who will use this book in their courses, we are pleased to offer *The Instructor's Manual*, which will be accessible in PDF format on the publisher's Web site. For information on obtaining the URL, please write to PHImanual@springer-ny.com.

Patrick W. O'Carroll, M.D., M.P.H., F.A.C.P.M.
William A. Yasnoff, M.D., Ph.D., F.A.C.M.I.
M. Elizabeth Ward, R.N., M.N.
Laura H. Ripp, R.N., M.B.A., M.P.H.
Ernest L. Martin Ph.D., M.B.A., F.L.M.I.

Acknowledgments

A work of this scope would not have been possible without the enthusiastic support and participation of numerous individuals.

We acknowledge with gratitude the support of Edward L. Baker, Jr., M.D., M.P.H., Assistant Surgeon General and Director, Public Health Practice Program Office, Centers for Disease Control and Prevention. Without Dr. Baker's continuing interest in and support of the project, we might still be struggling to assemble a book.

We also acknowledge with gratitude the contributions of Dan Schwartz, M.D., to the project. Early in the project, Dan imposed organization on our efforts and helped set us on a course that would lead to the publication of this book.

We are also grateful for the efforts of Amy James, Communications and Office Manager, Foundation for Health Care Quality, for her work in coordinating permissions, copyright agreements, and contributor information. Without Amy's important behind-the-scenes work, this book could not have gone to print. In addition, we are heavily indebted to Patricia A. Fulbright of the Public Health Practice Program Office at the Centers for Disease Control and Prevention for her extraordinary competence in handling hundreds of administrative details associated with the project, including manuscript compilation.

In addition, we acknowledge the extraordinary competence of our editor at Springer-Verlag, Michelle Schmitt, and of the executive editor, Laura Gillan, both of whom guided us through the publication stages and provided valuable advice.

Our production editor at Springer-Verlag, Louise Farkas, and her colleagues skillfully dealt with a number of challenges to make this book look better than it would otherwise be.

Finally, we acknowledge the chapter authors who played the most important roles in making this book possible. While continuing to undertake daily work duties, they found time to share their expertise by drafting the chapters, responding to inquiries, and reviewing and modifying edited versions of their drafts. We are fortunate indeed to have located and secured the participation of the preeminent authorities in numerous fields of public health informatics.

As editors, of course, we accept responsibility for any errors of omission or commission.

Patrick O'Carroll, M.D., M.P.H., F.A.C.P.M.
Executive Fellow in Public Health Informatics, Public Health Practice
Program Office, Centers for Disease Control and Prevention

William A. Yasnoff, M.D., Ph.D., F.A.C.M.I.
Senior Policy Advisor, Public Health Informatics Institute,
on assignment from the
Centers for Disease Control and Prevention

M. Elizabeth Ward, R.N., M.N.
Director, Community Health Information Technology Alliance,
Foundation for Health Care Quality

Laura H. Ripp, R.N., M.B.A., M.P.H.
Director, Business Development, Crystal Insights
Government Division of Metatomix, Inc.

Ernest L. Martin, Ph.D., M.B.A., F.L.M.I.
Technical Writer, Electronic Data Systems; Professor of English,
Truett-McConnell College

Contents

PART III   KEY PUBLIC HEALTH
INFORMATION SYSTEMS

PART IV NEW CHALLENGES, EMERGING SYSTEMS

PART V CASE STUDIES: APPLICATIONS OF INFORMATION SYSTEMS DEVELOPMENT

Contributors

Marion J. Ball, Ed.D.
Vice President, Healthlink Clinical Solutions; Adjunct Professor, Johns Hopkins University School of Nursing, Baltimore, MD 21210, USA

Christine C. Beahler, M.L.S.
Reference Librarian, Health Sciences Libraries, University of Washington, Seattle, WA 98118, USA

Bobbie Berkowitz, Ph.D., R.N., F.A.A.N.
Professor and Chair, Psychosocial and Community Health Department, University of Washington School of Nursing, Seattle, WA 98109, USA

Lewis E. Berman, M.S.
Branch Chief, Division of Health Examination Statistics, National Center for Health Statistics, Centers for Disease Control and Prevention, Hyattsville, MD 20782, USA

Donald J. Berndt, Ph.D.
Assistant Professor, Information Systems and Decision Sciences, College of Business Administration, University of South Florida, Tampa, FL 33620, USA

Guthrie S. Birkhead, M.D., M.P.H.
Director, AIDS Institute, and Director, Center for Community Health, New York State Department of Health, Associate Professor of Epidemiology, School of Public Health, University at Albany, State University of New York, Albany, NY 12237, USA

Claire V. Broome, M.D.
Senior Advisor to the Director for Integrated Health Information Systems, Office of the Director, Centers for Disease Control and Prevention, Atlanta, GA 30341, USA

Robb Chapman
Chief, Information Technology Branch, Division of Public Health Surveillance and Informatics, Epidemiology Program Office, Centers for Disease Control and Prevention, Atlanta, GA 30341, USA

John R. Christiansen, J.D.
Attorney, Preston Gates & Ellis, LLP, Clinical Assistant Professor, Oregon Health and Sciences University School of Medicine, Division of Informatics and Outcomes Research, Seattle, WA 98104, USA

Jac Davies, M.S., M.P.H.
Assistant Secretary, Division of Epidemiology, Health Statistics and Public Health Labs, Washington State Department of Health, Seattle, WA 98155, USA

Michael C. Davisson
HIV/AIDS Data/Program Manager, Bureau of HIV/AIDS Epidemiology, New York State Department of Health, Albany, NY 12237, USA

Linda K. Demlo, Ph.D.
Director, Division of Health Care Statistics, National Center for Health Statistics, Centers for Disease Control and Prevention, Hyattsville, MD 20782, USA

Larry L. Dickey, M.D., M.P.H.
Chief, Office of Clinical Preventive Medicine, Department of Health Services, State of California, Sacramento, CA 95814, USA

Stephen B. Fawcett, Ph.D.
Director, Work Group on Health Promotion and Community Development, University of Kansas, Lawrence, KS 66045, USA

William H. Foege, M.D., M.P.H.
Fellow, Bill and Melinda Gates Foundation, Presidential Distinguished Professor Emeritus, Rollins School of Public Health, Emory University, Atlanta, GA 30322, USA

Vincent T. Francisco, Ph.D.
Associate Director, Work Group on Health Promotion and Community Development, University of Kansas, Lawrence, KS 66045, USA

Mary Anne Freedman, M.A.
Director, Division of Vital Statistics, National Center for Health Statistics, Centers for Disease Control and Prevention, Hyattsville, MD 20852, USA

Jane F. Gentleman, Ph.D.
Director, Division of Health Interview Statistics, National Center for Health

Statistics, Centers for Disease Control and Prevention, Hyattsville, MD 20852, USA

Kenneth W. Goodman, Ph.D.
Director, Bioethics Program, Co-Director, Programs in Business, Government, and Professional Ethics, University of Miami, Miami, FL 33136, USA

Ivan J. Gotham, Ph.D.
Director, Bureau of Healthcom Network Systems Management, Information Systems and Health Statistics Group, New York State Department of Health; Assistant Professor, Department of Biometry, School of Public Health, University at Albany, State University of New York, Albany, NY 12237, USA

Carol L. Hanchette, Ph.D.
Assistant Professor, Department of Geography and Geosciences, University of Louisville, Louisville, KY 40292, USA

Tiffany Harris, M.S.
EVA Study Manager, Department of Epidemiology, School of Public Health and Community Medicine, University of Washington, Seattle, WA 98103, USA

Alan R. Hevner, Ph.D.
Salomon Brothers/HRCP Chair of Distributed Technology, and Professor, Information Systems and Decision Sciences Department, College of Business Administration, University of South Florida, Tampa, FL 33620, USA

Alan R. Hinman, M.D., M.P.H.
Principal Investigator, All Kids Count, Coordinator PARTNERS TB Control Program, Task Force for Child Survival and Development, Decatur, GA 30030, USA

Nancy L. Hoffman, R.N., M.S.N.
Deputy Director, Center for Health Information Management and Evaluation, Missouri Department of Health, Jefferson City, MO 65102, USA

Deborah Holtzman, Ph.D.
Sociologist/Section Chief, Epidemiology and Analysis, Division of Adult and Community Health, Centers for Disease Control and Prevention, Atlanta, GA 30329, USA

Daniel B. Jernigan, M.D., M.P.H.
Senior Medical Epidemiologist, Office of Surveillance, National Center for Infectious Diseases, Centers for Disease Control and Prevention, Atlanta, GA 30333, USA

Edwin M. Kilbourne, M.D., F.A.C.P., F.A.C.P.M.
Associate Administrator for Toxic Substances and Public Health, Agency for Toxic Substances and Disease Registry, Atlanta, GA 30329, USA

Ann Marie Kimball, M.D., M.P.H., F.A.C.P.M.
Director, MPH Program; Professor, Epidemiology and Health Services and Adjunct in Medicine, School of Public Health and Community Medicine, University of Washington, Seattle, WA 98195, USA

Pete Kitch, M.B.A.
KIPHS Project Director, Wichita, KS 67208, USA

Denise Koo, M.D., M.P.H.
Associate Director for Science, Epidemiology Program Office, Centers for Disease Control and Prevention, Atlanta, GA 30333, USA

Garland Land, M.P.H.
Director, Center for Health Information Management and Evaluation, Missouri Department of Health, Jefferson City, MO 65102, USA

Deborah A. Lewis, Ed.D., R.N., M.P.H.
Associate Professor of Nursing, University of Pittsburgh, Pittsburgh, PA 16066, USA

Robert W. Linkins, M.P.H., Ph.D.
Chief, Immunization Registry Support Branch, National Immunization Program, Centers for Disease Control and Prevention, Atlanta, GA 30333, USA

Nancy M. Lorenzi, Ph.D.
Assistant Vice Chancellor for Health Affairs, Professor of Biomedical Informatics, Vanderbilt University Medical Center, Nashville, TN 37232, USA

John R. Lumpkin, M.D., M.P.H.
Director, Illinois Department of Public Health, Springfield, IL 60605, USA

Perry L. Miller, M.D., Ph.D.
Professor and Director, Center for Medical Informatics, Yale University School of Medicine, New Haven, CT 06520, USA

Meade Morgan, Ph.D.
Assistant Director, Informatics Division of HIV/AIDS Surveillance and Epidemiology, Centers for Disease Control and Prevention, Atlanta, GA 30341 USA

Fran Muskopf, B.S.
Chief Administrator, Information Resource Management, Washington State Department of Health, Olympia, WA 98501, USA

Patrick W. O'Carroll, M.D., M.P.H., F.A.C.P.M.
Executive Fellow in Public Health Informatics, Public Health Practice Program Office, Centers for Disease Control and Prevention, Northwest Center for Public Health Practice, Seattle, WA 98105, USA

Yechiam Ostchega, Ph.D., R.N.
Captain, United States Public Health Service, Nurse Consultant, Survey Operation Branch, National Center for Health Statistics, Centers for Disease Control and Prevention, Hyattsville, MD 20782, USA

Rex Petersen
Chief, Office of Information Systems, Center for Health Information Management and Evaluation, Missouri Department of Health, Jefferson City, MO 65102, USA

John D. Piette, Ph.D.
Senior Research Associate, Department of Veterans Affairs and University of Michigan, Ann Arbor, MI 48106, USA

Kathryn Porter, M.D., M.S.
Medical Officer, Division of Health Examination Statistics, National Center for Health Statistics, Centers for Disease Control and Prevention, Hyattsville, MD 20782, USA

Eve Powell-Griner, M.A., Ph.D.
Associate Director for Science, National Center for Health Statistics, Division of Health Interview Statistics, Hyattsville, MD 20782, USA

Neil Rambo, M.L.S.
Associate Director, Pacific Northwest Region, National Network of Libraries of Medicine, University of Washington, Seattle, WA 98118, USA

Debra S. Reed-Gillette
Computer Specialist, Division of Health Examination Statistics, National Center for Health Statistics, Centers for Disease Control and Prevention, Hyattsville, MD 20782, USA

Janise Richards, M.S., M.P.H., Ph.D.
Director, Public Health Informatics Fellowship Program, Applied Sciences

Branch, Division of Public Health Surveillance and Informatics, Epidemiology Program Office, Centers for Disease Control and Prevention, Atlanta, GA 30341, USA

Robert T. Riley, Ph.D.
President, Riley Associates, Nashville, TN 37215, USA

David A. Ross, Sc.D.
Director, All Kids Count, The Task Force for Child Survival and Development, Atlanta, GA 30300, USA

Richard D. Rubin
President, Community Health Connection Division, Pointshare Corporation, Bellevue, WA 98004, USA

Kristin Saarlas, M.P.H.
Deputy Director, All Kids Count, Decatur, GA 30300, USA

Jerry A. Schultz, Ph.D.
Associate Director, Work Group on Health Promotion and Community Development, University of Kansas, Lawrence, KS 66045, USA

Ron E. Seymour
INPHO Project Manager, Washington State Department of Health, Olympia, WA 98501, USA

Alan Sim, M.S.
Health Informatics Scientist, Division of Public Health Surveillance and Informatics, Epidemiology Program Office, Centers for Disease Control and Prevention, Atlanta, GA 30341, USA

Perry F. Smith, M.D.
Director, Division of Epidemiology, New York State Department of Health, Assistant Professor, Department of Epidemiology, School of Public Health, University at Albany, State University of New York, Albany, NY 12237, USA

James Studnicki, Sc.D., M.B.A., M.P.H.
Professor and Director, Center for Health Outcomes Research, Department of Health Policy and Management, College of Public Health, University of South Florida, Tampa, FL 33620, USA

James A. Weed, Ph.D.
Deputy Director, Division of Vital Statistics, National Center for Health Statistics, Centers for Disease Control and Prevention, Hyattsville, MD 20782, USA

G. David Williamson, Ph.D.
Director, Division of Health Studies, Agency for Toxic Substances and Disease Registry, Atlanta, GA 30329, USA

William A. Yasnoff, M.D., Ph.D., F.A.C.M.I.
Senior Policy Advisor, Public Health Informatics Institute, Decatur, GA 30030, USA

Part I
The Context for Public
Health Informatics

Introduction

The term *public health informatics* is relatively new, but the concept of the systematic application of information and computer science and technology to health practice, research, and learning is not. Many health disciplines—including nursing and medicine—have developed their own concepts of informatics, and yet there is no textbook that treats the topic of public health informatics comprehensively. This work attempts to fill that gap in knowledge.

This section is intended to set the stage for other sections in this book—by placing the discipline of public health informatics in its context.

In Chapter 1, Patrick W. O'Carroll defines the concept of public health informatics and writes of the promise that implementation of a comprehensive informatics approach can bring to public health practice. Dr. O'Carroll also treats the basic principles of public health informatics, including discussion of the ways in which the focus of that discipline resembles and differs from the informatics of other health disciplines. He concludes the chapter by discussing the drivers of change that are pointing to the necessity for implementing a comprehensive public health informatics approach.

In Chapter 2, John R. Lumpkin provides a historical context for the discipline of public health informatics. Tracing the earliest emergence of public health practice, Dr. Lumpkin focuses on the evolution of technology as a supporting force for public health officers, emphasizing public health developments in the 19th and 20th centuries and concluding with modern developments that have necessitated a more systematic approach to the collection and analysis of public health information.

In Chapter 3, Marion J. Ball gets to the root of the issues driving public health practice to adoption of informatics as a formalized approach. She places public health informatics in the context of value creation, and she discusses the organizational factors that determine whether an informatics approach to any health practice will result in added value. As an overarching theme of the chapter, Dr. Ball points out that there is already strong evidence that a sound informatics approach improves the life of each individual through promoting better health.

This part of the book concludes with John Christiansen's Chapter 4, an examination of the governmental and legislative context of informatics. Mr. Christiansen points out that an understanding of this context is crucial for any public health employee. Defining the concept of a public health agency in two ways, he proceeds to discuss the implications of privacy laws affecting the handling of public health information, focusing in particular on the recently developed and implemented provisions of the Health Insurance Portability and Accountability Act. He concludes the chapter by discussing legal and practical implications of information sharing and by providing an overview of principles and practices governing a public health agency's use of a Web site to convey health information.

1
Introduction to Public Health Informatics*

Patrick W. O'Carroll

Learning Objectives

After studying this chapter, you should be able to:

- Define the concept of public health informatics and explain the aspects that it has in common with medical informatics.
- List and briefly explain the four principles that define, guide, and provide the context for the types of activities and challenges that comprise public health informatics and differentiate it from medical informatics.
- List and briefly discuss three major developments that have increased the importance and immediate relevance of informatics to public health.

Overview

The technology necessary for effective, innovative application of information technology to public health practice is available today at very reasonable costs. The barrier to the widespread application of such technology is that few public health professionals have received any formal training in informatics, and most lack even a basic understanding of the nature and purpose of informatics as a discipline. Although the discipline of public health informatics has much in common with other informatics specialty areas, it differs from them in several ways. These include (1) a focus on applications of information science and technology that promote the health of populations, rather than of individuals; (2) a focus on disease prevention, rather than treatment; (3) a focus on preventive intervention at all vulnerable points in the causal chains leading to disease,

*Some of the material in this chapter was originally published in "Public health informatics: Improving and transforming public health in the information age" (Yasnoff WA, O'Carroll PW, Koo D, Linkins RW, Kilbourne E. *Journal of Public Health Management and Practice* 2000;6(6):67–75).

injury, or disability; and (4) operation within a governmental. rather than a private, context. Drivers of change forcing public health professionals to be conversant with the development, use. and strategic importance of computerized health information systems include public health reform, the growth in managed care, and the information technology revolution.

Introduction

It is 8:30 AM, a few years from now. As the director of a local health department, you are looking forward to a relatively quiet morning working on an initiative to promote the use of bicycle helmets in your community. When you start your computer, the screen directs you to place your thumb on the small scanner attached to the monitor. After you have been recognized and logged in, the computer says, "Good morning," launches your calendar, and automatically opens the working draft of the initiative.

As you prepare to begin dictating, an alert pops up on your screen to the sound of a barking dog: "Rover has detected an unusual incidence of *Escherichia coli O157:H7*," the alert says. You are presented with several options: SURVEILLANCE DATA, LEARNING RESOURCES, and COMMUNICATIONS. You select SURVEILLANCE DATA and are presented with a table and a chart of recent cases of *E. coli*—both suspected and laboratory-confirmed—in your community. From there, you click on the MAP THIS button, and a "pin map" of the cases in your county is displayed. You click the ZOOM OUT button. and the pin map expands to show your county and adjacent counties—one of which is in the adjacent state. You click on the TIME SERIES button and are shown a classic epi-chart. with associated statistics at the bottom. It surely has the look of an outbreak.

In the next few minutes, without ever leaving your chair. you send an alert about the cluster of cases to the primary care clinicians and hospital infectious disease control staff in your community. as well as to your own epidemiology staff. You send an electronic food-borne illness questionnaire to your local "sentinel event" network of care providers (attaching a predefined case definition and other instructions). as well as to a standing community-based control group. You instruct your computer to schedule a priority videoconference with your fellow health officers and the state infectious disease epidemiologist; and you locate and download various prevention guideline documents from the Centers for Disease Control and Prevention (CDC). Finally, you turn to a list of on-line learning resources. noting the availability of several interactive, full-motion video courses, to brush up on the diagnosis, clinical presentation, epidemiology. and control of *E. coli O157:H7*.

To many in public health today, this scenario seems rather futuristic. After all, consider some of the elements that would have to be in place for this scenario to occur: biometric authentication of the user (via the thumb scan): software "agents" automatically searching distributed clinical and laboratory databases for apparent outbreaks of disease; software for epidemiologic analysis and geographic information systems to analyze and display the data; electronic alert systems capable of reaching community clinicians and others through well-maintained, distributed directories of health personnel; the ability to distribute preconfigured electronic forms that can be completed, returned, and automatically compiled and analyzed; ubiquitous video-conferencing capacity at all levels of the public health system; succinct, well-structured prevention guidelines from CDC on all public health–relevant diseases and conditions; and an on-line learning system that makes public health knowledge and know-how available on demand, at the desktop of every public health professional.

Yet, all of this technology is available today—off the shelf, at very reasonable and ever-decreasing cost. (The thumb scanner, for example, is available for less than $100 at the time of this writing.) In other words, if we want the kinds of public health detection and response capacity illustrated by the scenario, *technology is not the barrier.*

If the technology is available, and if the costs of that technology are within reach, why are we so far from this vision of public health practice?

The answer is that the effective application of information technology to public health or to any other discipline is very challenging. It is not a question of computer science or information technology *per se*; it is a question of *informatics*—harnessing the available technology to meet the information needs of health practitioners in general, and of public health practitioners in particular.

What Is Public Health Informatics?

We define public health informatics as the *systematic application of information and computer science and technology to public health practice, research, and learning.*[1,2] Public health informatics is primarily an engineering discipline. It is a practical activity, undergirded by science and oriented to the accomplishment of specific tasks. The scope of public health informatics includes the conceptualization, design, development, deployment, refinement, maintenance, and evaluation of communication, surveillance, information, and learning systems relevant to public health. Public health informatics requires the application of knowledge from numerous disciplines, particularly information science, computer science, management, organizational theory, psychology, communications, political science, and law. Its practice must also incorporate knowledge from the other fields that contribute to public health, including epidemiology, microbiology, toxicology, and statistics (see Figure 1.1).

Although public health informatics draws from multiple scientific and practical domains, computer science and information science are its primary underlying disciplines. Computer science, the theory and application of automatic data-processing machines, includes hardware and software design, algorithm development, computational complexity, networking and telecommunications, pattern recognition, and artificial intelligence. Information science encompasses

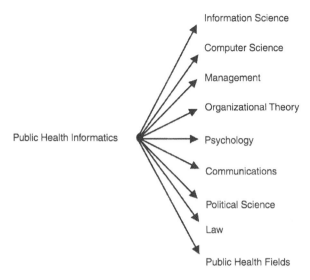

FIGURE 1.1. Disciplines underlying public health informatics. Source: author.

the analysis of the structure, properties, and organization of information, information storage and retrieval. information system and database architecture and design, library science, project management, and organizational issues such as change management and business process reengineering.

Public health informatics involves more than simply automating existing activities. It enables new approaches that were previously impractical or not even contemplated. (The automated detection of putative epidemics in our opening scenario is but one such example.) In the near term, most public health information systems projects will focus on improving the efficiency or effectiveness of traditional public health practice. In the long term, however, the promise and challenge of public health informatics will be in engineering innovative new ways to protect and promote the public's health using the power of information science and technology.

Principles of Public Health Informatics

Public health informatics is related to medical informatics in several respects.[3] Both disciplines seek to use information science and technology to improve human health, and there are subject matter areas of common concern (e.g., standards for vocabulary and information exchange). Moreover, lessons learned in medical informatics often apply to public health informatics. Further, there are informatics applications for which there is no real distinction between public health and medical informatics. Examples of such applications include systems for accessing public health data from electronic medical record systems or for providing patient-specific prevention guidance at the clinical encounter. An example of how informatics is transforming health care follows.

Building Physician–Patient Networks on the World Wide Web

Hook up the stock price of drkoop.com or Healtheon/WebMD to a heart monitor and any doctor would tag and bag it.

For privately held Medem, an on-line health network founded and financed by the American Medical Association and other medical groups, quarantining itself from public markets buys the time to build a business and market its greatest asset: trust.

"I don't think anyone in the e-health space would say they have better information than the American Academy of Pediatrics on pediatrics issues," says Dr. Edward Fotsch, Medem's CEO and a veteran of rival Healtheon. "I think the societies offer tremendous values."

Medem builds physician Web sites, and Fotsch says, "Our business model is to create a secure patient–physician network that has information [from trusted sources] and to facilitate communications between docs and patients." drkoop.com doesn't provide the latter. "I don't think secure messaging, for example, has much meaning for drkoop.com. It's absolutely critical for us."

Fotsch says it's too early to tell if the Web changes the balance of power among patients, physicians, and insurers, but he predicts interests will align. "It's not hard to imagine a scenario in which a pharmaceutical company and a health plan get together to fund an on-line information delivery program [approved by the medical societies]. And docs are happy to enroll their patients because they are confident in the clinical message. I think the patients are going to love it. I have yet to hear a patient say, 'I am tired of getting spammed by my doctor's office.'"

Source: Thomas Claburn, "Physician, Heal Thy Web Site," in *Ziff Davis Smart Business, December 2000*, page 70. Reprinted from *Ziff Davis Smart Business, December 2000*, with permission. Copyright © 2000 Ziff Davis Media Inc. All Rights Reserved.

Nevertheless, we believe that public health informatics is a new and distinct specialty area within the broader discipline of informatics, a specialty area defined by a specific set of principles and challenges.

Our view is that the various informatics specialty areas—for instance, nursing informatics and medical informatics—are distinguished from one another by the principles underlying their respective application domains (i.e., nursing and medicine), as well as by the differing nature and challenges of their informatics applications. In the case of public health informatics, there are four such principles, flowing directly from the scope and nature of public health, that distinguish it from other informatics specialty areas. These four principles define, guide, and provide the context for the types of activities and challenges that comprise this new field:

1. *The primary focus of public health informatics is on applications of information science and technology that promote the health of populations as opposed to the health of specific individuals.* As a discipline, public health focuses on the health of the population and the community as a whole, rather than on the health of the individual patient. In the healthcare setting, the primary focus of concern is the individual patient, who presents with a specific disease or condition requiring diagnosis and treatment. In public health, on the other hand, the primary focus of concern is on populations of individuals. One can think of the entire community as the patient. The community-patient requires "diagnosis" in terms of an assessment of the major threats to health and well-being facing the community. "Treatment" of the community-patient might involve the development of new policies, stepped-up enforcement of existing laws, the elimination of infected foodstuffs, efforts to modify behavior (e.g., to reduce smoking prevalence), and even such relatively extreme measures as quarantine or disclosure of the disease status of individuals to prevent further spread of infectious illness. It is true that some measures to protect the community's health do ultimately resolve to interventions involving specifically identifiable individuals (e.g., vaccination). However, public health practice also requires attention to factors that affect the health risk of entire populations rather than of individuals (e.g., water quality, food safety, working conditions, and automobile crash protection).

2. *The primary focus of public health informatics is on applications of information science and technology that prevent disease and injury by altering the conditions or the environment that put populations of individuals at risk.* Although notable exceptions exist, traditional health care largely treats individuals who already have a disease or high-risk condition, whereas public health practice seeks to avoid the conditions that led to the disease in the first place. This difference in focus has direct implications for the ways in which information technology might be deployed.

3. *Public health informatics applications explore the potential for prevention at all vulnerable points in the causal chains leading to disease, injury, or disability; applications are not restricted to particular social, behavioral, or environmental contexts.* In public health, the nature of a given preventive intervention is not predetermined by professional discipline, but rather by the effectiveness, expediency, cost, and social acceptability of intervening at various potentially vulnerable points in a causal chain. Public health interventions have included, for example, legislatively mandated housing and building codes, solid waste disposal and wastewater

treatment systems, smoke alarms, fluoridation of municipal water supplies, redesign of automobiles, development of inspection systems to ensure food safety, and removal of lead from gasoline. Contrast this approach with the approach of the modern healthcare system, which generally accomplishes its mission through clinical and surgical encounters. Although some of these healthcare system encounters can properly be considered public health measures (e.g., vaccination), public health action is not limited to the clinical encounter.

4. *As a discipline, public health informatics reflects the governmental context in which public health is practiced.* Much of public health operates through government agencies that require direct responsiveness to legislative, regulatory, and policy directives; careful balancing of competing priorities; and open disclosure of all activities. In addition, some public health actions involve authority to take specific (sometimes coercive) measures to protect the community in an emergency. Examples include medication or food recalls, closing down a restaurant or a contaminated pool or lake, and making changes to immunization policy (e.g., the recent change in recommended use of rotavirus vaccine[4]).

Table 1.1 provides an overview of the distinction between the attributes of medicine and public health. These distinctions drive differences in the nature of medical and public health informatics, respectively.

In addition to these principles, the nature of public health also defines a special set of informatics challenges. For example, in order for public health practitioners to assess a population's health and risk status, they must obtain data from multiple disparate sources, such as hospitals, social service agencies, police departments, departments of labor and industry, population surveys, on-site inspections, etc. Data from these various sources about particular individuals must be accurately combined. Then individual-level data must be compiled into usable, aggregate forms at the population level. This information must be presented in clear and compelling ways to legislators and other policymakers, scientists, advocacy groups, and the general public. At the same time, the public health practitioner must insure that the confidentiality of the health information about specific individuals is not compromised.

Together with the four principles that distinguish public health informatics from other informatics specialty areas, then, these and other special challenges define public health informatics as a distinct specialty area.

Drivers of Change

Three major developments in recent times make it increasingly critical that public health professionals be conversant with the development, use, and strategic importance of computerized health information systems. These developments are discussed below.

TABLE 1.1. Key differences between the attributes of medicine and public health

Attribute	Medicine	Public Health
Primary focus of concern	Health of specific individuals	Health of populations/ communities
Primary health improvement strategy	Treatment of disease or injury, with secondary emphasis on prevention	Prevention of disease or injury
Intervention context and scope	Clinical and surgical encounters and medical/surgical treatment; preventive interventions within the context of each professional discipline (e.g., pediatrics), with focus on one or a few points in the causal chain	Any and all vulnerable points in the causal chains: prevention approach not predetermined by professional discipline, but rather by the effectiveness, expediency, cost, and social acceptability of intervention
Operational context	Operation through private practices, clinics, hospitals, with governmental direction primarily in terms of quality assurance.	Operation within a governmental context requiring responsiveness to legislative, regulatory, and policy directives

Public Health Reform

Public health has always been an information-intensive field. Effective public health practice requires timely, accurate, and authoritative information from a wide variety of sources. For this reason, public health professionals have developed a wide array of information resources to help them perform their work.[5,6]

However, with the publication of *The Future of Public Health*[7] in 1988, the importance of information as both a critical currency and a product of public health practice was amplified enormously. This seminal report by the Institute of Medicine (IOM) launched a period of public health reform that continues to this day, refocusing the practice of public health around three core functions: assessment, policy development, and assurance. Information is central to each of these core functions. For example, the essence of community health assessment is the collection, analysis, interpretation, and communication of data and information. Timely and authoritative information is also at the heart of the development of well-informed public health policy. Finally, the assurance function described in the IOM report moves public health away from "clinical care provider of last resort" toward the role of monitor and communicator of information about community access to critical health services—another role for which information is the essential currency. Thus, each of the core functions at the heart of public health reform accentuates the importance of public health as "information broker," directly increasing the need for public health officials to be effective planners, developers, and users of health information systems. Some of the key recommendations contained in the document *The Future of Public Health* are listed below.

Among the report's 55 recommendations directed at state health departments as ways of improving public health practice in the United States were:

1. State health departments should improve community involvement in public health practice, including strengthening relations with physicians and other health professionals, voluntary health organizations, and legislators and other public officials.
2. State health departments should focus efforts on a wide range of environmental health issues, such as drinking-water quality and toxic exposure evaluation.
3. State health departments should expand responsibilities to include issues related to substance abuse, Medicaid, mental health, and regulation of public health professionals.
4. State health departments should increase support for local health services, using subsidies and technical assistance, while establishing standards specifying minimum services to be provided by local public health services and holding these local services accountable.
5. The public health system, including state health departments, should develop more effective leadership and greatly improved data gathering and analysis.

The public health reform launched by the publication of *The Future of Public Health* has led to the development of new partnerships and expanded expectations of the public health system. These partnerships and expectations require better and more efficient access to information as well as better means of communication. Finally, the changed and increased responsibilities associated with public health reform are occurring in an era of shrinking budgets for our nation's state and local health departments, coupled with a heightened focus on accountability and performance assessment. These additional aspects of public health reform demand the efficiencies of well-developed and professionally managed information and communication systems.

Growth in Managed Care

The American medical system has evolved rapidly in recent years, primarily because of the growth of organized healthcare delivery models, including health maintenance organizations. By 1997, nearly 70 million Americans were enrolled in health maintenance organizations, a 10-fold increase from 1978 that reflects the movement of employers and other plan sponsors toward cost-control measures.[8] These enrollees include mounting numbers of Medicare and Medicaid beneficiaries who are being shifted into managed care plans to control costs and improve access. In addition, membership in preferred provider organizations, another form of managed care, is increasing rapidly. Finally, continuing mergers and acquisitions among hospitals and medical practices, along with wider variability in the insurance products offered, have also led to fluidity in the size and composition of healthcare organizations.

These changes provide important opportunities for public health and managed care to collaborate in addressing shared concerns for cost-effective health care, prevention, and population health. The new arrangement of medical care service delivery means that for-profit provider organizations have a shared focus with public health on preventing disease and injury and promoting wellness. For example, some health plans have implemented practices geared toward improving the level of immunization and cancer screening among their enrollees.[9] The advent of standardized electronic medical records, coupled with the consolidation of electronic medical record stores, creates the potential for public health to access an unprecedented wealth of morbidity data in nearly real time—a potentially revolutionary improvement in our capacity to assess community health.

On the other hand, inherent in the growth of managed care is an intense focus on efficiency and cost-savings. If public health is to engage as a partner with managed care, it will necessarily do so only in a highly efficient and collaborative manner. In particular, public health professionals will need to design surveillance and data systems according to standards that allow for seamless interaction of public health data assessment processes with the clinical and business activities of managed care organizations. Developing these standards and appropriately incorporating clinical data into public health surveillance are among the primary public health informatics challenges of the coming decades.

The Information Technology Revolution

The final driver of change marking the increased importance of informatics to public health lies in the information technology revolution itself. Today's computer systems are both faster and less expensive than ever before, and prices are continuing to decrease rapidly. In fact, computer hardware is no longer the major cost it once was in information system development projects.

More important, the Internet has emerged as both a universal communications medium and the source of a universal graphical user interface—the World Wide Web, accessed with Internet browser software. In fact, the growth in use of the Internet has been little short of phenomenal in recent years.

The existence of the Web provides a powerful new paradigm for standardized implementation of the communication capabilities that are central to all information systems. A Web browser interface potentially allows universal access without the necessity for development or deployment of specific software or communications protocols for potential users. Updating information systems is greatly simplified, since new versions of Web-based applications are immediately available to users without distribution of new software. Most system development is now utilizing this paradigm, with the resultant creation of many new and powerful tools to streamline and simplify the process. As a consequence, information system development is now faster and easier than ever before. In this environment, the benefits of public health information systems are more obvious and more easily achievable, and thus much more compelling. Table 1.2 summarizes the effects of these drivers of change.

In the context of these societal trends, familiarity with at least the basic principles and practices of informatics is becoming essential. This may not be a welcome development for many public health practitioners, who already must be conversant with such wide-ranging fields as epidemiology and statistics, risk communication, community organization, legislative development, behavioral modification, emergency response, and of course program management. Nevertheless, facility in at least the use of key information technologies for public health (e.g., e-mail, the Web, and epidemiologic databases) is already a requirement for state-of-the-art public health practice. And more advanced informatics expertise is undeniably critical for the development of future information systems such as immunization registries, improved disease and epidemic surveillance, and so forth. Like it or not, informatics has already joined the long list of disciplines with which public health practitioners must be conversant. In the next chapter, we will trace the history of information systems and their evolution as crucial tools in public health practice.

TABLE 1.2. Drivers of change mandating that public health professionals be knowledgeable about computerized health information systems

Change Driver	Impact
Public health reform	Launched by publication of *The Future of Public Health* in 1988. Placed focus on three core functions of public health: assessment, policy development, assurance—all information-intensive
Growth in managed care	Emphasis on prevention, in common with public health, has created an increased need and opportunity for application of efficient information technology in partnership with health care
The information technology revolution	Faster, less expensive computer systems and the development of the Internet have dramatically increased both the potential and the rate of development of computerized health information systems

Questions for Review

1. What factors, other than a lack of education about informatics among public health professionals, might account for the fact that the field of public health lags far behind traditional health care in the effective deployment of information technology?

2. Explain why an intensive knowledge of traditional public health–specific fields—such as epidemiology, microbiology, toxicology, and statistics—is insufficient by itself for developing and applying information systems in public health practice.

3. The primary focus of public health informatics is on applications of information science and technology that promote the health of populations, whereas the primary focus of traditional medical informatics is on the promotion of the health of specifically identifiable individuals. To what extent does the public health informatics focus intersect with the focus of traditional medical informatics? What do the informatics specialties have in common?

4. It has been said that public health informatics applications explore the potential for prevention at all vulnerable points in the causal chains leading to disease, injury, or disability. Provide some examples of causal points that a public health professional might explore and a practitioner of traditional medicine would not.

5. It has been said that public health informatics reflects the governmental context in which public health is practiced. To what extent do practitioners of traditional medicine also operate within a governmental context? Is there any difference in the role that government plays in the practice of the two fields?

6. Compare and contrast the functions performed by public health professionals and practitioners of traditional healthcare. How do they differ in their approach to (1) the individual, and (2) the community? To what parties are these two categories of professionals accountable for their actions? How?

7. Discuss the relative impact of (1) public health reform, (2) the growth in managed care, and (3) the information technology revolution as drivers of change in the way that public health professionals view and use computerized health information systems. In your opinion, which of them will have the greatest impact on the use that public health professionals make of information technology over the next decade? Why?

References

1. Yasnoff WA, O'Carroll PW, Koo D, Linkins RW, Kilbourne E. Public health informatics: Improving and transforming public health in the information age. *J Public Health Manag Pract* 2001;6(6):67–75.

2. Friede A, Blum HL, McDonald M. Public health informatics: How information age technology can strengthen public health. *Annu Rev Public Health* 1995;16:239–252.
3. Greenes RA, Shortliffe EH. Medical informatics: An emerging academic discipline and institutional priority. *JAMA* 1990:263:1114–1120.
4. Centers for Disease Control and Prevention. Withdrawal of rotavirus vaccine recommendation. *MMWR Morb Mortal Wkly Rep* 1999;48:1007.
5. Friede A. O'Carroll PW. CDC and ATSDR electronic information resources for health officers. *J Public Health Manag Pract* 1996;2:10–24.
6. Gable DB. A compendium of public health data sources. *Am J Epidemiol* 1990;131:381–394.
7. Committee for the Study of the Future of Public Health. Division of Health Care Services, Institute of Medicine. *The Future of Public Health*. Washington, DC: National Academy Press; 1988.
8. National Center for Health Statistics. *Health, United States, 1998 with Socioeconomic Status and Health Chartbook*. Hyattsville, MD: National Center for Health Statistics; 1998.
9. Stoto MA, Abel C, Dievler A, eds. *Healthy Communities: New Partnerships for the Future of Public Health*. Washington, DC: National Academy Press; 1996.

2
History and Significance of Information Systems and Public Health

John R. Lumpkin

Learning Objectives

After studying this chapter, you should be able to:

- Clearly differentiate among the terms *data, information,* and *knowledge* and provide an example of each.
- Briefly trace the evolution of information systems, from the development of counting and counting machines to the development of computers.
- Explain and distinguish between the age of observation and the age of analysis in early public health practice.
- List and discuss the 19th century developments in Europe and the United States that led to the development of modern public health data collection and analysis.
- List the major principles underlying the Cornerstone system as a model of an integrated state public health system, and explain why these principles are important in the development of any modern public health system.
- List and describe the characteristics of the three waves of federal-state public health information systems.

Overview

From the earliest development of counting and counting machines to today's sophisticated public health systems, a fundamental problem of public health practice has been the development of systems that can collect and analyze data, then convert it to useful forms. The development of modern mechanical measuring devices was a quantum leap toward solving the problem, but even after the invention of the computer in the 20th century, there was a continuing need for systems that would maximize integration of system components and minimize duplication of data entry. The history of the automation of public health practice in the state of Illinois illustrates the complexities of optimizing public health system integration. A review of the three waves of modern federal-state public health system development reveals the progression toward the optimization goal.

In general, today's systems to manage public health data and information have evolved in step with the scientific basis underlying public health practice, a practice that integrates findings in the biomedical field with the sciences of epidemiology and biostatistics.

Introduction

Today's public health information systems are products of a partnership between state and federal public health officials. Federal agencies now fund development of many state information systems. Increasingly, these information systems permit states to exchange information rapidly and effectively with local public health officials and with other states and national organizations. The ongoing development of standards for public health information systems by such organizations as the Centers for Disease Control and Prevention (CDC) has paved the way for development and implementation of sophisticated applications and heightened interconnectivity with other information systems. It was not always this way. Only a few years ago, many state public health information systems were stand-alone products with little or no interconnectivity and relatively crude data collection and data processing capabilities.

Today's systems to manage public health data and information have evolved in step with the scientific basis underlying public health practice. Public health practice now integrates findings in the biomedical field with the sciences of epidemiology and biostatistics. As the need for knowledge integration has become more complex, so has the nature of the information systems necessary for acquisition and understanding of larger amounts of data, along with the analytical systems necessary for processing those data. Technological advances have allowed the automation of the systems that the practice of public health requires.

In this chapter, we will trace the history of the evolution of the science of public health informatics. We will begin by tracing the development of counting and counting machines in the human experience. In a brief examination of public health information management in the pre-computer era, we will then discuss the developments that created the need for increasingly complex data collection and analysis systems. We will next move to an examination of the experience of the Illinois Department of Public Health in automating public health practice. We will conclude the chapter with a look at the three waves of federal-state public health systems development, beginning with the first wave in the late 1960s and concluding with an examination of the third wave now under way. Before undertaking this history, however, we will define some commonly misused terms of information science.

Data, Information, and Knowledge

The terms *data, information*, and *knowledge* are often misused in discussions of public health informatics. Yet, if issues related to the development of public health informatics are going to be understood, a grasp of the precise meaning of these terms is essential.

The term *data* designates a measurement or a characteristic of the person or thing that is the focus of an information system. It can also be a clinical measurement, a laboratory value, a medication dosage, or even a listing of treatments. In isolation, data have little meaning. Consider, for example, the components of data in a vital records system used as part of a mission to monitor the health status of a nation. Each form in the system includes a notation of the deceased individual's age, race, and other demographic features. It also typically includes a description of the cause of death by a physician, a medical examiner, or a coroner. All of these data are the raw material of the vital records system. However, without context or analysis, these isolated bits do not convey much meaning.

Information, on the other hand, is data placed in context with analysis. Consider, for example, the data element indicating cause of death in a vital records system. If a public health official correlates this data element and generates a table categorizing the frequency of numerous causes of death, he or she has created information. A user of the table can identify the leading causes of death as well as the distribution of those causes in the nation.

Finally, *knowledge* in a public health system is the application of information by the use of rules. In our vital records system, for example, suppose that one leading cause of death identified in a locality is lead poisoning. In that locality, a toxicologist can review results of blood lead tests administered to the population and compare the outcomes to normal blood lead values. This process in itself yields information. At the same time, the toxicologist has access to action levels developed by experts working with the CDC. These action levels represent rules for action for managing blood lead levels in the affected population. The action levels, then, are an example of knowledge; they prescribe the rules to be used in the application of information. Table 2.1 summarizes the distinction among these three terms.

The Development of Counting and Counting Machines

"When you can measure what you are speaking about, and express it in numbers, you know something about it," said Lord Kelvin in his famous pronouncement equating measurement with knowledge. Indeed, the history of

TABLE 2.1. Data information and knowledge

Term	Definition	Example
Data	A measurement or characteristic of the person or the thing that is the focus of an information system	A public health assessor records the levels of thallium at various locations at a toxic waste site.
Information	Data placed in context with analysis	A public health assessor creates a table showing the proportion of the locations exceeding the appropriate maximum contaminant level for thallium at the site.
Knowledge	The application of information by the use of rules	The public health assessor consults the action levels for thallium as published by CDC/ATSDR and determines the appropriate remedial actions to be taken at the contaminated site.

information systems is in one sense a history of measurement. From the earliest known artifact associated with counting—a fibula of a baboon, with 29 clearly defined notches, dated approximately 35,000 BCE and found in a cave in the Lebombo Mountains in southern Africa—to the present day, information systems have concentrated on measurement. In addition, of course, they now perform sophisticated analytical work on large sets of data.

The earliest counting systems reflect the fact that the human brain has inherent limitations in its ability to comprehend quantity. The eye is not a very precise counting tool, particularly in comprehending quantities above four or five. Societies that entered the 20th century isolated from the rest of the world rarely had words for numbers greater than four. You can verify the limitations of the eye in counting with a simple experiment: Look at a number of marbles in a bowl very briefly, starting with one or two marbles and then adding a few marbles to the bowl. As you add marbles, try to determine the number without counting. If your visual limits are typical, you will have difficulty in determining the exact number of marbles without counting them once the actual number exceeds four or five.

That kind of limitation of the human brain to readily accommodate larger numbers led to the use of objects to implement one-to-one correspondence in measurement and to reliance on the property of mapping. We can see this human tendency to grasp the principle of one-to-one correspondence and to utilize the property of mapping in an infant who, at 15 or 16 months, has gone beyond simple observation of the environment. If we give such a child an equal number of dolls and little chairs, the infant will probably try to fit a doll on each seat. This kind of play is nothing other than mapping the elements of one set (dolls) onto the elements of a second set (chairs). But if we set out more dolls than chairs (or more chairs than dolls), after a time the child will begin to fret: it will realize that the mapping is not working.[1]

Application of the principle of one-to-one correspondence led early humankind to the use of objects to record the association of one thing to another. We have already mentioned the fibula of the baboon dated to approximately 35,000 BCE; it is marked with 29 clearly defined notches, and it resembles calendar sticks still in use by Bushmen clans in Namibia.[2] In a similar fashion, cave drawings with clear counting marks beneath the depicted animals may have represented an account of success at a hunt. In addition, tally sticks used from the earliest time for counting as well as for accounting represent one-to-one correspondence, as do other historic devices, including counting pebbles and using molded, unbaked clay tokens. Other examples include an early form of an abacus used in Sumer (lower Mesopotamia).

It is believed that the earliest counting tool was the human body, and specifically the hand. In fact, the earliest device used for calculation was the fingers of the hand. (This counting system would seem to have led to the development of numbering systems with a base of 5 in many locations throughout the world.) Funerary paintings from an Egyptian tomb at Beni Hassan dating from the Middle Kingdom (2100–1600 BCE) depict people playing the game of morra, a game that uses finger-based calculations to determine the winner.[3]

The Egyptians were noted for their early adoption of a written numerical system. A document carved on the Palermo Stone (circa 2925–2325 BCE) listed the current census of livestock and a 600-year history of the cycle of flooding of the Nile.[4] The Egyptian civilization was dependent upon the water from the Nile River that watered the fields when it flooded once per year. However, if the flooding was too great, the damage to the homes and irrigation systems would lead to poor crops. The government stored grain to abate any shortfall of grain production. By measuring the height of the flood, they were able to calculate the expected size of the crop and project a shortfall.[5]

The Egyptians of the Middle Kingdom were early users of numbers and counting to do more than just document their environment; they also used counting to predict and plan for the future.

Development of Mechanical Counting Devices

The success of the abacus, of finger-based calculation, and of other methods predominated until the 1600s CE. These counting methods were used primarily in commerce. It was the measurement of time, of the motion of stars, and of distance that sparked the development of mechanical calculating devices. Egyptians were among the first to use mechanical devices to measure the passage of time. They invented the water clock to mark the hours of the night (early 14th century BCE). The water clock used the passage of water from a carefully designed vessel to divide the night into 12 equal hours. This device had adjustments for the seasons, when the length of night and day varied. This water clock is one of the earliest known mechanical calculation devices.[6] In approximately 150 BCE, Hipparchus developed a device, called an astrolabe, to calculate the position of the stars.[7] Other Greek mechanical artifacts from the time indicated the use of gears and wheels to calculate the positions of the planets and stars.[6(p73)] In the same period, Roman documents indicated the development of a geared device to measure distance.[6(p121)] Such devices were also developed in China in the 3rd century CE. In 723 CE, I-Hsing, a Buddhist monk and mathematician, developed a water-driven mechanical clock, the first such known.[6(p126–127)]

The Development of Modern Mechanical Measuring Devices

Mechanical devices for arithmetic or other mathematical calculations were not developed until 1622 CE, when William Oughtred invented the rectilinear logarithmic slide rule. In 1630 CE, his student, Richard Delamain, developed the circular slide rule.[8] These devices used logarithmic theory to approximate complex mathematical calculations. Slide rules were used until the 1970s, when electronic calculators replaced them.

German scientist Wilhelm Schickard developed the first truly mechanical calculating device in 1623, a machine that used sprocket wheels to add numbers. Multiplication and division was possible with the use of logarithm tables.[9] In 1642, Blaise Pascal developed the first adding and subtracting device; it was able to carry or borrow digits from column to column automatically.[1(p382),8(p203)] Over the next 240 years, the fundamental principles developed by Oughtred, Schickard, and Pascal formed the basis of calculation machines.

Although these calculating machines and their increasingly sophisticated descendants were able to perform the basic arithmetic functions accurately, they were unable to perform more sophisticated analytical work on large sets of data. In 1820, a British mathematician, Charles Babbage, began the construction of a machine for calculating mathematical tables. He secured aid from the Royal Society and the British government to continue his work. He ran out of funding in 1856 without completing his device.[8(p204)] However, many of his concepts have formed the foundation of electronic computers in use today.[10]

While the mechanical calculators were effective in the business setting for accounting purposes, they were less effective for the analysis of large data sets. It was the 1880 US census that served as the occasion for the development of the first machine capable of performing analysis of such large data sets.

By 1880, the increase in the population in the United States created significant obstacles for the decennial census. In fact, the 1880 census took 8 years to complete. Under direction of Dr. John Shaw Billings, from the US Surgeon General's office, Herman Hollerith borrowed technology from Joseph-Marie Jacquard, the developer of the automated loom. Jacquard's loom was controlled by a series of cards with holes punched in them corresponding to the weave pattern. Hollerith developed a system that read holes punched into a card. Each dollar bill–sized card was able to hold a large amount of data. The card was read in a rapid fashion by a machine designed by Hollerith. The 1890 census was completed in half the time required for the 1880 census, with savings of $500 thousand (1890 dollars).[11] This innovation was the basis of many electric business and scientific machines well into the second half of the 20th century.

The military challenges of the First World War led to a greater focus on automated calculation. To hit the faster targets that existed on the mechanized battlefield, gunnery officers had to make quick adjustments for speed of the target, weight of the shell, and wind speed and direction. To assist the gunnery officers, the US Army sought to prepare firing tables. Those tables allowed the gunnery office to determine angulation and direction for the gun quickly. However, the time-consuming computations necessary for developing the tables completely overwhelmed the Ballistic Research Laboratory. Through a contract with the University of Pennsylvania, more than 100 students were working on the project without eliminating the backlog.

In response to the need to speed up this process, the Army funded the creation of ENIAC (Electronic Numerical Integrator and Computer). The project was started in 1943 and completed in 1945. When completed, it weighed 30 tons, contained 18,000 vacuum tubes, and was capable of 360 multiplications per second.[11(p115,116),12] The ENIAC, along with the Mark I, developed by Howard Aiken, were the first modern programmable computers.[9(p1,2)]

Although ENIAC was not the only computer of its time—the British computer Colossus, for example, had been designed to crack Nazi codes—it was the first multipurpose computer. It could be programmed to perform different functions, and it was also fast. For example, it could add 5,000 numbers or do 14 10-digit multiplications in a second. Although these feats are slow by modern standards, they were incredible for the 1940s. ENIAC was the brainchild of Professor John Mauchly, a physics teacher, and graduate student J. Presper Eckert, both of the University of Pennsylvania. Although the purpose of the design of ENIAC was assisting the army in performing the calculations necessary for gunnery charts, it was completed too late to be of use for that purpose during World War II. ENIAC, in fact, began its first task even before it was dedicated in 1945: performing millions of calculations associated with top-secret studies of nuclear chain reactions in connection with the eventual development of the hydrogen bomb.

Later, Dr. John von Neumann of the Institute for Advanced Study in Princeton contributed an enhancement to ENIAC. Before he worked with ENIAC, reprogramming the computer involved manually rewiring it. Dr. von Neumann suggested that code selection be made with switches, so that cable connections could remain fixed. This innovation saved considerable time in reprogramming ENIAC.[12]

Pre–Computer Era Public Health Information Management Systems

Pre–computer era public health information management systems have their roots in antiquity. The first phase of these systems reflected public health observations according to individual experience. A second phase reflected a movement beyond observation to analysis of the root causes of public health disturbances. Finally, a third phase, leading to the rise of modern public health informatics, featured advanced methods of data collection and analysis in public health practice.

The Age of Observation

Observations based upon individual experience marked the first phase of public health practice based on data. Observations by the great physicians of their times in China, Egypt, India, Greece, and Rome provided the foundation for preventive and curative practice, and the practice of vaccination is known to have existed as early as the first century BCE in China.[14] Of course, the most famous of the pre–computer era public health practitioners was Hippocrates, whose teaching reflects the way early health practitioners used observation to understand the relationship of health to living conditions. The observations of such practitioners led to the development and implementation of public health interventions. For example, the importance of sanitation was discovered early in the rise of civilization. Eventually, the age of observation in public health gave way to the age of analysis.

The Age of Analysis

The fall of the Roman Empire during the late 400s of the Common Era marked the end of an exchange of scientific learning between the hemispheres. For the next 1,000 years, social and political forces led to the isolation of Europe from many of the cultural and scientific developments in Africa, Asia, and other parts of the world. Much of the writings and the knowledge acquired during the Observation Era was lost. However, the Arab cultures of the Mediterranean preserved it to some extent and reintroduced it to the peoples of Europe during trade and the Moorish occupation. The European rediscovery of the Americas and the subsequent colonization resulted in a Eurocentric New World scientific community. The scientific and health systems that developed in the colonial and 19th century United States was dependent on the state of the art in Europe.

Certain events occurring during the Age of Analysis had profound implications for public health practice. These events included:

- The breakout of bubonic plague in Messina, Sicily, in October 1347, with the subsequent spread of the deadly disease to other parts of Europe, resulting in social upheaval.
- The great explosion in knowledge and learning accompanying the Renaissance in Europe. An important resulting enhancement to the evolution of public health practice was the adoption of the scientific method, a systematic approach that laid the foundation for collection and analysis of health-related data.
- General recognition of the importance of a healthy population to the national wealth and power. The philosopher William Perry, who invented the term *political arithmetic*, argued that the analysis of data could throw light on matters of national interest and policy, and he suggested that the control of communicable disease and the reduction of infant mortality would contribute the most to preventing impairment of the population. He was one of the first to calculate the economic loss caused by disease.[14]
- The establishment of basic principles for analysis of data and determination of data reliability by John Graunt, who in 1662 analyzed over 30 years of vital statistics and social data. Graunt's work demonstrated a method of developing useful information through the careful and logical interpretation of imperfect data.
- The work of Huygens in developing a precursor to mortality tables, work that was based on the findings of Graunt and his own earlier work on probability.
- Edmond Haley's merging of these concepts and his development of the first mortality tables to predict life expectancy in 1693. Haley's merger of data collection and probabilistic analysis established modern principles for the management and analysis of public health data.
- The contributions of scientists such as Laplace and Bernoulli in the application of mathematical principles to public health issues, work that set the stage for the major advances in data and information management that led to the development of the modern epidemiological approach.

The Roots of Modern Public Health Informatics

During the 19th century and the first half of the 20th century, developments in both England and the United States created the necessity for advanced methods of data collection and analysis in public health practice.

The Cholera Outbreaks in England

In England, the 19th century cholera epidemics led to major changes in the practice of public health. The cholera epidemics of 1831 and 1832 highlighted the role that neglected sanitation among the poor had in imperiling the health of all. The New Poor Law was passed, and the Poor Law Commission was formed in 1834 in response. Dr. Edwin Chadwick was appointed the secretary of the commission and became one of the leading forces in the sanitation movement. He proposed the formation of the Bureau of Medical Statistics in the Poor Law Office. Under his leadership, Dr. William Farr began to use data that became available under the 1836 Births and Deaths Act. Chadwick proposed that this act would lead to registration of the causes of disease with a view to devising remedies or means of prevention.[15] A vast amount of data was collected under these two acts. Analysis of these data by Farr led to the understanding of the role of sanitation and health. Farr's analysis represented one of the earliest examples of the presentation of a plausible epidemiological theory to fit known facts and collected data.

In 1859, Florence Nightingale, working with William Farr, confirmed the connection between sanitation and mortality by studying the horrendous death rate in the British Army in the Crimea. Not only did these public health workers compare death rates in the army for non-combat-related illness to a reference population, but they also published one of the first uses of graphics to present public health data. At this time, Adolphe Quetelet consolidated current statistical developments and applied them to the analysis of community health data compiled by observation and enumeration. He noted that variation was a characteristic of biological and social phenomenon and that such variation occurred around a mean of a number of observations. Further, he demonstrated that the distribution of observations around a mean corresponded to the distribution of probabilities on a probability curve. This work helped form the foundation of biostatistics as applied to the health of the public.

In 1854, cholera again struck London. Dr. John Snow conducted an investigation of this outbreak in the Soho section of London. He carefully mapped the location of each of the victims. The mapping revealed a pattern centered on the Broad Street pump. He then proceeded to convince local authorities to remove the handle from the pump, thereby stopping the outbreak. He continued the analysis of the outbreak and was able to associate the location of the water intake that supplied the Broad Street pump with other water companies and sewage outflows in the Thames River. His work led to future regulation of water supply intakes. The methodology that he used has become the foundation of all modern epidemiological investigations of a disease outbreak. He also was one of the first to use a rudimentary manual graphical information system (GIS)—a map and a pencil.[16,17]

The application of scientific learning began to have a positive impact on the health of the English population. In 1866, it was noted that cities without a system for monitoring and combating cholera fared far worse in the epidemic of that year.[18]

Public Health Data Collection in the United States

In the United States, independence led to the development of strong state and local governments. These organizations began to incorporate current scientific knowledge into protecting the health of their populations. The first local health department was formed in 1798 in Baltimore, Maryland.[19]

In the early 1800s, local health departments collected health data only sporadically. In Illinois, for example, sporadic data were collected in the City of Chicago starting in 1833, with the formation of the Chicago Department of Health.

Data collection problems in the seventh decennial census in 1850, however, resulted in more comprehensive public health data collection and analysis in the United States. The seventh census included gross death and birth rates that many considered inaccurate because of defects in the collection of this data. Changes in the methods of data collection were implemented for the eighth decennial census in 1860, and more reliable data were collected.[20]

One of the most profoundly influential 19th century data collection developments in the states was the publication in 1850 of Lemuel Shattuck's Report of the Sanitary Commission of Massachusetts. This report provided the basic blueprint for the development of a public health system in the United States. It outlined many elements of the modern public health infrastructure, including a recommendation for establishing state and local health boards.

By 1900, many state and local health departments had formed in the United States. An important role of these departments was the collection and analysis of reports of communicable diseases and vital statistics. In the early 1900s, the vital record system was still struggling. The Census Bureau worked with many states to encourage recording and reporting birth and death data. During the Depression and the Second World War, the importance of enumerating and documenting births became evident as more people needed to prove citizenship for eligibility for relief and other programs. In fact, during World War II, laws prohibited the employment of noncitizens in essential defense projects; for many job seekers, proof of citizenship through birth or naturalization was essential.

In 1933, Texas became the last state to begin reporting vital statistics to the federal government. Even so, in 1940, it was estimated that as many as 55 million native-born persons did not have birth records.[21] In response, the US Bureau of the Budget recommended moving the vital statistics office to the Public Health Service. In the 1960s, the vital statistics function became a part of the new National Center for Health Statistics, and the current cooperative system with states was in place.[22,23]

In the first part of the 20th Century, the system for collecting birth and death records was being established and standardized. However, data about nonfatal illness were difficult to obtain and were therefore sparsely available. The year 1933 marked the first attempt at a survey-based assessment of the health status of the US population. The survey was conducted through use of Work Projects Administration funds. The survey incorporated data from 750,000 households in 84 cities and several rural areas. It was conducted with the time's accepted methodology, which did not include probability sampling or standardized questionnaires. These data became the reference for policy development until the National Health Interview Survey (NHIS) reported its first results in 1957.[22] The design of the NHIS was one of the early tasks of the National Committee on Vital and Health Statistics (NCVHS) in 1953.[23]

The scientific discoveries of the 19th century laid the basis for making substantial progress in the control of infectious disease. The nature of public health challenges changed as the importance of data in policy and program decision making became better understood by organized public health agencies and researchers. Advances in immunizations, sanitation, and nutrition led to substantial improvements in the health of the public. By the middle of the 20th century, the leading causes of death became heart disease, cancer, and stroke. The increasing importance of these chronic illnesses in public health practice mandated a disease model capable of handling numerous factors, with longer intervals between cause and effect. The fact that interventions had become more complex and long term required the development of new approaches involving data collected about individuals over time and space. In turn, the need to analyze data in different locations and times led to the concept of data linkage.[24] Initially, attempts were made to develop a paper-based cross-index. The complexity of such a task became daunting and led to frustration and failure.

Better surveillance systems and enhancements to national and local vital statistics systems increased the data that were available to public health agencies, enabling programmatic decisions for the prevention and treatment of disease to be data and information driven. The increasing volumes of data and the increasing need to analyze that data created conditions that were ripe for technological advancement. In fact, many tasks, including record linkage on a large scale, were impossible, given the state of technology in the mid-20th century. The newly emerging automated information systems and the need for public health entities to manage large volumes of data and information were a perfectly timed match. The experience of the public health system of Illinois in collecting and analyzing public health data, the subject of the next section, is typical of the development process for public health information systems in the states.

The Automation of Public Health Practices: The Illinois Experience

Measurement of the population is one of the most basic of health statistics. As we have already seen, the need to measure populations has driven important innovations in data collection and analysis. In fact, it was the desire to speed up the US census process in the 1880s that led to the invention of the card reader. This technology had rapid adaptation in the business world. In the following years, statistical sampling techniques were developed to allow the provision of population estimates in the years between census counts. As the population of the United States continued to grow, the task of the Census Bureau in processing the data by using existing methods was daunting. In response, the Census Bureau began the first nonmilitary use of a computer in April 1951, when the first computerized system began tabulating data from the 1950 Census.

Many state public health agencies now have responsibilities for collecting data on vital events. Early on, the collection and reporting of vital events was the province of local administrators, such as county clerks. In the State of Illinois, the Illinois Department of Public Health (IDPH) assumed statewide responsibility for this activity in 1916. The IDPH had responsibility for collecting, tabulating, and printing summary tables on live births, stillbirths, and deaths. This responsibility was amended in 1951 to include marriages, divorces, and annulments. Initially, records were collected on written documents and tabulated by hand. In 1938, IDPH acquired IBM tabulation equipment and used it for vital statistics and other health data. It was the first automated system for data installed in state government in Illinois.[25] Eleven years after the national Census Bureau used the first computer in the US civilian practice in 1951, IDPH became one of the first state public health departments to adopt computer technology. In 1962, IDPH converted all existing applications from tabulation equipment to an IBM 1401 computer. Within two years of installation, the system was being used to manage data from the divisions of sanitary engineering, administration, laboratories, communicable disease control, dental health, and maternal and child health.[26]

The use of the new computer grew, and IDPH purchased a second computer, an IBM 360. By 1967, over 100 separate files and 500 programs had been written for the processing, storing, and retrieval of data. IDPH then created the Division of Data Processing, which ultimately had two operating units: the computer science section for the development of new systems and the maintenance of established systems, and the operations section for providing routine or ad hoc reports. A major project of the Division of Data Processing was to develop a Total Health Information System (THIS) that was designed to integrate demographics, public and private health resources, health status, and need data. It was envisioned that this system would enable large volumes of data to be analyzed in order to provide program administrators with support for planning, decision-making, investigative, and regulative functions. The first systems included in THIS were (a) long-term care licensing, (b) hospital licensing, (c) venereal disease control, (d) radiological health, (e) food and drugs, (f) clinical laboratories, and (g) the tuberculosis registry. Subsequent data management systems, including a computerized general ledger system, were completed in 1977. The new systems moved away from the concept of a single integrated system to separate stand-alone systems.[26(p175-176)]

In 1977, the department installed three dumb terminals in the Division of Vital Records with the adoption of the Entrex system. The Entrex system created a tape that was used to update records on the mainframe. The capacity to load records locally represented the IDPH's first excursion into distributed systems. Prior to that, paper records were taken to the Division of Data Processing for data entry. Reports and tabulations would then be returned to the user on paper. In 1984, direct access to the mainframe systems was added to the terminals in the Division of Vital Records.

In the early 1980s, all mainframe computer systems were centralized in the Illinois Central Management Services Agency system. IDPH staff continued to develop, implement, and operate public health systems on the centralized computers. A Wang minicomputer–based word-processing system was installed to form the basis of the first network in the agency. This system was modified in 1987 to establish an electronic mail system throughout the agency. An Ethernet-based local area network was soon established, and the Wang system was retired in 1992.

In 1985, Illinois suffered the largest milk-borne outbreak of salmonellosis in the nation's history. After the outbreak was brought under control, the interagency critique identified communication capability with local health departments as a major weakness of the response. The state legislature appropriated money to establish a microcomputer-based information system. This system was named the Public Health Information Network (PHIN). Each local health department had a PHIN computer placed in its offices. The PHIN computer was used by each local health department to dial into the state network on a regular basis. This modem-based system formed the backbone of communications between the IDPH and local health departments until 1999. In that year, the desktop computers were replaced to assure year 2000 compliance. Additionally, funds from the federal Centers for Disease Control and Prevention bioterrorism preparedness program became available to implement the Health Alert Network. This network used wide area network technology to incorporate each of the 94 local health departments into the IDPH network.

Cornerstone: Development of an Integrated Maternal and Child Health Case Management System

In the late 1980s, IDPH operated a number of categorical information systems related to maternal and child health. An earlier system added an immunization module to the US Department of Agriculture's Women, Infants, and Children (WIC) case management system.[27] The department had also developed a stand-alone case management system to assist in the delivery of services to pregnant women and children, the Case Management Information System. Recognizing that many Maternal and Child Health (MCH) functions used the same data, IDPH authorities made a decision to develop a comprehensive system, called Cornerstone.

Cornerstone was designed around a core functionality termed CASE (Coordinated Activities, Services, and Encounters). The CASE functionality passed data between the various modules. The WIC module managed the allocation of food supplementation. It managed the determination of need and the selection of appropriate food baskets, printed the WIC coupons, and managed their redemption and payment. Some of this function was achieved by integrating legacy systems into Cornerstone. The well-child module managed data collected during well-child visits to healthcare providers; these data included clinical data, biometrics (height, weight, etc.), health history, and physical examination results.

Additional modules were immunization and MCH case management. When fully implemented in the early 1990s, Cornerstone was functional in almost 300 sites, including local health departments, community health centers, rural health centers, and other community-based organizations.

Cornerstone represented the prototype for an integrated public health system designed with a strong set of underlying principles:

- The first principle was that data would be entered only once, at the point of service. Each case manager and service provider would have a personal computer at his or her workstation. Clinical information such as the results of a lead test would be entered in the well-child module. The results of the lead or hemoglobin test would also be incorporated into the WIC module. In the WIC module, decisions about the types of foods that are part of the benefit would be modified according to those clinical measurements.
- The second principle was that design and implementation would be focused on the point of service. For this reason, Cornerstone's developers interviewed frontline staff before developing system parameters and functionality. The developers also involved focus groups of frontline staff in field-testing to make sure the system met frontline staff needs. This approach assured that the functionality the case managers needed was available through Cornerstone, while at the same time the system documented their activities. In addition, management systems were designed to operate exclusively from frontline data, avoiding additional data entry requirements. The system also provided scheduling for case managers and referral sources, eliminating the requirement for most logs.
- The third principle was interoperability between the modules and the flexibility to add new modules. The sharing of data was a key operational feature of Cornerstone. In addition, the design was such that additional case management systems with their own sets of rules could be added on with greatly reduced costs and time. For example, a breast and cervical cancer screening and case management system was developed and operated through the CASE functionality with minimal development time and costs.
- The fourth principle was the utilization of decision support. This rule-based expert system assisted case managers in making appropriate assessments and decisions. For instance, a low hemoglobin test result in the well-child module would result in the WIC module's prompting the case manager to augment the standard food package.
- Finally, the system was designed in a modular fashion focused on the point of service. Each clinic would have its own local data set. Access was restricted at the element level and based upon centrally established rules. When consent was obtained, records could be transferred from one Cornerstone site to another. A master patient index was created at the state level to allow records to be located. An individual case manager designates each set of data as being sharable or not, depending upon the client's desires. Access to many data elements is restricted to the case manager. In

TABLE 2.2. The core principles underlying Cornerstone

Principle	Implementation
Data entered only at the point of service	Each case manager/provider provided with a personal computer and access to the WIC module
Focus of Cornerstone is the point of service	Management systems designed to operate exclusively from frontline data
Interoperability between the modules and the flexibility to add new modules	System provided for sharing of data among modules. New case management systems could be added with greatly reduced costs and time.
Utilization of decision support	Rule-based expert system assisted case managers in making appropriate assessments and decisions.
System designed in modular fashion and focused on the point of service	Each clinic provided with its own local data set, with access restricted at the element level and based on established rules. A state-level master patient index allowed records to be located.

this way, Cornerstone maintains privacy and confidentiality at the data element level.

Table 2.2 summarizes the core principles underlying Cornerstone and how each principle was implemented. The result of these system design principles was an integrated MCH case management system that allows the case managers to function in a paperless environment. Management had access to a rich data set to monitor outcomes and performance of the system and individual staff. Although the system now needs reengineering to take advantage of current technology, many of the design principles stand as the basis for public health information systems of the future.

The Three Waves of Federal-State System Development

At the beginning of this chapter, we pointed out that many of today's public health information systems are products of a partnership between state and federal public health officials. The evolution of this partnership occurred in three waves, representing, respectively, independent systems development, with federal systems imposed on the states; federal funding of state-level systems; and integration of the benefits of state-level system development with the tools of software reuse.

The First Wave: Independent Systems Development

In the early days of system development, states and the federal government developed information systems independently. Standards developed through the cooperative system in vital statistics assured that data that were delivered to the National Center for Health Statistics (NCHS) were comparable from one state to another. The NCHS developed the cooperative system in vital statistics in cooperation with state registrars. Any changes made to this system occurred according to a process of agreement among the many partners.

Similarly, the CDC and the Council of State and Territorial Epidemiologists collaboratively developed standards for reports of communicable diseases. States actively developed stand-alone systems to manage their own programs. Federal systems were also developed and made available to states. Some federal systems used standardized data definitions, whereas others did not. However, as is common in public health, because resources for system development were hard to come by, states considered these federal systems as major enhancements to their own capacity to meet their missions.

Early state systems included newborn metabolic disease screening. Screening newborns for phenylketonuria began in 1969; severe mental retardation can be avoided if a child is diagnosed soon after birth and placed on a diet low in phenylalanine.

Laboratories were the earliest users of computers to keep track of newborn screening test results. The challenge was to assure that every positive laboratory test was followed up and the baby was put on the low phenylalanine diet. The earliest newborn screening systems were developed in California, Illinois, Oregon and Texas.[28-30] By 1984, 19 states had such systems in place.[31] These systems were developed in each state separately.

In the same time frame, the CDC and other federal agencies were developing information systems for use in states. One example is the system developed by the CDC to automate the data collection for the AIDS/HIV registry. It was designed in 1987 to take completed surveillance forms and read them with an optical scanner. The optical scanner converted pencil marks on a specially designed document into an electronic database. On a monthly basis, state data were transferred to the CDC for national surveillance programs. The system worked very well for the purpose for which it was designed. However, state health agencies needed to modify their operational systems to use it. Clerical staff had to review each form by hand for completeness before the forms were inserted into the scanner. If the data were incomplete, the form could not be scanned. State health department staff had to contact the local health department to complete the form. Organizationally, the state health department staff would be able to work more efficiently if the system could be modified to read the form and kick out the records with incomplete data.

Because CDC designed the turnkey system, modifications could not be made at the state level. The system was designed to meet the needs of the program at CDC, not the needs of those who would be collecting the data. Despite the frustrations felt by state health agency staff, this arrangement had a clear ability to be cost effective. Because the CDC developed the program and then provided it to the states, the development costs were paid only once.

The Second Wave: Federal Funding of State-Level Systems

Over time, state agencies became concerned about the number of systems existing in each program, and they became concerned that the number of systems was increasing. At the same time, the systems were unable to communicate with each other. What had initially been a blessing became a curse as state and local health agency staff had to enter the same data into multiple systems.

During this time frame, data standards had been under development for health care. For example, the College of American Pathologists developed a standard nomenclature for pathology in 1965.[32] Similarly, the NCVHS proposed standards for a Uniform Hospital Discharge Data Set in 1979.[33] Systems that were independently developed by CDC centers, institutes, or offices each used the data definition that seemed to be the best for their own purposes. Those definitions were frequently different from those developed by other units of the CDC, by the Health Resources and Services Administration (HRSA), by the Health Care Financing Administration, or by other federal agencies. States also developed their own definitions and scoring systems. Consequently, most of the systems were unable to share data. As an example, in the HIV/AIDS program at the Illinois Department of Public Health, there were eight different information systems that transferred and monitored laboratory data, operated the AIDS registry and the HIV registry, provided AIDS service delivery under the Ryan White program and state-funded programs, delivered data to the CDC, and operated the AIDS Drug Assistance Program.

Because each system was independent, data had to be entered separately into each system, and individual data elements had to be entered multiple times.

In the early 1990s, state and local health departments, the Association of State and Territorial Health Officials (ASTHO), and the National Association of County and City Health Officials (NACCHO) opened a discussion of their system problems with Phil Lee, the Assistant Secretary for Health, US Department of Health and Human Services. Dr. Lee was noted to comment, "I knew that *data* was a four letter word. I just never knew it was spelled T-U-R-F." State and local health departments were looking for the ability to build more integrated information systems along the lines of the Illinois Cornerstone and the Georgia Information Network for Public Health Officials and Host systems.[34] In response, CDC and HRSA began allowing state and local health departments to use categorical funding to implement information systems integrated across programs. In addition, funding became available for the development of information systems at the state and local level. The immunization registry program is an example. Using a combination of state and federal funding, many states created state-based information systems. In Illinois, the system has been designed to use multiple information technologies, including telephone, fax, modem, and electronic data interchange (EDI). The new Tracking Our Toddlers' Shots (TOTS) system was designed to exchange information with the legacy Cornerstone system. This tracking system allows the integration of immunization information for both public-funded and private patients. The TOTS system was designed to accommodate EDI with providers and other states. With leadership by the CDC, the Health Level 7 (HL7) Committee's standard for immunizations was extended to include public health–relevant information. The success of such efforts to integrate systems is illustrated by the following example: In July of 1999, an immunization record was developed in Arizona, transmitted to Illinois, and then transmitted on to Georgia by use of EDI.

With federal agencies funding state information system development, state information systems could be developed with a focus on state and local operations. The automated processes could reflect the nature of the public health environment in each state. The adoption of standards for health information developed by national standards development organizations will allow data to be exchanged between states. This is a crucial issue because of the highly mobile nature of the population. This wave of state–federal development had the clear advantage of assuring that information systems could be developed to fit the needs of each individual state. The disadvantages were that the cost of development had to be paid 50 times—each time one of the states developed a specific system. In addition, there was no assurance that each state would build the system to be consistent with national standards.

The Third Wave: Integration of the Benefits of State-Level System Development with the Tools of Software Reuse

The third wave of system development integrates the benefits of state-level system development with the tools of software reuse. Software reuse is possible, given the current state of system development. Current system development uses such tools as object-oriented software development and the Web-enabled environment. Further, an axiom of third-wave system development is that each system that is developed must be standards based.

In the third-wave approach, federal funds are granted to a limited number of states to develop prototype systems. Those systems are designed in a modular fashion to facilitate easy modification for use in other states. After the prototype systems are completed and validated, the federal government makes funding available only for the costs of modifying the prototype system to meet the unique needs of each state. An example of this principle is the adaptation by Illinois of a laboratory information system developed in North Carolina in 2000.

The third wave of state–federal system development is also dependent upon the development of standards for public health data. The CDC has been playing a leading role in this process with the formation of the Health Information and Surveillance Systems Board (HISSB) in 1993. In 1995, HISSB released a landmark report, "Integrating Public Health Information and Surveillance Systems."[35] Working with other federal agencies—ASTHO, NACCHO, and the National Association of Local Boards of Health—the CDC has developed a conceptual model for public health data.[36] The collaborating organizations have also developed the Common Information for Public Health Electronics Reporting (CIPHER)[37] standard that is based upon the record structure of the National Electronic Telecommunications System for Surveillance.[38] These documents will be an integral part of the proposed National Electronic Disease Surveillance System.[39] With these standards and those developed by other SDOs like HL7, a new era in state–federal information systems development can begin.

Conclusion

Public health information management has been an important aspect of protecting the health of the public since prehistoric times. Public health practice has used currently available science in mathematics, chemistry, and biology to carry out its mission. In the last 200 years, public health has made dramatic advances. Building on discoveries in other fields, public health has constructed a unique science base with the development of biostatistics and epidemiology. This science base facilitates the analysis of large sets of data to describe and understand health problems. Through analysis, data are converted into information to drive effective interventions. The advent of the computer and the development of automated information systems have increased the effectiveness of public health analysis. Using these approaches, public health interventions have accounted for the bulk of the spectacular increases in life expectancy experienced in the United States in the 20th century.

Questions for Review

1. What factors account for the fact that early public health information systems developed as stand-alone products?
2. What distinguished the Age of Observation from the Age of Analysis?
3. What characteristic distinguished the computer ENIAC from all the other computers developed during World War II?
4. In what sense did the cholera epidemics in 19th-century England serve as a watershed in public health practice and public health information systems?
5. To what extent can it be said that the needs of the US Bureau of the Census

laid the foundation for the development of modern state public health
information systems?

6. Can any of the principles underlying the development of the Cornerstone
   system by the Illinois Department of Public Health be eliminated without
   causing harm to the remaining principles? If so, what is the sacrifice?

7. To what extent is the third wave of state-level public health system
   development a continuation of the second wave? In what respect does
   federal funding for the third wave differ from the federal funding for the
   second wave?

References

1. Smith DE. *History of Mathematics*. Vol. I. New York: Dover Publications;1951:
   6–7.
2. Bogashi J, Naidoo K, Webb J. The oldest mathematical artifact. *Mathematical
   Gazette* 7:294.
3. Ifrah G. *The Universal History of Numbers: From Prehistory to the Invention of
   the Computer*. New York: John Wiley & Sons; 2000:51–52.
4. Britannica.com. Palermo Stone. Available at: http://www.britannica.com/seo/p/
   palermo-stone/. Accessed March 13, 2002.
5. Garndiner A. *Egypt of the Pharaohs*. Oxford: Oxford University Press; 1961:62.
6. James P, Thorpe N. *Ancient Inventions*. New York: Ballantine Books; 1994.
7. "Hipparchus." *Microsoft® Encarta® 98 Encyclopedia* [CD-ROM]. Redmond, WA:
   Microsoft Corporation.
8. Smith DE. *History of Mathematics*. Vol. II. New York: Dover Publications; 1951:
   205.
9. IEEE-IFIP TC3 and TC9 Joint Task Group. History in the computing curriculum.
   IEEE Annals of the History of Computing. 1999:21(Appendix A1):2.
10. Bromley AG. Charles Babbage's analytical engine, 1838. *IEEE Annals of the His-
    tory of Computing*. 1998:20(4):29–45.
11. Burke J. *Connections*. Boston: Little, Brown and Co.; 1995.
12. Polachek H. Before the ENIAC. *IEEE Annals of the History of Computing*.
    1997:19(2):25–30.
13. Brown S. A Dissertation on Small-Pox, Varioloid, and Vaccination. *American
    Medical Reporter* 1829;45:45–88.
14. Rosen G. *A History of Public Health*. Baltimore, MD: Johns Hopkins University
    Press; 1993:184–192.
15. Chadwick E. *Report...from the Poor Law Commissioners on an Enquiry into the
    Sanitary Condition of the Labouring Population of Great Britain*. London: Clowes;
    1842.
16. Ginsberg R. John Snow is remembered with a pump–At the scene. *Nations Health*.
    1992:22:31.
17. The Committee for the Future of Public Health. *The Future of Public Health*.
    Washington, DC: National Academy Press; 1988:62.
18. Turnock BJ. *Public Health: What It Is and How It Works*. Gaithersburg, MD:
    Aspen Publishers; 1997:5.
19. Rawlings ID, Evans WE, Koehler G, Richardson BK. *The Rise and Fall of Disease
    in Illinois*. Springfield, IL: Illinois Department of Public Health; 1927.

20. Hetzel A. *US Vital Statistics System: Major Activities and Developments 1950–95*, National Center for Health Statistics. Centers for Disease Control and Prevention, US Department of Health and Human Services; 1997:PHS 97-1993.
21. Rice DP. Health statistics: Past, present, and future. In: Perrin EB, Kalsbeek WD, Scanlon TM, eds. *Toward a Health Statistics System for the 21st Century: Summary of a Workshop.* Washington, DC: National Academy Press, 2001.
22. Melnick D. *Building Robust Statistical Systems for Health.* Report to the National Committee on Vital and Health Statistics; November 11, 1999. In press.
23. National Committee on Vital and Health Statistics. *45th Anniversary Report of the National Committee on Vital and Health Statistics.* 1995.
24. Smith ME. Record linkage: Present status and methodology. *J Clin Comput* 1984;13: 52–71.
25. Richardson BK. *A History of the Illinois Department of Public Health 1927–1962.* Springfield, IL: Illinois Department of Public Health; 1963:39.
26. Wittenborn EL. *A History of the Illinois Department of Public Health 1962–1977,* Springfield, IL: Illinois Department of Public Health; 1978.
27. History of WIC. US Department of Agriculture Food and Nutrition Services Web site. Available at: http://www.fns.usda.gov/wic/MENU/NEW/WICHistory.PDF. Accessed March 13, 2002.
28. Meaney FJ. Computerized tracking for newborn screening and follow-up: A review. *J Med Systems* 1988;12:69–75.
29. Mordaunt VL, Cunningham GC, Kan K. Computer assisted management of a regionalized newborn screening program. *J Med Systems* 1988;12:77–88.
30. Therrell BL, Brown LO. Computerized newborn screening in Texas–A multiple microcomputer approach. *J Med Systems* 1988;12:115–120.
31. *Newborn Screening: An Overview of Newborn Screening Programs in the United States.* Springfield, IL: Illinois Department of Public Health; 1985.
32. National Committee on Vital and Health Statistics. *Report to the Secretary of the U.S. Department of Health and Human Services on Uniform Data Standards for Patient Medical Record Information.* Available at: http://www.ncvhs.hhs.gov/hipaa000706.pdf. March 13, 2002.
33. Larks M. State systems gather more health care data but lack uniformity. *Bus Health* 1986;3:49–50.
34. Chapman KA, Moulton AD. The Georgia Information Network for Public Health Officials (INPHO): A demonstration of the CDC INPHO concept. *J Public Health Manag Pract* 1995;1:39–43.
35. Health Information and Surveillance Systems Board. "Integrating Public Health Information and Surveillance Systems." Available at: http://www.cdc.gov/od/hissb/docs/katz.htm. March 13, 2002.
36. Health Information and Surveillance Systems Board. "Public Health Conceptual Data Model (PHCDM)." Available at: http://www.cdc.gov/od/hissb/docs/phcdm.htm. March 13, 2002.
37. Health Information and Surveillance Systems Board. "Common Information for Public Health Electronic Reporting (CIPHER) Guide (DRAFT)." Available at: http://www.cdc.gov/od/hissb/docs/cipher.htm. Accessed March 13, 2002.
38. Division of Public Health Science and Informatics, Centers for Disease Control and Prevention. "National Electronic Telecommunications System for Surveillance." Available at: http://www.cdc.gov/epo/dphsi/netss.htm. Accessed March 13, 2002.

39. Health Information and Surveillance Systems Board. "SupportingPublic Health Surveillance through the National Electronic Disease Surveillance System (NEDSS)." Available at: http://www.cdc.gov/od/hissb/docs/NEDSS%20Intro.pdf. Accessed March 13, 2002.

3
Better Health Through Informatics: Managing Information to Deliver Value

MARION J. BALL

> *In the correct formulation of the question lies the key to the answer*
> —*Nobelist Max Planck*

Learning Objectives

After studying this chapter, you should be able to:

- Explain why the effectiveness of health informatics is dependent on human factors, including the integration of informatics with the business plan and work processes, the existence of teamwork in the health enterprise, and the development of core competencies in the use of informatics.
- Define value creation as it relates to the use of information technology in the health enterprise.
- List and discuss at least three ways in which use of the Internet is reducing costs while improving the effectiveness of healthcare delivery.
- Explain how health informatics is improving health in the areas of (1) disease management, (2) telehealth, (3) patient safety, and (4) decision support.

Overview

The effective use of health informatics involves much more than implementation of hardware and software. It is dependent on human factors, including the development of competencies by those who would employ health informatics and the development of teamwork by information technology (IT) professionals and health professionals. Effective health informatics creates value. It is an enabler that maximizes its potential when its users work as a team to integrate health informatics with the business strategy and work processes. Already we are seeing Internet applications begin to drive down healthcare costs while improving the delivery and effectiveness of health services. This trend will continue in coming years. We are beginning to amass proof that informatics actually improves health through aiding in disease management, providing specialist support, improving patient safety, and serving as decision support for practitioners. Over the next decade, we will see many more advances in the use of technology in support of the shared missions of health care and public health to improve the life of each individual.

Introduction

In the preface to the *Yearbook of Medical Informatics 1999*, Hans E. Peterson states, "The new challenge is to learn what fundamental values in health care are supported by information technology and how they can contribute to its continued development." The intent of the *Yearbook* is clear: "To take a critical look both backwards and forwards. What were the early expectations and what was the outcome? What is to be expected for the next decade? In what way and to what extent can health care benefit from the accomplishments of medical and health informatics?" [1]

In this chapter, we take up Peterson's challenge, but from a different vantage point. To begin, we enlarge the context to include the full range of health-related activities, from wellness and population-based programs to illness and patient-focused care. At the heart of our discussion is a simple question: Can informatics improve health? In seeking to answer this question, we do not look to academia or to theoretical models. Rather, we look to health practices as they are today and draw evidence from actual informatics applications, which to date have been more generously supported in traditional healthcare institutions. At the same time, we note that the changes brought about by the Internet and by patient empowerment are already beginning to affect the broad set of functions, practices, disciplines, and other factors that affect how well people live their lives.

Drilling Down

As we proceed, we will drill down to a series of specific questions:

- What is health informatics and what are its components?
- What factors affect organizational success in using health informatics?
- How is the Internet affecting the provision of health services?
- What evidence is there that informatics actually improves health?

What Is Health Informatics and What Are Its Components?

In Chapter 1, we defined public health informatics as "the systematic application of information and computer science and technology to public health practice, research, and learning." However, it is important to note that, as an evolving discipline at the intersection of rapidly changing fields, health informatics in general lacks a single definition. In some quarters, it is viewed as a management and engineering discipline, and in others, as a science that may be theoretical, applied, or both. For our purposes in this chapter, we define health informatics as the demonstration of how organizations can use IT to bring their strategic goals from theory into practice. Within this context, IT serves as an enabler.

While success in the 21st century will be predicated upon harnessing and managing information, it will require a focus on value and the elements contained therein. Value resides in the relationship between cost containment, customer service and satisfaction, and superior clinical results or outcomes. Expressed conceptually,

value is a function of (cost, service, outcome).

Achieving this value proposition is no simple task. Supporting and measuring its components require that we receive and generate data, transform data into useful information, and transform information into knowledge. The capabilities provided by information technology function as key enablers in this process, supporting information management and knowledge creation. Informatics addresses these areas through its four cornerstones, described by Nancy Lorenzi and Bill Stead.[2] These involve the "systematic integration ... from intellectual development of how information assets are organized and managed, to what work processes should look like and how information systems should be implemented to support them."

Specifically, these cornerstones include the following:

- "Producing *structures to represent data and knowledge* so that complex relationships may be visualized."
- "Developing methods for *acquisition and presentation of data* so that overload can be avoided."
- "*Managing change* among people, process, and information technology so that the use of information is optimized."
- "*Integrating information* from diverse sources to provide more than the sum of the parts, and integrating information into work processes so that it can be acted on when it can have the largest effect."[3]

As Lorenzi notes, these cornerstones "extend well beyond the skills associated with traditional data processing and information systems." They stress the need to transform data into information and from accumulated information to create knowledge. They also acknowledge that human factors, not technical considerations, constitute the greatest obstacles to informatics success. As Reed Gardner stated in his 1998 Davies Lecture, "The success of a project is perhaps 80% dependent upon the development of the social and political interaction skills of the developer and 20% or less on the implementation of the hardware and software technology!"[4]

The International Medical Informatics Association Working Group 1 recently published competencies for different categories of health informaticians.[5] Further, Janise Richards has defined informatics competencies in public health informatics in her doctoral dissertation at the University of Texas.[6] (Ms. Richards' definitions form much of the subject matter of Chapter 6 of this textbook.) Well-defined competencies are increasingly important, as the emphasis shifts from the *how*—the technique and/or technology—to the *why*—what can be accomplished with health informatics, and how information can be managed and used to improve health.

What Factors Affect Organizational Success in Using Health Informatics?

Optimizing information management requires a focus first on values. Successful organizations understand that their strategy, set by their business plan, is the driver. Informatics is the enabler, and information technology provides the tools. As Paul Strassman remarks in his book, *The Squandered Computer*, "The principle purpose of investing in IT is not overhead cost reduction but value creation. Cutting costs can contribute to profitability, but in the long run one does not prosper through shrinkage. The objective of all investments is to improve overall organizational performance."[7]

To improve performance, IT and health professionals need to work as a team. Both need to understand the problem being addressed; both need to contribute their expertise toward its solution. Increasingly, trained health informaticians are playing a critical role in developing, selecting, and implementing applications. This role includes helping health professionals understand what informatics can offer in order to make wise decisions about IT.

Although allocations for IT in healthcare sectors reached record levels at the close of the 1990s, expenditures do not guarantee solutions. Investment analysts Volpe Brown Whelan and Co. estimate that health care wastes as much as $270 million a year on inefficient computer systems.[8] We do not dispute there is waste, but we question whether it is the result of inefficient computer systems. It is more likely, we believe, that ineffective *use* of those computer systems is the cause.

One striking example comes in the aftermath of year 2000 (Y2K). To avert problems associated with older systems, many institutions installed new applications without leveraging them to add value to their core business. Recent studies show this to be a common failing in health care and in industry in general.[9] Institutions need to make concerted efforts to target objectives and processes as they acquire and integrate IT. Those with newly installed and incompletely leveraged systems should revisit such critical activities and establish a clear agenda for change.

This need to establish and measure value is manifest in another area, specifically that area involving work processes. We mentioned the importance of human factors earlier, and the need for both organizational skills and technical know-how. In the broadest sense, human factors extend to include organizational and professional development, both of which imply redesigned work processes. Such efforts must be ongoing. If staff are to learn new skills, use new tools, and make optimal use of new technology, "unlearning" old ways is critical—and even more difficult than learning the new.

New ways of doing work are the end point of the classic three-stage model for technology adoption: substitution, innovation, and transformation. Medical imaging provides an excellent example of this model: the old radiology departments disappeared gradually and are gone forever, and new tools support diagnoses and interventions previously impossible. Changes in informatics of the sort we discuss here will proceed in the same fashion. After being used in specific places for special uses, new technologies will become more widespread, and the changes they enable will become more commonplace.

How Is the Internet Affecting the Provision of Health Services?

The Internet can help control costs; more importantly, it can change information flow in health-related areas. In industries such as banking, the Internet has cut costs and transformed the way business is carried out. While a teller transaction costs between $1.25 and $1.50, an Internet transaction costs only $.015. Healthcare organizations choosing the Internet for simple business processes also stand to realize major cost reductions, estimated at 10:1 to 100:1, in routine transactions, both business to business and business to consumer.[10]

However, as John Naisbitt states, "The new source of power is not money in the hands of a few, but information in the hands of many."[11] In health care, where information can literally be a lifesaver, the power of the Internet lies in its unprecedented capability to make information available when, where, and how it is needed. Given the number of Americans on the Web, this capability is staggering. In 1999, almost half of US adults, or 97 million, were on-line, and three out of four of these had used the Internet to search for health and medical information.[12] Another estimate, by Harris Interactive, a research firm, puts the number of people visiting Internet health sites at 60 million or more.[13]

The National Cancer Institute is developing a Cancer Informatics Infrastructure (CII) that will optimize Web technology and enterprise systems to translate cancer research into clinical care.[14] The CII will create a knowledge environment that serves multiple stakeholders, including consumers, and supports the continuum of cancer research: basic, clinical, translational, and population-based research.[15] The initial focus of the CII will be on easing and speeding the clinical trials process, which reaches across sectors. Another federally supported site introduced in early 2000, www.clinicaltrials.gov, reflects the emphasis on consumer needs for valid health information.[16]

In the private sector, health plans and integrated delivery networks are developing e-health offerings, using the Internet to improve consumer services and business-to-business processes. In early 2000, most organizations were still in the early stages of development but had ambitious plans for the near future, according to unpublished First Consulting Group surveys.[17] According to Figure 3.1, most such organizations had reached Stage 1 of the five stages in Internet business development/maturity; they published information online. Others had advanced to Stage 2 by allowing the community to interact with their organizations—for example, with member services. Fewer had deployed online transactions—Stage 3—while none had entered fully into Stages 4 and 5 by integrating multiple transactions and transforming the entire process. Most healthcare organizations will shortly be or already are in the later stages of development and revisiting the work they did in the early stages to reflect their business transformations.[18]

As traditional healthcare settings move toward wellness and population-based health, they are using the Internet to link consumers and various organizations across health care. Web-enabled applications will soon become the new standard. They are already proving of value in bridging the gaps between existing legacy applications to create enterprise-wide patient records and in linking computing and communications technologies to provide state-of-the-art call centers. As these applications grow, they will support data reposi-

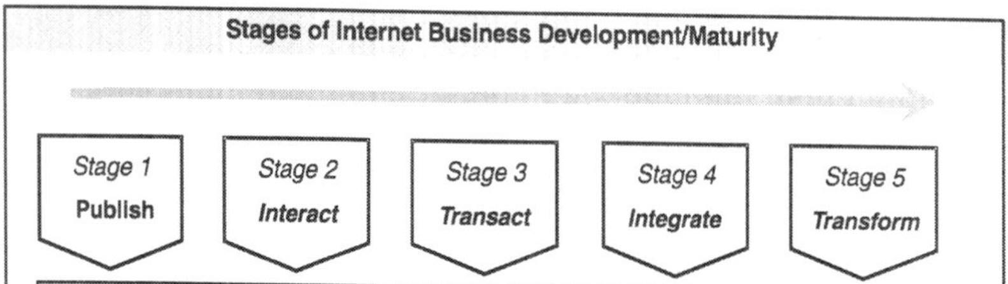

Publish	Build Web ***awareness*** and presence with customers and employees primarily by ***publishing*** static information (e.g., company profile, marketing information, news).
Interact	***Engage*** the community by providing relevant information and enabling the community to ***interact*** with the site and the organization (e.g., on-line provider directory, search formulary, interact with member services).
Transact	Deploy robust self-service capabilities and on-line ***transactions*** (e.g., on-line enrollment, on-line referral processing, claims submission).
Integrate	***Integrate*** the automation of numerous transactions in an effort to automate entire business functions (e.g., on-line medical management).
Transform	***Transform*** the entire enterprise through seamlessly integrating all processes through ***end-to-end*** Web-based interactions with customers and business partners.

FIGURE 3.1. Stages of Internet Business Development/Maturity (*Source:* First Consulting Group and Cisco Systems. Used by permission.)

tories to serve patients and providers and support activities in epidemiology and prevention, facilitating the interface between medicine and public health.

Estimates by CyberDialogue in early 2000 put the number of health-related Web sites at about 17,000, including a growing number of consumer-oriented sites. In addition to simply seeking information online, consumers can seek consults and post their medical records on the Web. Such sites offer new capabilities, but they also pose new problems.[19] For example, consumers can opt to make personal health records available to authorized professionals during emergencies, but those consumer-controlled records may not always be up-to-date, or they may not include all relevant health information. Similarly, sites may provide consumer advice, but they may not identify their sponsors or potential conflicts of interest, and consumers may not be able to validate a given site's credentials.[20]

One of the early organizations to recognize the transformational potential of the Web—and the need to validate information appearing on it—was the Geneva-based Health On the Net (HON) Foundation. In 1995, 60 participants from 11 countries, including representatives from the World Health Organization, the European Commission, and the National Library of Medicine, among others, concluded an international conference by voting unanimously to create a permanent body to "promote the effective and reliable use of the new technologies for telemedicine in healthcare around the world."[21] Six months later, www.hon.ch became one of the very first URLs to guide both lay users and medical professionals to reliable sources of healthcare information in cyberspace. Today, HON offers two widely used medical search tools and the HON Code of Conduct (HONcode) for the provision of trustworthy Web-based medical information. The statement that a site adheres to this code appears on a number of US-based sites.

Through all this innovation, certain factors hold constant. Although the Internet is changing the terms on which physicians and patients interact, their relationship remains primary. Anecdotal accounts abound of the patient arriving at the physician's office with printouts. For these to have a positive influence on care, however, patients have to understand the complexity and variability of information online, and doctors have to adjust to a new role as information mediators. As patients gain access to health information, they look to their physicians for help in evaluating and acting upon the information available. A recent report indicates that this is indeed happening. According to Saurage-Thibodeaux Research, "74 percent of online health site users would be more likely to trust a Web site recommended by their doctor or pharmacist."[22]

An innovation such as recommending a Web site to a patient enhances the role of the physician, rather than diminishes it. Yet, such a change in role requires a change in attitudes and in the doctor/patient relationship itself. The learning curve will be steep for both parties, once again underscoring the importance of human factors to the development of health informatics.

Patient health records are one tangible expression of these changing roles. Now available on a limited number of Web sites, essentially for personal record keeping, these records represent the next generation of the computer-based patient record. Institutions will continue to maintain their own records, which will increasingly be available across the healthcare enterprise as Web applications provide linkages to legacy systems. Clearly, consumer-owned records on a banking model represent the best hope for maintaining comprehensive information over time.[23] The true coordinators of patient care—the patients—will manage their own records. They will control who accesses what in their record, while healthcare institutions maintain their own records, just as financial service organizations do today.

We cannot leave this look at Internet resources, however, without noting two instances in which they have delivered financial benefits. According to United Healthcare, Optum Online, that organization's Web-based nurse line and call center, yielded savings of $4.50 for every dollar invested in the project.[24] In Seattle, Swedish Medical Center worked with an on-line solution provider to build a sophisticated Web site that has attracted over $50,000 a month in referrals.[25] We expect more such documented successes as dot.com hype subsides and health offerings on the Web mature.

What Evidence Is There That Informatics Actually Improves Health?

We are beginning to amass proof that informatics can deliver value and improve health. Although multiple factors have made hard data difficult to come by, the primary reason for the lack of hard data is simple. Until recently, most large-scale implementations targeted administrative aspects of facility-based care. Clinical applications tended to be much smaller in scale and did not extend to address evidence-based medicine or population-based health. Today, applications do more. The Health Plan Employer Data and Information Set (HEDIS) measures widely used in managed care, for instance, have the potential of improving health in two respects: first, by giving plans an incentive to improve services, especially preventive services, and second by giving consumers and purchasers information to guide their choice of health plans. More specifically in the public health area, a 1997 Institute of Medicine (IOM) report, "Improving Health in the Community: A Role for Performance Measurement," extends these ideas to community health settings.[26] Informatics is essential to either of these strategies having an impact on health. Today we are beginning to see the impact of informatics on clinical systems, as they begin to address the need for decision support, for both healthcare providers and patients, whatever the care context.

Disease Management

Consider disease management programs that capture and manage information to better support intervention and thereby prevent or minimize the impact of chronic conditions on the patient and the health system. With chronic disease accounting for 80% of all deaths, 90% of all morbidity, and 70% of all medical expenses in the United States, these attempts can have measurable results.[27] For example, one program for diabetes patients reported that none of its enrollees had been hospitalized over a four-year period, and net savings for one year totaled $510,133.[28] One program for congestive heart failure patients reduced the 30-day readmission rate to zero and cut the 90-day readmission rate by 83% through a combination of telemonitoring and patient education.[29]

Telehealth

Consider also the provision of specialized services, where telehealth capabilities offer savings. The Veterans Administration (VA) has consolidated its imaging services in the state of Maryland; radiologists at the VA's Baltimore facility read digital transmissions of procedures conducted by technicians at multiple facilities.[30] As of this writing, IC-USA is launching efforts to provide specialist support for intensive care units (ICUs). Estimates put the number of intensivists needed to staff all the ICUs in the country all the time at 35,000, while there are only 5,500 physicians specializing in this area. The concept of providing specialist support for ICUs was tested in a four-month clinical trial that covered more than 200 patients. The test found that adding telemedicine coverage around the clock to normal staffing reduced patient mortality by 60%, complications by 40%, and costs by 30%.[31] IC-USA claims that a hospital utilizing telemedicine can realize gross savings of $150,000 per year per intensive care bed, and net about half of that amount.

Patient Safety

The landmark study by the IOM reported in *To Err Is Human: Building a Safer Health System* highlights issues of value through its focus on patient safety. In addition to citing horrific cases of and staggering statistics on medical errors, the IOM reviews the literature documenting the ability of computerized information systems to identify and prevent such errors.[32] According to David Bates et al., from 53% to 89% of adverse drug events were identifiable, and a small but significant number of them were judged "preventable by using such techniques as guided-dose, drug-laboratory, and drug-patient characteristic software algorithms."[33]

The IOM cites other work by Bates, estimating cost savings attributable to the prevention of adverse drugs events at more than $4,000 per event, totaling over $500,000 at one teaching hospital. Even more significantly, this study of automated physician order entry showed "an overall savings from all decision support interventions related to order entry of between $5 to 10 million per year."[34] The IOM concludes, "A computerized system costing $1 to 2 million could pay for itself in three to five years, while preventing injury to hundreds of patients per year."[35] Still another study by Bates showed that decision support systems reduced the number of adverse events by 55%.[36]

In a second report released in 2001, *Crossing the Quality Chasm: A New Health System for the 21st Century*, the IOM intensified its focus on the use of information technology to improve health care, while simultaneously identifying specific strategies for doing so. This second report clearly underscored the significance of informatics and related issues such as organizational development and priority conditions.[37]

Decision Support

More than 30 years ago, Larry Weed prefaced his book *Medical Record, Medical Education, and Patient Care* with the following words:

"The medical record must completely and honestly convey the many variables and complexities that surround every decision, thereby discouraging unreasonable demands upon the physician for supernatural understanding and superhuman competence; but at the same time it must faithfully represent events and decisions so that errors can be detected and proper corrective measures taken when lapses in thoroughness, disciplined thought, and reasonable follow-up occur."[38]

As father of the problem-oriented medical record, Weed did much to advance his theories and to improve care, serving as an advocate of the empowered patient decades before the concept began to find its way into the mainstream. Certainly the structured record is the *sine qua non* for the computerized record, as are the consistency and maintenance of the database that he stressed in his work was critical to the care of the individual patient health.

According to Jonathan Teich, clinical decision support (CDS) systems are "up and running in several different healthcare environments," from acute care to ambulatory practice.[39] Teich continues:

"Right now, [some] physicians are using CDS systems to enhance their decision making and to be more efficient in their everyday clinical practices... Furthermore, CDS systems are not only a tool for physicians; they can also be used by patients who are active participants in their own care and who will appreciate having a technological partnership with their physicians."[39(p46)]

As CDS systems become more commonplace, they will feed the clinical data repositories that are key to evidence-based medicine by the individual practitioner, the institution, and ultimately the scientific community. They will also, through intelligent linkages, make it possible to identify and respond to epidemics and bio-threats. Indeed, such a system exists now, constructed by the US Air Force by using commercially available technologies: laptop computers in the field linked by satellite to centralized databases back in the United States.[40] Called Desert Care, the system maintains records on individuals, tracks illnesses, and analyzes illness trends area-wide in the hope of preventing another Agent Orange or Gulf War Syndrome. This application, as Bill Gates notes,

"provides a good template for civilian applications. With digital records we'll be able to study illness in a variety of population groups to help discover long-term correlations in environment, genetic predisposition, age and gender, without having to institute special studies."[40(p351)]

Initially developed with only $200,000 in four months and incrementally enhanced, this application serves as a remarkable example of the value health informatics can deliver.[41]

Desert Care is far more than a military application. It demonstrates how information can function to improve care for individuals by permitting an understanding of the context in which their symptoms occur. By supporting evidence-based medicine, Desert Care furthers population-based health. Expanded beyond the military setting, it could change our understanding of disease and of wellness among populations.

Looking Ahead

Can informatics improve health? The answer, we believe, is yes. Information is key to the science that underlies health, and technology can—and clearly does—improve the flow of information, making it accessible, usable, and meaningful. Over the next decade, we expect to see many more advances, as the worlds of health care and of public health support one another in their shared mission of improving the life of every individual.

Questions for Review

1. Value is said to be a function of cost, service, and quality. What is the interrelationship between these variables? How does changing one (e.g., cost) affect service or value? To what extent does an increase in investment in IT result in an increase in the value of healthcare services?
2. Why does effective utilization of information technology in support of a healthcare concern's strategic plan inevitably require (a) changes in work processes, (b) increased teamwork, and (c) emphasis on well-defined competencies?
3. Aside from the obvious benefits of use of the Internet to improve customer services and business-to-business processes, what major challenges does the use of the Internet for such purposes pose to physicians and other health practitioners?
4. What factors are now causing health concerns to consider information technology as a route to increasing the value of their services?

References

1. Peterson H. Preface. In: van Bemmel JH, McCray AT, eds. *Yearbook of Medical Informatics 1999: The Promise of Medical Informatics.* Stuttgart, Germany: Schattauer; 1999:1.

2. Lorenzi N. Preface. Proceedings of the AMIA Symposium. *J Am Med Inform Assoc* 1999;(Suppl):vii–viii.
3. Lorenzi N. The cornerstones of medical informatics. *J Am Med Inform Assoc* 2000;7:204–205.
4. Gardner R. Never fail evaluation methods. Unpublished speech at: Davies Symposium; July 9, 1998; Washington, DC.
5. International Medical Informatics Association. Recommendations of the International Medical Informatics Association (IMIA) on Education in Health and Medical Informatics. Available at: http://www.imia.org/wg1/rec.htm. Accessed March 14, 2002.
6. Richards J. *Public Health Informatics: A Consensus of Core Competencies* [dissertation]. Austin, TX: University of Texas at Austin; 2000.
7. Strassman P. *The Squandered Computer: Evaluating the Business Alignment of Information Technologies*. New Canaan, CT: The Information Economics Press; 1997.
8. Menduno M. Prognosis: wired. Why Internet technology is the next medical breakthrough. *Hosp Health Netw* 1998;72(21):28–30, 32–35.
9. Turisco F. *Valuing IT Investments: Justify the Purchase. . .Realize the Value*. Long Beach, CA: First Consulting Group; 1999. Available at: http://www.fcg.com/webfiles/WhitePaper/white_paper_files/wpValueIT.asp. Accessed March 14, 2002.
10. First Consulting Group. *Managing Healthcare Value: Strategies That Work*. Long Beach, CA: First Consulting Group; 1999:33.
11. Naisbitt J. Aburdene P. *Megatrends 2000: Ten New Directions for the 1990s*. New York: William Morrow & Co; 1990.
12. Internet increasingly used to find health care information. *Healthc Financ Manage* April 1999:Vol 52(4).
13. Nua Internet Surveys. How many online? Available at: http://www.nua.com/surveys/how_many_online/index.html. Accessed March 14, 2002.
14. Silva J. Fighting cancer in the information age: An architecture for national scale clinical trials. *MD Comput* 1999;16:43–44.
15. Silva J. Informatics: NCI's cancer informatics infrastructure. *Oncology Issues*. 1999;14:21–22.
16. Silva J, Ball M, Chute C, Douglas JV. *Cancer Informatics: Essential Technologies for Clinical Trials*. New York: Springer-Verlag; 2002.
17. First Consulting Group. *Health Systems on the E-Health Path*. Long Beach, CA: First Consulting Group, 2000. Available at: www.fcg.com/knowledge/first_reports.asp.
18. First Consulting Group. *Health Plans on the Road to E-Health*. Long Beach, CA: First Consulting Group, 2000. Available at: www.fcg.com/knowledge/first_reports.asp.
19. Anderson J. The business of Cyberhealthcare. *MD Comput* 1999;16:23–25.
20. Freudenheim M. Advice is the newest prescription for health costs. *New York Times* April 9, 2000;Section 1, pg. 1.
21. Health On the Net Foundation. Unpublished materials prepared for the HON board. Additional information available at: http://www.hon.ch/.
22. Rodsjo S. Prescribing information: No waiting on the Web. *Healthc Inform* 2000;17:132–134, 136–138, 140–141.
23. Ramsaroop P, Ball M. The "bank of health": A model for more useful patient health records. *MD Comput* 2000;17:45–48.
24. Kimball-Baker K. What's the ROInfo (return on information) in MCOs (managed care organizations)? *Healthc Inform* 1998;15(4):50–52, 54, 56–58.
25. Yamamoto H. What works. Swedish Medical Center website attracts $50,000 a month in referrals. *Health Manag Technol* 1999;20(3):44–45.

26. Institute of Medicine. Measurement tools for a community health improvement process. In: Durch J, Bailey L, Stoto M, eds. *Improving Health in the Community, a Role for Performance Monitoring*. Washington, DC: National Academy Press; 1997;126–165.

27. Bringewatt R. The metamorphosis of chronic care. Healthcare's next big hurdle. *Healthc Forum J* 1998;41(5):14–16, 18, 21.

28. Petrakos C. Finding a cure: Disease management aids the search for better outcomes. *Modern Physician*. September 1, 1998. Available at: www.modernphysician.com.

29. Roglieri JL, Futterman R, McDonough KL, Malya G et al. Disease management interventions to improve outcomes in congestive heart failure. *Am J Manag Care* 1997;3(12):1831–1839.

30. Flagle C. Economic analysis of filmless radiology. In: Siegel E, Kolodner R, eds. *Filmless Radiology*. New York: Springer-Verlag; 1999:113–136.

31. Salganik W. Telemedicine business is launched by 2 doctors. *Baltimore Sun*, April 6, 2000, Business section Page 1D.

32. Kohn L, Corrigan J., Donalson M, eds. *To Err Is Human: Building a Safer Health System*. Washington, DC: National Academy Press; 2000.

33. Bates DW, O'Neil AC, Boyle D, Teich J, Chertow GM, Komaroff AL, Brennan TA. Potential identifiability and preventability of adverse events using information systems. *J Am Med Inform Assoc* 1994;1:404–411.

34. Bates DW, Spell N, Cullen DJ, Burdick E, Laird N, Petersen LA, Small SD, Sweitzer BJ, Leape LL. The costs of adverse drug events in hospitalized patients. Adverse Drug Events Prevention Study Group. *JAMA* 1997;277:307–311.

35. Kohn L, Corrigan J., Donalson M, eds. *To Err Is Human: Building a Safer Health System*. Washington, DC: National Academy Press. 2000:191.

36. Bates DW, Leape LL, Cullen DJ, Laird N, Petersen LA, Teich JM, Burdick E, Hickey M, Kleefield S, Shea B, Vander Vliet M, Seger DL. Effect of computerized physician order entry and a team intervention on prevention of serious medication errors. *JAMA* 1998;280:1311–1316.

37. Institute of Medicine. *Crossing the Quality Chasm: A New Health System for the 21st Century*. Washington, DC: National Academy Press; 2001.

38. Weed LL. A preface to the 1969 edition of *Medical Records, Medical Education, and Patient Care*. Reprinted in: Weed LL. *Knowledge Coupling: New Premises and New Tools for Medical Care and Education*. New York: Springer-Verlag; 1991:316–317.

39. Teich JM, Wrinn MM. Clinical decision support systems come of age. *MD Comput* 2000;17:43–46.

40. Gates B. *Business @ the Speed of Thought*. New York: Time Warner; 1999:348–351.

41. Schafer K, Kline E, Williams R, Hardie B, et al. Force health protection through global medical surveillance. In: Ramsaroop P, Ball M, Beaulieu D, Douglas J, eds. *Advancing Federal Sector Healthcare: A Model for Technology Transfer*. New York: Springer-Verlag; 2001.

4
The Governmental and Legislative Context of Informatics

John R. Christiansen

Learning Objectives

After studying this chapter, you should be able to:

- Define a public health agency by (1) function and (2) delegated governmental authority, and discuss the complexities of applying legal and regulatory constraints on public health agencies with regard to information management.
- Discuss the obligations of a public health agency with respect to the management of information by a contractor under the "applications services provider" (ASP) business model.
- List the provisions of the Health Insurance Portability and Accountability Act (HIPAA) with regard to (1) the definition of a "Covered Entity," (2) the scope of the health information covered by HIPAA, (3) the requirements that a Covered Entity must meet in giving consumers control over their health information, (4) the extent to which a Covered Entity may release protected health information without the consent of the affected individual, and (5) the principal steps a Covered Entity must take to ensure the privacy of personal health information.
- List two major challenges in public health information sharing, and discuss the provisions that must be present in a prospective information sharing arrangement between a public health agency and a business partner.
- Differentiate between "passive" and "active" public health information Web sites, and discuss the risk management principles that such a Web site's owner must exercise in offering an interactive health communication system (IHC).

Overview

An understanding of the governmental and legislative context of public health informatics is crucial for any public health employee dealing with health information of individuals, whether as patients, health plan enrollees, or the subjects of collected data. Whether a public health agency is defined by function or by delegated governmental authority, the agency itself and its contractors are subject to state and federal laws defining the privacy rights of patients. The single most important federal law governing the use of information by public health agencies and their contractors is the Health Insurance Portability and Accountability Act of 1996 (HIPAA),[1] which applies to or must be taken into account by all healthcare organizations in the United States. The regulations issued by the US Department of Health and Human Services under HIPAA impose comprehensive restrictions on the use and disclosure of individual health information, whether that information appears on a computer device, exists in paper form, or is contained in an oral communication. Federal public health agencies must also comply with and take into account the requirements of the Privacy Act of 1974, which does not apply directly to private organizations but may be applied to agency contractors, vendors, or researchers by agency policies or contractual provisions. Most states have laws controlling the collection and use of information by public health agencies that are equivalent to the federal Privacy Act, which by the same principles apply directly to state agencies and indirectly by policy or contract to private organizations. Many states have also enacted or are considering health information privacy laws applicable to both public and private organizations. While federal Privacy Act requirements are likely to be harmonized with and integrated into HIPAA's privacy requirements, state law privacy protections that are more stringent than HIPAA will continue to apply. Finally, a public health agency operating a Web site must be aware of privacy issues related to user data it collects and of risk management principles connected to the operation of interactive health communications systems. Emerging consumer protection principles make it necessary to disclose information collection activities, while in some cases federal Food and Drug Administration (FDA) regulations may limit the ways information may be provided to the public.

Introduction

Understanding the governmental and legislative context of public health informatics is fundamental to its competent use. After all, even the best-intended informatics projects and systems serving great public good must be managed and operated in compliance with a wide variety of legal constraints and within the boundaries of the legal authority granted the agency or agencies in question. One overriding constraint on the nature of public health informatics is the need to safeguard individual privacy. Public health agencies frequently gather and manage large quantities of very sensitive personal information. A failure to protect that information properly can lead to a breach of both the public trust and of individual privacy. In some cases, such a failure can even lead to criminal charges.

Public health occupies a special, complex niche in the US healthcare system. An understanding of this niche is crucial to an understanding of the legislative and governmental context of public health informatics. This niche is best defined functionally—according to traditional public health purposes and operations—as well as jurisdictionally—according to the laws, regulations, and other governmental enactments that establish an agency's authority.

Legal and Regulatory Constraints on Public Health Agencies

Public health information collection, use, and disclosure activities are not generally exempt from the laws and regulations that apply to other kinds of healthcare organizations that work with personal information. Some laws do include exceptions for some public health functions, but these exceptions need to be analyzed carefully to insure an accurate understanding of their implications and limitations. Such analyses are complicated by the fact that healthcare information laws and regulations are currently undergoing fundamental revision at both the federal and state levels. In this changing environment, healthcare information systems managers have an obligation to monitor legal developments constantly and be ready to update policies and procedures to adapt to changing laws and standards of care.

The complexity of the analysis is aggravated by the fact that both federal and state laws may simultaneously apply to a given agency, to an information system, to a data set, or to a practicing individual. At the same time, such laws probably were not drafted in a coordinated fashion, and they need not (and frequently do not) impose the same standards or obligations. For example, the fact that a given use of sensitive information is acceptable under federal law does not necessarily mean that it is also acceptable under applicable state law, and vice versa.

Professional obligations further complicate the picture. A licensed healthcare provider, such as a physician in a clinic employed by a public health agency in her professional capacity, is subject to professional obligations of confidentiality to her patients quite apart from the obligations imposed by any of the laws applicable to the agency that runs the clinic. For example, it is possible that federal law might allow a public health agency to disclose information about a patient under circumstances in which the licensed healthcare provider is prohibited from doing so by her professional standards of care.

Finally, common law standards for the competent management of information systems are beginning to emerge. A very few standards already apply as a matter of law to some governmental agencies or contractors; nongovernmental bodies are formally developing others; and still others are emerging from litigation or regulatory actions. All of these governmental, legislative, and regulatory standards affect the implementation and use of informatics in public health, and a failure to take them into account may put an important project or a function at unnecessary risk.

The applicability of any given law or standard typically hinges on both the legal status and activities performed by an organization. The definition of a public health agency is therefore crucial to the determination of applicable law. As we will see in the next section, that definition can differ, depending on whether the term is defined by function or by delegated governmental authority.

What Is a Public Health Agency?

A *public health agency* is not necessarily easy to define, as a legal matter. We may, to paraphrase a famous definition of pornography, "know public health when we see it," but the boundaries of public health services are blurry. They fade into private hospital and clinical care, health insurance, and private research without any clear border. *Agency* is perhaps easier to define, but in an era of outsourcing and privatization of public health functions, this term too has become slippery.

Nevertheless, accurate definition is important because the laws regulating the use and disclosure of information frequently depend upon the intended purposes and functions and whether the user or disclosure is within a private or a governmental agency. Most of the time, the question whether an organization is a public health agency will be easily answered, but there will also be gray areas and hard cases. In these cases, answers will have to be determined by an analysis of the informatics functions in question and the relation of the organization to governmental oversight bodies.

Definition by Function: The Prevention of Disease and Promotion of Health

Public health had its start in conceptual if not formal opposition to private medicine, and the tension between the two has never been entirely resolved. As we have seen in Chapter 2, state and local health departments in the United States were developed and instituted during the latter half of the 19th century for the primary purpose of controlling outbreaks of epidemics and promoting public sanitation, and are also to some extent rooted in the "dispensaries" that provided clinical care to the destitute in many American cities from the late 18th through the early 20th centuries. These dispensaries relied upon small charitable budgets, and they utilized free services provided by part-time physicians and medical students.

However praiseworthy and valuable the efforts of public health entities, from their beginning they generated a certain degree of opposition in the private sector. As one author writes,

> But just as doctors did not want hospitals or dispensaries to steal patients from them, so they did not want public health agencies to interfere in their business. While they favored public health activities that were complementary to private practice, they

opposed those that were competitive. This opposition became even more strenuous in the early twentieth century.[2]

As a result of the opposition, "wherever public health overreached the boundaries that the [medical] profession saw as defining its sphere, the doctors tried to push it back," though this attitude was also "consistent with prevailing beliefs held by public officials."[2(p196)]

Historically, this tension led to a difficult distinction between "preventive" and "curative" functions; in principle, prevention was a legitimate public health function, whereas curative functions were reserved for private physicians or hospitals. Whether or not this is a viable distinction—it is difficult to see how an effective public health campaign to prevent the spread of highly contagious diseases could work in the absence of treatment for at least some disease victims—it continues to be one of the defining elements of public health.

The preventive function as a defining element in public health can be seen as well in the Centers for Disease Control and Prevention (CDC), whose stated mission is "to promote health and quality of life by preventing and controlling disease, injury, and disability." The CDC had its start shortly after World War II. Its preventive functions have included epidemiological studies, conducting and funding research into disease causation and prevention, the promotion of preventive care, and other prevention-oriented activities. Many, if not most, state health departments and a number of local health departments and agencies have conducted and continue to conduct similar programs.

The line between prevention and cure has not been easy to maintain, however, and over the years programs for child and maternal care, the diagnosis and treatment of sexually transmitted diseases and substance abuse, and other services intended to prevent the spread of diseases or promote health have been instituted in a variety of clinical public health settings. Until the advent of Medicaid in 1965, public health clinics were frequently the provider of last resort for the indigent, and while the private sector assumed much of this burden, many public health providers have continued to serve this function as Medicaid participants.

Public health functions therefore span the spectrum from individual clinical diagnosis and treatment through population-wide epidemiological studies. The common thread among these functions is that they are in some sense preventive—even individual clinical care, in the public health setting, is primarily intended to prevent the spread of disease or the worsening of a condition, or to promote some healthy behavior. At the same time, the diversity of public health functions means that the legal context of public health informatics is quite complex, requiring careful analysis to determine which laws a public health information system must comply with, and how.

Definition by Delegated Governmental Authority

In addition to being defined through its service of providing preventive functions, a public health agency can be characterized as an organization dependent upon public funding and delegated public authority by a governmental

TABLE **4.1.** Typical contrasts between public health agencies and private health organizations: Definition by delegated governmental authority

Public Health Agency	Private Health Organization
Authority basis:	Authority basis: Nongovernmental
A. Established by statute	
B. Established by existing governmental body, within scope of statutory authority	
C. Under contract to (A) or (B)	
Funding: Government funds	Funding: Private donations or commercial revenues
Constraints: Constitutional and other government-level constraints	Constraints: Subject to governmental regulatory authority and sometimes government licensing

body. These characteristics are crucial to the definition of a public health agency. Private organizations such as foundations, teaching hospitals, and other educational institutions perform many of the same kinds of research, preventive care, and health promotion functions as public health agencies; such private organizations, however, typically receive their support from private donations or commercial revenues. Most critically, such private organizations do not wield governmental power, and while they are typically subject to governmental regulatory authority, they are not subject to constitutional and other government-level constraints. Table 4.1 highlights the primary differences between public health agencies and private organizations.

The tightening of governmental budgets in recent years has caused a trend toward public health agency delegation of functions to private organizations. All too frequently, legislatures direct a public health agency to undertake an activity without allocating adequate funding, or cut budgets for established activities. Through such processes, health departments and other public health authorities may be given considerable authority—and even specific public health mandates—without corresponding resources.

The ASP Business Model

The resulting search for resources adequate to public health missions has led to some substantial reconsideration of what constitutes an appropriate public health function. In particular, a number of agencies have begun privatizing various clinical services. The search for adequate resources has also had implications for public health informatics. The "application services providers" (ASP) business model, in which a company provides outsourced information storage, processing, and/or transmission functions through the Internet or through a proprietary network, may provide some advantages to such agencies. An ASP can make information functions available at a reasonable rate on a leased or subscription basis that otherwise could be acquired only by purchases of hardware and applications that are beyond the agency's acquisition budget.

ASP contracting, and any other privatization or outsourcing of the management of information functions by a public health agency, requires that a public health agency take care to insure that the contractor is bound to strong, appropriate information disclosure and use restrictions consistent with the agency's own obligations in this area. Contractors should be subject to routine audit for compliance with their contracts. They should also be qualified as trustworthy before they are delegated any task involving sensitive information. Privatization and outsourcing can provide an avenue for the fulfillment of public health obligations in a more cost-effective fashion, but the public health agency must retain a strong oversight role.

Privacy Laws and Public Health Informatics

Many studies indicate that public concern over the potential invasion of health information privacy by use of computer technology is high and increasing. This concern is far from unique to public health. Rather, it is a general reaction to genuine risks arising from use of computer technology in many sectors. The result is an increasing number of new laws and regulations concerning privacy. Many of these laws and regulations apply to public health agencies or to public health functions in general.

Anyone acquiring or managing information technologies in public health should be acquainted with these laws. Any public health agency that operates a system that stores, processes, or transmits information about the health status or claims of individuals needs to have one or more officers charged with knowing and overseeing compliance with these laws. For example, HIPAA specifically requires a health organization to designate an individual to serve as a privacy officer to insure that the law's information privacy requirements are followed.

Even if a law does not apply directly to a public health agency, the law may need to be taken into account when a public health agency is working with other organizations to which the law does apply. For example, HIPAA may affect a hospital's ability to provide certain kinds of information to other participants in some kinds of public health activities, or may otherwise impose restrictions that need to be taken into account in a project.

Public sensitivities should also be taken into account, even if they are not clearly spelled out in the law. There is always potential for public distrust of "big government" projects that gather sensitive personal information, especially when the reasons for the project, the potential benefits, and the precautions that will be followed are not well understood. Because public health agencies are dependent upon public funding, it is prudent to make sure that the public is informed of privacy safeguards that a public health agency will use. It is also essential that a public health agency be aware of the laws that might apply to the handling of health information.

Federal Mandates and Restrictions

Federal public health agencies have long been bound by the Privacy Act of 1974, which requires them to protect personal information about individuals. As noted above, most states have equivalent laws that apply to state public health agencies and need to be reviewed when a public health employee is considering activities at the state level.

The Privacy Act and its subsequent amendments are highly generalized. The Privacy Act essentially requires agencies to make informed judgments about what information they can disclose without violating individual privacy, though the courts have held that the Act specifically does apply to individual medical records. The Act applies to information in all media, including both paper and electronic, and has been interpreted by the Centers for Medicare & Medicaid Services (CMS, formerly Health Care Financing Administration) to apply to non-governmental Medicare contractors. In particular, the CMS Internet Security Policy prohibits such contractors from transmitting Privacy Act–protected information over the Internet without using encryption and some reasonable means of authenticating the identity of the parties to the transmission. Some key provisions of the Privacy Act of 1974 are as follows[3]:

1. Prohibits an agency or its contractor from disclosing any record that is contained in a system of records by any means of communication to any person, or to another agency, without the prior written consent of the individual to whom the record pertains. Exceptions are provided for disclosures to certain agency employees, the Bureau of the Census, research studies, law enforcement officials, and others.
2. Requires an agency to document the date, nature, and purpose of a record disclosed and the name and address of the person or agency to whom the disclosure is made, and to keep the documentation for a period of five years or the life of the record, whichever is longer.
3. Requires that an agency allow any individual to have access to his/her own record and to request amendment of the record.
4. Specifies that an agency may maintain only such information about an individual as is relevant and necessary to accomplish the purpose of the agency.
5. Establishes certain standards for maintaining individual health records.
6. Requires an agency to establish agency rules for carrying out the provisions of the act.

7. Provides civil remedies and criminal penalties for knowingly and willfully violating provisions of the act.

Information Privacy Protection in HIPAA

HIPAA is of more general significance to the use, disclosure, and protection of health information. Under HIPAA, the US Department of Health and Human Services (HHS) was granted the authority and duty to craft the necessary privacy protections by regulation. After years of work, the final privacy regulation was issued and became final on April 14, 2001. Because HIPAA provides for a two-year period between the date a regulation becomes final and the date compliance is mandatory, compliance will therefore be legally required as of April 15, 2003. (Other regulations pertaining to healthcare claims processing and information security are being issued on different schedules. These may have important implications for some public health functions but are beyond the scope of this discussion.)

The provisions of the final privacy regulation apply directly to "Covered Entities," a term that applies to health plans, healthcare clearinghouses, and those healthcare providers who conduct certain financial and administration transactions—including electronic billing and funds transfers—electronically. Inasmuch as virtually all healthcare providers do conduct such transactions electronically already, it should be assumed the privacy regulation applies to a provider unless it is proven otherwise.

The terms of the regulation are very broad, so that activities of a public health agency are frequently also covered by HIPAA. As HSS states, "The provisions of the final rule generally apply equally to private sector and public sector entities. For example, both private hospitals and government agency medical units must comply with the full range of requirements, such as providing notice, access rights, requiring consent before disclosure for routine uses, establishing contracts with business associates, among others." For instance, a public health agency that provides any health care, serves in any capacity as a health plan or as a plan administrator, or processes health claims data fits the definition of a Covered Entity. The regulations also apply indirectly to other kinds of companies and organizations that are otherwise not directly subject to the regulations. Such entities are called "Business Associates."

Comprehensive Coverage of Individual Health Information by HIPAA

Compared with traditional paper documents, information in standardized electronic formats is very vulnerable to surreptitious copying, transmission, and modification. Congress recognized this problem in enacting HIPAA and therefore authorized and directed HHS to promulgate comprehensive privacy and security regulations.

However, in establishing the final regulation, HHS went beyond covering individual health information contained only in electronic formats or even in paper documents originally contained in electronic format. The final regulation covers oral communications and paper records in their entirety, regardless of whether those records originally appeared in electronic form. HHS states, "The final regulation extends protection to all types of personal health information created or held by covered entities, including oral communications and paper records that have not existed in electronic form."[4] The information subject to this regulation is defined as "Protected Health Information," and it encompasses not only information that includes identifying elements, but also information "which is reasonably believed could be used to identify an individual." HHS has characterized the effect of this regulation as follows: "This creates a privacy system that covers all health information held by hospitals, providers, health plans and health insurers."

Public health agencies and public health providers, then, must take HIPAA into account if they are responsible for handling or processing *any* health information related to an individual, whether that information appears in written or in oral form.

Provisions in HIPAA

The final privacy regulation issued by HHS contains privacy provisions covering four areas. These areas are (1) consumer control over Protected Health Information, (2) boundaries of Protected Health Information use and disclosure, (3) ensuring the security of Protected Health Information, and (4) accountability for Protected Health Information use and disclosure.

HIPAA's Requirements for Consumer Control over Health Information

HHS's final regulation gives patients significant new rights to understand and control how their own health information is used. Specifically, the final regulation:

- Requires healthcare providers and health plans to give patients a clear written explanation of how those providers and plans can and do use, keep, and disclose health information.
- Requires healthcare providers and health plans to permit a patient to see and get copies of the patient's records and to request amendments to those records. Moreover, these providers and health plans must make a history of disclosures of such records accessible to a patient. For example, a public health agency handling Protected Health Information must generally provide a requesting patient with the identity of any entity to whom the agency has released information about the individual, along with the release date and the nature of the information released.
- Specifies that a Covered Entity must obtain patient consent before sharing Protected Health Information for treatment, payment, and healthcare operations purposes. In addition, a Covered Entity must obtain comparable

consent, called an "authorization," when the healthcare information is to be used for nonroutine and most non-healthcare purposes, such as releasing information to financial institutions determining mortgages and other loans or selling mailing lists to interested parties such as life insurers. Patients have the right to request restrictions on the uses and disclosures of their information.

- Specifies that, except for uses or disclosures for purposes of treatment, payment, or healthcare "operations" (administrative functions directly associated with organization management), patient consent to use and disclosure of Protected Health Information may not be required and must not be coerced by providers and health plans. Providers and health plans are entitled to condition a patient's treatment or payment for care on the patient's consent to the disclose and use of health information for treatment, payment or operations purposes, but may not require or coerce authorization for any other purposes.
- Provides a patient the procedures to remedy when a Covered Entity violates the patient's rights under HIPAA or under the Covered Entity's own policies and procedures. Such recourse includes a patient's right to complain to the Covered Entity and to report violations to the Secretary of HHS.

Following are some situations in which a Covered Entity would be required to obtain authorization from an individual prior to release of health information about that individual:

1. A licensed physician treating a patient requests blood test results concerning a patient from a health assessor who has arranged to administer blood tests to community members living near a toxic waste site. Both the physician and the health assessor would be considered Covered Entities. However, despite the treatment relationship between the physician and patient, the health assessor would not be permitted to release the information without the patient's written consent.
2. A health insurance plan operator requests details and verification regarding a physical examination administered to a prospective plan enrollee by a public health agency's medical services contractor as part of the continuing contract with the agency. Both the plan and the medical services contractor would be considered Covered Entities. The contractor would nonetheless be required to obtain the prospective enrollee's written authorization before disclosing information about the examination to the plan.
3. A commercial company offers to pay a Covered Entity a fee in return for use of a list of patients who have been treated for diabetes in the last five years. If the Covered Entity provides the list without first obtaining the written authorization of all the patients, both the Covered Entity and the officers of the entity who participated in the sale of the list could be charged with criminal violations of HIPAA, and face penalties of up to 10 years in prison and a $250,000 fine per individual on the list.
4. A state health department operates a cancer registry as part of its

information services division, in which it collects and analyzes the incidence of various cancers reported by providers throughout the state as required by state law. A newspaper reporter files a request under the state's public disclosure laws seeking the records from the registry. Because the health department division is not acting as either a health plan or healthcare provider, it is not a Covered Entity under HIPAA. Unless there is some state equivalent of the Privacy Act or some other statutory protection providing more protection than HIPAA in this case, the information may have to be disclosed by law even if it contains personal health information.

5. A life insurance company wants a Covered Entity to provide verification of health information provided by an applicant for a life insurance policy. The Covered Entity must have a written authorization for the disclosure from the patient.

Boundaries of Protected Health Information Use and Disclosure

Health care is a complex sector, and health plans, healthcare providers, and their contractors and vendors must constantly share Protected Health Information for many legitimate reasons. Because HIPAA reaches only Covered Entities directly, there is a risk that the protection of information will be lost when it is disclosed by a Covered Entity to a vendor or contractor that is not a Covered Entity. To close this loophole, HHS included a requirement in the privacy regulation that Covered Entities implement specific forms of agreement with their "Business Associates" before disclosing Protected Health Information to them. (In governmental settings, this document may take the form of a memorandum of understanding between an agency or division in its role as Covered Entity, and another agency or division acting on behalf of the Covered Entity agency.)

A "Business Associate" is any organization or individual to which a Covered Entity discloses HIPAA-protected information in order to perform some function or activity on behalf of the Covered Entity. Specific examples include claims processors, data analysts and aggregators, utilization review, quality assurance, consulting, legal counsel, accountants, actuaries, and so on. This category could also include other Covered Entities, as when a health plan processes claims data for a clinic, or a physician examines a prospective enrollee on behalf of a health plan.

The contract between a Covered Entity and its Business Associates must include the following provisions at a minimum:

- A prohibition against the Business Associate using or disclosing the protected information in any fashion not permitted to the Covered Entity. The contract may provide for greater limitations, but not lesser.
- A requirement that the Business Associate use "appropriate safeguards" to protect the information.
- A requirement that the Business Associate report any violation of the privacy or protection of the information to the Covered Entity.

- A requirement that the Business Associate not further disclose the information, or if it does (e.g., to a subcontractor), that the Business Associate implement an equivalent or more protective agreement with that party.
- Requirements that the Business Associate make the information available to subject individuals, allow them to copy and seek amendment of it, and receive an accounting of any disclosures of the information made by the Business Associate.
- A requirement that the Business Associate permit the inspection of its books and records by HHS to audit the Covered Entity's compliance.
- A provision requiring the return or destruction of all protected information on termination of the contract, "if feasible," and, if not feasible, providing that the information shall be used or disclosed only for purposes connected with the reason why return or destruction is not feasible.
- A provision permitting the Covered Entity to terminate the contract if the Business Associate breaches it.

Ensuring the Security of Personal Health Information Under HIPAA

The final HIPAA privacy regulation contemplates the issuance of a final security regulation as well. A draft security regulation was published in August 1998, and the final version is expected sometime in late 2002. Informed sources indicate that the final form of the security regulation should not be drastically different from the draft version.

Under both the final privacy and the draft security regulation, Covered Entities have some discretion in establishing detailed policies and procedures for meeting the information protection requirements of HIPAA. Specific implementation is intended to be "flexible and scaleable, to account for the nature of each entity's business, and its size and resources."[4] However, all Covered Entities, regardless of size and resources, must

- Adopt written privacy procedures, including specifying who has access to protected information, how the information will be used within the entity, and when the information will or will not be disclosed to others. In addition, as noted above, covered entities must take steps to insure that their Business Associates protect the privacy of information.
- Train employees to understand the new privacy protection procedures and designate an individual—a privacy officer—to be responsible for insuring that the procedures are followed. A public health agency whose activities are subject to HIPAA must therefore provide its employees with the training necessary for them to understand all the privacy protection procedures in HIPAA and designate an employee to monitor privacy-protected information use within the agency.
- Establish grievance processes by means of which patients can make inquiries or complaints regarding the privacy of their records.

The obligations of a Covered Entity under HIPAA may be summarized as follows:

1. A health plan or healthcare provider must publish a notice of privacy practices and should obtain and retain for use and disclosure executed consents by enrollees and/or patients regarding protected health information for treatment, payment, and healthcare operations purposes.
2. Must release only the minimum amount of information authorized and necessary for the purpose of the disclosure. For instance, a patient's consent to release details of a treatment for a diabetic condition does not authorize release of the patient's entire medical record covering other treatments or conditions.
3. If a health plan or healthcare provider, records of executed authorizations by patients and/or enrollees must be obtained and retained for any nonroutine disclosures (e.g., disclosures to financial institutions) and must be obtained in such a way as to be informed and voluntary.
4. Must identify all Business Associates, and implement and retain records of executed Business Associate agreements with all those identified.
5. Must appoint a privacy officer, and establish job descriptions, internal policies and procedures, and training to insure that all individuals working with protected health information understand and comply with all requirements.

Accountability for Protected Health Information Use and Release

Most Covered Entities will be required to comply with the final privacy regulation two years after their issuance—in other words, in April 2003. (Certain small healthcare organizations will be permitted three years to come into compliance.) HHS has made that department's Office for Civil Rights responsible for civil implementation and enforcement of the privacy regulation. By statute, Covered Entities that violate the standards in the regulations are subject to civil penalties of $100 per incident, up to $25,000 per person, per year, per standard.

The regulations also provide for federal criminal penalties for health plans, providers, and clearinghouses that knowingly and improperly use, disclose, or obtain Protected Health Information. These criminal penalties are up to $50,000 and one year in prison for the most basic level of the offense; up to $100,000 and up to five years in prison for obtaining Protected Health Information under false pretenses; and up to $250,000 and up to 10 years in prison for obtaining or disclosing Protected Health Information with the intent to sell, transfer, or use it for commercial advantage, personal gain, or malicious harm.

Balancing Public Responsibility with Privacy Protections Under HIPAA

The final regulation issued by HHS recognizes that there are certain instances in which the welfare of the public may take precedence over the privacy rights of individuals. It recognizes that certain existing disclosures of Protected Health Information without the consent of the individual(s) affected have legitimacy. Specifically, the final regulation permits, but does not require, a Covered Entity to disclose Protected Health Information without the consent or authorization of the individual(s) affected if the purpose of the disclosure is for:

- Oversight of the healthcare system, including quality assurance activities.
- Public health. HIPAA permits Covered Entities to disclose Protected Health Information to "Public Health Authorities" without the consent of the individual affected. "Public Health Authority" is quite broadly defined as "an agency or authority of the United States, a State, a territory, a political subdivision of a State or territory, or an Indian tribe that is responsible for public health matters as part of its official mandate."[5] Disclosure without patient or enrollee consent or authorization is specifically permitted to organizations authorized by law to collect or receive Protected Health Information for vital statistics, disease, injury, disability reporting and prevention, public health surveillance and investigation, etc.,[6] and to "appropriate authorit[ies] authorized by law to receive reports of child abuse or neglect,"[7] as well as certain other authorities and purposes specified in the regulation.

Disclosures to Public Health Authorities are permitted based upon verification of their identities by in-person presentation of official credentials, a letter on agency letterhead, or if "to a person acting on behalf of a public official, [by] a written statement on appropriate government letterhead that the person is acting under the government's authority or other evidence or documentation of agency that . . . demonstrates that it is acting on behalf of the public official."[8]

The privacy regulation includes the following further specific cases where Protected Health Information may be used or disclosed without specific consent or authorization:

- To individuals who may have been exposed to, or are at risk of, contracting or spreading a communicable disease, where notification is otherwise authorized by law.
- For reporting of diseases, injuries, and conditions, and reporting of vital events such as birth and death to vital statistics agencies.
- For public health surveillance, investigation, and intervention, including activities undertaken by the FDA to evaluate and monitor the safety of food, drugs, medical devices, and other products.

These terms probably effectively cover all or almost all public health activities carried out by federal, state, and local public health authorities. The actual authorities and terminology used will vary under different jurisdictions.

Disclosures may also be made to a government agency or a private entity acting on behalf of a government entity for the purpose of inclusion in a governmental health data system or for research purposes, either based on subject authorization or when a waiver of such authorization has been independently reviewed and accepted by a privacy board or an institutional review board. Many public health agencies conduct research on human subjects or make their records and databases available for such research. Many federal agencies and organizations that conduct research on human subjects using federal funding have been subject for some years to the Federal Policy for the Protection of Human Subjects, or "Common Rule."

The Common Rule requires that any such research receive prior review and approval by an "Institutional Review Board" (IRB), made up of institutional and community representatives. An IRB is intended to minimize or eliminate risks to human subjects in the research, including privacy risks. The final regulation of HIPAA extends comparable research subject protections to all Covered Entities, whether or not they are governmental agencies or receive federal funding. For example, a healthcare provider would have to submit proposed research protocols to a "privacy board" before beginning the project. The privacy board would then analyze the project for possible risks to privacy and might impose additional conditions intended to increase protections. Finally, disclosures are authorized by regulation.

- for judicial and administrative proceedings
- for limited law enforcement activities
- in emergency circumstances
- for identification of the body of a deceased person, or the cause of death
- for facility patient directories, provided that patients must be permitted to "opt out" of inclusion
- for certain identified activities related to national defense and security

Many of these exceptions are somewhat vaguely worded. A healthcare agency would be well advised to seek legal counsel before acting on an apparent exception. Table 4.2 provides examples of situations in which a Covered Entity would and would not be required to obtain informed and voluntary patient consent before releasing the patient's medical information.

Privacy Protections of HIPAA as a Floor

The final regulation specifies that privacy protections under HIPAA serve as minimums that Covered Entities must meet. The aim of the final regulation, according to HHS, is to establish a "national 'floor' of privacy standards that protect all Americans."[4] The regulation specifically acknowledges that stronger state laws, such as those covering mental health, HIV infection, and AIDS information, continue to apply. In addition, the final regulation permits states that have enacted laws requiring disclosures of health information for civic purposes to continue to enforce such laws.

However, HIPAA preempts any state laws that are "less stringent" in their privacy protections, so that the stronger of the privacy provisions in HIPAA or state law will apply. Table 4.3 presents a hypothetical set of situations, along with an indication of the federal or state law that would prevail according to the HHS final regulation.

TABLE 4.2. Situations in which a covered entity under HIPAA would and would not be required to obtain a patient's informed and voluntary consent for release of the patient's medical information

Situation	Patient Consent Required?
A licensed physician requests a state health department to release information related to his patient from a cancer registry.	Probably yes. The health department cancer registry function is not a Covered Entity function under HIPAA. However, under the Privacy Act and its state equivalents, patient-identifiable registry information should be protected against unconsented disclosure.
A law enforcement official presents a court order signed by a judge for release of complete medical information on a patient.	No.
A hospital needs to construct a telephone listing of patients in the hospital.	No, as long as the patients are permitted to "opt out" of the listing.
As part of a security background check for a defense worker, the FBI requests the worker's medical record.	No.

Implications of HIPAA for Public Health Agencies

Previously, we have listed and discussed certain exceptions provided by HIPAA for public health agencies. However, it is important to understand that, in general, the final regulation issued by HSS does not differentiate between public and private sector health plans and providers in terms of applicability of the law. According to HHS, "[t]he provisions of the final rule generally apply equally to private sector and public sector entities. For example, both private hospitals and government agency medical units must comply with the full range of requirements, such as providing notice, access rights, requiring consent before disclosure for routine uses and establishing contracts with business associates, among others."[4]

The specific terms of a public health agency's HIPAA privacy and security compliance will depend on the functions that agency performs. If the agency is a Covered Entity, or if it has divisions or programs that perform Covered Entity functions, it will need a comprehensive compliance program that either covers the entire agency, or else applies to the covered division or program as if it were a separate entity. If the agency it is not a Covered Entity, it will still need to establish policies, procedures, and contracts that allow it to interact with Covered Entities effectively. If a public health agency outsources

TABLE **4.3.** Hypothetical situations illustrating the prevailing law governing covered entities according to HIPAA

Situation	Prevailing Law
The privacy laws of State X require that a patient sign a notarized authorization for release of medical information, accompanied by the patient's initialing of passages stating his/her privacy rights and the implications of information release, whereas HIPAA requires only a signed and dated authorization, together with some verification of informed and voluntary consent, for the release of information.	State X
State X does not require a patient to authorize release of medical information to be exchanged between licensed physicians for research purposes, whereas HIPAA requires a signed and dated authorization.	HIPAA
State X does not require a Covered Entity to designate a privacy officer and to train employees in the handling of patient information, whereas HIPAA does.	HIPAA

protected health information functions or privatizes them, that agency will have to take careful steps to make sure its contractor is compliant as well and understands its own obligations.

Privacy Protections and Information Sharing

One of the fundamental functions of a public health agency is the collection, analysis, and distribution of disease and health status information. This information may come from many sources, including healthcare provider clinical records, health plan data, and research conducted by or for the agency.

Generally speaking, the most valuable information source is provider records, because these include detailed professional observations of individual clinical indicators. The aggregation of such information in disease registries or the sharing of such data through other mechanisms and systems could provide valuable insights into disease prevention or effective health promotion. Robust, well-designed, and broadly available information systems could prove very valuable in tracking disease outbreaks.

Most of the technological barriers to the development of such systems have already fallen or have been substantially reduced, and this trend is likely to continue. The real barriers to the implementation of registries and other comparable systems are the questions of funding and privacy.

Privacy may prove less intractable than funding. Legislatures find it all too easy to underfund or cut public health programs, so that even if a viable system is developed, its continuity may not be assured. At the same time, private organizations such as health plans and hospitals have not proven very willing to fund systems that primarily benefit the community and only secondarily benefit the organization as a member of the community. A few commercial ASPs have emerged to serve this kind of purpose. This model may prove a viable solution since system funding can come from private investment and user fees spread across the community, but it is not yet clear whether public health agencies trust the model sufficiently to allow widespread acceptance.

On the other hand, there are reasonably clear principles for the resolution of privacy issues. The primary applicable law will be HIPAA, though state law should be analyzed carefully in the establishment and management of any information-sharing program. HHS has explicitly recognized that public health activities require information sharing between governmental and private agencies. On the one hand, as discussed above, Covered Entities will "be permitted to disclose protected health information to public health authorities for the full range of public health activities."[4] On the other hand, the privacy regulations "would further provide that disclosures may be made not only to government agencies, but also to other public and private entities as otherwise required or authorized by law."[4]

Examples of permitted disclosures to other public and private entities include disclosures to private medical device manufacturers or to cancer registries operated by private universities. HHS has recognized that

> the reality of current public health practice is that a variety of activities are conducted by public health authorities in collaboration with non-governmental activities. Federal agencies also use a variety of mechanisms including a contract, grants, cooperative agreements, and other agreements such as memoranda of understanding to carry out and support public health activities. These relationships could be based on specific or general legal authorities.... Limiting the ability to collaborate with other entities and designate them to receive protected health information, could potentially have an adverse impact on public health practice.[4]

A reasonable interpretation is that public health information sharing is a permitted function that can be conducted by, through, and among a wide range of public and private organizations. The underlying function must be public health–related, and the activity must be under governmental authority either by statute or by contracts with an authorized public health agency. If contracts are used, required Business Partner agreement provisions should be included.

Web Site Principles and Practices

Web sites are one of the fundamental tools in electronic commerce. A good Web site can provide genuine public services by providing a range of services and content. Many governmental agencies, including public health agencies, already have Web sites. Web sites may serve useful marketing or educational functions. In addition, they sometimes include functions such as scheduling, which are of administrative value to both patient and organization. In many cases, Web sites are created and run ("hosted") by ASPs or Internet service providers (ISPs). This kind of application, in particular, might be appropriate for outsourcing, and a number of companies have emerged to serve this market niche.

Web Site Interactivity and Jurisdiction

Before establishing a Web site, a public health agency needs to assess its functionality needs carefully. An "active" Web site could create an unexpected exposure to the laws of jurisdictions outside the state where the agency is physically and jurisdictionally located. Web sites by their nature communicate across jurisdictional boundaries, so if they include functions that could be deemed "doing business" elsewhere, such sites may subject the agencies to other states' jurisdictions. (The same consideration may apply to activities involving multijurisdictional information networks and telemedicine.) Under current law, relatively passive, informational Web sites should not trigger jurisdictional concerns, but any interactive Web site functions should be reviewed in this light before being implemented.

Web Site Privacy Issues

Many, perhaps most, Web sites collect information about visitors, sometimes in considerable detail. This kind of information is not subject to HIPAA or other medical or healthcare privacy laws. The scope of acceptable information collection and the kinds of notices that may be required are topics of some controversy, and in some areas self-regulatory "better business practices" are being developed. There have already been lawsuits filed when Web sites failed to disclose their information collection practices accurately, and the Federal Trade Commission is aggressively pursuing a number of regulatory initiatives. Any public health agency Web site should include an appropriate privacy policy statement that the agency should adhere to. If any Web site applications are outsourced, the agency should take steps to insure that the contractor also adheres to the published policy.

Web Site Content Issues

One of the more potentially valuable services some Web sites offer is health information content for consumers. A number of companies and professional organizations provide such content, and an organization may create its own. Before publishing any content on a Web site, the site owner must be sure it has the right to do so. If, for example, the content is copyrighted, the site owner should obtain a license to publish the content.

A potentially valuable, but also potentially risky, Web site content application is interactive health communication systems (IHCs). Typically, ASPs provide IHC content and systems. An organization contracting for an IHC agency will typically lease or subscribe to the right to link that site to the outside system, usually incorporating the organization's own "branding" graphics and text. While the vendor's logo and some attribution is usually present, a consumer accessing an IHC site may not really know that the content does not originate with the primary organization. If something goes wrong from use or reliance on that content, then both the organization and the vendor may be exposed to liability.

Offering health information content therefore brings risks along with its potential benefits. It also raises novel questions of liability and the management of risks to consumers. While it is likely to be many years before the full implications of these systems are well understood and adequately addressed, any public health agency that wants to provide health information content to consumers needs to (1) be aware of the risks and (2) take steps to manage them.

The starting point is with the three basic legal domains that might apply to the regulation of consumer health information. Oddly enough, these are a disparate group:

- medical practice
- medical device regulation
- constitutional freedom of speech.

Justifying providing health information content to consumers by application of the domain of medical practice principles would be a mistake, although it may be an understandable one. The real question for any given content-providing system is whether the system is a "medical device," and therefore regulated, or "free speech," and therefore protected against regulation. There is a fine line between the latter two, and it takes some care to walk it.

HHS has defined IHC as "the interaction of an individual—consumer, patient, caregiver, or professional—with or through an electronic device or communication technology to access or transmit health information, or to receive or provide guidance or support on a health-related issue."[9] Consumer use of IHC in particular brings the issue of disintermediation in the healthcare sector into sharp focus, because it empowers consumers to search out information that previously had been available only to, or with the assistance of, medical professionals.

Disintermediation is an important point of focus in the regulation of IHC. One of the fundamental concepts in electronic commerce, *disintermediation* is the notion that the Internet does away with the "middlemen" who are needed to enable transactions and provide information in the "bricks and mortar" world. The paradigmatic example is travel agents who are being "disintermediated" as consumers buy plane tickets on-line directly from airlines. However, the same process is occurring in many sectors.

Comparably, the Internet and other systems through which individuals can obtain health information serve to disintermediate healthcare providers partially. Consumers no longer need to depend upon professional intermediaries to obtain medical information. For the first time in the history of medicine, lay individuals are able to gain access to much of the medical information formerly available only to their doctors quickly and easily, without their doctors' help or support.

IHC therefore reduces or may in many circumstances eliminate the traditional doctor's role as learned intermediary between patient and medical information. This development is not an unmixed blessing. The sheer volume of information available through the Internet often makes it difficult to find information that is truly useful. This difficulty is even greater for lay individuals who seek but may not be able to fully understand medical information. In the absence of some kind of intermediary that can filter out irrelevant, erroneous, and misleading information, consumers may become confused; there is therefore a risk they will make misguided healthcare decisions with harmful effects. To deal, in part, with this problem and others, the international organization HON (Health On the Net) has developed a voluntary code of conduct to which many medical and health-related Web site owners subscribe.

The HON Code of Conduct (HONcode) for Medical and Health Web Sites

PRINCIPLES

1. Authority
   Any medical or health advice provided and hosted on this site will only be given by medically trained and qualified professionals unless a clear statement is made that a piece of advice offered is from a nonmedically qualified individual or organization.
2. Complementarity
   The information provided on this site is designed to support, not replace, the relationship that exists between a patient/site visitor and his/her existing physician.
3. Confidentiality
   Confidentiality of data relating to individual patients and visitors to a medical/health Web site, including their identity, is respected by this Web site. The Web site owners undertake to honor or exceed the legal requirements of medical/health information privacy that apply in the country and state where the Web site and mirror sites are located.
4. Attribution
   Where appropriate, information contained on this site will be supported by clear references to source data and, where possible, have specific HTML links to that data. The date when a clinical

page was last modified will be clearly displayed (e.g. at the bottom
of the page).

5. Justifiability

Any claims relating to the benefits/performance of a specific treatment, commercial product, or service will be supported by appropriate, balanced evidence in the manner outlined in Principle 4.

6. Transparency of Authorship

The designers of this Web site will seek to provide information in
the clearest possible manner and provide contact addresses for
visitors that seek further information or support. The Webmaster
will display his/her E-mail address clearly throughout the Web site.

7. Transparency of Sponsorship

Support for this Web site will be clearly identified, including the
identities of commercial and noncommercial organizations that have
contributed funding, services, or material for the site.

8. Honesty in Advertising and Editorial Policy

If advertising is a source of funding it will be clearly stated. A brief
description of the advertising policy adopted by the Web site owners will be displayed on the site. Advertising and other promotional
material will be presented to viewers in a manner and context that
facilitates differentiation between it and the original material created by the institution operating the site.

Source: Health On the Net. Available at: http://www.hon.ch/
HONcode/Conduct.html. Accessed March 21, 2002. Used by permission of HON.

Nonetheless, the value of such information is great enough that a number
of electronic intermediary solutions to this problem have been developed,
and there are a number of vendors in this niche. Information indexing systems
on Web sites may allow consumers to browse for documents or links that
appear to be of interest. On a more sophisticated level, electronic "agents" on
Web sites may accumulate information about a consumer's search and viewing choices during a number of sessions and use it to make future searches
more customized. If a consumer elects to store personal data at a Web site—a
service that has become available through a number of companies that also
provide health information content—neural networks and fuzzy logic may
allow health profiling tools to develop additional assumptions about the
consumer's needs and interests.

The use of these technologies can also raise a number of difficult questions
about the changing nature of the doctor-patient relationship. It is technologically possible to develop an IHC system that uses highly developed "expert
systems" and related agents to draw on vast electronic medical libraries and
detailed, individualized health records to deliver precise, detailed, and personalized diagnostic and healthcare information to consumers. It is at least

theoretically possible that in some cases such a system will outperform human doctors in diagnosis and treatment recommendations. What will these possibilities mean for the definition of the practice of medicine and the future of the doctor-patient relationship? Only time will answer that question, but the fact that it is raised almost automatically means it needs an answer.

Putting IHC Systems in Perspective

What does it mean to say a computer "practices medicine"? The only real answer is that the question itself is a mistake. The established paradigm for the practice of medicine is that it is a personal relationship between individual doctors and patients. In real life, of course, this paradigm is more the ideal than the practice. The frequency with which patients change doctors because they move or change insurance companies, the emergence of payment intermediaries in the medical care decision-making process, and the fact that many courses of treatment require teams of professionals have all conspired to complicate and interfere with genuinely personal relationships.

Nonetheless, the established paradigm is the foundation for existing law and medical ethics. As a consequence, neither current law nor traditional medical ethics address the status of a computer system that performs sophisticated consumer IHC services. This failure has important implications for the regulation of IHC systems, especially IHC systems that include any diagnostic or care recommendation functions and those IHC systems storing consumer health records.

By the same token, it would be a fundamental error to try to analyze IHC functions according to the legal principles applicable to the practice of medicine. Because these principles are rooted in the concept of an interpersonal relationship, they presume that both parties are human beings. This is no small presumption: it means that the practice of medicine is regulated primarily by the licensing of individual practitioners, whose standards of practice are determined by the standards of their licensed (human) peers. This concept has expanded to permit the application of medical malpractice standards, for example, to licensed nonhuman "healthcare providers" such as hospitals and other regulated health businesses and entities, but these are all regulated as legal "persons."

But so far, not even the most sophisticated computer systems are considered legal "persons," and they are not likely to be recognized as such any time in the reasonably foreseeable future. Until that time, if it ever comes, existing legal principles applicable to medical practice cannot be applied to regulate IHC systems.

Appropriately, because they are not "persons," IHC systems may, and in many cases should, qualify as regulated "medical devices" subject to federal FDA jurisdiction under the Food, Drug and Cosmetic Act (FDCA).

Under federal law, a "medical device" is defined very broadly, as any "instrument, apparatus, machine, contrivance . . . or other similar or related article, including any component, part or accessory . . . intended for use in the diagnosis of a disease or other conditions, or in the cure. mitigation, treatment, or prevention of disease . . . [or] intended to affect the structure or any function of the body of man[.]"[10] The FDA has stated that it considers medical expert systems, defined as "'knowledge-based' computer software applications designed to assist doctors in the medical diagnostic process," as "medical devices" within this definition.[11]

The question whether any given IHC should qualify as a medical device turns on the personalization of the content it provides. On the one hand, the First Amendment protects the free dissemination of information to the public, so an IHC that essentially serves as a sophisticated indexing system or search engine should be protected. On the other hand, First Amendment protection is limited where the "speech" has the potential to cause harm, and FDA regulation is premised on the avoidance of harm from medical devices.

A knowledge-based computer software application that crosses the line from sophisticated search functions to assisting consumers in making diagnostic or treatment decisions without the assistance of a professional intermediary has a very real potential to cause serious harm. According to the FDA:

> While [medical expert systems] allow medical diagnosis with the touch of a finger, the widespread use of medical expert systems carries the risk of product-caused injuries to users. The most obvious danger of patient at-home use is incorrect diagnosis by [medical expert systems], resulting in patients who improperly treat their ailment. This danger will be a great concern if [medical expert systems] are used by patients without doctor supervision, as may be the case in the near future [sic]. Confronted with this prospect, [as of 1985] the FDA . . . considered imposing regulations on [medical expert systems] . . .[11]

What was a prospect in 1985 is now emerging as reality, in a fashion that could not have been foreseen prior to widespread consumer use of the Internet. And although there are no current regulations specifically regulating consumer IHC, existing law could already be applied to enjoin the use or marketing of a potentially dangerous IHC system, impose penalties, and probably render the IHC owner and/or operator liable for civil damages. Thus, both the vendor of a consumer IHC system that crosses the line into action as a "medical device" and the agency that acquired the right to use that system on its Web site may be exposed to substantial penalties.

Any given IHC system may include functions that run the gamut from constitutionally protected speech to highly risky. presumptively regulated diagnosis and treatment information. It is therefore not possible to determine whether such a system might be considered a "medical device" without specific analysis of the form and phrasing of its content.

Recognition of the risk, however, is the necessary first step to its management. Content can then be assessed and modified if necessary, and appropriate disclaimers and warnings implemented. In some contexts. it might be both necessary and desirable to have consumers enter into use agreements before granting access, perhaps by means of a click-wrap link. A click-wrap link is an on-screen process in which an individual viewing a Web site can access certain pages only by first viewing another page, stating the conditions under which access is permitted, and then placing the cursor on an icon and clicking the mouse to indicate acceptance of the conditions. However, a mere recital that "information is not to be used for diagnostic or treatment purposes" is probably insufficient protection, if the content itself is not properly phrased and structured.

Questions for Review

1. Arcadia Hospital, a privately held corporation, derives most of its support from private donations and commercial revenues. Recently, Arcadia's board of directors has entered into a contract with the federal Agency for Toxic Substances and Disease Registry (ATSDR) to test residents living near a toxic waste site for possible metallic mercury poisoning and to treat those residents found to have blood levels of mercury above the maximum contaminant level established by ATSDR. Arcadia has negotiated a fee of $500 per resident for the testing and $5,000 for each resident treated. All of Arcadia Hospital's other activities and revenues are connected to examination and treatment of private patients.
   a. To what extent is Arcadia Hospital a "public health agency" functionally?
   b. To what extent is Arcadia Hospital a "public health agency" if that term is defined according to delegated governmental authority?
2. As an officer in a public health agency, you are negotiating with Comdata Corporation, a closely held corporation, to provide data processing services under the "application service providers" (ASP) business model in connection with an epidemiological study your agency is about to undertake. Comdata has no other connections to a public health agency.
   a. What characteristics will you look for in determining Comdata's qualifications to enter such a contract?
   b. To what extent do the provisions of the Privacy Act of 1974 apply to Comdata, assuming you enter into the contract?
   c. To what extent do the provisions of HIPAA apply to Comdata under such a contract, and what are your agency's responsibilities with respect to Comdata under HIPAA?
   d. After Comdata has met the terms of the contract and the contract ends, to what extent, if any, do the provisions of HIPAA apply to Comdata with respect to data it has collected during the term of the contract?
3. As a U.S. public health agency employee in the year 2004, you have been designated the project officer in connection with a study of physical examination results of more than 1,000 individuals who may have been exposed to asbestos fibers as a result of working at a now-closed asbestos plant. Your agency had recently contracted with a physician group in the vicinity of the former plant to conduct the physical examinations. The

physician group has refused to disclose information to you without a Business Associate Contract.

   a. Under HIPAA, what were the obligations of the contracting physician group to the individuals examined?

   b. If one of the individuals examined demands to see the health information you possess regarding him and submits a signed and dated request to see the information, what are your obligations under HIPAA?

   c. If a physician not connected to the contracting physician group submits to you a signed request for a copy of the physical examination results related to an individual whom that physician is treating, what are your obligations under HIPAA?

4. As a US public health agency officer, you head a project under which you have assembled hundreds of medical records with the consent of the individuals to whom those medical records pertain. You have received a number of requests from parties other than the individuals for release of these records. For each situation listed below, determine whether, *in general*, under the Privacy Act or HIPAA, you are required to obtain voluntary and informed consent of individuals before releasing medical records.

5. As a licensed public health physician, you specialize in the field of examination and rehabilitation of amputees injured in public transportation

Request	Authorization Required?
A county child health services agency investigating a case of possible child abuse requests the medical record of a 12-year-old girl.	
A state health department investigating an outbreak of sexually transmitted disease requests the medical records of five individuals believed to have been exposed to the disease.	
The head of a public health project approved by an Institutional Review Board and a "privacy board" submits a request to view certain records.	
A private law firm requests the disclosure of all medical records for individuals diagnosed with a certain condition in a specified geographic region, for use in a class action lawsuit.	
A mortgage company requests verification of medical treatment for one individual who has applied for mortgage life insurance.	
The father of a hospitalized 25-year-old male requests to view his son's medical record in connection with a potential liability suit.	

accidents. A manufacturer of prosthetic devices has submitted a request to view your patients' medical records to determine the potential marketability of a prosthetic device now in the research phase. What are your obligations under HIPAA with respect to sharing this information?

6. Your health agency, which is not government-sponsored, has a Web site with the purpose of informing the public about the functions of your agency and providing advice about detecting and reporting the presence of metallic mercury near the site of natural gas registers that have been removed from certain homes. The Web site has been created and is now hosted by an Internet service provider (ISP). An individual can log into your site and navigate it from any location in the United States. The site provides no treatment advice for mercury poisoning, and it functions in a "read only" mode. Your agency is located and conducts all its business in the state of New York.

    a. Is your Web site an "active" or a "passive" site?
    b. What are your obligations with respect to collecting information about Web site visitors? What are your obligations about your ISP's collecting such information?
    c. You contract with the Medifax Company, an interactive health communications system (IHC), to add that system to your Web site, using your own branding graphics and text. This IHC collects information from site visitors and provides, through an expert system, a probable diagnosis of prior exposure to mercury along with recommendations for self-treatment. Is this component of your Web site an "active" or a "passive" system? In the event a Web site visitor's reliance on information obtained from this expert system results in physical harm to the visitor, to what extent are your liable? In the case of physical harm caused to the visitor as a result of reliance on the IHC, is the legal jurisdiction with regard to the IHC system limited to New York? Under federal law, is the use of the expert system governed by the legal domain of (a) medical practice, (b) medical device regulation, or (c) constitutional freedom.

References and Notes

1. The actual act is quite lengthy and most of it concerns matters not relevant to this discussion, such as health insurance reforms. The relevant portions of HIPAA are found in the "Administrative Simplification" section, HIPAA Title II Subtitle F. This section does not set out many details, but instead authorizes and directs HHS to issue regulations on a variety of information-processing oriented matters, including privacy and security protections.
2. Starr P. *The Social Transformation of American Medicine.* New York: Basic Books; 1982.
3. Privacy Act of 1974, 5 USC §552a.
4. Protecting the Privacy of Patients' Health Information; Summary of the Final Regulation [press release]. Washington, DC: Department of Health and Human Services; December 20, 2000.

5. Standards for Privacy of Individually Identifiable Health Information. 65 Fed. Reg. 82462, 82805, 45 CFR 164.501 (2000).

6. Standards for Privacy of Individually Identifiable Health Information, 65 Fed. Reg. 82813, 45 CFR 164.512(b)(1) (2000).

7. Standards for Privacy of Individually Identifiable Health Information, 65 Fed. Reg. 45 CFR 164.512(b)(1)(i) (2000).

8. Standards for Privacy of Individually Identifiable Health Information, 65 Fed. Reg. 82820 45 CFR 514(h)(ii) (2000).

9. Eng TR, Gustafson DH. *Wired for Health and Well-Being: The Emergence of Interactive Health Communication.* Washington, DC: US Department of Health and Human Services, US Government Printing Office; 1999.

10. USC § 321(h) (1996).

11. Nguyen FD. Regulation of Medical Expert Systems: A Necessary Evil? *Santa Clara Law Review* 1994;34:1187.

Part II
The Science of Public Health Informatics

Introduction

Part I of this book placed the science of public health informatics in its context. In Part II, we attempt to explore some nuts-and-bolts issues and aspects.

Part II opens with Patrick O'Carroll's discussion of the topic of information architecture. How does one go about building enterprise-wide information systems that meet the needs of the enterprise and its stakeholders, while at the same time avoiding an inefficient, piecemeal approach? The answer to that question forms the content of Chapter 5, in which Dr. O'Carroll emphasizes planning, including clarification of business processes; an orientation to a component approach; an emphasis on compatibility and interoperability of present and future systems; and executive control over the distribution of information systems.

However, even the most advanced concept of information architecture is of little use to an enterprise if the right people are not available to conceive and build the systems to serve the public health enterprise. In Chapter 6, Janise Richards defines the core knowledge components and competencies required of public health informaticians. Working with a model that emphasizes the interrelationships of the informatics curricula with knowledge domains, skills and knowledge, and the development of competencies, Richards focuses on those competencies that are crucial in a public health informatics environment.

In Chapter 7, Pete Kitch and Bill Yasnoff focus on the topic of managing an information system project. They emphasize the importance of looking beyond the typical hierarchal structure of an organization in business process analysis; examining desirable linkages of systems at the federal, state, and local level; and selecting a sound strategy. They also emphasize the importance of developing a complete requirements definition for a system, using effective principles of cost and benefits estimation, and of knowing when enough is enough—when the effort expended on an information system project is greater than the marginal benefit to be derived.

In Chapter 8, Kitch and Yasnoff look at managing information technology (IT) projects—and personnel—from a different perspective. Moving from a conceptual to a skills-based approach, Kitch and Yasnoff examine the nature of IT project management in a public health environment, focusing on such practical issues as identifying desirable skills for project team members, attracting the right candidates for positions, forming the project team, involving users in the project, using the right tools to ensure project success, knowing when and how to involve consultants in a project, and dealing with political opposition within the organization.

In Chapter 9, Nancy Lorenzi and Robert Riley focus on how an information system project manager can guide and help manage the organizational change that inevitably occurs with the development and implementation of systems. They emphasize the need for a project manager to recognize and deal with the inevitable resistance to change occurring in the organization. Using both small-group and field theory as the basis for change management, Lorenzi and Riley present a practical change management model that can help a manager of an informatics project overcome organizational resistance and achieve buy-in to a system.

In Chapter 10, William Yasnoff focuses on the important issue of maintaining privacy, confidentiality, and security of public health information, with a discussion of the practical and legal necessity for maintaining this confidentiality, Yasnoff provides some guidelines to govern the release of aggregate public health information. After discussing the need for confidentiality agreements between the public health organization and the users of health information, Yasnoff points to some practical steps that the public health organization can take to safeguard information, including use of passwords, smart cards, biometrics, and cryptography. He concludes the chapter with a discussion of the issue of preventing unauthorized access to information via the Internet and detecting potential intruders of systems.

In Chapter 11, Dan Jernigan, Jac Davies, and Alan Sim stress the necessity of adopting data standards as a means of avoiding development of redundant information systems that do not communicate with other systems. They proceed to define data standards by use of the metaphor of a vocabulary and a grammar. After examining the nature of flat, relational, and object-oriented formatting of data, they provide an overview of the standards-setting process and of standards-setting organizations. Jernigan, Davies, and Sim conclude the chapter with a discussion of the trade-offs involved in a public health organization's choosing between national and local standards.

In Chapter 12, Deborah Lewis covers the issue of how to evaluate a public health information system, explaining the purposes of evaluation and the typical phases. Differentiating between formative and summative characteristics of an evaluation, she focuses on subjectivist and objectivist evaluation strategies and methods, describing the characteristics of each. After a discussion of the need to consider the audience and the purpose of the evaluation,

Lewis provides guidelines for developing sound evaluation reports. She concludes the chapter by stressing the need for public health systems evaluators to go beyond traditional evaluation models.

Part II concludes with Chapter 13, in which Kenneth W. Goodman focuses on the issue of making ethical choices with respect to handling and releasing public health information. Beginning with the basis of an "electronic standard of care" in public health information systems as a guide to differentiating between appropriate and inappropriate uses and users of information technology, Goodman points out that failing to use appropriate IT tools in public health practice and using tools inappropriately are equally blameworthy. He then employs the concept of "progressive caution" as a guide in the ethical application of information technology to public health. He concludes the chapter with a discussion of key ethical questions facing public health scientists—questions relating to the emerging field of bioinformatics, of the appropriate use of computers in public health interventions, and of the challenges inherent in the use of such tools as meta-analysis and data mining in making public health decisions.

5
Information Architecture

Patrick W. O'Carroll

Learning Objectives

After studying this chapter, you should be able to:

- Define the concept of *information architecture*, and name at least three ways in which this metaphor can be helpful in designing, planning, and maintaining information systems.
- Discuss the Zachman framework, and indicate the level(s) of the framework at which public health managers can make the most useful contribution.
- Incorporate the technology-focused chapters of this textbook into the larger conceptual model of information architecture.

Overview

Too often, information systems developed by public health agencies have been developed in isolation from enterprise-wide needs and the needs of stakeholders. Such systems have tended, as a result, to lack interoperability with other systems, to be difficult to maintain, and inefficient to develop and support. Implementation of the concept of information architecture provides a solution to the problems created by such piecemeal systems development. Information architecture is a metaphor for a systematic, planned approach to building enterprise-wide information systems. It offers a myriad of benefits, including enhanced system interoperability, ease of support, efficiency, and reduced redundancy of data entry. It also returns the locus of control of information systems development to the executive level. Information architectures can be developed though a process called information resource management (IRM) planning. Although it is ultimately concerned with the management of an enterprise's information resources, IRM planning may be considered synonymous with business planning itself. IRM planning in public health involves understanding, simplifying, and integrating the public health enterprise itself. IRM planning uses information resource models and development of an implementation/migration plan as tools to help a public health organization develop and build its coherent systems, gradually moving toward an improved information architecture. While public health agencies have taken a largely piecemeal approach to information systems development in the past, many agencies are now using the concept of information architecture as a guiding metaphor in developing coherent and well-integrated information systems.

Introduction

Imagine building a house without any architectural plans. You have selected a lot for your home, and you are anxious to get started—why wait for plans? You know you will need bedrooms, a kitchen, bathrooms, and so forth, so why not just start building it and design it as you go along? Alternatively, if you feel that architectural plans might be useful, then imagine building your house with only very general sketches as to how the house is supposed to look from the street. Conversely, imagine building your new home after having seen only detailed diagrams for wiring, plumbing, etc., with no idea of how the house will look when it is finished.

Imagine that your subcontractors—for plumbing, electrical work, foundation construction, heating and air conditioning installation, and other components—each do their work according to their own ideas, without ever consulting with the owner, the architect, or any of the other participants in the construction, and without any guiding instructions. Further imagine building a house with no specialized functions for any of the rooms, a house in which every room has its own little stove, bed, bathtub, television, commode, etc. Finally, imagine building this improbable house in such a way that the entire house has to be torn down to remodel even one room.

This approach, self-evidently absurd, provides an analogy to the way that most public health data and information systems have been built since the advent of the personal computer. Typically, an epidemiologist or other public health professional with no formal training in computer science would have an idea for using computers to help accomplish some task—to record and transmit surveillance data, for example, or to manage a disease treatment and prevention program in a health department. After developing a general idea of what was needed, this person would often rush to begin coding the project, essentially beginning construction of his "house" with entirely inadequate plans. Such projects, even if carefully planned, would generally be designed with little or no consideration given to how the new information system would work with other public health information systems already in use or in development. As such, each project necessarily adopted or developed its own user interface: its own approach to data security; its own data model (specifying, for example, how to code data for age, race, and sex); its own underlying database engine; its own system for backups and data integrity; its own protocols for transmitting the data electronically; its own system for user support, system documentation, and user training; and its own system for updates and bug fixes. Finally, because these systems were not typically designed and developed by information systems professionals, they were usually very difficult to update—often necessitating complete rewrites of program code to add new or enhanced functionality or to take advantage of new technologies.

The result, of course, was a set of public health data and information systems that neither looked nor worked at all alike. Such systems required redundant data entry across systems, did not easily share data between systems, and were difficult to install and maintain. From the developer's perspective, this incoherent approach resulted in multiple development teams who were generally unaware of each other's existence, multiple user support systems; and lengthy development cycles.

Enter Information Architecture

Such piecemeal systems development in public health has been abating in recent years, in part because of the widening recognition of the value of conducting systems development in the context of a guiding information architecture.

Information architecture is a metaphor for a systematic, planned approach to building enterprise-wide information systems. The term refers not only to the use of information technology, but also to the totality of the data, processes, and technology used in a given enterprise and the relations between them. As such, information architecture includes the databases, applications, standards, procedures, information use and confidentiality policies, hardware, software, and networks for a given public health enterprise.

The elastic concept of a public health *enterprise* is important here. A public health enterprise may be, for example, the local public health department, a particular division within a large metropolitan health department, a state health department, or the entire local-state-federal public health system. The scope of the enterprise is defined by the nature of the information system being developed. For some information systems (e.g., a system for tracking publications in progress), the enterprise might be appropriately defined as the epidemiology research unit in a given health department. However, for any information system in which data are likely to be shared with other organizations or with other parts of an organization, or in which data are likely to be entered and stored redundantly with other existing systems (e.g., patient names), the nature of the enterprise should be defined much more broadly. For certain applications (e.g., public health surveillance of reportable infectious diseases), the public health enterprise for which the architecture is designed might properly be considered to include local health departments, state health departments, and the federal Centers for Disease Control and Prevention (CDC).

Benefits of an Information Architecture

There are myriad benefits to be derived from developing public health information systems using the concept of information architecture. First, of course, the architecture provides a guiding plan across development projects. Second, an information architecture promotes a *component* orientation to the development process, so that larger pieces of the system are built out of smaller units. This component orientation allows for easier development (in that big problems are broken down into manageable chunks—so-called "functional decomposition"), easier upgrades, and easier incorporation of new information technologies. Third, an information architecture simplifies systems by decreasing redundancy of data entry and storage, and by providing a coherent approach to cross-cutting systems issues like security and data backup. Fourth, an information architecture usually promotes efficiency and interoperability through the incorporation of *standards* (e.g., for data representation and user interface) and through solving common challenges once instead of many times in many ways. Fifth, an information architecture also necessarily promotes planning and clarifies business processes, as discussed further below.

Sixth, and perhaps most importantly, an enterprise-wide public health information architecture returns the locus of control and decision making to the executive level and takes it away from the information technology community. Simply put, using a coherent information architecture provides the basis for business control over the distributed development of information systems. To return to our house-building metaphor, the prospective homeowner does not closely supervise and interact with all the builders, electricians, plumbers, and so forth. Instead, the homeowner specifies the nature of the home to be built via architectural plans developed with the help of an experienced architect. These plans, clearly communicated to the general contractor, form the basis for the homeowner's control over the building process. In the same way, public health executives can direct the development of information systems by means of the clear business specifications inherent in a well-developed information architecture. These specifications are developed through a variety of formal and informal processes, including a process called joint application design (JAD). Table 5.1 provides a comparison of the features of systems developed with and without a guiding information architecture.

Of course, architectural plans come in many levels of detail. Only certain levels of architecture detail, or *views* of the architecture, are the appropriate concern of the owner-designer, whether of homes or of information systems. Information system development requires multiple levels of architectural plans, from general 'business' views (representing overall public health processes and objectives) to specific technical views (indicating specific technology and implementation details). The business views of the information architecture represent *what* processes need to be automated, whereas the information technology views of the architecture represent *how* these processes should be automated. It is important, however, to recognize that the specific (i.e., tech-

TABLE 5.1. Comparison of information systems developed with and without a guiding information architecture

System Attribute	Independent Development	Development Guided by Information Architecture
Planning for development projects	No guiding plan across development projects	A single plan guides development across development projects.
Whole vs. component orientation	Oriented to one application or system built as an integral whole	Uses component orientation so that larger pieces of the system are built from smaller units, allowing easier development, easier upgrades, and easier incorporation of new technology.
Approach to common tasks	Each system built independently, necessitating (at the agency level) redundant data entry and storage, multiple security and data backup systems, etc.	Integrated approach to common tasks yields simplified systems, decreasing redundancy of data entry and storage, and provides a coherent approach to crosscutting systems issues like security and data backup.
Utilization of standards	Independent development does not necessitate use of standards. "Home-grown" standards proliferate, leading to a lack of interoperability, multiple approaches to data representation, multiple user interfaces, etc.	Established standards employed, promoting inter-operability, ease of use across systems, and efficiency.
Planning and clarification of business processes	Independent development proceeds in the absence of detailed planning, as the (limited) scope of the single application does not appear to warrant thorough planning processes.	The development of the information architecture requires a clear and relatively comprehensive description of business processes, which promotes planning and critical examination of business processes.
Control of system development	Control is local without regard to enterprise-wide needs; decision making is often in the hands of the IT community.	Control is at the executive level; policy-makers control the distributed development of information systems.

Source: Author

nical) views of the architecture should be based on higher, business-level views. In other words, the information technology architecture should be tightly tied to the business processes and objectives represented in higher-level views.

Some argue that, given the pace of technological change, it is impractical to attempt the development of a coherent, enterprise-wide information architecture—that, by the time the architecture is developed, the rush of technological advancement will have rendered the plans obsolete. However, the business views of an information architecture are relatively stable. After all, despite an ever-widening emphasis on public health reform consequent to the publication of *The Future of Public Health* in 1988,[1] the business of public health does not change all that rapidly. Information technology views, on the other hand, can and should adapt to take advantage of improvements in technology, while still serving these higher-level business goals.

Developing an Information Architecture

Information Resource Management (IRM) and IRM Planning

Information resource management (IRM) is, as you might expect, a set of principles and practices by which an organization manages its information resources. Inherent in IRM is a disciplined approach to the development and management of an organization's information resources: data, applications (software, programs, code) and technology (hardware, networks, telecommunications). The true importance of IRM, however, lies in its central, underlying ethic: *information is one of a public health organization's key strategic assets*, along with financial resources and human resources. Yet the value of information is not evident from observing the practices of many public health organizations. The value that such organizations place on dollars and people is easily inferred from the careful, high-level way in which these resources are managed: there is usually a chief financial officer overseeing a budgeting and accounting operation, and a chief personnel officer overseeing a department of human resources. In contrast, relatively few public health agencies can boast of a chief information officer who oversees a similarly well-staffed and well-supported information resources management operation. The principles and practices of IRM can help a public health organization effectively harness and deploy the information that is one of the organization's most valuable assets.

IRM *planning* is the process by which an information architecture is developed. IRM planning also specifies how to achieve the agreed-upon architecture. The goal of IRM planning is to provide business guidance to those in the public health organization who develop its information systems and to provide a framework (in terms of policies, standards, and tools) for an agency's

TABLE 5.2. Information resource management planning

- Is *business* planning—it is *not* just about IT planning.

- Requires a high-level review of the business—its goals, procedures, customers, organizational structure, etc.

- Requires ongoing *executive level sponsorship*. Failure of IRM planning is guaranteed without this element.

Source: Author

information technology development and management. However, in a larger sense. IRM planning is synonymous with business planning itself. To be most effective, IRM planning requires a high-level, comprehensive review of the business. For a public health agency, it requires a thorough review and prioritization of the agency's goals, procedures, customers, organization, and so forth. These are the high-level "business" elements that determine the development of the technical levels of the information architecture, as described above. Table 5.2 summarizes the nature of IRM planning.

Given the scale, importance, and sometimes-lengthy nature of IRM planning, it should be undertaken only when there is informed, ongoing, executive-level sponsorship of the process. Such support is not always easy to achieve and maintain in a government setting, but it is nevertheless critical: IRM planning will predictably fail without this key ingredient. After all, it is the high-level executives who conduct the business planning of which IRM planning is a part, and it is also these executives who undertake the review of the business in the planning process.

Stakeholders in a Public Health Organization's IRM Planning

To be effective, IRM planning also requires in-depth stakeholder involvement. A common shortcoming in IRM planning comes from defining *stakeholders* too narrowly (e.g., as all senior managers and information users in a particular public health agency). A public health agency, in fact, has many stakeholders, considering that a stakeholder is anyone or any group affected in some way by the actions of the organization. For example, for a state health department, stakeholders in the department's information resources planning might include partners in local health departments, community groups, clinical care professionals, allied state and federal agencies, and especially the general public being served by the organization. Such stakeholders are all affected in some way by the manner in which a public health agency manages its information, and they need to be considered and often involved in IRM planning.

Steps in IRM Planning

There are three key steps in IRM planning for a public health agency or for any other enterprise. These steps are (1) understanding the business, (2) simplifying the business, and (3) integrating the business.

The first step in IRM planning is to *understand* the business—to elucidate in concrete terms exactly what the public health agency does. This step, seemingly straightforward, can in fact be the most difficult and time-consuming element. It involves the development of models of the business by use of formal modeling techniques. It may also involve reexamination and rewriting of the organization's mission statement.

The second step in IRM planning is to *simplify* the business, through reorganization, the use of information technology, or both. Usually, the process of modeling the workings of a business (including the workings of a public health agency) reveals a variety of obvious redundancies, outmoded work processes, and other problems that can be addressed through simplification.

The final step is to *integrate* the business. With regard to information resources, integrating the business of public health means arranging public health information systems so that data, software code, and technology can be shared across the agency, and so that "one fact is stored in one place."

Information Resource Models: Views of the Architecture

As noted, understanding the business of public health involves modeling its many processes. These models represent the enterprise and the information resources that support it. The models represent different types of information (data, applications, technology) at different levels of abstraction (conceptual, logical, physical). These different levels of abstraction are analogous to the different levels of architectural diagrams, the different architectural "views" we have discussed.

Perhaps the most famous of the architectural diagrams used for such modeling is John Zachman's Enterprise Architecture Framework, first published in 1987.[2] Zachman developed the diagram after observing how the architecture and construction industries as well as the engineering and manufacturing industries managed change. The Zachman framework provides a model of how enterprise managers and their information technology (IT) departments can work together to design and change enterprises and the computer systems that support them and to develop the capability for rapid organizational change. The Zachman framework is shown in Figure 5.1.

For all practical purposes, the Zachman framework of business models and information types uses a two-dimensional structure to describe the information architecture of an enterprise. The first dimension describes the roles

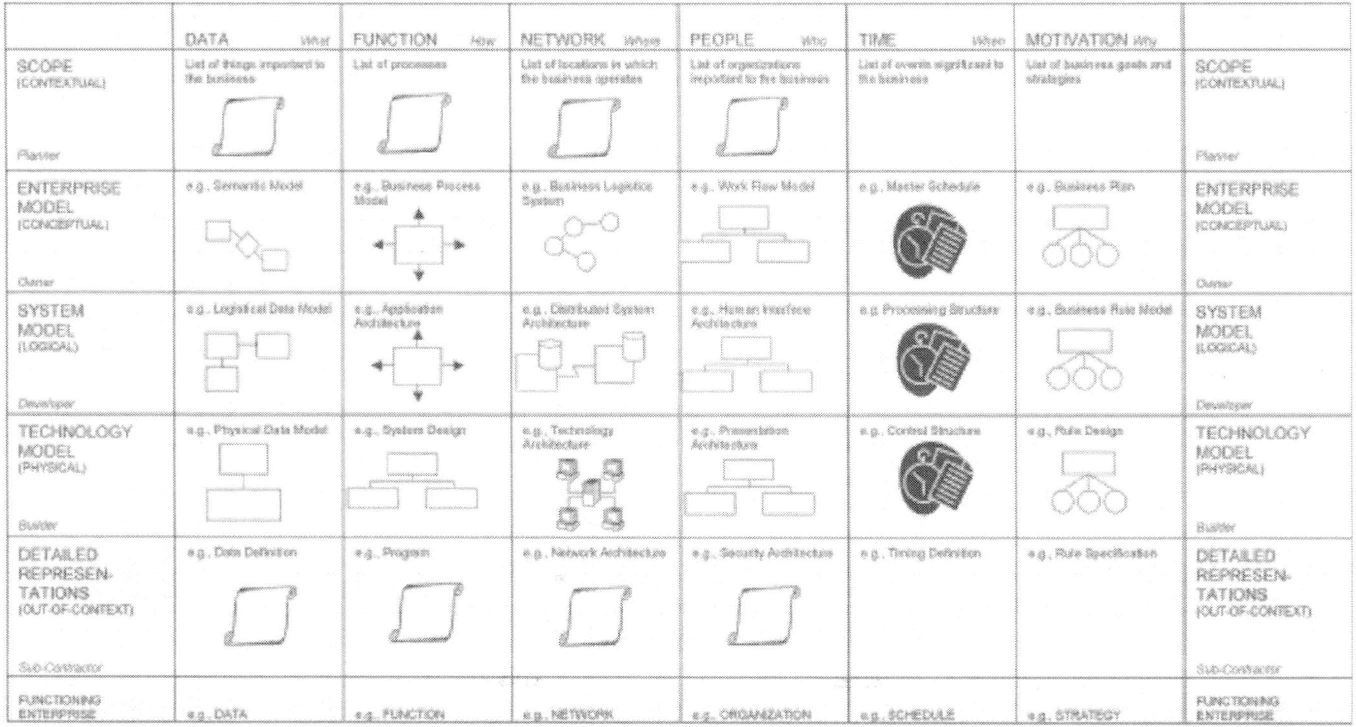

Figure 5.1. The Zachman Enterprise Architecture Framework. (Adapted by permission of ZIFA—Zachman International. Available at: http://www.zifa.com/frmwork2.htm.)

TABLE 5.3. The two-dimensional framework of the Zachman model

Participant	What (Data)	How (Function)	Where (Network)
Planner/Owner			
Designer			
Builder			
Subcontractor			

Source: Author

involved in information systems design, while the second dimension specifies various attributes of the system. Table 5.3 is a representation of this two-dimensional framework.

Employing slightly different terminology from that used in Figure 5.1, we can further describe the levels in this model as they apply to a public health agency.

The *enterprise (functional)* model describes what the enterprise does (or should be doing) to meet its missions and objectives, and describes what the enterprise needs to know to do it. The *information* model identifies and defines the subjects (entities) about which the enterprise keeps information and also identifies the significant relationships between those entities (entity-relationship diagrams). This information model provides the basis for later database development. The *application* models identify and define a set of applications that support the enterprise and information models. The *distribution* model specifies the physical distribution of entities and applications of the models to physical locations. Finally, the *technology* model specifies the blueprint for the development and integration of the information technology resources of the enterprise, now and for the future.

Public health executives should be intimately involved in the development of the first (enterprise) level of the framework. In addition, public health officials involved in defining the databases needed to support public health action should be closely involved (along with database designers) at the second (information) level of the framework. As one proceeds toward the lower levels of the framework, the lead responsibility shifts from public health officials to information systems specialists. For example, IT professionals should take the lead role in the technology model, although executives at the enterprise level will necessarily be involved.

Next Steps: Implementation/Migration Plan

Modeling the business of a given public health agency and then determining how that business can be simplified and integrated by use of information technology is the essence of developing an information architecture. This process defines where you are, both in terms of your agency and the information systems that support it, and where you want to be.

However, the planning process requires one final ingredient before a public health organization can determine how to begin moving toward the desired architecture. This ingredient is an *implementation and migration plan*. This plan (or set of plans) needs to lay out a stepwise process for moving from legacy information systems to the new systems called for in the IRM plan. The implementation/migration plan defines, scopes, and sequences a comprehensive set of projects that will design and build or otherwise acquire the data structures, applications, and IT represented in the models. This plan needs to account not only for the technical challenges, but also for the human and organizational challenges inherent in all information systems development projects.

Getting There: Toward Information Architecture in Public Health

The potential benefits of an information architecture for public health are clear and compelling, but the development of this architecture is an arduous task. This chapter has described how one process (IRM planning) can be used to develop an information architecture for a given enterprise, but this formal approach is not feasible organizationally or politically in every public health agency. Different state health departments have, in fact, taken approaches of varying formality. However, almost all state health departments are working at some level to articulate a guiding architecture for their information systems development. The inefficiencies and frustrations associated with the heretofore "Wild West" approach to public health information systems development have convinced many that a more coherent approach is long overdue.

Questions for Review

1. Public health officials in the epidemiology division of a large state health department have decided to develop an information system that will allow them to collect and analyze data related to an outbreak of a new virus in their state. Although the state health department operates integrated information systems developed for epidemiological studies, the planned system will not have any compatibility or interoperability with those systems, nor will enterprise management be involved with development of the new system.

   a. Will this system be developed more quickly than it would be if it were developed as part of the state health department's integrated information systems? Will it be more difficult to build? Will it be more difficult to maintain?

b. Given the existence of a guiding enterprise-level information architecture, is it ever appropriate to develop such independent systems? If so, under what circumstances is it appropriate?

2. Explain the difference between "business" views and information technology views of an enterprise's information architecture.

3. Most public health agencies and organizations have not managed their information assets as strategically as they have their personnel and financial assets. Why is this so?

4. Explain why IRM planning is so closely linked to business planning. In what ways are a public health organization's mission, organization, and processes connected to IRM planning?

5. A state health department is engaged in IRM planning. For each of the activities listed in the first column below, indicate whether an activity is most directly related to (1) understanding the business, (2) simplifying the business, or (3) integrating the business by putting a checkmark in the column corresponding to the IRM planning step to which the activity relates.

Activity	Understanding the Business	Simplifying the Business	Integrating the Business
The department implements plans to ensure that all divisions within the agency share the same data, software code, and technology.			
The department reorganizes its divisions to eliminate duplication of effort.			
The department develops a strategic plan, including a mission statement, to recognize the nature of its activities.			
The department streamlines procedures to be used by all divisions in undertaking the department's mission.			

6. In a public health organization's application of the Zachman model, leadership for the higher-level views of the architecture resides among public health officials, whereas leadership for lower levels tends to shift to information systems specialists. Why this shift in leadership? What features differentiate lower levels of the model from higher levels?

7. Why is modeling the "business" of public health an important feature in a given public health organization's effort to develop an information architecture?
8. How does an implementation/migration plan for information technology differ from the general business planning that is part of IRM planning?

References

1. Institute of Medicine. *The Future of Public Health*. Washington, DC: National Academy Press; 1988.
2. Zachman JA. A framework for information systems architecture. *IBM Systems Journal* 1987;26:276–292.

Suggestion for Further Reading

Cook MA. *Building Enterprise Information Architectures: Reengineering Information Systems*. Upper Saddle River, NJ: Prentice Hall PTR. 1996.

6
Core Competencies in Public Health Informatics

Janise Richards

Learning Objectives

After studying this chapter, you should be able to:

- List the core disciplines of public health informatics and describe the areas of management that they comprise.
- Describe the knowledge domains of public health informatics.
- List the key public health informatics competencies for public health practitioners.
- List the key public health informatics competencies for public health informaticians.
- Explain why management skills are more important than technical skills for a public health informatician.
- Explain how public health organizations can promote the acquisition of public health informatics skills by employees.

Overview

What competencies in public health informatics should a public health practitioner possess? What competencies should a public health informatician possess? How can public health provide the educational and skill-building experiences that both public health informaticians and public health practitioners need? These are some of the questions that need to be asked early in the development of this discipline. Defining the core knowledge is necessary for an understanding of what competencies are needed. There are two methods for identifying core knowledge—watching experts doing their jobs, or asking them about what it takes to do their jobs. Because of time and travel constraints, it is difficult to watch informaticians and public health practitioners do their jobs, but asking them is feasible. From the identified knowledge, four domains of public health informatics knowledge that encompass the skills and knowledge public health practitioners and informatics specialists need to possess become apparent. To determine how these skills and this knowledge may be turned into educational interventions for use by public health organizations and academic institutions is a challenge the discipline of public health informatics must face.

Introduction

In Chapter 1, Patrick O'Carroll defined public health informatics as "the systematic application of information and computer science and technology to public health practice, research, and learning." Still, a definition by itself does not answer several questions:

- What should public health informaticians know in order to assist public health practitioners in applying information and computer science and technology to public health practice, research, and learning?
- What should public health practitioners know in order to apply public health informatics appropriately to public health practice?
- What specific competencies should public health informaticians have in order to apply the necessary knowledge to assist practitioners in such tasks as collecting, organizing, manipulating, and reporting data and information?
- What informatics competencies should public health practitioners possess?
- How can public health provide the educational and skill-building experiences that both public health informaticians and public health practitioners need?

The principal purpose of this chapter is to develop answers to these questions. Developing these answers will require us first to establish a process for defining core knowledge. We can then move to consideration of the knowledge domains of health-related informatics in general. With this framework established, we can focus on the knowledge domains specific to public health informatics. Finally, we will isolate the public health informatics competencies—the skills and knowledge—that are important for public health informaticians, on the one hand, and for public health practitioners, on the other. We will conclude the chapter with a brief discussion of how public health can provide the educational and skill-building experiences that both public health informatics specialists and public health practitioners need.

Defining Core Knowledge

For our purpose, we will use a four-step cyclic process to define the core knowledge of public health informatics and, for that matter, of health-related informatics in general, as illustrated in Figure 6.1.

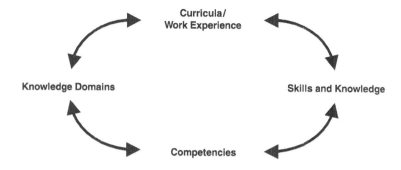

FIGURE 6.1. The knowledge determination process.

The process begins with an examination of the curricula—whether the curricula relate to formal educational exposure in a public health school or to direct experience and training—that lead to the acquisition of knowledge of a field. The curricula, in turn, suggest knowledge domains, or fields of knowledge. These knowledge domains, in turn, provide the basis for the development of competencies—the general abilities that an individual needs to possess in order to apply knowledge. The competencies then lead to the skills and knowledge—the specific abilities—required for exercise of the competencies. Finally, these skills and knowledge provide the basis for what needs to be taught in a curriculum that is designed to convey the core knowledge. Although an arbitrary end is placed here at curriculum design, this cyclic process is continuous.

Public Health Informatics Knowledge Domains

What are the key knowledge domains in public health practice in general and in public health informatics in particular? We will answer this question in two parts, focusing first on knowledge domains in public health practice and later on knowledge domains specific to public health informatics.

Knowledge Domains in Public Health Practice

The Public Health Foundation and its Council on Linkages between Academia and Public Health Practice have identified eight public health knowledge domains required of public health practitioners, as listed in Table 6.1.[1]

These knowledge domains apply to all public health workers, not merely to public health informaticians, and their soundness is self-evident. Without analytic/assessment skills, for instance, a public health practitioner is unable

TABLE 6.1. Core public health knowledge domains

> ➤ Analytic/assessment skills
> ➤ Basic public health science skills
> ➤ Cultural competency skills
> ➤ Communication skills
> ➤ Community dimensions of practice skills
> ➤ Financial planning and management skills
> ➤ Leadership and systems thinking skills
> ➤ Policy development/program planning skills

Source: Public Health Foundation. *Refining and Validating Public Health Competencies: A Proposal for Next Steps.* Washington, DC, 1999.

to apply appropriate methods to address outbreaks of disease. Without basic public health science skills, a practitioner lacks the background to conduct an analysis or an assessment of a public health problem. Without cultural competency skills, the same practitioner lacks the basic framework for addressing the public dimensions of a health problem and for understanding the associated behaviors. Without communication skills, a practitioner lacks the ability to communicate with the public and to publish findings, etc. Although these domains do not address informatics, there is a subset that contains some informatics-related competencies (i.e., managing information systems for collection, retrieval, and use of data for decision making). Just as with these public health knowledge domains and related competencies, we need to make public health informatics competencies more explicit to assist in training programs and curricula development. To accomplish this, we must determine the knowledge domains and underlying competencies, along with the supporting skills and knowledge in public health informatics.

Knowledge Domains in Public Health Informatics

What are the knowledge domains specific to public health informatics? An acceptable method to answer this question is to identify and interview public health informatics experts to determine what they think are the important skills and knowledge in the discipline. Once the data are collected, sorted, and classified, we can begin to define knowledge domains and key competencies and create a competency model that is confirmed with other experts. [2-4] We interviewed experts in informatics in general and in public health informatics in particular.[5]

These interviews revealed, first of all, that the emphasis in public health informatics should be on *methods*, rather than on specific software applications or technology. The basis of this emphasis is that a public health informatician may be called upon to undertake many different tasks and to focus more on the development, implementation, management, and evalua-

TABLE 6.2. The core disciplines of public health informatics

Sciences	Management	Skills
Computer science	Technology management Database management Network management	Knowledge representation skills
Information science	Information management	Technical skills
Behavioral science	Personnel management	People skills Communication skills Interpersonal skills
Organizational science	Organizational management Transition (change) management	Facilitation skills Leadership skills
Management science	Resource management Program management Project management Process management	Management skills Planning skills

tion of the overall information system than on a specific technology. In fact, specific software applications may be the responsibility of epidemiologists, biostatisticians, or others in the public health office, rather than of the informatician.

The experts emphasized that public health informaticians need to have knowledge in five core disciplines of public health to understand the unique problems associated with public health practice. In addition to having core public health knowledge, public health informaticians must have knowledge in five other science-related areas, understand the related management implications, and be able to perform the associated skills. Table 6.2 shows these core disciplines and associated skills.

The experts stressed the overriding importance of a public health informatician being able to exercise *management skills*, with a heavy emphasis on people skills, communication skills, interpersonal skills, and planning skills. These skills were deemed more crucial than the acquisition of specific expertise in a particular science. In short, the skills that the experts emphasized were those associated with being able to *apply* knowledge effectively. They agreed that public health informaticians should be able to understand how to capture information more efficiently, how to manipulate it, how to disseminate it, etc., through an essential understanding of information systems and information technology. Although several experts suggested other,

TABLE 6.3. The knowledge domains of public health informatics

Domain I	Domain II	Domain III	Domain IV
Organization and systems management	Information systems	Information technology	Public health

more specific knowledge areas—standards, evaluation or outcomes assessment, Web design, hardware, and software—most emphasized the acquisition of comprehensive understanding as more vital.

Further analysis of the interview results revealed that all the knowledge areas can be collapsed into four main knowledge domains, as shown in Table 6.3. We will briefly define and discuss the nature of each of these domains.

Organization and Systems Management

This domain includes the competencies needed to manage projects, programs, and organizational and technology systems. For example, it includes the competencies discussed by Kitch and Yasnoff in Chapters 7 and 8—the ability to assess business processes in public health, the ability to manage information technology personnel, and the ability to manage information technology projects. It also includes such competencies as managing organizational change (see Chapter 9).

Information Systems

This domain contains the competencies needed to design, develop, implement, and evaluate information systems. It essentially includes tasks such as identification of the appropriateness of using information technology to solve the public health problem being addressed, examination of the needs of users, and integration into existing systems. It also includes the ability to exercise knowledge of data standards (see Chapter 11) and to evaluate the effectiveness of a system, once it is implemented (see Chapter 12).

Information Technology

This third domain differs from the information systems domain in that the emphasis of information technology is on the hardware and software aspects—the computers, networks, communication technology, software applications, etc. It includes the technology used to complete a task, whereas information systems are overall methods and technology used to complete the task or solve the problem.

Public Health

This domain concentrates on the acquisition and exercise of knowledge in the five core public health disciplines: (1) behavioral sciences, (2) biostatistics, (3) environmental health, (4) epidemiology, and (5) health services. Without knowledge of these disciplines, a public health informatician is unlikely to be able to apply systems and technology effectively to support public health practice. In particular, the experts emphasized that public health informaticians must possess more than a knowledge of informatics: they must also possess a knowledge of the disciplines within which all public health practitioners function.

Public Health Informatics Competencies for Public Health Practitioners

The knowledge domains we have discussed set the stage for the next step in our process—determining the critical competencies, skills, and knowledge within those knowledge domains for both public health informaticians and for public health practitioners. We will begin with a focus on public health informatics for public health practitioners.

Friede et al. provided an early definition of public health informatics that includes several competencies associated with the application of information science and technology to public health practice and research.[6] These authors suggested the definition should include developing innovative ways to use inexpensive and powerful computers, on-line databases, and the capacity for universal connection of people and computers, together with multimedia communications, to support the mission of disease prevention and health promotion. Among the skills and knowledge needed to perform the functions of public health informatics are:

- Skills and knowledge in computer science, together with competency in the use of computers, as a means of developing innovative ways to apply computers to public health practice
- Skills and knowledge in information systems management and technology in order to implement effective database design and development
- Skills and knowledge in information science sufficient to develop a universal connection among people, computers, and multimedia communications
- Currency in the theories and skills related to the five core areas of public health and the information resources available within these core public health areas

The question here is why are these skills important for public health practitioners? One major reason for obtaining and maintaining these skills and the associated knowledge is that public health information resources are rapidly expanding, both for public health practitioners and for consumers.[7] Besides knowing how to access, store, and share information, the knowledgeable public health practitioner also must contribute to consumer health networks and participate in consumer health bulletin boards and mailing list servers (e.g., LISTSERV) as means of helping to keep information accurate and current. As the general public becomes more knowledgeable about personal information technology, a competent public health practitioner will need to use this electronic connection to promote the core functions of public health—assessment, policy development, and assurance. Secondly, practitioners who understand how to use information technology effectively and who can implement its potential will be innovators in the delivery of public health delivery systems.[8]

Competencies

Before we continue discussing competencies, we need to ask the question: what is a competency? Although the term *competency* has been defined differently by nearly everyone who has developed competencies, three terms are usually included: (1) knowledge, (2) skill, and (3) attitudes or values. In this chapter, we discuss both core competencies and other competencies. Here, *core competency* is defined as the fundamental knowledge, ability, or skill for the specific subject of public health informatics. The "core" part of the term indicates that it the basis from which additional competencies—a subset of core skills and knowledge—are derived by the individual to perform a specific task. A *specific competency* indicates a mastery of the knowledge and skills to perform a specific task; such a competency is often used to measure performance, or outcomes. The focus here is on the broader competencies that would be common throughout all public health organizations.

To determine the importance of the identified competencies, a Web-based Delphi survey—an iterative questionnaire that refined opinion—was administered to a larger group of experts, including those who had participated in the interview. The survey elicited judgments about the critical (or highest priority) and the important (second highest priority) competencies and skills and knowledge for public health informaticians and for public health practitioners.

Critical and Important Competencies for Public Health Practitioners

The surveyed experts suggested that public health practitioners need only a moderate level of knowledge of public health informatics. Table 6.4 provides a listing of the informatics competencies that the experts believed a public health practitioner should possess.

Although the experts did not view any of these competencies as critical for a public health practitioner, they saw the ability to use resource management

TABLE 6.4. Delphi survey opinion of informatics experts about informatics competencies required of public health practitioners

Important competencies

Use resource management skills and knowledge to provide efficient support for public health information systems.

Apply information management knowledge and skills to support public health efforts.

Moderately important competencies

Apply project management skills and knowledge to develop public health information systems.

Use change management skills and knowledge to encourage adaptation of current methods and adoption of new methods of information management.

Demonstrate skills and knowledge to plan, design, and develop information systems that meet the needs of public health practice and research to create effective and efficient public health systems.

Use information systems skills and knowledge in the implementation of public health systems.

Use information systems skills and knowledge to evaluate implemented public health information systems.

Apply skills and knowledge about information technology hardware to assist in the development and adoption of appropriate information technology in public health.

Apply skills and knowledge about operating systems, software, and applications when developing or consulting on a public health information system.

Apply public health science theories, principles, and methods when developing public health information systems.

---

skills and knowledge to provide efficient support for public health information systems as important. Equally important was the ability of the practitioner to apply information management knowledge and skills to support public health efforts.

Of moderate importance were such competencies as a public health practitioner's ability to apply project management skills and knowledge to the development of public health information systems; to apply change management skills within a public health organization; to know how to plan, design, and develop the right kinds of information systems; to understand how to implement and evaluate public health information systems; and to develop/adopt information technology in public health.

Thus, the survey results clearly indicate that there should be no effort to transform public health practitioners into informatics specialists. Rather, the aim should be for public health practitioners to be knowledgeable in information systems and information technology, so that they can be effective managers and users of these resources.

In fact, the specific skills and knowledge that experts regarded as critical for public health practitioners include those that one would expect them to possess if they were involved in public health, even if no information systems were involved. Table 6.5 lists these critical skills and the associated knowledge.

The critical items include leadership; political aptitude; knowledge of the theory, principles, and methods of public health core disciplines; and good communication skills. Among these items, there are only two information technology–related items: (1) practitioners should be able to search the Web to find public health information, and (2) practitioners should be able to use presentation and communication applications. In summary, the experts indicated that the emphasis for public health practitioners in the field of informatics should be on the basics, or literacy, in informatics, computers, and information.

TABLE 6.5. Critical skills and knowledge for public health practitioners

Critical Skills and Knowledge

Develop strategic plans that reflect future needs of public health and information technology.

Apply leadership and advocacy skills within all levels of the public health system.

Demonstrate good communication skills to interact with a variety of technical and health professionals interpersonally, in public speaking and through writing.

Identify situations when public health and technical experts should be asked for advice.

Identify, participate in, and be sensitive to office, local, state, and federal politics.

Maintain security, privacy, and confidentiality of personal and public health information within local and enterprise systems.

Use presentation applications (e.g., PowerPoint) and communication applications (e.g., e-mail, mailing list servers such as LISTSERV) to effectively communicate.

Use different Web browsers and search engines to effectively find public health information.

Apply biostatistics theory and methods.

Apply environmental and occupational health theory, principles, legislation, and methods.

Apply epidemiology theory and methods.

Apply health service administration theory, methods, principles, and models.

Critical and Important Competencies
for Public Health Informaticians

The public health informatician must possess numerous critical informatics competencies and several important competencies. Table 6.6 provides a listing of the competencies that the experts believed a public health informatician should possess.

Interestingly, the critical competencies predominately are from the management domain, Domain I, organization and systems management. Competencies from the technology knowledge domains (Domain II. information

TABLE **6.6.** Competencies necessary for public health informaticians

Critical competencies

Apply project management skills and knowledge to develop public health information systems.

Use change management skills and knowledge to encourage adaptation of current methods and adoption of new methods of information management.

Apply information management knowledge and skills to support public health efforts.

Apply basic information systems and information systems theory to create effective and efficient public health systems.

Demonstrate skills and knowledge to plan, design, and develop information systems that meet the needs of public health practice and research to create effective and efficient public health systems.

Use information system skills and knowledge in the implementation of public health information systems.

Use information system skills and knowledge to evaluate implemented public health information systems.

Apply skills and knowledge about information technology hardware to assist in the development and adoption of appropriate information technology in public health.

Apply skills and knowledge about operating systems, software. and applications when developing or consulting on a public health information system.

Important competencies

Use resource management skills and knowledge to provide efficient support for public health information systems.

Apply skills and knowledge to develop software for unique public health needs.

Apply public health science theories, principles. and methods when developing and implementing information systems.

systems; and Domain III, information technology) are secondary. The critical competencies include project management skills, change management skills, planning and design skills, implementation and evaluation skills, and consultation skills. It is important to note that many of these critical competencies are related to general management skills, rather than to any specific knowledge of technology. In short, the experts viewed those higher-level skills as considerably more important for a public health informatician than the development of purely technical expertise. The important competencies for public health informaticians include the ability to exercise resource management skills and the ability to apply skills and knowledge in the development of software for unique public health needs.

This opinion strongly reinforces an underlying fact: Public health informaticians are the managers, designers, developers, implementers, and evaluators of public health information systems. They are not merely better database builders. Although databases are important to the practice of public health, the people who create and populate them are not necessarily engaged in informatics; rather, they are using information science and computer science skills and knowledge. Public health informaticians work at a considerably broader and more encompassing level, emphasizing overall management of the system. They have competencies in all four of the knowledge domains.

Providing Educational and Skill-Building Experiences for Public Health Practitioners and Informaticians

How can public health provide the educational and skill-building experiences that both public health informaticians and public health practitioners need? Clearly, public health informaticians and public health practitioners could obtain informatics education at schools of public health. However, for public health practitioners, it is impractical to leave full-time employment to enroll in a school or graduate program of public health. Public health management, however, can open other avenues of informatics training for practitioners. These avenues include continuing education programs and in-service courses.

Continuing Education Programs

The most effective method to reach public health practitioners in need of education in public health informatics is continuing education programs. Many schools and graduate programs in public health offer continuing education programs. These can take the form of evening courses at a school, courses taught by faculty at a public health work site, and even distance education courses. Delivery of these educational programs can be accomplished in a variety of ways. Such programs can take the form of regular college courses, short seminars, or nontraditional courses, including Web-based courses, teleconferences, or self-instructional media programs.

In any case, such programs and courses need to focus on the critical and important public health informatics skills and knowledge. They will also require organizational support and sponsorship from the organizations to which public health participants belong. Such sponsorship of education and training in public health informatics is critical if public health is to meet current and future challenges.

In-Service Courses

In-service courses are another way that public health organizations can meet the needs of public health practitioners for education and training in informatics. Such courses may be offered individually, focusing on specific topics related to critical and important competencies, or as part of a series. In larger public health organizations, an employee with advanced public health informatics knowledge and competencies could teach the courses. Such in-service courses could serve not only to develop an understanding of the principles of public health informatics, but they could also develop individuals who in turn can help co-workers to learn how to use and manage information systems and technology. The internal support network created by this sharing of knowledge may be invaluable for increasing the skill level of public health practitioners and the improvement of public health practice.

Schools and Graduate Programs of Public Health

In schools and graduate programs of public health, the differences in training between informaticians and public health practitioners can be expressed at three different levels: (1) introductory informatics training that every master of public health (MPH) or master of science in public health (MSPH) student receives prior to graduation; (2) advanced training for those who have a public health discipline, but want to increase their informatics skills and knowledge; and (3) informatician training that focuses on the all of the informatics competencies.

Introductory Training

At this level, the emphasis should be on an understanding of (1) what informatics is, (2) computer literacy, (3) information literacy, (4) basic information management, and (5) basic software programs.

Advanced Training

Advanced training would include some of the competencies, skills, and knowledge found to be critical and important for public health informaticians (see

Table 6.6). This level would emphasize the organizational and system management competencies in informatics. This training could not occur in the confines of one course. A series of courses would need to be developed to support this level of learning.

Informatician Training

Informatician training should be made available to MPH/MSPH students who want to pursue professional careers in public health informatics. Courses should focus on all the competencies and the skills and knowledge that are critical and important for public health informaticians. This level of training would need a series or track of courses specifically designed to produce competent public health informaticians.

Faculty

Who would teach these courses? Most graduate programs and schools of public health currently offering courses in public health informatics have only enough resources to offer an overview course or courses that cover only some of the needed competencies.[9] At this point in the development of the discipline, there are very few faculty who have the training and background in public health informatics to teach the courses needed for advanced training of public health informaticians. Partnerships with other disciplines, informatics professionals. or other public health schools or programs may be a solution to this problem.

Academic Residence

Where should this training for public health informaticians and advanced training for public health practitioners take place? One argument is that an informatician is first and foremost an informatician and is only secondarily a public health professional. According to this argument. public health informaticians should be trained in established health informatics programs. The supplemental public health theory and experiences could be acquired at a school or graduate program of public health. Until there is a cadre of faculty in public health who have the background to teach public health informatics in the work place, this model of academic residence may be the most realistic. For some graduate programs in public health with limited faculty and students, this may always be the realistic model.

The argument for housing the public health informatics track in the schools and graduate programs of public health is based on the idea that public health informatics is an integral component of public health. If public health activities truly are based on the use of information. it is especially important for public health faculty and students in schools and graduate programs of public health to have exposure to the models, theories, and activities of the faculty and students in the informatics department. Collaboration on research projects would push the innovative envelope for public health informatics. Furthermore. it would be an avenue to encourage other public health faculty and students to participate in public health informatics research.

Conclusion

The challenge facing public health informatics is educating the public health workforce in the knowledge domains that are the framework for public health informatics. This chapter is an initial step. It sets forth baseline, or broad, informatics competencies that public health practitioners and public health informaticians, respectively, need to possess. Efforts to further test and improve these competencies need to be made. Clearly, the experts think that public health practitioners should have, at a minimum. competency, or basic literacy, in computers, information. and technology. For public health informaticians, competency must include a host of management-related skills. not merely specialization in technology. These skills include project management skills and knowledge. change management skills and knowledge. and skills in planning, designing, and developing information systems.

The next step is to create educational experiences that are easily accessible for practitioners and informaticians. Public health schools and graduate programs, professional organizations, public health agencies, and private industry need to collaborate in developing educational programs that provide practitioners opportunities to increase their informatics skills without leaving their jobs. The academic experiences of MPH/MSPH students need to provide informatics competencies either through existing courses or the development of an informatics track. The experiences for the public health informatician could come from specialized tracks within schools and graduate programs of public health or from other sources.

For both groups. attaining and maintaining these skills is crucial if public health is to address future challenges. In addition. addressing these challenges will require the leadership in public health to recognize the need for these skills—indeed. for public health informatics—and to provide the necessary training for employees to acquire them.

Questions for Review

1. Explain why experts assert that the emphasis in public health informatics should be on methods, rather than on specific software applications or technology. Why isn't an understanding of software or technology enough?
2. The experts indicated that they thought management-related competencies

were important and critical to both practitioners and informaticians. In what sense can it be said that management skills are more important than technical skills in public health informatics?

3. Why are leadership and advocacy skills critical to public health practitioners in the area of public health informatics?

4. Briefly delineate the key differences between the critical informatics competencies for a public health practitioner and the critical informatics competencies for a public health informatician.

5. What benefit would public health practice derive from the inclusion of public health informatics in the established public health curriculum?

6. List and describe at least two possible methods that could be used to increase informatics competency in the public health workforce.

7. Differentiate among a) introductory training, b) advanced training, and c) informatician training in public health education. To which level should every public health professional be exposed?

References

1. Public Health Foundation. *Refining and Validating Public Health Competencies: A Proposal for Next Steps.* Washington, DC: Public Health Foundation; 1999.

2. International Medical Informatics Association. Recommendations of the International Medical Informatics Association (IMIA) on Education in Health and Medical Informatics. Available at: http://www.rzuser.uni-heidelberg.de/~d16/rec.pdf. Accessed December 2, 2000.

3. American Health Information Management Association. *Model Curriculum Project.* Chicago, IL: American Health Information Management Association; 1996.

4. Meyer GS, Potter A, Gary N. A national survey to define a new core curriculum to prepare physicians for managed care practice. *Acad Med* 1997:8:669–675.

5. Richards J. *Public Health Informatics: A Consensus on Core Competencies* [unpublished doctoral dissertation]. Austin, TX: The University of Texas; 2000.

6. Friede A, Blum HL, McDonald M. Public health informatics: how information-age technology can strengthen health. *Annu Rev Public Health* 1995;16:239–252.

7. Rees A. *Consumer Health USA: Essential Information from the Federal Health Network.* Phoenix AZ: Oryx Press; 1995.

8. Yasnoff WA, O'Carroll PW, Koo D, et al. Public health informatics: Improving and transforming public health in the information age. *J Public Health Manag Pract* 2000;6:67–75.

9. Richards J. *Informatics Training in Schools and Graduate Programs of Public Health* [unpublished masters thesis]. Houston, TX: The University of Texas–Houston, School of Public Health; 1998.

7
Assessing the Value of Information Systems

PETE KITCH AND WILLIAM A. YASNOFF

Learning Objectives

After studying this chapter, you should be able to:

- Explain why an information system project must begin with a thorough analysis of the business process the project is to support, and list four questions a project manager should ask in this analysis.
- Explain why the typical hierarchical organizational structure limits the understanding of business processes in an organization, and describe the nature of the additional parallel structure in a public health organization that further hinders process understanding.
- List the elements that a model for public health informatics should possess and the linkages that an information system should provide for federal, state, and local public health organizations.
- List the three options for selection of an information system project strategy, and describe the nature of the consideration that an information system project manager should give to each.
- Explain why a sound requirements definition for a new information system is crucial, and describe the steps that a project manager should take in developing the requirements definition.
- List and discuss seven questions that an information system project manager should be able to answer in applying creative thought to process reengineering.
- Explain why using the strategy of comparing a vendor's product to the organization's needs is superior to a strategy of comparing one vendor to another in evaluating vendor responses to a request for proposal.
- Identify the three goals associated with information systems effectiveness auditing and the work activities associated with each.
- List and describe the principles of effective cost estimating for an information system project, and explain why (1) preparing estimates for many elements is likely to produce a more accurate project cost estimate

than preparing estimates for only one or two elements, and (2) a project cost estimate becomes progressively more accurate as an information system project proceeds.

- Differentiate between direct and indirect benefits of an information system project, and list at least seven ways that an effectively developed and implemented information system can provide value to an organization other than monetary value.
- Discuss the principles involved in determining when an information system project is completed, and explain why effort and completion are not directly correlated for such a project.
- List and discuss five questions that an information system project manager can ask in determining the completeness status of stages in an information system project.

Overview

How does one go about managing an information system development project, and how can the value of such a project be assessed? This chapter provides some answers to this dual question. Effective information system project management begins with an assessment, and sometimes a reengineering, of the business process or processes that a new system will support. Effective project management also requires use of a comprehensive public health informatics model that recognizes an emphasis on business processes rather than on programs and employs both horizontal and vertical integration. Only after the process analysis and possible reengineering does a project manager choose a strategy for the project implementation.

Introduction

Information systems development in private industry has gone through a number of stages over the past 30 years. In many respects, the use of information systems in public health has traveled only about half that distance and lags behind other medical disciplines, as Patrick O'Carroll indicates in Chapter 1. True, public health uses modern hardware and communications technology extensively, but the application of informatics for the purpose of improving productivity and business practices is piecemeal and spotty at best. In contrast, private industry has used key discoveries in the application of information systems within business environments made in the late 1980s and popularized in academic and consulting circles in the 1990s. These discoveries, often marketed under the guise of business process analysis or reengineering, produced a wave of information system integration and expansion in private industry.

The principles derived from this private sector activity are also critical to the application of informatics in public health. Understanding these principles and how they apply to public health begins with an understanding of business processes and the need to analyze those processes carefully before undertaking an information system project. After all, as Marion Ball has pointed out in Chapter 3, the value of informatics is in part derived from the opportunity to examine and modify work processes.

In this chapter, we will define and discuss the nature of business processes in public health and the way in which organizational structure needs to support and reflect those processes in the development of a public health information system. We will next present an overall model for public health informatics. We will then proceed to discuss the nature and methodology of information system projects, including coverage of how to define requirements for such a project, how to reengineer processes as part of the project activity, how to evaluate and select vendors, the steps involved in development and implementation, and how to conduct post-auditing. After discussing cost estimation for an information system project, we will conclude the chapter with coverage of how to define the benefits to be derived from the project, how to assess the project's value, and how to establish a conceptual framework for management of information system project activities.

Business Processes

We begin with the definition of a business process. The term itself suggests a process that is in some way associated with a business activity, as opposed to some other framework, such as a chemical process. Within the context of a business framework, the published literature associated with the concept of business process reengineering has defined a business process in several ways:

- "A process is a structured, measured set of activities designed to produce a specified output for a particular customer or market. It implies a strong emphasis on how work is done within an organization, in contrast to a product focus's emphasis on what."[1]
- "A business process is a series of steps designed to produce a product or service. A process can be seen as a 'value chain.' By its contribution to the creation or delivery of a product or service, each step in a process should add value to the preceding steps. Processes are the way in which work gets done within organizations."[2]
- "A business process is a collection of activities that takes one or more kinds of inputs and creates an output that is of value to the customer."[3]

All these definitions are fairly consistent in terms of a basic definition, but each emphasizes a slightly different aspect because of the author's particular emphasis in defining business process reengineering or improvement. Davenport, for example, links reengineering to its roots in industrial engineering, thus emphasizing task flow and the analysis of work activities.[1] Rummler and Brache are also interested in task flow, but from the perspective of managing hand-offs from one organizational unit to another.[2] In fact, the subtitle of their book is *How to Manage the White Space on the Organization Chart.* Finally, Hammer and Champy emphasize the goal or result obtained from the performance of a business process.[3]

We believe that in its most basic and complete form, a *business process* can be defined as a collection of tasks that are performed for the purpose of achieving some specific set of business purposes or objectives. Each execution of the task set is triggered or initiated by one or more initiators that cause the set of tasks to be executed. Just as every kid has set dominos or blocks on end in a line, then knocked the first one over in such a way as to hit the next, setting off a chain reaction until all the dominos have tumbled, the initiator transaction(s) set in motion the execution of the tasks in the process until all have been performed and the business objective has been achieved. In essence, a business process can be defined by use of the diagram in Figure 7.1.

The diagram suggests that if we are to define a business process totally, there are four basic things we need to understand. They are encapsulated in the following questions:

1. *What are the tasks in the task set that defines the business process?* (shown as tasks 1 through N in Figure 7.1.) In this context, a task is defined as a continuous work activity that a single individual or a group can perform without interruption or without the need for additional inputs once the task has begun. In a sense, it is the equivalent of the activity that occurs between the "In" and "Out" baskets on a desk.

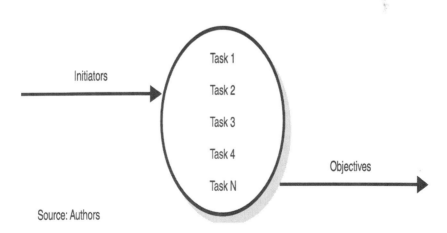

FIGURE 7.1. Defining a business process.

2. *How are the tasks related in execution?* In most business processes, the task set constitutes a network of activities with many parallel and branching paths. The relation of the tasks to one another is as important as the identification of the task set, inasmuch as the tasks are never simply performed as a random set of actions. In fact, the definition is incomplete if the objective is simply to identify the tasks involved. Further, for any single execution of the process, only a *subset* of the tasks may be required, depending on the characteristics of the initiator transactions. However, over the course of a large number of executions of the process, all the tasks will be performed in conjunction with at least one execution. In essence, if a task was never required to be executed in conjunction with one or more cases, it would not be a part of the given business process.
3. *How is the process initiated?* Each of the trigger mechanisms must be identified and defined in terms of the way in which they trigger the execution of the process defined.
4. *What is the goal/objective associated with the performance of the process?* In essence, the result of the last task to be performed constitutes a definition of the goal or objective of the process. If not, then there would have to be other, subsequent tasks to be performed to complete the work required under the definition of the process.

We must obtain answers to all four of these questions to have a full understanding of the business process to be supported by information systems technology. The absence of any of the four component answers will preclude a proper analysis and hinder subsequent attempts to support the work.

Assessment of Business Processes

In public health, it is common to use the Institute of Medicine's model of assessment, policy development, and assurance as a guide. It is important to note that how one goes about business process assessment is itself a business process. There are certain key initiators, a number of assessment tasks, and certain objectives the analysis should achieve. Generally, assessment is associated with having data available. In fact, the assumption is that the more data we have, the better the assessment. How do we know? Obviously, the process should be more than simply collecting and tabulating data.

But where and how do we find the answers to the questions we have presented? Are they readily evident in the way in which we traditionally think about organizations and the way in which work is accomplished? Private business has discovered that they in fact are not. In general, we in public health have not even asked the questions.

We must begin the exploration of process assessment with the topic of organizational structure, for business processes are tied to organizational structure.

Organizational Structure and Business Processes

Much has been written about the modern business organization and its origins. Basically, the management concept of *span of control*—focusing on the desirable number of subordinates that a superior can manage effectively—has caused organizations to evolve along vertical lines, with most organization charts looking like hierarchy diagrams branching from the top to the bottom. A typical organization chart highlights reporting structure and might look like Figure 7.2.

One can clearly see the "chain of command" associated with any position in the chart. A person holding a specific job within the organization can quickly determine the reporting structure. It follows that it is important for any manager to understand and oversee the work performed by the portion of the structure reporting to him. It is also important for that manager to understand something about the way in which work is done and the decisions that are made in the portion of the organization above him. For example, the individual occupying position A2 needs to be aware of the work processes and activities undertaken by positions A3, A4, and A5, who report to him. At the same time, position A2 needs to be concerned with the decisions made and the work performed by the person holding position A, to whom A2 reports. This kind of orientation automatically produces a specific focus within each distinct branch structure in an organization. Who is to the left or the right of you in the chart quickly becomes irrelevant; it is who is below and above that counts.

Such a hierarchical structure, then, is analogous to the use of blinders on a horse. Blinders were used on horses back in carriage days to prevent the horses from seeing what was to the left or right of them. These devices pre-

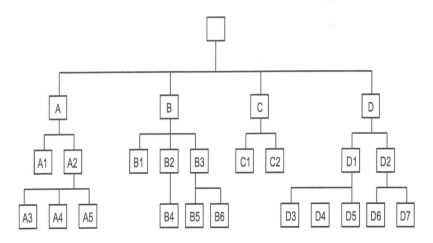

FIGURE 7.2. Reporting structure in a traditional organization chart.

vented the horses from being spooked or distracted by anything not immediately in front of them. It was the job of the carriage driver to see to the left or right of the path of travel. It was the horse's job to concentrate on pulling the carriage down the path indicated by the driver. The reins were the medium by which the directions for the course of travel were communicated to the horses as well as the mechanism by which the horses were controlled. A one-horse carriage required that a driver hold two reins. Add a horse, and the driver held two more reins. This reality set a practical limit on the number of horses one could use to pull a carriage or a wagon. Expert drivers could sort out eight pairs of reins in their hands and still send individual signals to each horse. But that became about the practical limit, or the maximum span of control. After that, adding horses became a liability, rather than an asset. Traditional organizational theory, concentrating on span of control, produces the same result, as illustrated by the following modification to the organization depicted in Figure 7.2. This modification is presented in Figure 7.3.

The vertical orientation produced by the concept of span of control naturally led to the evolution of horizontal "blinders," shown as walls in Figure 7.3. In this modified structure, it was not an individual's job to be concerned with what went on in command structures next to him, let alone to be concerned with activities of some remote corner of the organization. The individual was to concentrate instead on responding to the commands coming to him or her via the "reins" as these commands were passed down through the organization by the "drivers." who have the responsibility for looking out to the right and the left.[4] The horizontal "blinders." or barriers, are sometimes referred to as producing a "silo effect." Most silos, epitomized on the grand

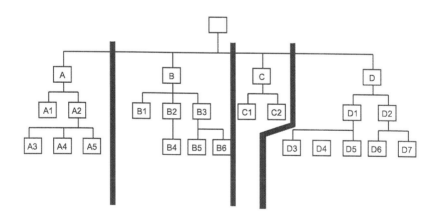

FIGURE 7.3. The evolution of horizontal "blinders" in the organizational structure: the silo effect.

scale by the giant grain elevators that dot the landscape in farming regions of the country, have thick, strong concrete walls in order to contain the high vertical pile of grain, where the weight of the pile produces tremendous outward pressure at the bottom. In Figure 7.3, these walls or barriers are represented by the vertical lines delimiting each major branch of the organizational structure. This organizational structure carries a distinct message regarding what is important. What is important is not what is going on in the neighboring department. Rather, the organizational structure effectively concentrates the energies and efforts of the occupants of each box by providing a vertical orientation. Obviously, there is merit in this orientation, just as there was merit in using blinders on a horse. There are, for example, fewer distractions, fewer opportunities to digress from the goals and direction of the organization, and fewer opportunities to panic or become overly concerned with something out of one's jurisdiction or beyond one's span of control.

Although this compartmentalized orientation is useful for controlling work, it tends to run counter to an employee acquiring a good understanding of how work actually gets done in the organization. This fact brings us back to the original issue regarding how the four questions posed in the definition of a business process can be answered within the context of an organization. Quite simply, understanding the relationship of work tasks associated with the achievement of goals and objectives for a given business process requires a horizontal, rather than a vertical, perspective. The reason is that the flow of work cuts across the vertical silos, requiring a radically different perspective for analyzing the flow of that work. Figure 7.4 illustrates the way that the work flow of a business process penetrates the silo walls.

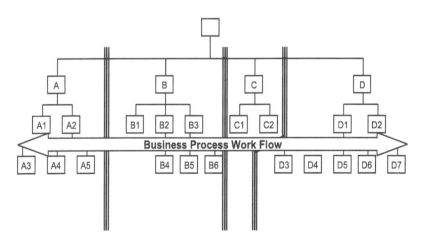

FIGURE 7.4. Business process work flow and the compartmentalized organizational structure.

Given that a business process is defined as a set of interrelated tasks performed in a specific sequence, and that these tasks are performed by a variety of entities within the organization, the typical organizational structure of a company mitigates against any given manager having a sound understanding of an entire business process, let alone control over it. In fact, because each manager has control over and a focus on only a subset of the process activities, the way in which a process evolves within an organization tends to have some distinct characteristics:

- Change in the process instituted by one participant may produce unexpected problems in other work tasks, inasmuch as the manager initiating the change likely has an imperfect view of the entire task set associated with the process. This fact practically prevents the natural occurrence of any sweeping modernization of a business process. Yet when managers associated with a business process get together and start developing a good framework and an understanding of the entire business process, we are always amazed at the number of suggestions for improvement that arise simply because these managers start to understand each other's area of responsibility. We are often tempted to ask the question "Don't you people ever talk to each other?"

- Second, and as a by-product of the first point, any natural evolution of a business process tends to be limited to independent efforts to improve performance within a given manager's span of control. This micro-optimization may make a single area of responsibility within the process more efficient, but often the same effort expended from a more global perspective produces considerably greater impact on the overall process. Traditionally, information systems development efforts have concentrated on meeting the needs of individual or small subsets of managers, and the systems have been built within their boundaries, thus creating systems to support portions of processes controlled by specific "user sponsors". Interestingly, the information engineering data modeling efforts of the 1980s was supposed to overcome this system isolation problem by modeling the data requirements for the whole organization before building any one particular component. However, the overconcentration on data rather than on business process modeling severely limited the effectiveness of these efforts. In fact, efforts now seem to have shifted to trying to create appropriate technology for tying these systems and their databases together in a cohesive manner. The data warehouse movement is at least partially fueled by this need. These topics, loosely knit together under the title of "integration," are very popular as we enter the 21st century.

- Third, within each manager's span of control, there is a tendency to add work to the process flow. One major reason for this phenomenon is that there is a tendency to overcompensate for any work errors or procedural omissions that occur in executing a process. For example, if someone makes a mistake and the research indicates that the mistake occurred because the particular situation was not well covered in the existing work procedures, the suggested remedial action inevitably includes the modification of an existing work task or the addition of one or more additional tasks to the work flow. Often, these recommendations focus on making sure the "expert" who, if consulted, would have realized that a mistake was being made now becomes a regular part of the review routing in the work flow. Thus, processes tend to expand like an overgrown bush, with occasional pruning done by one or more of the process managers. Further, if a task is eliminated from a process, one runs the risk that it was eliminated because of a lack of memory of the reason that the task was added in the first place, thus making managers less inclined to eliminate tasks. Finally, as the business rules change, certain tasks may become obsolete, but rarely are these tasks eliminated from the process as a natural by-product of the business rule change. Rather, the natural tendency is for processes to grow in complexity over time, instead of evolving naturally to fit the current, ever-changing business environment.

- Fourth, as a generalization of the third point, it seems that any time there is a doubt about the adequacy of the existing process task set, the tendency is to add more tasks until the doubt disappears.
- Fifth, most organizations do not have an effective mechanism for determining when a task is no longer required. Good managers will be able to identify irrelevant tasks in their own units when an organization is making major changes in the way work is done in an organization. However, such managers have jurisdiction over only their own units: their insight will not apply to analysis of tasks performed by other units.

Thus, business processes tend to be static, to become more complex over time, and to have no natural mechanism for remaining relevant to the way in which business should be conducted today. At some point, every task identified as a part of a business process made sense when it became a part of the definition of the process. In most cases, however, processes change over time, but the process change does not always result in task set change.

What does it mean that process flow occurs horizontally through an organization? In the literature of business process reengineering, one of the base criteria for identifying a process as a candidate for reengineering is that the process must involve multiple departments or organizational entities within the company. Further, many have estimated that the typical organization has no more than 30 or 40 business processes. In a recent study done for a major meat processing company, 13 business processes associated with the procurement, slaughter, processing, and sale of pork products were identified. All of these processes involved many departments within the organization. Typical order processing, for example, normally involves sales, customer service, accounting, credit, engineering, and manufacturing or inventory management. When one actually starts tracing the set of tasks associated with a business process through an organization, the horizontal orientation becomes obvious. Figure 7.5 illustrates the typical horizontal flow.

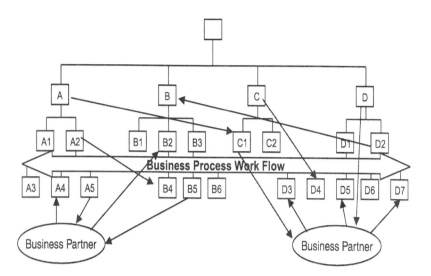

FIGURE 7.5. Typical horizontal work flow of a business process.

This is the same organization chart we have been using, with a mythical process flow overlaid on it. The arrows represent the "flow" of the process. We will define *flow* in more detail in a minute, but first note several relevant points that Figure 7.5 attempts to illustrate:

- First, there are organizational entities from all four major organizational structures involved in the illustration.
- Second, the flow will never be in a single direction, nor will it contain any logic as it relates to the organization chart. Primarily, this feature reflects the fact that organization charts are rarely constructed with process flow in mind.
- Third, in certain instances, there are multiple arrows pointing to and/or away from a given entity. One cannot make the assumption that all the work required to be done by a given entity will be done in a contiguous fashion. That is, the flow may visit the given entity numerous times, with intermediate work required elsewhere before the next segment of the work can be performed by the given entity.
- Finally, and most important, there are a number of arrows pointing beyond the limits of the organization chart and connecting the organization to a number of "business partners." A typical business process, if properly described, will contain tasks performed by organizations other than the one being examined. We refer to these participants in the business process as external entities. During the performance of a process, there may be multiple points at which these external entities play an important role. For example, customers initiate most customer-facing processes (a customer is

an external entity), and the achievement of the goals or objectives of such processes normally requires an interaction with the customer as the final step in the process work flow. In addition, many other interactions with the customer occur between the initiation and the completion of a process.

Business Processes and Public Health

The organizational structure of public health is remarkably similar to the vertical organizational structure of private business. Simply replace the word *department* with *program*. Figure 7.6 depicts the typical organizational structure of a public health department.

As a result of a rigid enforcement of the silo effect, many health departments today cannot even calculate the number of unduplicated clients being served. Instead, it is much easier to get a simple count of participants in each program. Employees become even more uncomfortable when a discussion turns to outcome analysis. Does participation in prenatal care *and* WIC (Women, Infants and Children program) produce better birth outcomes than participation in one or the other program? It should, but the statistical data to prove it is hard to come by, for obvious reasons. Ideally, the business process should be defined to include all aspects of improving birth outcomes, and the various program activities should be viewed as an integrated whole. The rigidity of the silo walls, however, helps make such a comprehensive view difficult.

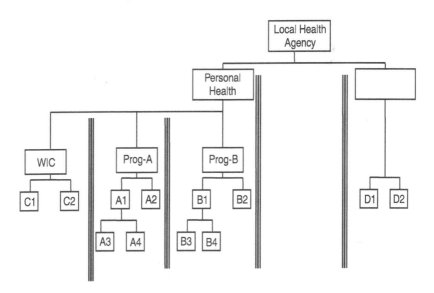

FIGURE 7.6. Typical organizational structure of a public health department.

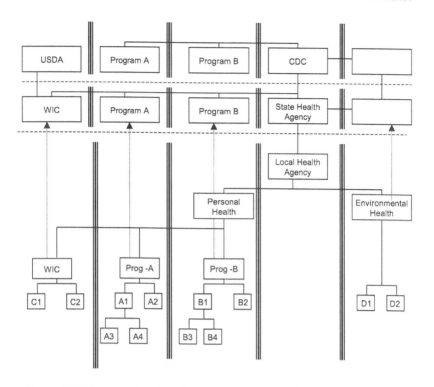

FIGURE 7.7. Hierarchical and parallel structures in the public health organization.

The situation is even worse in public health than in private business because of the overall organizational structure of public health in the United States. The silos do not stop at the health department level. Rather, Figure 7.7 reflects another public health reality.

In private industry, the three levels roughly equate to plant, division, and corporate, rather than local, state, and federal (mainly the Centers for Disease Control and Prevention [CDC]). In addition, there is a "parallel" structure across the three layers in public health that does not generally exist in private industry. There are program offices (or their equivalents) at each level in the structure. Thus, there are essentially two lines of authority. For example, not only does the WIC director at the local level report to the local department director, but he or she also has to be accountable to the WIC program office at the state level, and to a certain extent to US Department of Agriculture. Thus, it is no wonder that this structure (reflecting programmatic funding) tends to produce programmatic-oriented information systems. In most instances, these software products reflect the need for reporting up through the structure. They rarely reflect the business process needs at the local level within individual silos, let alone begin to address the needs of a horizontal, or client-centered, perspective.

This analysis is not intended to place blame. However, it is obvious that programmatic funding from Congress has produced an orientation toward programmatic organizational structure in public health. Thus, WIC information systems tend to be separate from public health program systems because of differences in funding sources, not because they deal with distinctly different client populations (there is at least a 70% overlap, in our opinion).

An Overall Model for Public Health Informatics

A simple analysis of the nature of the current public health organizational structure and the nature of public health business processes leads to the conclusion that an overall conceptual framework for public health informatics should include the following elements:

1. Emphasis on business processes rather than programs
2. Horizontal integration across program boundaries
3. Vertical integration across local, state, and CDC levels, so that the system applications recognize and account for the differences in business process tasks performed at each level
4. Recognition of the need for standardized data exchange between the local and state layers, and between state and CDC layers

In Kansas, these framework elements have led to the conceptual model for the development of public health information systems shown in Figure 7.8.

The recently developed CDC model structure is similar. In the Kansas model, the blank building blocks recognize the fact that at this point (as of mid-2002), we do not even know the names of all the items that ought to be included, let alone the definitions of all the business processes involved in public health. Still, these models are useful as a framework within which to make individual information system project decisions.

The Turning Point Collaborative on Excellence in Information Systems, a project started in mid-2000, is pursuing another way of conceptualizing public health information system needs. Over the next two years, the collaborative is hoping to develop a three-dimension application matrix by use of the structure appearing as Figure 7.9.

The work of the collaborative is intended to identify the set of information system applications required to support (1) public health business processes (the application framework), (2) associated ideal data architecture models, and (3) existing systems that meet best-practice criteria associated with the data architectures and application framework. In private business, these relationships are fairly well known for any industry, and a full set of applications exists. In public health, we do not even know which pieces exist today, let alone understand which pieces are missing. However, from a public health informatics practice standpoint, it is useful to think of any application in terms of these three dimensions.

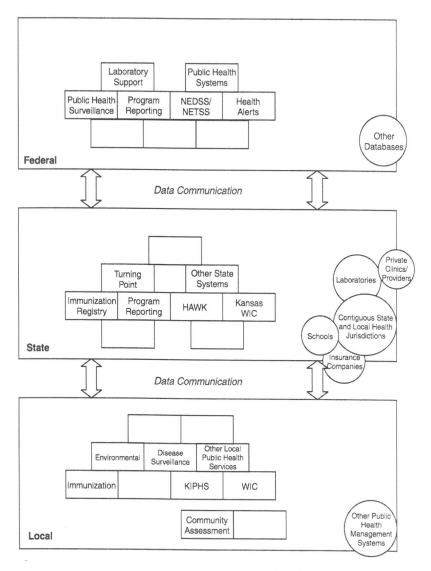

FIGURE 7.8. The Kansas Conceptual Model for public health information systems.

With these principles and conceptual frameworks in mind, we are now in a better position to start a more specific discussion of information system projects.

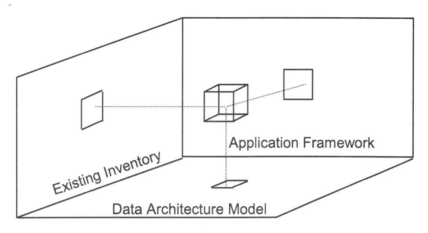

FIGURE 7.9. The three-dimensional application matrix of the Turning Point Collaborative on Excellence in Information Systems. (*Source:* Adapted from Turning Point Infotech Collaborative.)

Strategies for Information System Projects

Although we have talked a great deal already about information systems, we have not yet introduced the topic of information system projects. However, it should be readily evident by now that an information system project is undertaken to provide support for a business process. Often, people believe that the information system is itself the end objective. In fact, it is never more than a support mechanism. Thus, information system projects should be defined as efforts to enhance the support of task performance within a business process. Another way of stating it is that the organization will be better equipped to meet the given business process's goals and objectives and perform the process tasks more efficiently due to the new information system support mechanism.

In this context, enhanced support of business process tasks can be defined in three general categories. First, and most common, the project is undertaken to replace outdated information system support. Second, it can be initiated to expand and/or upgrade an existing support system. Such expansion or upgrading is normally achieved through the purchase of additional modules in a vendor-supplied system, or through in-house or contractor development of custom code. Third, support of business process tasks through information system projects can occur in situations in which no current information system technology support is utilized in association with an existing or proposed business process or task set. Projects in each of the three categories have different characteristics and management concerns that will be discussed later.

In addition to direct task support, an information system project should include consideration of the associated communication layer or layers as depicted on the Kansas conceptual model. If at the CDC level, the system should include consideration of the communication layer between CDC and the state level. If at the state level, both the local–state and the state–CDC communication layers should be considered. If at the local level, the project must include the communication layer with the state. This segment of the project must address the need for moving data sets up or down in a standardized format and within a Health Insurance Portability and Accountability Act (HIPAA)-compliant manner. As John Christiansen has pointed out in Chapter 4, the final regulation for HIPAA applies to all levels of public health practice, making compliance with HIPAA in the movement of data critical. In general, it should be CDC's responsibility to create the standardized formats for data communication.[5]

There are three distinct strategies that can be employed for an information system project. The primary decision is whether to purchase an existing software package or to develop the application internally. This is generally described as the "build/buy decision." Within the context of this decision, there are several strategies that can be employed. The specific strategy choice depends on the organization's resources and capabilities in the area of information system development and implementation. Organizations with low skill levels may be forced to purchase an existing software package or contract out all the work, whereas organizations with high resource and capability levels may choose to perform all project activities in house. Even in these situations, the organization may choose to contract for some or all of the project activities. These strategies are reflected in the flowchart shown in Figure 7.10.

The two decision boxes denote the three basic options. The first major break is determining whether to build the system with internal information system development resources (or contractors) or to buy an existing system in the commercial marketplace. Building the system with existing resources is often called creation of a "custom" system. In many senses, this option is parallel to hiring a mechanic to build a car to one's exact specifications, rather than buying a commercially manufactured model from one of many automobile dealers. Certain consequences follow from this decision. First, it may be difficult in the future to find a mechanic to repair or modify the car if the mechanic hired to build it is not around any more. Finding the willing mechanic, however, is not the only potential consequence. An owner may be very dissatisfied with the cost associated with the repairs. In the same way, custom code generally costs more to create and maintain than purchasing a commercial software product. Second, there is no way to determine whether the car really meets the prospective owner's needs until after it is built. If it does not meet those needs, then the owner must start modifying it. Custom software projects often suffer significant cost overruns for the same reason.

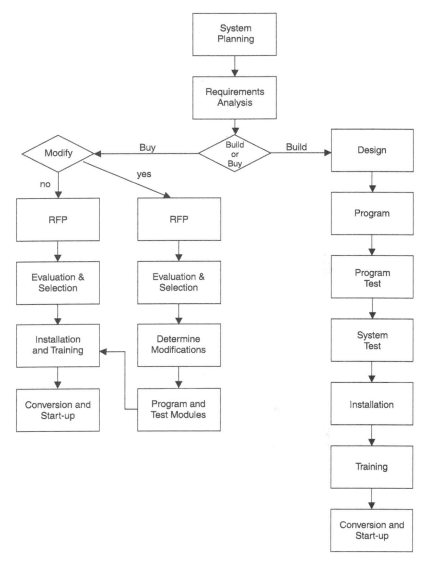

Figure 7.10. Flowchart of alternative strategies for an information system project.

With a negotiated purchase of a commercial software product, it is possible to determine the estimated total cost of a project much more accurately.

The second decision box is a subset of the decision to purchase. The two options are (a) installing the system as is without any modification, and (b) having the vendor modify or expand the package to include more of the buyer's requirements. The purchased product may not meet all desirable specifications. If the vendor is willing, one can choose to have the commercial product modified, a process that generally results in a customized system once it is installed, even if the vendor provides the modifications. Such modifications will, of course, cost more than simply purchasing the existing product, unless the buyer can convince the vendor that inclusion of the additional requirements would make the product much better. In the latter case, the modifications would become part of the vendor's offering, and the buyer is not stuck with a custom system that will cost more to maintain. If the buyer modifies the system, the buyer can forget any vendor warranties or help. Further, the buyer will likely be unable to load vendor upgrades and enhancements. In other words, the buyer will have converted to a build strategy for the remainder of the life of the system.

A decision-maker should always explore the buy options first, even if the decision-maker has access to information system development expertise within the organization. However, exploration of the buy options may result in the conclusion that there are no appropriate solutions meeting the requirements definition in the marketplace. At that point, the only option will be to build the support. If so, the decision maker needs to determine whether any other public health entity has built a system for support of a similar business process. If the decision maker finds any custom solutions, then he or she needs to conduct what is commonly called in the private sector "industrial tourism" by visiting one or more sites before starting the project, taking along technical people to gather information on how to design the system based on the other organization's experience.

Specific System Development Project Steps

Making the buy, build, or buy/modify choice affects the project content, tasks, cost estimating, and management. However, the general project steps must be performed regardless of the chosen implementation strategy. Each of the activities are described below.

System Planning

The term *system planning* simply relates to the process by which a manager decides to undertake a given information system project. Obviously, one wants to make the decision based on assessment of need and benefit, as well as the estimated cost. At the same time, one needs to minimize the amount of work expended (i.e., cost incurred) defining the project before the decision has been made as to whether or not to do the project. In many instances, elements of the cost/benefit analysis discussed later in this chapter are used in the planning process.

Requirements Definition

Defining the requirements for a new system is the most important step in any information system project. The reasons are many, but the key lies in the fact that any information system project is basically an analytical process: if you don't get the requirements correctly defined, the resultant system will not meet your needs. Systems analysis work is really not much different from many other disciplines involving analysis. Are you good at working jigsaw puzzles? We are convinced that good strategies for working jigsaw puzzles are similar to good strategies for definition and design of business application systems requirements. Both have to do with building logical frameworks that then lead an analyst through the rest of the process. Developing a requirements definition is best done through a process similar to that used to put a jigsaw puzzle together. How do you solve a jigsaw puzzle? If you think about it awhile, you will discover that there is an almost universally accepted way of approaching the problem. In general, the process is broken out into the following sequential steps:

1. Sort out all the pieces with straight edges
2. Find the four corner pieces
3. Working out from the corners, assemble the outer edge of the puzzle
4. Look at the picture of the puzzle on the box cover (unless you are an expert and are convinced that technique is cheating) and gather pieces relating to some theme or color near the edge of the puzzle
5. Assemble the gathered pieces into subassemblies
6. Connect the subassemblies to the outer framework
7. Repeat steps 4 through 6 until the puzzle is completely filled in and no pieces remain

The analytical process here is one of building a framework and then progressively filling in the details. The edge pieces define the boundary or limit of the puzzle. Once that boundary is established, all the remaining pieces fit *within* this boundary, and the interior pieces are grouped into subsets for further analysis. Compare this to simply picking up a piece at a time and looking for one that connects to it. Which approach is better?

Good approaches to systems design do the same thing. They set a boundary, subset the problem, and solve each problem subset until the design is completed. A requirements definition should define the business process to be supported by the proposed information system project (the framework). This definition should include the identification of the tasks associated with the business process. From this information, the way in which the information system will support the performance of the task can be defined. Normally, the way in which the system will support each task is defined as the data set (screen, report, etc.) required by the user to perform the task. In essence, a requirements definition establishes the framework or boundary for the project. All the subsequent project activities are associated with "filling in the pieces" inside the boundaries. Each subsequent step in the project should be formulated according to the requirements definition and the strategy (buy, build, buy/modify) chosen for the project.

Obviously, a key objective of the requirements definition process is the delineation of the project scope. Traditionally, scope has been difficult to establish, or constrain, because projects tend to grow and expand during the development process. Because of this phenomenon, a requirements definition should specifically address the issue of scope. Delineating the scope of a project is not a single activity, but a progression of activities that define and refine the project scope. It starts with a broad definition, but that definition tightens as the requirements definition unfolds.

In essence, the first, broad scope statement is embodied in the problem statement developed as a part of the project proposal in system planning. This "loose-bounded" scope implies that project activities and resultant system development efforts will have an identifiable relationship with the problem statement.

The next activity in defining the scope of the project limits the project boundary to the business process tasks delineated as candidates for system support.

Finally, the identification of the output set required to support the specified business process tasks within the user domain sets the scope in terms of system capability. If this scope is too large to handle within the context of a single project, it can be segmented into logical phases that will lead to further reduction in scope—down to one or more of the phases delineated.

Thus, by the time the requirements definition is complete, the system scope will be specifically delineated. It will be stated in terms of the system capability to be designed, programmed, and implemented. Later in this chapter, we will argue that benefit is determined by the impact of the output set on the business process involved. Thus, the activity undertaken to define the scope in a requirements definition aligns with the determination of cost/benefit and is critical for the management of data processing system development activities.

A project manager may have also thought of better ways to organize the work while working through the requirements definition. Such thinking constitutes business process engineering. Just how should the organization achieve the process objectives? Why and how should the new set of business tasks be different from those currently performed? Development of the new vision is a creative process. How one engages in this creative process is the subject of a divergence of expert opinion.

For example, Thomas Davenport, in his book *Process Innovation,*[6] cites the need for a "clean slate" as the starting point in the creative process and emphasizes the use of brainstorming techniques as an effective means of surfacing creative process designs.

Mike Hammer correctly points out that "at the heart of reengineering is the notion of discontinuous thinking—of recognizing and breaking away from the outdated rules and fundamental assumptions that underlie operations."[7] He has postulated a number of principles that can be applied to the creative process of reengineering. Each of these principles is based on insights into how the current task set evolved within the organization over time. Application of Hammer's principles can lead to improvement in the required tasks. For example, applying his principle of capturing information only once and at its source leads to the elimination of tasks associated with the manual recording of the data and later capture of the data in the company's database. These tasks would be replaced by immediate data capture and the elimination of the paperwork previously required. However, application of design principles generally leads to streamlining the process tasks, rather than a radical change in the definition of the way in which the process objectives are achieved. Streamlining existing processes can be a useful result, but it falls short of the real potential of reengineering. Our experience indicates that one can take an even more formal approach that helps trigger the formulation of creative ideas and process task alternatives.

The core issue involved in process reengineering is whether one can stimulate and direct the creative thinking process. After all, to start with a blank slate in a brainstorming environment provides little framework for directing the effort towards a *feasible* creative solution, and it provides very little stimulus for creative thinking. Exceptionally creative people might succeed in this environment, but people generally have been frustrated in blank-slate sessions, either because they lack creativity or because they dislike the lack of a specific structure or framework in which to work.

On the other hand, too much structure will prevent radical solutions from evolving. Examination of existing task sets within the context of design rules can have the effect of channeling the effort into streamlining an existing environment, producing incremental improvement instead of radical change.

Most task sets used in business environments have evolved over time to meet the needs of the organization. Often, the specific tasks were never intentionally designed; rather, they were defined within the boundaries of an existing paradigm or within principles stating the way in which the process objective(s) ought to be achieved. For example, in a famous Ford Motor Company accounts payable example, the task set was constructed around the generally accepted principle that payment would be made after receipt of an invoice. The principle underlying the process had a great deal to do with the way in which the task set evolved over the years at Ford. The new vision in this case, on the other hand, replaced the underlying principle with a new one: Payment will be made after receipt of the goods. As a result, the task set required to support the process objective of payment changed dramatically.

We believe that a different reengineering strategy from either a blank slate or the application of design principles can unlock the door to a new vision. In essence, understanding the way in which the current task set achieves the process objective(s) is the starting point for discovery of a new vision. In this way, one can use the knowledge gained to identify the underlying paradigms or principles that controlled the development of the task set and the relationship of each task to another. The problem with past methods of approaching reengineering has been that underlying paradigms or principles consist of accepted models of how to perform specific functions, structural constraints that prevented or forced the task set to evolve the way it did, and standard accepted principles regarding the way in which business should be conducted. Many of these paradigms, principles, and structural restraints are no longer valid in a modern business environment as a result of the intrusion of information systems technology. Examining these potential roadblocks to creative thinking is a necessary first step in reengineering processes. Once these underlying forces have been identified, the reengineering team can examine each one for validity in the current environment.

For example, in a paper-based environment, the document being processed was in essence a database, and each task basically added new information that was required in order for a subsequent task to be performed. Further, only one task could normally be performed at a time, because the database was integrated with the document being processed (it was contained on it.) Thus, it was natural to perform the task set in sequence. Once the sequential nature of such a process is recognized, the need for it can be challenged in a world where on-line, interactive information systems provide a new definition of the database as well as of the term *document*. It is in this sense that information systems technology becomes a key enabler of business process reengineering.

But what kinds of questions will lead to the identification of the underlying paradigms, principles, and structural restraints driving the current task set? We have developed a set of questions that represent perspectives, or angles, with which to examine the current task set for the purpose of identifying the underlying factors driving the organization of the task set. These perspectives are, in essence, keys that unlock the door to a new vision. They lead to a challenge of the underlying factors and set in place a framework for exploring alternative models for the achievement of the process objectives. Rather than leading to a reorganizing or streamlining of the task set (which would not be all bad), they lead to an opportunity for controlled, directed creativity in process reengineering.

We have found it useful to ask a series of seven questions about the tasks in the current environment as a means of identifying the underlying factors driving the organization of the work. These questions represent perspectives with which to evaluate the task set. Many of them relate directly to basic work design principles but are asked for the purpose of understanding the driving factors behind the organization of the work. Once identified, each of these factors can be challenged as to their validity. New visions evolve from the exploration of replacement paradigms, principles, and structural restraints. In many cases, the new vision is feasible only because of the application of current information systems technology. In this sense, information systems technology is a key enabler in the reengineering process. A brief discussion of each question follows:

1. *Can other subsequent tasks be performed parallel to this one?* This question is designed to attack the rationale behind sequential processing. In most

environments modeled after a manual processing flow, the work is strung out sequentially because of the need to pass the manual file information from one location to another. Parallel processing based on subsets of the required data (either through copying or providing the needed subset data via the information system support) can lead to the creation of a new paradigm that radically decreases the overall processing time.

2. *Why can't unconnected tasks performed by the same department be grouped into a single task—what causes them to be separate?* Many times, for the purpose of work task verification, management control, and work task specialization, logical units of work are broken into multiple separate tasks. This question encourages a perspective that challenges the need for work segmentation in a modern work environment.

3. *Why is a given task required?* Can it be combined with another task? Why is it done this way? Many tasks may continue to be performed long after their reason for existing has disappeared. They once contributed to the achievement of one or more process objectives but are no longer relevant because of other changes in the way in which the objectives are being achieved. Further, each task should always be examined to determine whether the task structure is based on old, inefficient assumptions regarding how the work must be performed. Many of these assumptions, discovered within the context of a single task, will explain a great deal about the overall organization of the work and create challenge opportunities.

4. *Why can't the task be automated? Why must this task be performed manually?* Often, tasks are still performed manually because the tasks providing input into the task are performed manually. Supporting previous tasks through the computer system may make it feasible to automate a subsequent activity, because the required data has now been captured as a by-product of the support provided to a prior task. Further, changes in technology may now invalidate previous assumptions about the economic feasibility associated with computer support.

5. *Could the task be performed in a different sequence, given current information systems technology?* Current capabilities of technology may invalidate prior assumptions regarding the sequence in which work must be performed. Many times, tasks are placed later in a sequential flow in order to minimize the number of times rework is required, or because the task takes too long to perform earlier in the task sequence.

6. *Could a group of individual tasks be combined as a single task?* Again, this question attacks prior assumptions regarding the logical content of individual work tasks. Are the prior assumptions still valid, or would grouping tasks into a single work activity produce processing economies or work enrichment?

7. *Does everything have to be processed in the same manner?* In many old task environments, everything was processed through an environment in the same way, because the group performing each task had to see every item to determine whether action was required. Even if only 10% of the

items required a performance of a given task, every item had to be passed through the group to identify the subset requiring action. This question suggests the possibility of creating multiple processing paths, each tailored to the specific needs of a unique subset of the items. The information system support can perform the logic checks required and route items to a particular task area only if action is required.

Although applied to individual tasks, these questions are designed to explore the underlying factors controlling the way in which the process objectives themselves are achieved within the business environment. Once discovered, these factors can be challenged and replaced with new paradigms that represent the heart of a new vision. The understanding of the controlling factors provides a springboard for the creative process. Why do we still do it this way? What are the operative factors in the current environment? What new controlling factors should be substituted for the old? These questions lead to the discovery of new and exciting visions for the way in which the work can be performed. Once a vision has been formed, however, the supporting work environment must still be designed, tested, and implemented.

The Request for Proposal and the Evaluation and Selection Processes

Why is a requirements definition relevant for all strategies, rather than just the build strategy? Private industry discovered that if an organization is going to purchase, rather than build, the system support, there are only two basic strategies in selecting a product. First, the request for proposal (RFP) can be based on comparing one vendor to another, along with a comparison of the products. Second, the RFP can be based on comparing a vendor's product with the organization's needs, as delineated by the requirements definition. Companies that chose the first strategy often found that when they tried to implement the selected product, it really did not meet their specific requirements. Those choosing the second strategy were able to hold the vendor responsible for meeting all the company requirements stated in the RFP. In essence, trying to select a product based on external comparisons rather than on the organization's own requirements is the best way to set a project up for failure.

Thus, the RFP process should reflect the system requirements stated in the requirements definition document. Of course, that document can add all the usual specifications about vendor stability, client references, pricing, etc., but the key to effective evaluation and selection of bids must be the degree to which the vendor's bid meets the organization's needs.

The Remainder of the Project Steps

If a project manager has chosen to build an information system, the systems group or contractor should be able to describe the methodology to be used for the design, program, program test, system test, installation, conversion, and training stages of the project. This information should be in writing, and the approach to project management should be built around it. One reason for getting deliverables in writing is that many vendors use an impressive-looking methodology when they begin a project; later, the project often degenerates into chaos when a vendor gets into difficulty. The project manager and the vendor should be able to agree on "deliverables" from each step of the methodology. The project manager should get samples of each and hold the vendor accountable for actually producing complete sets of deliverables for every step of the process. These methodology steps are generally known as "phases" in information systems parlance, and ideally they should be linked to a concept of phase-limited commitment that will be described in the cost discussion later in this chapter.

Design is the stage that involves translating the requirements definition into program specifications. This translation should include detailed mockups of each screen and report, as well as specification of the system navigation (the ways in which a user can move from one screen to another). In addition, this phase includes the specification for any hardware and network requirements, as well as the deployment configuration or architecture (Web-based, client-server, local-area network [LAN], wide-area network [WAN], etc.). However, designers should not be permitted get carried away in trying to design the perfect system. After all, only implemented systems are of use to the organization; a great design never implemented is worse than no design at all! These comments apply to the *determine modifications* phase in the *buy and modify* strategy flowchart as well.

Programming, program test, system test, and *installation* work should all be done in accordance with the methodology agreed upon with the contractor or information services staff. There are a number of different, equally valid strategies for performing these phases. The key for the project manager is understanding the approach selected, and then making sure it is followed throughout the project.

In an information system project, it is impossible to overestimate the need for *training*. Initial training must be carefully worked out and provided. Depending upon the complexity of the system being installed, it may be necessary to relieve the users from their regular responsibilities in order to concentrate on learning the new system. It is also necessary to give careful attention to help-desk support. In many organizations, informal networks of "super users" evolve that help others gain proficiency in a system. Regardless of the training delivery method to be used, a project manager should make sure that the vendor or information system staff has worked out a thorough training program.

Finally, *conversion* and *start-up* must be carefully planned. Conversion from an old system to the new system may be a major undertaking. A project manager should push for trial conversions, whereby the data can be verified for accuracy against the output of the existing system. Many people stress the need for parallel operation of the old and new systems. This activity, however, places considerable strain on the organization, because it essentially means doubling the workload. As information systems support becomes more comprehensive and complex, parallel operation becomes more difficult. When pressed to perform parallel operation, a project manager should try to suggest installing the new system in a single department or group before organization-wide roll out as an alternate option.

Project Post-Auditing

The typical system user employs only a fraction of the functionality of a system, and, in fact, usually attempts to perform new tasks within the context of the subset with which he or she is already familiar. The reason lies in human nature. Most of us prefer the familiar to the unknown. We will take the familiar, longer route of travel in lieu of the new "shortcut." We convince ourselves that we don't have time right now to learn the "shortcut," but will certainly try it out sometime in the future. For most of us, the future never arrives. With information system usage, familiarity leads to essentially exclusive use of a subset of the available functionality. Familiarity and comfort are linked. Usage reinforces itself in that people will go out of their way to solve new problems within the context of what they already know. In fact, even when shown that there is a better, easier way, they will persist in using the familiar path unless there is considerable reinforcement of the new way.

This human tendency to stay with the familiar and the comfortable can be illustrated by a simple example. Think of the word processing software you use. Do you use all the functionality? Have you reached a level of proficiency (comfort) where you can "figure out" how to do almost any task within the portion of the software functionality you understand? Would you intentionally look for a new way to do some task? If you answered no–yes–no to these three questions, you are in the majority.

The same tendency exists with regard to using a newly installed system, and it runs counter to the opportunity that a system presents for deriving greater productivity from a system at very low cost. In other words, even though the project is "completed," there is still the need to make sure it is being utilized properly. The following paragraphs outline an analytical approach to increasing system utilization and efficiency. We have coined the term *information systems effectiveness auditing* to describe this process.

Information Systems Effectiveness Auditing

There are three goals associated with information systems effectiveness auditing. These goals are to:

1. Identify changes in procedures, system usage, and user job tasks (descriptions) that will produce incremental productivity gains and match the intent of the initial project, particularly if the users have reverted to old ways.
2. Evaluate the overall system usage to identify (a) potential changes in system functionality provided (available to) specific users, (b) additional training needs, and (c) requirements for increased system access within the user environment.
3. Assure optimal usage of existing information system technology as a prerequisite to introduction of new technology into the operational environment.

Accomplishing these objectives requires the following three major work activities:

1. Evaluate the extent to which the information systems technology supports users in the accomplishment of their various tasks and responsibilities. This work activity will:
   a. Evaluate the degree to which the system outputs are integrated into the tasks rather than simply overlaid on them
   b. Evaluate the extent to which secondary actions are required to make system outputs useful to the users—the extent to which the user must "recast" the data outside the system in order to make it useful
   c. Evaluate the appropriateness of system functionality available to each user
2. Determine the efficiency with which the system is being used. Tasks within this work activity include:
   a. Evaluating the general level of user proficiency
   b. Evaluating data input efficiency and accuracy
   c. Evaluating the adequacy of hardware (terminals and printers) available to the users
3. Determine the extent to which the system supports the entire spectrum of user activity. This is an evaluation of the system's breadth in relation to the user environment and the need for functional support. This work activity will include:
   a. Determining whether the system supports all tasks that could reasonable be supported by the information systems technology
   b. Determining whether the system provides cohesive, integrated usage across the spectrum of user activities
   c. Evaluating the degree of dependence on system files. Have users adopted the computer records as the official record, or do they continue to maintain other files outside the system?

Even a nonprofessional can often come up with some very good ideas about how to further enhance the value of information system support to the organization. In essence, the old adage that "if all you have is a hammer, then everything starts to look like a nail" is true. In information systems, the parallel is that users may try to continue to do their tasks the same way they always did them and will be very creative at forcing the new system to support old habits.

Cost Estimating

As Marion Ball points out in Chapter 3, the value of information technology is a function of service, quality, and cost. In this section, we will also point out that value is possible even if the benefit of a system cannot be quantified.

An information system should add value to the organization, but determining that value is difficult. The assessment of an information system's value begins with the topic of cost. Obviously, it is impossible to know the exact cost of a system until the development project is completed and all the bills are paid. Even purchasing an existing system may result in an initial cost estimate that is considerably lower than the final cost, because potential modifications and other factors may drive the final cost up.

Much as initial estimates for building a house are likely to prove inaccurate by the time construction is completed, the actual cost of an information system project at the proposal stage cannot be estimated with certainty. The first estimate is likely to vary from the actual cost by as much as plus or minus 40%. Usually, a project manager must base the initial estimate on some set of macro parameters, because there is not enough information about the actual work required to make a closer estimate. Thus, at the project proposal stage, a project estimate of $100 really means that the actual cost will probably be in the range of $60 to $140. Because of the potential for the actual cost to vary so much, it is a major mistake to interpret the estimate as an actual, specific cost; in such a case, the actual cost may turn out to be $140, and management will interpret that cost as an "overrun," when in actuality it may have been a tremendous bargain for the results produced. A good project manager will add a "contingency" to the base estimate in order to position the estimate closer to the $140 cost. The contingency should be visible, rather than buried in the estimate; in other words, the base estimate should include a $40 contingency as a line item in the estimate, rather than merely stating the estimate as $140. In this way, a project manager will be able to alert others to the fact that the initial estimate cannot possibly have a high degree of accuracy.

In addition, a project manager should prepare estimates by aggregating estimates for specific elements of the project. After all, probability theory suggests that an estimate prepared from 10 factors, each of which might have a plus or minus range of 40%, will have greater overall accuracy than an estimate prepared from two factors with the same accuracy range, simply because overestimates in some factors are likely to be offset by underestimates in other factors. The more factors used, the higher the probability that the aggregate estimate will be more accurate than the accuracy associated with each factor. Further on in this section, we will present a "template" that should be helpful in identifying the factors to use in the preparation of an information system project's cost estimate.

The estimate should also be updated after completion of each phase of an information system project. As the project progresses, the estimate will become more concrete. There will be fewer and fewer unknowns. For example, after 50% of the project work is completed, a project manager will know 50% of the actual cost. In fact, once even the requirements definition phase is completed, the accuracy of the estimate should increase dramatically. In some situations, in fact, it is a good strategy to fund the requirements definition phase separate from the overall project. In other words, the organization should make a "phase-limited" commitment to expend the necessary money to complete the requirements definition and only then make the project funding decision on the basis of the estimate prepared as a part of the requirements definition final report. We have seen organizations fund the requirements definition work as an overhead cost center, thus eliminating it as a project cost. In such a case, project budgets are prepared on the basis of the requirements definition results. A summary of these estimation guidelines for more accurate cost estimations for information system projects follows:

1. Use and state as a separate item a contingency figure that explicitly recognizes that an estimate can vary as much as plus or minus 40%.
2. The project cost estimate should be an aggregate of estimates for specific elements of the project, each explicitly stating a contingency figure.
3. The greater the number of project element cost estimates included in the total project cost estimate, the greater the likelihood that the project cost estimate will be accurate.
4. Update the project cost estimate after completion of each stage of the information system project. Recognize that as project completion progresses, the cost estimate for the project will become increasingly more reliable.

Managing the cost estimate is one of the key project management activities. It consists of looking forward from the present to modify or impact incomplete activities as necessary. Such a forward look may mean seeking alternative solutions for implementation tasks according to current knowledge of the project details, reducing system scope, or utilizing a portion of the contingency fund to cover unavoidable cost overruns on specific activities or changes.

Key estimate elements must align with the proposed project phases from requirements definition to implementation. The buy, build, or buy and modify strategy chosen should drive the overall structure. Further, the organizational resources available will have an impact on the estimate tasks, and such resources should be consulted and utilized to establish the specific line items of an estimate in each phase. For example, if an organization will have an in-house systems help desk, this help group should provide input into user training needs. In short, the project manager should not prepare the estimate in isolation; rather, the estimate should be a joint effort of the project stakeholders. As the project progresses, individual line items can be further subdivided as project details are defined. For example, after work on the design phase, it may be possible to break programming efforts out into categories such as modification to existing programs, database construction, screen programming, report programming, etc., under the general line item category called programming. In addition, we have included a category of non-phase-specific costs that must be included in the estimate in the following table, presented as Table 7.1. This table also includes certain costs that are not specific to any project phase.

Other costs unique to a particular project must also be included. As the project progresses, a project manager moves from summary line items to more detailed line items for larger cost items. Generally, use of a spreadsheet package will enable a project manager to present comparisons and changes in the estimate more easily and accurately.

Defining Benefits of an Information System Project

Private industry uses a number of ways to calculate value that have an impact on cost/benefit or return on investment calculations. We believe the impact of application software goes far beyond the typical traditional considerations; this impact adds both direct and indirect value not normally included in the calculations. Further, in public health, there are some unique indirect benefits that must be considered because of public health's unique mission and purpose.

Just as cost is likely to be the first question asked of a project manager, benefit is likely to be the second. From the very beginning, management is going to want to know the benefits to be derived from the expenditure of money on the proposed project. Just as with cost estimating, the first calculation of a proposed project's benefit will not be correct. However, this initial estimated benefit should nevertheless be more accurate than the initial cost calculation. This is so because projects are undertaken as a result of organizational needs, which often can be articulated specifically; those needs are associated with a fault in the existing way in which a business process is supported, or because no support is being supplied at all. Correcting a fault in existing support or supplying support lends itself to calculation of a benefit.

Still, the calculation of a system's benefit can be significantly improved after the completion of the requirements definition. The requirements definition will delineate the way in which the fault will be corrected or new support provided where none existed before. In addition, the requirements definition

TABLE 7.1. A template for estimating the costs of an information system project

Category	Item	Item Definition
Requirements definition		
	Consultants	Hiring of outside experts to help perform the requirements definition work
	Facilitators	Retain the services of group facilitator(s) to aid in the requirements gathering activity
	Staff	Personnel assigned to work on the requirements
	Travel	Cost for visiting other organizations ("industrial tourism")
	Miscellaneous	Miscellaneous expenses
Design		
	Consultants	Hiring of outside experts to help perform the system design activities
	Training	Train staff to use new tools or databases
	Staff	Personnel assigned to work on the design
	Travel	Travel for off-site training
	Miscellaneous	Miscellaneous expenses
Programming		
	Consultants	Hiring of outside programmers to assist in the system programming
	Training	Train staff to use new tools and languages
	Staff	Travel for off-site training
	Travel	Personnel assigned to work on the programming
Program testing		
	Staff	Personnel assigned to test the programming
System testing		
	Staff	Personnel assigned to work on the system integration testing
	Other staff	Nonprogramming personnel utilized to aid in testing
Installation		
	Consultants	Outside resources hired to install system software (operating system, etc.)
	Staff	Personnel assigned to install system and application software
	Travel	Travel costs if installation must be done at multiple sites
Training	Consultants	Outside resources for training (could be vendor-supplied)
	Staff	Training provided by in-house trainers (include time for training the trainers and preparation of training materials)

TABLE 7.1. (*Cont.*) A template for estimating the costs of an information system project

Category	Item	Item Definition
	Travel	Travel costs if training must be done at multiple sites
Conversion and start-up		
	Programmers	Development of conversion programs to convert database files to new system
	Staff	Trainers and others to support "first" day operation
	Travel	Travel costs if installation must be done at multiple sites
RFP preparation		
	Consultants	Outside resources to assist/write RFP
	Materials	RFP documents
	Staff	RFP preparation and pre-bid activities
	Travel	Travel costs for visiting vendors and users
	Miscellaneous	Postage and other expenses
Evaluation and selection		
	Consultants	Outside resources to assist in reviews
	Staff	Personnel assigned to perform evaluation and demonstrations
	Travel	Travel to vendor reference user sites
Other costs not specific to phases		
	Project manager	Cost of project management staff
	Hardware	Additions to company hardware configuration (computers, printers, communications, etc.)
	Software	Operating system software, etc.
	Presentations	Communications with stakeholders and team meetings
	Marketing	Project materials and promotional pieces
	Reviews	Special costs associated with periodic management reviews and progress reporting
External factors		
	Staff	New system may create increased demand from external users, thus increasing need for support staff and program staff (increased flow of information may create imperative to act, e.g., collecting surveillance data)
	Hardware	Same issue as staff increases
Contingency		May want to break out by hardware, software, etc.

process can uncover other opportunities for benefits not previously articulated. In many cases, a slight expansion in the scope of the project can produce incremental benefits far in excess of the incremental cost. Thus, an important element of the scoping task in the requirements definition is to explore the work tasks on the project boundary for incremental benefit. In many instances, in fact, the case for the project's benefit is weak precisely because of inadequate effort in the requirements definition task.

As indicated earlier, the process of streamlining the task set may shift work from one area to another. Although there will be a net gain overall, the work may increase in some areas. It is helpful to document these shifts as a part of the benefit analysis in order to justify the increased overall benefit to be derived. For example, increasing the work associated with client check-in to require current verification of Medicaid and Medicare IDs may reduce the need to process rejected claim submittals.

Not only might a well-constructed requirements definition shift work within the organization, but it is also possible that it will shift work to or from external partners. For example, automation of immunization records in such a way that school nurses could have direct access to them might reduce the pre-school rush to obtain immunization records from a health department. The new system might allow a school nurse to look up the records and print out the certifications at the school site. Obviously, such a change will reduce the workload at the health department and increase it in the schools. The trade-off will have to be evaluated to determine the net benefit. At the same time, the nurses might get used to using the system and increase the overall transaction load, forcing the health department to increase server capacity and thus increasing costs for the health department. Additional costs may come about when other partners have to initiate their own information system projects in order to interface with the new system. For example, a project to institute Health Level 7 standards for transmission of immunization data to other registries may force one or more of the other registries to rewrite their interfaces in order to continue to receive data from the new system.

Thus, the benefit calculation must go far beyond monetary items within the organization. The calculation should include the following categories in order to measure the impact of an application software project adequately:

- *Impact derived from revisions to the business process task set.* Good systems design results in changes to the way in which the business functions that are being supported are performed. Such changes may impact on benefit by enabling the same staff to serve more clients faster and more efficiently. In addition, these changes may allow a reallocation of staff resources and even increase the ratio of service providers to support staff (a change in this ratio of 10% would have a major cost benefit).
- *Value acceleration.* Value often accrues more quickly to the organization when a new system is in operation. For example, a new user-friendly invoice

presentation format might reduce client questions about monthly statements and thus reduce the length of time from service provision to receipt of payment.

* *Value linking.* The installation of the system may have ripple effects in other areas of the organization, bringing benefit to operations outside the immediate system support area. For example, the installation of a new, more readily accessible immunization registry may be of considerable value for immunization verification to the WIC or Child Care Licensure programs, even though that was not the intent of the project.

* *Value restructuring.* Providing appropriate functional support may not eliminate a given job, but may in fact cause the job content to change from work that is of lower value to the organization to work that is of greater value. For example, if the new system automates WIC appointments and eliminates the need for the clerical support staff to track them manually, the staff might be able to spend more time making sure the clients keep the appointment, thus reducing no-shows and subsequent underutilization of nursing staff.

* *Innovation opportunity.* Installation of the new system creates the opportunity for enhancing the specific services being provided when it enables higher quality, better outcomes, and other improvements. For example, a department performing latent tuberculosis treatment services might benefit from the inclusion of or reference to clinical treatment guidelines embedded in the clinic support software.

* *Strategic match.* The project aids in achieving one or more strategic objectives important to the organization. In public health, that could mean increasing capacity to utilize the Institute of Medicine's model of Assessment, Policy Development, and Assurance through the provision of community assessment information.

* *Compliance enhancement.* The project may enable the organization to be compliant with one or more state, federal, or grant requirements. A prime example in public health is projects oriented toward HIPAA security and confidentiality requirements.

* *Management information.* The project contributes to management's need for information about its core activities.

* *Operational efficiency.* Utilization of new technology may reduce infrastructure cost by eliminating high-cost maintenance of old technology and by reducing staff time required to monitor and run a system. For example, most workstation vendors now provide three-year warranty agreements. The old computers being eliminated may be covered by rather expensive maintenance agreements, and staff will probably spend far less time troubleshooting the new network compared with the old one. In addition, system availability (the percentage of time the system is usable) may radically increase, impacting on overall productivity.

Measures of value can be stated in terms of both direct and indirect benefit. Those with direct benefit can be translated directly into dollar savings or increased revenue. Those with indirect benefit cannot be directly tied to dollar amounts, although from a business perspective they may be just as important. For example, a project that primarily addresses compliance enhancement may not be translated directly into dollars, but it may help avoid future lawsuits. Such intangible benefits have value to the organization, even if the benefits cannot be translated to dollar amounts.

Because all benefits cannot be quantified as dollar amounts that offset the cost of a project, there is never a simple formula for arriving at value. In the calculation of the value of a system, it is best first to delineate potential dollar savings that are direct offsets to the project cost estimate, followed by statements of indirect benefit. A project manager should involve the stakeholders in the indirect benefit assessment. Many stakeholders may even be willing to assign a dollar value to the indirect benefits they believe will be of value to them, and such stakeholders can become very active advocates for the project as a result of these benefits.

The Project Management Framework

Although we have given hints about project management throughout this discussion, we have not delineated a conceptual framework for this important activity. There is a certain extent to which project management remains an art. There are people who are intuitively good at it, and others who are not. However, our experience indicates that having a good perspective or framework in which to perform project management activities is one of the characteristics that distinguish good information system project managers. The framework presented in the following paragraphs is specifically oriented toward information systems projects and is not intended as a universal framework for all kinds of projects.

All our intuition and most of our experience have taught us that a direct relationship exists between effort expended on a task and the completion of the task. For example, when the lawn needs to be mowed, we know the accomplishment of the task basically involves the expenditure of a relatively known amount of effort. The keys to getting it mowed are simply getting started (often the most difficult part) and then exerting the required effort. When we have expended all the required effort, we are done, and there is usually no question about whether we are really done because the *physical evidence* (the mowed lawn) allows us to conclude rationally that the task is complete. We see a farmer harvesting a field and can estimate at a glance how close he is to being done. In fact, if he tells us how long it has taken so far, our childhood training in algebra allows us to calculate quite accurately when he will probably be done. We intuitively understand that in any task there is a direct correlation between effort expended and percentage complete. Figure 7.11 illustrates our algebraic understanding of this concept.

Generally, all approaches to information systems work delineate specific work tasks associated with each phase of a project. After all, even systems

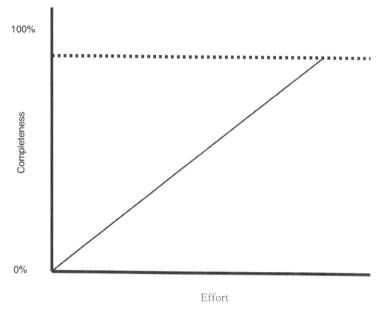

Figure 7.11. A graphical illustration of the common perception of the relationship between task completion and effort.

work is a business process. Any logical and workable approach to a software project must be based on the establishment of a consistent, logical set of work tasks.

Unfortunately, the delineation of tasks inevitably leads to the project management assumptions reflected in the Figure 7.11. The most basic of the assumptions is that effort and completeness have a direct correlation. This subtle, sometimes unconscious, conclusion shapes the way in which project management often approaches software projects. Its influence often results in less than optimal management results. Our experience indicates there is another, more reasonable, set of assumptions that yield superior results with respect to management of an information system project.

The need for this different set of assumptions can be illustrated by an example of the difference between completing a fairly simple task and completing an information system project. In the case of mowing the lawn, completion provides objective evidence provided by a few questions. Did the mower mow? Is the lawn edged adequately? Is the lawn cut evenly? From simple observation, the mower can immediately conclude whether the task is complete *and* whether it was done with sufficient quality to pass inspection. In information systems project environments, on the other hand, it is more difficult to assess task completion, and in many instances the simple declaration of completion carries the stamp of completion regardless of the actual state of the task. Further, it is far more difficult to correlate expended effort with percentage completion, particularly in the requirements definition and design phases.

In information system project management, a task is never really completed. There is always an opportunity for incremental improvement. Writing a report is the same way; at some point you simply have to declare it complete. Potentially, system development could go on forever. The real issue with regard to task completion involves an assessment (or judgment) regarding the potential benefit to be derived from investing additional effort in the task, and there is rarely a magical point at which one can pause and know that the project is 100% complete in the same sense one can when mowing a lawn. This conclusion leads to the rejection of Figure 7.11 as a representation of an information system project task completion. Further, because of the diverse nature of tasks in information system projects, there is no one curve that adequately expresses the relationship between effort and completion. However, one can describe the boundary curves, or envelope, for the probable set of curves that would be representative of information system project tasks. Most information system development tasks consist of a conceptualization or an idea formulation state, followed by the

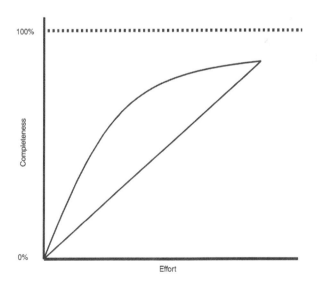

FIGURE 7.12. A graphical presentation of the relationship between effort and completeness in an information system project—front end progresses rapidly.

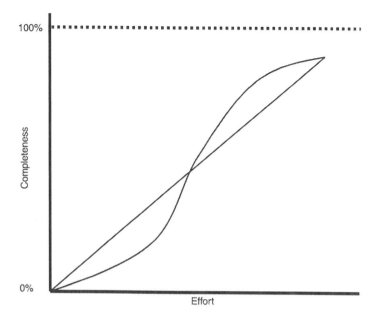

FIGURE 7.13. A graphical representation of the relationship between effort and completion in an information system project requiring a great deal of conceptualization work
followed by rapid detail support.

development of the necessary supporting detail. Figure 7.12 describes the
curve for a task in a situation in which the conceptualization stage advances
relatively rapidly, and rapid progress is reported at the front end of the task.
Progress generally slows when the concept has to be "fleshed out." Notice
that the task is portrayed as never being absolutely 100% complete. In other
words, it would take an infinite amount of effort to achieve absolute perfec-
tion in the work product.

On the other hand, for certain other tasks, a great deal of conceptualization
work is required before the idea or answer becomes apparent, followed by the
development of the adequate detail support. Obviously, the amount and level
of detail will vary from task to task. Figure 7.13 reflects a curve where the
details are easy to develop after a great deal of conceptualization work.

However, in many cases the conceptualization-intense curve will be a mirror opposite of Figure 7.12. Thus, the overall "boundary" set of curves would
look like Figure 7.14. The main point is that these curves illustrate the fallacy
in our intuitive belief that there is a direct correlation between effort and
completeness.

Figure 7.15 is the same curve as appears in Figure 7.14, but with some
additional information overlaid. It reflects the key issue in task management:

At any given point in time during the execution of a task, the relevant question must address the issue of whether an incremental investment of effort (delta E) will produce a worthwhile gain (delta C). That is, when is enough, enough?

The completeness question can be addressed in the following five specific ways that constitute an evaluation of the status of a given task:

- *How critical is the given task to the overall success of the given project?* There is general agreement that not all tasks are of equal importance in a project. Further, the particular importance of a given task can vary from project to project. It follows that more effort ought to be expended on the more critical activities. In scheduling and project management theory, it can be proven that only about 10% of the total number of activities will have an impact on the length of the project. These activities are called the *critical path*. In the same way, we believe that significantly less than 50% of the tasks in a particular requirements definition will control the shape of the end system. These tasks should be identified, and the project manager should make sure that more effort is expended on them—i.e., make sure that they come closer to being 100% complete—than on the noncritical tasks.
- *Is enough done so that the project manager can see how to do the next task?* Because tasks are sequentially related, and each task builds upon the

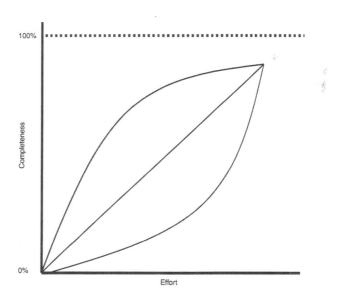

FIGURE 7.14. An alternative illustration of the relationship between effort and completeness for a conceptualization-intense information system project.

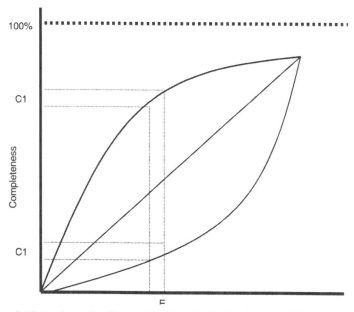

FIGURE 7.15. An alternative illustration of the relationship between effort and completeness for a conceptualization-intense information system project—additional information overlaid.

result of one or more previous tasks, a good way to evaluate a task's
completion status is to ask whether it is possible to see clearly how to
approach the next task. If so, the benefit to be derived from the current task
has been obtained, and it may not serve any useful purpose to pursue it
further. For example, an initial task in requirements definition may be to
"map" the business process environment, identifying the key players and
the ways in which they interact. In this task, the goal is *not* to draw the
perfect representation of the environment in a form suitable for framing
and hanging in the boardroom.

• *How vulnerable is the project manager if he or she has made a mistake or
left something out?* Often, we are driven to perform excess work on a
task by the fear of leaving something out. Each task can be evaluated in
terms of whether the result will be set in concrete or whether it will impact
on the quality of the overall system. For example, identification of the
output set is extremely critical to the whole process; it requires a high
degree of completion. On the other hand, if the definitions of the business
process tasks *not* included in the system scope definition are not

accurate, those definitions are not likely to have much impact on the overall system quality.

- *Will subsequent tasks tend to confirm the adequacy of the work done in the current task?* Many tasks in any approach to requirements definition and design actually provide a certain level of confirmation regarding the accuracy of the work done previously. In a good methodology, each step of the process will logically build on the previous work. If the subsequent task cannot be done because of lack of information from a previous task, then there is a need for more work on the latter. Experienced analysts have a good feel for when the work done in the current task is sufficient for subsequent use.
- *How easy would it be to add an element missed in the current task at a later stage?* Certain tasks are more "forgiving" than others. For example, if the definition of a data element is wrong, the definition can be corrected later without much impact on the design. However, failure to complete a task associated with an important area of functionality that *must* be supported for the system to be a success can create real problems later.

A project manager can use these questions to evaluate the work being done in an information system support project and increase the level of confidence that the project is proceeding at a reasonable pace.

However, if the project manager has a sense that the project is getting bogged down, there is one additional strategy that can be employed. We call it the Patton approach. After the D-Day landings in France, the allies found the going very tough, sometimes measured one hedgerow at a time. General Patton became impatient and devised a strategy of breaking through the enemy lines and seizing key strategic points with his tanks. Troops would then mop up the territory between the strategic points they had captured and the original battle line. A project manager can use the same principle whenever there is an impression that a project is getting bogged down. He or she can simply ask the project team to go to the next project steps and visualize what the results of these steps should look like. Often, this procedure will clarify the remaining work associated with the current tasks that are bogged down by providing focus for the remaining work in a sequential set of steps.

Summary and Conclusions

From community assessment to disease surveillance to operating immunization clinics, an information system project manager in public health must understand the underlying business process to be addressed by the project. Technical resources function best when they have a sound understanding of how a project manager wishes to organize the work associated with the business process as the starting point in an information system project. This understanding is derived from the requirements definition process, which must include representatives from staff who are actually involved in performing the public health tasks, from information system technical resources who will be building the support, and from the project manager.

It logically follows that the cost and benefit analysis used to derive an understanding of the project's value to the organization is built on the business process definition derived in the requirements definition. And although there are no magic formulas in informatics, the purpose of this chapter has been to present a framework for management of an informatics project and guidelines for estimating its value.

Questions for Review

Read the following short case and answer the questions that are based on it.

An information systems officer with considerable experience in information system project management in private industry has recently joined the staff of the public health department of State X. She has been asked to manage an information system project by which the department will significantly change the process by which it captures data related to sexually transmitted diseases (STDs) from county health departments and both public-sector and private-sector medical providers. At present, county health departments transmit this information in various ways. Some counties provide the department with paper forms containing the data; others use either personal or minicomputers to provide the department with the data electronically, either through tapes mailed to the department or through direct transmission via modem.

Under the present system for capturing STD data, workers in one unit of the STD Division enter all data from paper forms into the department's STD system. Data transmitted by computer is checked and then posted in the same system by another unit of the STD Division. The STD Division head is responsible for developing reports on the month's STD activity and transmitting those reports to the Bureau of Disease Control and Intervention, to which the STD Division reports. The Bureau of Disease Control and Intervention reviews these reports and then provides trend analysis reports to the department's chief administrator.

Last year, the legislature of State X enacted a law that all STD data reporting and processing will be automated. The law applies to both private and public health providers, to county health departments, and to the public health department of State X. The project that the newly hired information systems officer is expected to manage will result in a system that requires all data-reporting entities to provide STD data to the state health department in the form of computer data that are captured automatically. The new system will fully automate the production of monthly reports and trend reports.

1. If the organizational structure of the public health department of State X is typical, explain why the new information systems officer is likely to

find analysis of the STD data collection and reporting process more difficult than the analysis of a process in a private organization.

2. What are the challenges inherent in interviewing process participants about the nature of the current process? Why are personnel in the STD Division likely to have an incomplete picture of the entire process?

3. To what extent will the new system be required to emphasize vertical integration? Horizontal integration?

4. Assume that three vendors have produced and marketed systems that accomplish most, but not all, of the goals that the new system is expected to meet. How should the new information systems officer evaluate the competing systems, as provided in response to the request for proposal? Should the officer explore in-house system development first? Why or why not? In the event that she finds one of the three vendor systems easily modifiable, how should she approach the modification?

5. How should the new information officer go about developing the requirements definition for the project? What activities should precede the development of the requirements definition document?

6. What reengineering of the process will the new system necessitate, assuming the system is developed to meet the goal established by the legislature?

7. Explain why training in the use of the new system will be essential.

8. How should the new information officer develop the estimated cost for the new system? What principles should she follow?

9. Explain why project post-auditing will be necessary after the new system is completed and installed. If you were the heading the system development project, what behaviors of users would you be analyzing closely?

10. What direct benefits to the public health department can be expected from the new system? What are the likely indirect benefits?

11. Is there any cost or work shifting involved in this project?

12. Identify any value restructuring that is likely to arise from the new system.

13. Explain why the effort devoted to this project is unlikely to be proportional to the degree of its completion?

References and Notes

1. Davenport T. *Process Innovation*. Boston: HBS Press; 1993.
2. Rummler G, Brache A. *Improving Performance*. San Francisco: Jossey-Bass; 1990.
3. Hammer M, Champy J. *Reengineering the Corporation*. New York: Harper Business; 1993.
4. It has become popular to give the drivers more reigns by empowering the horses to make some of the decisions. Thus the demise of middle management.
5. The National Immunization Program at CDC has produced a wonderful guideline for the creation of immunization transactions for exchange of immunization data utilizing HL-7 message structure. We believe this should serve as a guide for the creation of communication standards for other data sets.

6. Davenport T. *Process Innovation.* Boston: Harvard Business School Press; 1993.
7. Hammer M. Reengineering work: Don't automate, obliterate. *Harvard Business Review* July-August 1990.

8
Managing IT Personnel and Projects

PETE KITCH AND WILLIAM A YASNOFF

Learning Objectives

After studying this chapter, you should be able to:

- Explain why information technology (IT) projects are especially challenging to manage.
- List the criteria by which an IT project manager can identify computer expertise in candidates for project positions and what general expertise is indicated by degrees and certification.
- Identify at least three job attractions other than pay that a public health project manager can provide in competing with the private sector for candidates for IT positions.
- Define the ideal composition of a good IT project team and of an IT project steering committee, and explain the roles of (a) company management, (b) users, and (c) IT technical staff in an IT project that is likely to succeed.
- List the skills that an IT project manager should exercise in managing a project.
- Explain rapid prototyping as a tool in IT project management and its advantages.
- Explain why a manager of an IT project often encounters political opposition within the company, and identify strategies that a project manager can use to minimize the effect.
- Define the roles that consultants should and should not play in an IT project, and list potential sources of qualified consultants.
- Explain why it is important for an IT project manager to include the input of users at every stage in an IT project.

Overview

Managing information technology (IT) personnel and projects is a challenging undertaking. A public health manager charged with developing and implementing a new information system must identify and recruit technical staff and consultants possessing the right kinds of educational qualifications and experience. In addition, the project manager must organize the technical team and use effective strategies for communication with every stakeholder, including company management, users of the proposed new system, and IT personnel assigned to the project. Along the way, the project manager must secure appropriate funding, analyze current processes, identify user needs, manage the expectations of every stakeholder, address the inevitable political opposition, analyze processes to be affected by the new system, determine the appropriate technology to be employed, and educate management about the costs of the proposed new system. Although IT projects have a history of very high failure rates, there are strategies that a project manager can use to help insure project success. Through use of such tools as rapid prototyping, a project manager can identify user needs and involve users from the beginning in the project. Through a careful review of business processes, a project manager can define the appropriate technology to be applied. Finally, through knowing and recognizing the characteristics of successful and unsuccessful IT projects, a project manager can minimize the probability that the IT project will fail.

Introduction

Imagine that you are operating a successful health insurance company. One of your board members, a dentist with considerable experience in operating an imaging system in his office, approaches you with the observation that your company seems to be involved in excessive paperwork. He points out that by digitizing all the paperwork, as he does in his office, your company could realize significant improvements in productivity and work flow. It strikes you as a great idea, and you and your board decide to put this man with experience in using an imaging system in charge of a project to develop an imaging system suitable for your company. Now imagine yourself a while later, writing off $100 million in system development expenses, with no implemented system to show for such a massive investment. It turns out that the dentist/board member had no experience in managing large-scale system development, and therefore he was unable to organize and implement such a complex project successfully.

A fable? No, this disaster really happened. The company was a large, well-known health insurance company in the United States. The company and the dentist/board member will remain nameless here. The experience remains a classic illustration of what can happen when the wrong people are hired to manage an IT project, and it emphasizes the importance of project management skills in developing and implementing systems based on technology.

In this chapter, we will review some of the most important issues in managing IT projects and personnel. Project management, of course, is a discipline unto itself. Many books are devoted exclusively to this single topic. Clearly, one chapter is insufficient to explore all aspects of this complex field, but we hope to emphasize some of the more important aspects with respect to management of IT projects.

IT projects represent a special challenge within project management. Unlike other projects, such as those involving construction, it is often difficult to see concrete progress in IT projects. Also, it is difficult to separate IT projects from other aspects of the operation of the organization. That quality alone makes IT projects different from others. For example, in a space-planning project, general-purpose office space can be constructed without regard to the specific work being performed in each office. Such is not the case with information systems, which can affect numerous offices and departments. Finally, IT projects are different from many other types of projects because they are always political; organizational challenges occur because of the inevitable shift in power through changes in access to information.

This chapter is divided into two major sections: managing personnel and managing projects. The personnel section deals with issues concerning hiring, retaining, and organizing technical personnel. The management section reviews key strategies for maximizing the probability of project success; it specifically highlights many pitfalls that an IT manager should avoid. Although there is no substitute for experience when it comes to managing IT projects, this chapter should provide you with a basic framework for approaching this very challenging management task.

Managing IT Personnel

Successful IT projects depend greatly on a project head's ability to identify and select the right people to work on the project, to communicate with technical people, to hire consultants appropriately, and to organize technical teams.

Identifying Computer Expertise

It is a fundamental principle that IT projects require the identification and selection of the right people to perform the work. The identification process necessarily requires a manager to determine whether candidates for project team positions have the right computer expertise.

One key problem managers have in recognizing computer expertise is that the technology is relatively new. Contrast this situation with automobile technology, which is now over a century old. In automobile technology, there is widespread familiarity with the differences between an inexperienced driver, an experienced driver, a race car driver, a weekend mechanic, and an engine designer for a major automobile manufacturer. No one would consider it reasonable to ask an experienced driver to design a new internal combustion engine. However, the equivalent is often attempted in the computer world. Asking an experienced user with no credible expertise to design and manage a complex information system is just as likely to result in failure as an automobile manufacturer's asking a driver to design an engine. The health insurance imaging system disaster discussed at the beginning of this chapter highlights the folly of relying on users of systems to manage the development of an IT system. IT projects require the core members of the project team to possess solid credentials in computer science.

But what are the key factors to look for in identifying computer expertise?

First, there is education. There are now many undergraduate and graduate programs in computer science awarding bachelor's, master's, and doctoral degrees. But it is necessary for a manager to know what these various degrees signify about the computer expertise of individuals. Someone with a bachelor's degree in computer science can be expected to have programming skills, some knowledge of database design, and some experience with project tools. A candidate possessing a master's degree in computer science will have completed at least one major IT project. However, that master's project may have been an individual project rather than a team effort, so a manager must still determine whether the candidate has project team skills. A doctorate in computer science indicates the degree holder's development of a significant new approach to solving a computer science problem. Typically, at this level, the focus is on research rather than on implementing systems. There are also numerous certifications available from vendors with respect to specific products and systems. A manager should inquire about relevant certification when hiring a network manager and give preference to any candidates who have achieved it.

The most important qualification for technical personnel, of course, is experience. It is critical to assess whether the experience is related directly to the current task. A candidate who has previously done exactly what a manager is now trying to do (and has been successful) is clearly most desirable. In addition, a manager should be familiar with the different roles to be performed in a project and select the appropriate personnel to fill those roles. For example, a *programmer* typically receives specific instructions about what needs to be developed and writes the code. An *analyst* determines what programs need to be written and generates the instructions for the programmer. A *system designer* develops the architecture for the entire system, including the relationships of all the various parts and the subsystems that are needed. The *project manager* orchestrates the entire team and is responsible for supervising and coordinating all the activities. Of course, in evaluating the qualifications of a candidate for an IT project team position, a manager needs to understand what role is suitable for the experience represented by an applicant.

As is always the case in selecting personnel, checking references is extremely important. A manager needs to check as many references as possible, especially those related to the relevant experience of the candidate. Although it is no easier

TABLE 8.1. Key factors to look for in identifying suitable computer expertise

Factor	Relevant Characteristics
Education in computer science	Bachelor's level: possession of programming skills, knowledge of database design, experience with project tools
	Master's level: all skills of bachelor's level plus completion of at least one major IT project
	Doctoral level: all skills of master's level plus development of a significant new approach to solving a computer science problem; primary emphasis is on research
	Certification: indicates possession of expertise with regard to specific products and systems
Experience	Should be related to current task
	Should be relevant to role the candidate will perform on the project team
	Should indicate cooperative service on a project team
References	Should be multiple
	Should include inquiry about the success of projects on which the candidate has worked

with technical than with other personnel to get candid information from references, it is possible to ascertain whether any systems that a candidate was involved with became operational or not. Even if the direct supervisor of the candidate is not available, the person currently responsible for the system that was developed will often provide very useful comments about its effectiveness.

Table 8.1 summarizes the factors that an IT project manager should consider in identifying computer expertise among candidates for IT positions.

Recruiting

Is no secret that the demand for computer personnel is so high that recruiting them is a difficult task. As in every other field of expertise, offering competitive compensation levels is extremely important in attracting high-quality personnel. In fact, it is not unusual for the most qualified technical personnel in a program to have a higher level of compensation than the program manager. This is simply a matter of supply and demand—good technical folks are very scarce. In the ideal world, a governmental public health organization would be able to offer market-level compensation for computer personnel. In the real world, however, government agencies often find it very difficult to match offers made by organizations in the private sector. Nevertheless, it is worthwhile for a public health manager to expend substantial effort to convince the public health agency to provide attractive compensation. After all, although technical personnel are certainly costly, failed IT projects are orders of magnitude more costly.

Luckily, compensation is not the only tool available to attract high-quality personnel. Other tools related to a candidate's career development and lifestyle are also extremely important. For example, a system designer may be able to earn at an Internet start-up company twice what a public health organization is offering, but he or she may be required to work twice as many hours at the start-up company. A public health agency manager's ability to offer a position involving fewer work hours may tip the scales in the system designer's decision. After all, many technical personnel are not workaholics, and they would like to have a normal life that includes remaining closely acquainted with their families.

Another advantage a manager may be able to offer a candidate is a desirable work environment. Nice office space, good equipment, and state-of-the-art software and hardware tools can go a long way to attract good people. Another important attraction is a manager's willingness to maintain the cutting-edge skills of personnel by providing time and funding for continuing training. Of course, such training opportunities benefit both the technical personnel and the organization.

Finally, public health can often provide more meaningful work than other sectors of the economy. Much of what public health does is very appealing to the altruistic side of job candidates. The combination of work that helps the community, pleasant working conditions, and reasonable hours often can provide an attractive enough package to offset below-market compensation.

Communication with Technical Personnel

To manage technical personnel effectively, a manager needs to be able to communicate with them. IT, like most other specialized fields, has its own peculiar jargon and vocabulary. It is important for a manager to be familiar with the basic terminology of information systems. One of the most painless ways to accomplish this familiarity is to read the computer trade literature. Publications such as *InfoWorld* and *Computer World* regularly contain simple, easy-to-understand explanations of technical terms. A side benefit of such reading will be an increased awareness of trends in the information industry.

Is also important for a manager to avoid being intimidated by the expertise of technical employees. Of course, he or she should be pleased that these employees have extensive technical expertise; such skills are why they were hired. At the same time, it is important for a manager to insist on clear explanations of technical terms. Computer personnel should be able to explain what they are doing in plain English. If a manager does not understand what he or she is being told and cannot get a clear explanation, it is time to hire a consultant.

Hiring Consultants

Consultants are an important part of an IT team. When there is a very specific issue or question that is beyond the expertise of an in-house staff, it is time to strongly consider bringing in a consultant. Finding available consultants is not terribly difficult: A manager can simply talk to other individuals who have been involved in similar projects and have had similar problems that were solved by the use of consultants. In addition, vendors of systems and software will be able to refer a manager to potential consultants.

When a manager is hiring a consultant, it is important to interview potential consulting candidates just as carefully as a potential full-time staff hire. The references provided should be checked carefully, and the check should be extensive. When engaging a consultant, a manager should also be certain that the tasks to be performed are well defined and understood in advance. After all, the most effective consulting engagements are those in which a very specific, thoroughly described problem is being addressed.

Organizing Technical Teams

Experience has shown that small interdisciplinary teams are the most effective for handling IT projects. Such a team should represent a spectrum of organizational interests. It should include users, program staff, managers, and technical personnel. In most cases, the management of an organization should lead the team, but this does not mean that decisions should be unilateral. It is important for a team manager to consider carefully the input of all team members, and especially of potential users of the system to be developed. After all, it is especially important to have the support of users, because they will be the ultimate consumers of any information system and the judges of its effectiveness.

Communication is probably the most important element in the success of IT teams. A project team manager should utilize every means available to facilitate communication. Holding regular meetings, making frequent e-mail contact, issuing progress reports regularly, and locating team members in close proximity to facilitate informal contact are all good communication strategies. In addition, a team manager needs to document everything: When an issue comes up during the development process, it is extremely helpful to have good documentation of the process that has brought the team to that particular issue.

Managing IT Projects

IT projects are high-risk. In a 1994 study of over 8,000 large information system development projects in the private sector and in government, the Standish Group found that only 16.2% (one in six) of the projects were fully successful: on time, on budget, and with all features implemented. More than half (52.7%) of the projects were partially successful: the system was delivered, but was either over budget, late, or missing expected features. Most important, 31.1% of the projects were total failures: the project was canceled, and all the investment of time and money was lost. A later (1998) study by the Standish Group found that although there was some improvement in the portion of IT projects completed fully successfully—to 26%—still, the overwhelming majority of IT projects were either "challenged" or else complete failures.[1] Needless to say, these are not encouraging findings for information systems developers.

The largest known information system development failure to date was at the Internal Revenue Service (IRS), where $3.5 billion in IT system investment was lost, according to congressional testimony by agency officials. The IRS worked for a number of years to try to revamp its information systems, and through a long series of mishaps aided by bureaucratic obstacles, ended up with this massive disaster.

The government is not alone, however, in experiencing IT disasters. When Sabre, the airline reservation system formerly owned by AMR Corporation, the parent of American Airlines, teamed up with a major rental car firm and a major hotel firm to create a unified air, hotel, and automobile reservations system, the result was a $125 million loss and no system.[2] This disaster, known as the CONFIRM Project, was the result of poor communications, mismanaged expectations, and mismanagement. It is sobering to see such a failure from an organization that clearly has such long-standing and high-level IT expertise.

The fact is that the current state of the art in IT project management does not allow for development of information systems with a high probability of success. The reason is that we really do not understand this activity well enough to prescribe a set of techniques that will always be successful. As might be expected, the expense and visibility of IT failures has prompted extensive inquiries into the aspects that predispose a project to failure. By learning about the factors that lead to success and failure, we should be able to improve the odds of success.

In addition, a basic concept in IT projects is the " triangle " relationship of the three key elements of time, features, and budget. You may remember from high school geometry that triangles are rigid figures—one side cannot be changed without affecting at least one of the other sides. It is this characteristic of interrelationship that applies to the key elements in IT projects: Not one of the elements of time, features, and budget of an IT project can be changed without affecting another element. The central relationships of time, features, and budget provide the context for all other discussions of IT project management. Table 8.2 illustrates these relationships.

TABLE 8.2. The interrelationship of IT project time, features, and budget

Project Component	Impact of Component Increase or Decrease
Time	If increased, will increase budget and may allow increase in system features
	If decreased, will reduce budget but also reduce system features
Features	If increased, will increase both project time and budget
	If decreased, will reduce both project time and budget
Budget	If increased, may increase features and reduce project time
	If decreased, will increase project time and reduce system features

Managing Expectations

Managing expectations is the most important skill for an IT project manager. It is essential that an IT project manager promise only what can be delivered and deliver what is promised on time. Of course, it is also important for a project manager to be very cautious about making commitments. In particular, a project manager must educate higher management in the process of system development, so that higher management will have reasonable expectations about progress. This education process is both slow and expensive.

It is also very difficult for a project manager to predict how long the project will take and how much it will cost, as we discussed in Chapter 7. One key element in project management experience is developing an understanding of what can be done and how fast it can be accomplished. An experienced project manager can better estimate future progress and therefore do a better job of managing expectations. One approach to this is "managing the estimate"—conducting periodic iterative refinements of the time and budget estimates for a project. The process of iterative refinement of a project's time and budget estimates is described in Chapter 7.

Involving Users

The other central element in successful IT project management is to engage the users in the systems development processes. Involving users is a uniform characteristic of successful information system development efforts, as Table 8.3 indicates.

It is important to give the users meaningful involvement from the inception of the project to its completion, for involvement of users not only serves to solve real user problems, but it also fosters a sense of ownership of the

TABLE 8.3. IT project success factors according to a Standish Group survey of IT executive managers

Project Success Factors	Percentage of Responses
User involvement	15.9%
Executive management support	13.9%
Clear statement of requirements	13.0%
Proper planning	9.6%
Realistic expectations	8.2%
Smaller project milestones	7.7%
Competent staff	7.2%
Ownership	5.3%
Clear vision and objectives	2.9%
Hard-working, focused staff	2.4%
Other	13.9%

Source: CHAOS, The Standish Group International, Inc., Copyright 1995. Available at: http://standishgroup.com.

system by the ultimate users. Of course, it is also important for a project manager to identify fully informed process users for involvement in a system development project. It is a frequently made mistake to engage the supervisors of the users, instead of the users themselves. Supervisors, although they have a legitimate interest in IT projects affecting their subordinates, often are not cognizant of the real problems and challenges in day-to-day work faced by the front-line workers. In fact, to insure that all interested parties to an IT project are involved, a project manager should consider establishing a steering committee for a project. This steering committee should be composed of users, managers, and the system developers. All major decisions affecting the project should be made by the steering committee. As in any group, there will be some decisions made by a steering committee that are not unanimous; however, a project manager needs to keep in mind that uniform opposition from the users to any major decision greatly increases overall project risk.

Communicating Project Benefits

Throughout the development process, it is important to focus on delivering real benefits to the real users. Often, systems are developed for the primary purpose of collecting information for use by higher levels of management. While there is nothing wrong with such a project goal, additional burdens placed on the users solely for this purpose will not be welcome. In addition, the perceived benefits of a new system should include improvement of the work flow of users. A manager can help insure achievement of this benefit by arranging for meaningful user participation in the project. In fact, participation itself should be structured as a user benefit. Rather than making project participation an added burden on the users, management should arrange for compensatory relief from regular day-to-day work in exchange for project participation. Finally, providing for small benefits to the intended users early in the project development cycle is extremely helpful in securing user participation. Such benefits help establish the overall good intentions of the development team and build trust in the user community that the real focus of the project is on users.

Rapid Prototyping

One of the most effective methodologies for IT system development is *rapid prototyping*. Rapid prototyping is the quick development of a nonfunctional test version of the ultimate system for discussion and review by users. It is a very effective mechanism for soliciting meaningful user input throughout the development cycle.

When users are assembled and questioned about their information needs, it is often very difficult for them to articulate those needs in a comprehensive fashion. If a system were to be built based on only one such session with users, inevitably the user reaction would be, " Yes, that's what we asked you to build, but no, this really doesn't meet our needs." Such a reaction is not a result of any inherent inability of users to communicate. Rather, it is a result of the extreme complexity and high level of abstraction of information system needs. Very few people can even visualize and articulate the details of an entire information system that they know, much less the details of an information system that has not yet been developed.

Rapid prototyping aids in the requirements specification process by presenting users with a framework that captures the current level of understanding of their needs. It is much easier for users (and others) to correct and amend an existing framework than to develop a coherent description of their system requirements. It is very rare for any individual to be able to articulate the totality of a complex system from scratch. The rapid prototyping process minimizes risk by making very small incremental investments in system developments to refine the requirements.

The traditional development process for information systems involves initial specification of requirements, design of the system, coding of the programs, testing of the programs, release of the system, and then maintenance. Often, when this approach is used, the time delay between assessing the requirements and delivering the system is so long that both user needs and technology have changed, and the resultant system is obsolete at its introduction.

Rapid prototyping, on the other hand, starts with a quick overview of user needs, with an initial prototype developed as quickly as possible. The project manager then reviews the initial prototype with users and discusses needed changes with them. The process is repeated, usually many times, until the users are satisfied. Then, the final prototype can be used to build a working system. Because that final prototype already implements a substantial portion of the system, the remainder of the development process can usually be concluded rapidly.

Why does rapid prototyping work? First, it maintains contact with users throughout the process of system development. Second, it shortens the development cycle, particularly the time between finishing analysis of requirements and delivering a working system. Third, and perhaps most importantly, it reduces the conceptual difficulty of developing requirements of complex and abstract information systems.

Use of rapid prototyping requires new and different tools and skills than traditional system development methods. Prototyping tools are somewhat different from standard development tools, inasmuch as the focus of rapid prototyping is on presenting an "apparent" system to users, rather than a complete working system. However, technical staff must be willing to develop and discard many prototypes, a requirement that can be a problem with technical personnel who have traditional "pride of authorship" in the code that they write. In particular, technical staff must be willing to view the prototype as a communication tool with the users, rather than as a product. It is important for a manager to emphasize that discarded prototypes are not "wasted effort," but rather the cost of important user feedback that will ultimately save tremendous amounts of development time and effort.

Managing Political Challenges

As pointed out early in this chapter, IT projects are inherently political. They cause shifts in power by creating shifts in access to information. They also create changes in processes, often impacting process owners. Recognition and management of political challenges is another important skill in successful IT project development. Part of the challenge for a project manager is overcoming the inertia—the desire to maintain the status quo—that is inherent in organizations, particularly at the management level. Inertia is probably the most difficult obstacle in implementation of new information systems. Stakeholders in the status quo will inevitably oppose the new system, while support for the new system from other quarters will be lukewarm at best. It is important to understand who will benefit from a failure of the new system development and to work to minimize the benefits of such failure to these individuals. Naturally, any change in business practices threatens the existing power structure. The employees who will lose power as a result of the new system inevitably will work against it. Therefore, a project manager must recognize, expect, and manage hidden agendas within the organization. One very specific strategy that a project manager can use to gain acceptance of a new system is to ensure job placement for any person whose position will be adversely affected by the new system.

Securing Funding for an IT Project

Funding a new information system development is always a difficult issue. It is very important to recognize that inadequate funding usually is a manifestation of political opposition within the organization. For this reason, it is very unwise to pursue underfunded projects. Although it is tempting to try to develop a badly needed system by extremely careful management of an inadequate budget, the reward is likely to be additional budget reductions and imposition of other obstacles. A project manager should recognize that if the decision makers holding the purse strings are not willing to pay for a new system, they don't really want it.

It is also important for a project manager to educate senior management about the true costs of information systems, which are often unappreciated. Also, strategic decisions about investing in information systems are difficult for an organization's top management to make.[3] For example, when AMR Corporation made the decision to build the Sabre airline reservation system, the project was considered a huge risk and was widely opposed. At the time, few, if any, would have predicted that this information system would prove more profitable in the long run than American Airlines itself.

Managing Change Created by a New System

As Lorenzi and Riley point out in Chapter 9, IT projects create many changes—changes that a project manager must manage. In fact, a key element in deploying new information systems is changing employee behavior. For most employees, change is extremely uncomfortable, even if it is for the better. The more rapid the change, the more the discomfort increases. Recognition of information system development as a process of change is a very helpful paradigm. The implication of this process of change is that behavior modification is a key part of system development. One of the most powerful tools for behavior modification is intermittent positive reinforcement, which should be used to help encourage the needed changes. Although using intermittent positive reinforcement to gain acceptance of change may seem manipulative, it really represents a legitimate change-management strategy needed to overcome the discomfort from the new procedures that will be required for use of a new information system. At the same time, it is also important for a project manager to respect the affinity that users have with the old system and the "grieving" process for its loss.

Using Technology Appropriately

In the development of information systems, technology must be used appropriately. It is important for a project manager to recognize that technology does not solve all problems. It is easy to be overzealous in the application of technology-based solutions; this tendency must be avoided. Sometimes a low-tech solution to an organizational problem is more effective than applying sophisticated technology. A good example of a low-tech solution to an IT problem is the case study comprising Chapter 32, which and describes the development of a paper-based input system for private-provider immunization data.

A careful review of business processes helps to define where technology can best be applied. As we emphasized in Chapter 7, examining existing business processes is the starting point in information system design. Merely automating inefficient processes is not a good business strategy. In fact, simply reengineering processes may eliminate the need for automation and reveal new and different information system needs. In short, it is absolutely critical for system developers to understand the business processes that underlie the need for an information system. There is no substitute for spending time in the user environment trying to experience the existing system from the user or customer viewpoint. For example, before addressing the information systems needs for a clinic, it would be very helpful for a system developer to register as a patient and experience that clinic from the customer viewpoint. In addition, time spent with the clinic's staff observing and perhaps participating in the actual work will prove very valuable.

Project Success and Failure

Over the years, studies have explored and identified factors associated with success and failure of IT projects. Although in this chapter we have pointed out many of the things that an IT project manager *should* do, we also need to emphasize those things that a project manager should *not* do. In short, in this section we choose to emphasize those strategies that lead to project failure. By understanding how disasters are created, it is possible for a student of public health informatics to effectively utilize this knowledge to maximize the probability of IT project success.

There are both management and technical strategies for creating IT disasters. We will review the management strategies first.

Management Strategies That Promote Project Failure

1. *Trust the vendor.* This failure strategy involves selecting a single vendor for all purchases and relying on that vendor for all IT advice. It also includes ignoring standards and open systems. Another variant of this approach is to purchase a system without a clear specification of its application within the organization.
2. *Delegate.* In this failure strategy, responsibility for IT is fully delegated to lower levels of management without providing for appropriate supervision and control. Another approach to failure is to delegate operational responsibility while retaining financial control. The use of separate groups to purchase IT systems and manage them also contributes to project failure. Finally, developing very rigid job specifications worsens the problem by limiting personnel flexibility.
3. *Impose rigid controls.* Opportunities for achieving innovation and business process reengineering can be markedly reduced by eliminating exploratory work. In conjunction with this failure strategy, enforcement of absolute conformity with current in-house standards will further limit creativity. Other control approaches guaranteed to lead to project failure include requiring justification for every computer system expenditure, no matter how small, and eliminating any operational managers who take an organization-wide view of system needs.
4. *Divide and rule.* The essence of this approach is to separate business and IT functions and personnel, creating separate career tracks and reporting lines. It is remarkable how pervasive this failure strategy has been. It is possible to enhance this failure strategy by encouraging competition within the organization, while discouraging collaboration. Also, maintaining management ignorance of IT and refusing to fund IT continuing education will enhance this tactic. Finally, providing inadequate compensation for IT staff will help insure failure by making it extremely difficult to recruit and retain high quality personnel.
5. *Use IT as a tool for finance.* This common failure strategy places IT under the director of finance, who often has no IT background or experience. The resources of IT are then primarily focused on financial control and executive information systems. It is possible to enhance the failure-promoting effects of this strategy by moving the corporate staff to a remote site and the IT staff to a different remote site. The negative impact of such separation on communications virtually insures project failure.
6. *Use consultants inappropriately.* Of course, the mere use of consultants is in no way a project failure strategy. However, sole reliance on external consultants for IT can be a serious problem, especially if the external consultants are not familiar with the business of the organization. In this failure strategy, use of the same consultants for providing general management and IT advice eliminates a potential source of balance and

independence in the approach to IT management. The effect of overreliance on external consultants can be accentuated by eliminating any in-house staff who have expertise in the areas of IT covered by the consultants.

7. *Set rigid objectives.* Another road to failure involves imposing rigid quarterly financial performance objectives with required cost-benefit analysis of all IT expenditures. The use of IT to support and reinforce vertical patterns of management reporting will further enhance the effect. Another component of this approach is avoiding detailed IT project planning that supports general business objectives.

8. *Control information.* Communication is absolutely critical to project success. Therefore, restricting contacts between departments, penalizing criticism of IT systems, and avoiding discussions of failures or conflicting views will greatly increase the probability of project failure. Minimizing communication between management and staff will add to the problem. Finally, overcentralization of IT operations and development can also reduce needed communication between IT and operational staff and thus contribute to project failures. This does not mean that centralization should always be avoided. Some IT operations—for example, network management—should be centralized.

9. *Avoid user input.* As we have emphasized earlier in this chapter, securing meaningful user input is the most critical factor in project success. Therefore, failure to consult with staff members who will use or be affected by new systems is a sure road to project failure. Providing inadequate training for users of the new IT system will also enhance the probability of a disaster. Another mechanism for ensuring a lack of user cooperation is to announce (or imply) that the goal of a new system is to automate all possible functions and eliminate the maximum number of staff. Even if this indirectly appears to be a system goal, although unannounced, it clearly will discourage the user cooperation that is essential to project success.

Technical Strategies That Promote Project Failure

Next, we will discuss technical factors that can lead to project failure. It is notable that there are not as many technical approaches as management strategies that create IT disasters. This fact alone highlights the overriding importance of management in determining IT project success or failure.

1. *Technical leadership.* The probability of project failure can be greatly increased by appointing a technical project leader with complete authority and ensuring that the project team consists only of programmers. The effect of this approach can be further accentuated by giving this technical team complete financial and decision-making autonomy without any user or management input.

2. *Resources.* Obviously, providing inadequate resources is a very effective

strategy for causing project failure. In fact, it is probably the most common strategy used by political opponents of projects. However, project failure can also be promoted by providing whatever resources are requested without appropriate controls. For example, an organization could provide the latest state-of-the-art equipment, software, and tools without regard to the actual needs of IT systems to be developed. The problem could be aggravated by not involving managers or users in the resource allocation decisions, leaving those decisions exclusively to the technical project team.

3. *Planning.* Planning is a key element in IT projects. However, too much planning can contribute to project failure. Insisting on a complete specification of a system in advance, including all deliverables, tasks, and sub tasks, can be a failure-promoting strategy. This failure strategy can be especially effective if no revisions are allowed as the project progresses. Similarly, requiring strict adherence to a timetable completely defined in advance also increases the probability of failure. On the other hand, allowing continuous modification of requirements throughout the project is also a dangerous strategy.

4. *Avoiding feedback.* This is the technical equivalent of the management strategy of avoiding user input. Avoiding any discussion of technical issues with users and not allowing the users to test system operational concepts increases the likelihood of failure substantially. Of course, developing complete working systems without user involvement and insisting on user cooperation in the use of these new systems, even if the systems do not benefit the users, will almost guarantee the failure of an IT project.

5. *Technology.* We deliberately mention the technology area last. Its potential contribution to project failure is vastly overestimated; in fact, it is rarely an issue. However, encouraging the development of custom software and tools rather than the use of commercial packages; using the latest technology, especially if it is unproven in operational systems; and avoiding purchases of any capability that can be developed in-house are definitely strategies that promote project failure.

Overall, the key reasons for project failure are mismatched expectations and poor communication. Other common reasons for project failure include forcing project delivery dates and assigning underskilled managers. Lack of high-level business sponsorship and lack of a comprehensive but flexible plan also contribute to failure. Finally, a project may fail simply because it is the execution of a bad idea that is not consistent with the operation of the business. It is important to remember that IT is not the answer to every business problem.

Recognizing the Warning Signs of a Project in Trouble

As projects progress, it is important for a project manager to be aware of the warning signs of projects in trouble. Given the relatively high probability of failure of IT projects, anyone managing IT projects is highly likely to be involved in such a situation. By recognizing the warning signs, a project manager can minimize the resultant failure costs.

The most important warning signs of failure are a lack of agreement on goals and continuously changing requirements. Another key indicator is a lack of a written project implementation plan. Other major danger signals include a rapidly growing budget, repeated contract modifications, and delays in major deliverables. Projects that have evolved to be managed solely by contractor personnel also are likely to be in serious trouble.

On the other hand, successful projects have been found to consistently exhibit a number of factors. Most prominent among these are extensive user involvement and strong management support. Other strategies associated with success are leadership by a skilled, experienced project manager and both a clear requirements statement and a comprehensive, realistic work plan. Use of sound development methodology, such as rapid prototyping, extensive testing, and a thoughtful and detailed transition plan, including comprehensive user training, are also characteristics of successful IT projects.

Conclusion

Successful management of IT projects is very difficult. There are seven important techniques for maximizing the probability of success that can be learned from the hard-earned experience of others:

1. Start with clear goals supported by management
2. Be sure adequate time and resources are available
3. Involve users throughout the process
4. Use education and planning as change management tools
5. Use proven methods and technology, such as rapid prototyping
6. Minimize the increments of change
7. Use behavior modification

Although no management approach can guarantee IT project success, intelligent application of these principles will greatly increase your ability to develop and deploy information systems effectively in public health organizations.

Questions for Review

Read the following short case and answer the questions that are based on it.
Paula Mazzini has recently been hired to head the IT branch at the Department of Public Health of State X. Members of the department have expressed

concerns to Ms. Mazzini that the department has fallen well behind the public health departments of other states in the application of technology to public health activities, and they expect her to help lead the effort to automate the department's functions.

There has been sharp disagreement among top managers regarding what the priorities for new systems development should be. The politically appointed head of the department has expressed a preference for a decision-support system that will provide reports about the department's activities and help to monitor progress in carrying out the department's strategic plan. The department's powerful director of accounting and finance has argued strongly for a new accounting system. The department's director of information systems has insisted that the department should purchase and apply the most advanced IT products available and use them for all systems that will be developed, regardless of which system is developed first.

Top management has finally settled on development of a system for monitoring the incidence of contagious diseases in the state. The head of the Department of Public Health has reluctantly agreed to this choice, although she has shown little enthusiasm for the project. The same is true for the director of accounting and finance, who has announced his intentions to monitor the project's expenditures closely. The choice, however, has been strongly opposed by the chief of the Office of Contagious Diseases, who is comfortable with the existing manual system for collecting data about the incidence of contagious diseases and also fears that automating his office's functions will cost the jobs of many of the office's employees and possibly reduce the scope and compensation of his own job.

Ms. Mazzini's preliminary project plan calls for a project budget of $4.0 million, although she has warned that the actual cost of the new system could vary significantly from this amount. The director of information systems has cut this budget in half. He has also insisted that Ms. Mazzini prepare detailed justifications for every project expenditure exceeding $10,000. Finally, he has insisted that Ms. Mazzini purchase and adapt two commercial state-of-the-art products and base the new system on them, although Ms. Mazzini has pointed out that the technology needs cannot be determined until the system's requirements definition is completed.

The department's director of accounting and finance works in an office almost 30 miles from the site where the new system will be built and installed. He does not understand why Ms. Mazzini cannot commit in advance to a fixed budget for the new project. He also insists that the compensation level for IT staff remain in the lowest quartile for all IT workers in the combined private and public sectors, pointing out that the department's budget is very tight.

Ms. Mazzini inherited only four IT staff members when she accepted the offer to lead the IT branch. She has received permission to hire two additional system designers, four additional programmers, and two additional system analysts to work on developing and testing the new system.

Ms. Mazzini has been analyzing existing processes in the Office of Contagious Diseases and is about to meet with users of the existing system.

1. Identify the political obstacles that Ms. Mazzini faces.
2. How should Ms. Mazzini proceed to deal with the budgeting constraints that she faces?
3. How should Ms. Mazzini deal with the opposition of the chief of the Office of Contagious Diseases to the new system?
4. Explain why Ms. Mazzini cannot commit to a firm budget at the outset of the project.
5. How can Ms. Mazzini attract good candidates to the new IT positions, in light of the fact that salaries are unlikely to be competitive with those paid in the private sector?
6. What qualifications should Ms. Mazzini look for in candidates to fill the new positions?
7. Assuming that employees in the Office of Contagious Diseases share their director's opposition to development of the new system, how can Ms. Mazzini win their support for the new system?
8. How can Ms. Mazzini insure that the new system will meet user needs?
9. How should Ms. Mazzini form her project team? Should she use a steering committee, and if so, what should be the composition of that committee?
10. Explain why the insistence of the director of information systems that Ms. Mazzini base the new system on two commercial produces is both premature and unwise.
11. What warning signs of project failure already exist?

References

1. CHAOS. The Standish Group Report. 1995. Available at: http://www.scs.carleton.ca/~beau/PM/Standish-Report.html.
2. Case Facts: CONFIRM: Computerized Reservation System. 1995. Available at: http://www.scit.w/v.ac.uk/~cm 1995/cbr/cases/case ø6/FOUR.HTM.
3. Clemons E. Evaluation of strategic investments in information technology. *Communications of the ACM*. 1991;34:22–36.

9
Public Health Informatics and Organizational Change

NANCY M. LORENZI AND ROBERT T. RILEY

Learning Objectives

After studying this chapter, you should be able to:

- Describe the four types of organizational change and the impact of each on levels of the public health organization.
- Describe the two types of resistance to change in an organization, and give an example of each type.
- Differentiate between *microchanges* and *megachanges* as classifications of the magnitude of changes.
- Identify the major tenets of small group theories and discuss the usefulness of small group theories as tools in gaining employee buy-in to change brought about by a new or significantly modified information system.
- Define *field theory* and discuss its usefulness in identifying conflicts about change in a public health organization.
- Identify the tasks involved in the stages of (1) assessment, (2) feedback and options, (3) strategy development, (4) implementation, and (5) reassessment in the practical change management model.

Overview

Effective public health informatics requires a project manager to be as conscious of the attitudes and needs of employees as of technical determinations associated with information technology in a public health organization. Bringing informatics to bear on a public health organization necessarily involves change in the way work gets done, and, in general, the natural tendency of people is not always to welcome change. An implementer of an information system must be aware of the types of change typical in an organization and of the impact of those types on various levels of the organization. In addition, a project manager needs to expect, identify, and deal with resistance to change.

To do so, a project manager needs to be conscious of the magnitude of change that a system will create. A knowledge and application of small group theories and field theory can be very useful to a project manager who wants to secure employee commitment to changes resulting from a new or significantly modified system. Finally, a change manager can greatly facilitate the task of guiding employees toward the changes brought about by new systems through involving employees in the changes by the use of practical change management strategies.

Introduction

Effective management of public health informatics projects requires more than making a technical determination of how information technology is to be applied to support an organization's mission. It also requires, for example, an understanding of the employees who will be affected by a new system or a combination of new systems and how they will react. In particular, it requires an understanding that any new information system involves organizational change, perhaps one of the most difficult areas of endeavor in public health management. As Kitch and Yasnoff point out in Chapter 7, developing an effective new public health information system inevitably involves assessing and making changes in business processes with which employees have become comfortable. Imposing organizational changes, particularly in the form of process changes, challenges that comfort level. As a result, many employees will attempt to revert to previous, known ways of completing work. The fact is that many employees are uncomfortable with change and tend to resist it.

A classic example of resistance to the changes brought about by the implementation of public health informatics is the development and implementation of automated immunization registry systems by the Centers for Disease Control and Prevention (CDC). Today's levels of immunizations for preschool children are very high. However, as many as a quarter of the nation's children still do not complete their basic immunization series on time. The societal consequences of this lapse were directly illustrated in the late 1980s, when an epidemic of 50,000 cases of measles resulted in some 11,000 hospitalizations and the death of 130 children nationwide.[1] Such problems motivated The Robert Wood Johnson Foundation to launch the national All Kids Count childhood immunization initiative in 1991. This program sought to identify communities and states that were capable of developing immunization monitoring and follow-up systems to "improve and sustain access to immunizations for preschool children."[2]

Despite this evidence of progress, however, estimates derived from the National Immunization Survey by the Centers for Disease Control and Prevention's National Immunization Program (CDC/NIP) indicated that in 1995, approximately 25% of preschool-age children had not received at least one dose of the recommended series of vaccines.[3] The failure to meet the minimum levels of immunization for preschool-age children—90% coverage for measles; diphtheria and tetanus toxoids and pertussis (DTP); polio; and *Haemophilus influenzae* type b (Hib); and 70% coverage for hepatitis B—is cause for serious concern.[4] Such failures impose not only a public health risk but also financial costs that are associated with diagnosing and treating the illnesses. It is estimated that every dollar spent on measles, mumps, and rubella vaccine can result in a saving of 21 dollars in future medical care costs.[5]

There were many strategies for addressing this issue, but comprehensive, computer-based information systems, at the state or local level, to monitor the immunization status of individual children and to trigger efforts to assist children who are not being immunized was a key change strategy. Public health people said that the information technology systems should be accessible to, and involve the participation of, all immunization providers. The systems should be used to facilitate service delivery through coordinated outreach and follow-up measures. Finally, the systems should be used to determine coverage rates for individual and institutional providers and to target populations in need of more attention.[1]

While the CDC piloted automated immunization registry systems between 1979 and 1985, there was no organized extension of this concept until the measles outbreaks in the early 1990s. Even when the extension did begin, there was no consensus regarding the technology that should be used to support the registry systems, and the cost of starting and maintaining the systems was relatively unknown. Imposition of a national standard was not permitted. Grant applicants were allowed considerable latitude in the direction their efforts would take, in the shape and scope of the immunization registries they would develop, and in the technology they would use.

Why? Quite simply, the imposition of a uniform change—even of a change that many healthcare providers agreed was necessary—is very difficult in public health. Such a change disturbs old work processes and comfortable ways of carrying out the public health mission. As an article concerning the extension of the registry concept explains,

"This initiative illustrates how an idea that is simple in concept can be complex and difficult in practice. The technology and protocols needed to develop registries may be routine in some fields, but they were not easy in public health. The task was complicated by the American system being built around a loose (and often ineffective) intersection of public- and private-sector responsibilities for child health care. These sectors must cooperate in the process of monitoring a series of immunizations for each child over a period of at least two years, during which child and family names, child guardianship, and residences may change. The great data management and technological challenges are compounded by the numerous providers using, entering, and accessing the systems. Also, some groups are suspicious of computerized monitoring of individuals, even for a good cause, and have occasionally objected to immunization registries as invasion of privacy. This tension between the public good and the individual rights of citizens is being played out in other, more publicized and generally more controversial arenas; it may continue to be an issue as the registries reach full operation and if (or when) data linkages are instituted between registries."[1]

Bringing change to public health's established and complex systems is difficult, but such change can be accomplished by application of techniques for skillful change management in public health informatics.

In this chapter, we will discuss the principles of change management in public health informatics. We will begin with a discussion of the four basic types of organizational change. We will then point out how to recognize organizational resistance to change and how to overcome it. In the course of the discussion, we will discuss classic change theories. We will end the chapter with a discussion of practical change management strategies and the presentation of a change management model that we believe is useful to the public health informatics manager interested in implementing and gaining organizational commitment to new systems.

Types of Change

Making the organizational change starts with understanding change and the change process. Changes within an organization can often be identified as one of four types, with the definite possibility of overlap between two or more:

- *Operational change:* one or more changes in the way that the ongoing operations of the business are conducted, such as the automation of a particular area or process
- *Strategic change:* a change in the strategic business direction, such as moving from an inpatient to an outpatient focus
- *Cultural change:* a change in the basic organizational philosophies by which the business is conducted (e.g., implementing a continuous quality improvement system)
- *Political change:* a change or changes in staffing or leadership occurring primarily for political reasons of various types, such as those changes that occur at top levels in government agencies at the patronage job levels

These four different types of change typically have their greatest impacts at different levels of the organization. The following four figures illustrate this point.[6]

Figure 9.1 shows that operational changes tend to have their greatest impact at the lower levels of the organization, right on the firing line. Those working at the upper levels may never notice changes that cause significant stress and turmoil to those called upon to implement the changes in their work.

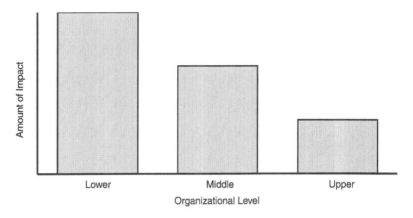

FIGURE 9.1. The relative impact of operational changes by organizational level.

Figure 9.2 illustrates that changes in the organization's strategic direction have potentially significant impact at all levels of the organization. Some similar activities will continue despite the changes; the accountants will still be doing financial reports, for example. Still, the nature and type of virtually everyone's work will be noticeably affected.

Figure 9.3 illustrates that cultural change typically affects all levels, but it has the strongest impact on the middle levels. This phenomenon has occurred countless times in recent years as organizations have introduced cultural

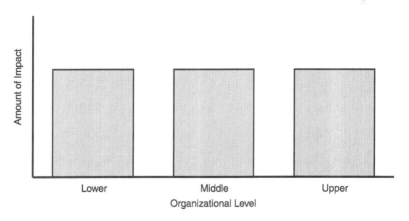

FIGURE 9.2. The impact of strategic changes by organizational level.

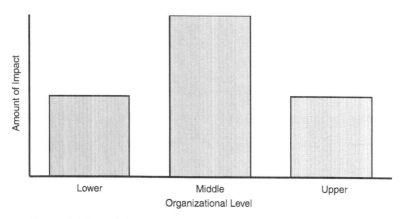

FIGURE 9.3. The relative impact of cultural change by organizational level.

changes that stress values such as employee empowerment, open communications, etc. As a result of cultural change, the traditional roles of middle managers have been changed completely. Mid-level management jobs now call for new skills, attitudes, and behaviors. This transformation of the role of middle managers explains why resistance to cultural change has often been higher in the middle than at lower levels of the organization.

Figure 9.4 shows that the impact of political change is typically felt most at the higher organizational levels. As the term implies, these changes are

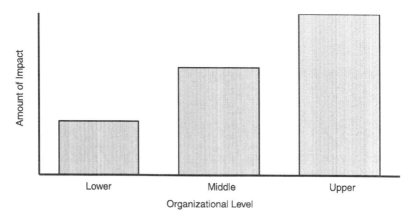

FIGURE 9.4. Impact of political change by organizational level.

typically not made for results-oriented reasons but for reasons such as partisan politics or internal power struggles. When these changes occur in a relatively bureaucratic organization—as they often do—the bottom layer of employees often hardly notices the changes at the top. For such lower-level employees, patients are seen and the floors are cleaned exactly the same as before. After all, performance itself is not the basis of political change within an organization; consequently, the ones who perform the work are not affected that much by it.

In a public health organization, then, as in every other type of organization, the impact of change depends upon (1) the type of change and (2) the organizational level of employees. For example, the impact of an operational change, such as the installation of a new system requiring a revision of business processes, will fall most heavily on the lower level of workers who perform the affected operations. On the other hand, strategic changes hit all organizational levels equally hard, whereas cultural changes most affect the middle level of an organization. Finally, the impact of political change is greatest on upper-level workers. Recognizing these principles, a public health information manager engaged in the installation of a new system will need to concentrate most on overcoming resistance from the operational employees most affected by the changes that the new system brings. Dealing with resistance to change is the subject of the next section of this chapter.

Resistance to Change

Someone once said that the only person who welcomes change is a wet baby. It seems to be part of the human makeup to be most comfortable with the status quo unless that status quo is inflicting discomfort. Even then, people will often resist a *specific* change. This kind of resistance to a specific change is probably part of the phenomenon known as the "devil you know is better than the devil you don't know." Quite often, it is a shock for inexperienced managers to see subordinates resist even a change that these subordinates requested.

Resistance Against What?

There can be countless reasons for resistance to change in a given situation, and the term *resistance to change* is often used very broadly. In order to clarify the term, it is necessary to differentiate between (a) resistance to a particular change, and (b) resistance to the changer, that is, the individual initiating the change.

In resistance to a particular change, the resistance is actually directed against the changes in the system. For example, an employee might resist a new system because the system eliminates his role as the gatekeeper of health information or because the new system requires him to develop additional computer skills to use it.

In resistance to the changer, on the other hand, the resistance occurs because of negative feelings toward the organization in general, toward specific units, toward specific managers, or toward the change agent (the changer). For example, an employee might resist a new system because he perceives that it will permit the organization he has come to dislike to respond more promptly and effectively to a public health emergency, or even because he perceives that a manager whom he dislikes will become more important to the organization after the new system is in operation. We can deplore the employee attitude that fosters such resistance to change, but the fact is that employees are human beings with the capacity to harbor and act on many complex emotions.

A public health organization must address both types of resistance, but first it is critical for the organization to identify the primary type of resistance it is facing.

Moreover, in introducing a new health informatics system, a project manager must recognize the general organizational climate in which the system must function. This climate is shaped both by the present state of organizational dynamics and by the previous history of informatics projects within the organization. In general, a project manager should ask the following questions:

- What is the general organizational climate—positive or negative, cooperative or adversarial, etc.?
- What has been the quality of the *process* used to implement previous informatics systems?
- What has been the technical quality of the informatics systems previously implemented?

Even project managers who are new to an organization inevitably inherit to some degree the organizational climate and history. If that climate and history are negative, the negative "baggage" can be a frustrating burden that adds significantly to the challenge of successfully implementing a new system. On the other hand, the ability to meet this type of challenge is a differentiating factor for truly skilled implementers.

Intensity of Resistance

A skilled implementer of a new system must recognize that resistance can differ significantly in intensity, from the trivial and relatively passive to the ferocious. In addition, the very perception of resistance can vary widely from one observer to another. One manager might perceive that an end user who asks many questions about a new system is very interested and aggressively seeking knowledge about it. Another manager might see the same person as a troublemaker who should just "shut up and listen."

It is a safe assumption that every significant health informatics implementation is going to encounter some resistance but that the intensity of the

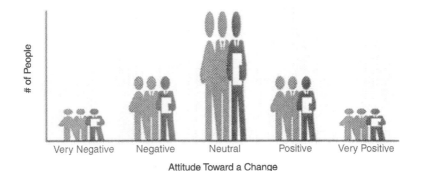

FIGURE 9.5. An organization with a basically neutral attitude toward change

resistance will vary significantly within the organization. Experience has shown that most employees are neutral-to-positive about a change. At the same time, there is always a definite negative component to be managed. The existence of some negativity about a change is not an atypical situation in an organization with decent morale and a history of managing changes reasonably well. The challenge in such organizations is to use sound organizational processes to overcome the negative factors. At the very least, this negative component must be prevented from enlarging. Figure 9.5 depicts a situation in which significant numbers of employees are initially neutral toward a proposed systems change.

Figure 9.6, on the other hand, depicts a very different situation. Here, the proposed change faces a strong negative bias that could arise from various sources. Such a situation is unfortunately common, and it constitutes a strong challenge for systems implementers.

If Figure 9.6 describes an implementer's hell, Figure 9.7 depicts sheer heaven. There is a high positive attitude toward the change, with only a low portion of employees having feelings of resistance. If Figure 9.7 represents an *initial attitude* toward the proposed change, then the organization has done a lot of things right in the past. The general morale must be good, and the aftertaste left by past systems implementations must be quite positive. We can think of these figures—or an even more positive distribution—as our goal. Obviously, if the initial attitude we face is something like Figure 9.6, then our work is cut out for us.

Using Change Attitude Models

Merely identifying the types and levels of change that a systems implementer faces will not solve the change management challenges encountered in imple-

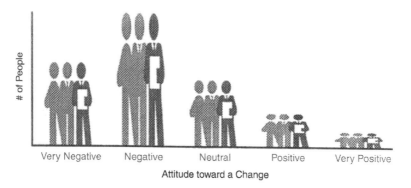

FIGURE 9.6. An organization with a basically negative attitude toward change

menting health informatics systems. However, it is a first step in organizing
an implementer's thinking about these challenges. Identifying and defining
the types and levels of prospective change adequately enables an implementer
to use more effectively the change management strategies described in the
final portion of this chapter.

Magnitudes of Change

Finally, a systems implementer should recognize that resistance is also a function of the magnitude of change[6] that a new system will create.

One useful and simple classification scheme for designating the magnitude of change to be created by a new system is to use the two categories of
microchanges and *megachanges*. Without elaborate efforts to differentiate
between the two, we can define these categories as follows:

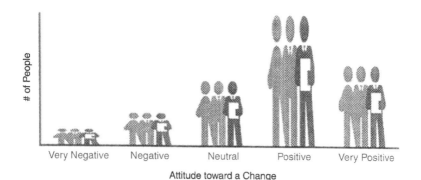

FIGURE 9.7. An organization with a basically positive attitude toward change

- microchanges: differences in degree
- megachanges: differences in kind

As an example of a microchange, consider modifications, enhancements, improvements, and upgrades to an existing system. Such changes are not likely to affect the fundamental nature of the system, nor are they likely to create major changes in existing processes.

On the other hand, a megachange might take the form of a completely new system or a very major revision of an existing system. The changes that either form of megachange would create would fundamentally alter the way work is done.

Although this classification scheme is very simple, it works surprisingly well in communicating within organizations about systems implementation. At the same time, a systems implementer should remember that one person's microchange is another person's megachange.

Classic Change Theories

The literature of change management provides two basic categories of change management theory. These categories are small group theories and field theory.

Small-Group Theories

The *primary group* is one of the classical concepts of sociology, and many sociological theories focus on small-group analysis and interaction process analysis. These theories outline and delineate small-group behavior. Small-group theories help us to understand not only how to make things more successful, but also how to analyze problems when things go wrong. Bales presented one practical application of small-group research in the *Harvard Business Review.*[7] In that article, Bales applies small group principles to running a meeting and makes the following suggestions:

- If possible, restrict committees to seven members.
- Place all members so that they can readily communicate with every other member.
- Avoid committees as small as two or three if a perceived power problem between members is likely to be critical.
- Select committee members who are likely to participate in varying degrees. A group with all highly active participants or all lowly active participants will be difficult to manage.

We have all seen small-group behavior at work. For example, a job candidate is interviewed by a number of people. Information is then collected from the interviewers and shared with a search committee. The search committee selects its top candidate and that person is hired. If the person hired does not work out, a member of the search committee may very well say, "I knew that Mary would not work out, but I didn't say anything because everyone seemed to like her."

Small-group behavior is also at work in employee discussions, reviews, and debates about the introduction of new technology within an organization. If, for instance, if a group opinion leader reveals negative sentiments about a product or service, the group's less-vocal employees will often not challenge those sentiments. For example, a medium-sized organization was selecting a local-area network (LAN) system. While the senior leader wanted one system, some of the other people not only had suggestions about, but also documentation of the superior qualities of another system. During the meeting to decide which system to purchase, the senior leader stated his views first and quite strongly. A couple of the lower-level staff members started to confront the senior person; however, when there was no support from any of the other people present, they did not express their strong preferences for the other system. When the system finally arrived, the senior leader's initial enthusiasm had dwindled. He then confronted the other members of the team as to why they had not made him aware of the shortcomings of the system selected.

Such an example leads us to a change management principle: to manage change effectively, it is imperative for change agents—the people who are seeking to implement a change—to understand how people behave in groups, and especially in small groups. It is especially necessary for the implementer of a new system to identify and cultivate group opinion leaders and to encourage less vocal employees to contribute to discussions of proposed changes.

Field Theory

Kurt Lewin and his students are credited with combining theories from psychology and sociology into field theory in social psychology.[5] Lewin focused his attention on motivation and the motivational concepts that underlie an individual's behavior. Lewin believed that there is tension within a person whenever a psychological need or an intention exists, and the tension is released only when the need or intention is fulfilled. The tension may be positive or negative. These concepts of positive and negative forms of tension were translated into a more refined understanding of conflict situations and, in turn, into what Lewin called "force fields."

Lewin indicated that there are three fundamental types of conflict:

1. The individual stands midway between two positive goals of approximately equal strength. A classic metaphor is the donkey starving between two stacks of hay because of the inability to choose. In information technology, if there are two "good" systems to purchase or options to pursue, then we must be willing to choose.
2. The individuals find themselves between two approximately equal negative goals. Such a choice certainly has been a source of conflict within

many organizations wishing to purchase or build health informatics systems. A combination of the economics, the available technologies, the organizational issues, etc., may well mean that the organization's informatics needs cannot be satisfied with either of the available products—whether purchased or developed in-house. Thus, the decision makers must make a choice of an information system that they know will not completely meet their needs. Their choice will probably be the lesser of two evils.

3. The individual is exposed to opposing positive and negative forces. This conflict is very common in health care organizations today, especially regarding health informatics. It usually occurs between the systems users and the information technology or the financial personnel.

As an example of field theory at work, one hospital decided to implement a new computer system for its clinical laboratory. The hospital chief executive officer (CEO) decided on the maximum price for the system before the planners began calculating system capabilities to meet user needs. The hospital's clinical laboratory was a very complex and busy organization. Consequently, when the needs of the laboratory were fully outlined, the basic hardware and software were more costly than originally budgeted by the CEO. Faced with the positive (an automated laboratory system) and the negative (an underpowered system because of finances), the members of the planning group and the chief information officer (CIO) recommended purchasing a smaller-than-needed laboratory system. As soon as the system was operational, everyone was understandably upset with it. The system did not meet the needs of the clinical laboratory, it did not meet the needs of the physicians and nurses, and ultimately, it did not meet the needs of the total organization. The CEO blamed the head of the clinical laboratory, and eventually that person was replaced. We wonder to this day if that CEO ever understood his role in the creation of this disaster.

Another type of positive-negative conflict occurs frequently between a clinical system's end users and the needs of the total organization. In one hospital, representatives from an obstetrics department did extensive research on the type of clinical information system that would best meet the needs of the department's patients, especially because those patients visit clinicians before, during, and after the birth of the child. On the basis of this research, the department's representatives selected a system (positive force) and then presented their decision to their parent organization's CIO. The hospital's information technology staff could not decide whether the system desired by the obstetrics professionals would blend into the system that they were designing for the total hospital. Therefore, instead of saying yes or no, the CIO said nothing (negative force), greatly increasing stress levels within the organization.

All of these social science theories assist change management leaders in understanding some of the underlying behavior issues as such leaders bring health informatics technology into today's complex health systems.

What Do These Theories Mean
to Change Management?

People can easily be overwhelmed by change, especially within large organizations where they may perceive they have little or no voice in or control over the changes they perceive are descending upon them. The typical response is fight or flight, not cooperation. Managers often interpret such human resistance to change as "stubbornness" or "not being on the team." This managerial reaction solves nothing in terms of reducing resistance to change or gaining acceptance of it. Many managers do not accept that they are regarded as imposing "life-threatening" changes and establishing "no-win" adversarial relationships between management and those below in the organization.

Small-group theory is highly applicable to change in public health organizations because of the way that medical environments are organized. The care of the patient or the education of students entails many small groups. These groups converse and share information and feelings, and strong opinion leaders can sway others to their way of thinking relatively easily.

Kurt Lewin's field theory is also very applicable to implementing changes in public health organizations. It allows the diagramming of the types of conflict situations commonly found in health care. A practical illustration of Kurt Lewin's original force field approach is shown in Table 9.1.

There are several critical points in this force field diagram:

- Every change, whether actual or proposed, is characterized primarily by the goal or termination point intended as a result of the change. The goal is often multiple and in series, such as a change intended to (1) implement a new information system in order to (2) improve patient care.
- Every change creates effects upon people and existing systems, some intended and some unintended.
- In most change processes, the forces operating will be either positive (moving people to accept and cooperate with the change) or negative (driving people to resist, fight, and work against either the change or its manner of implementation.) These forces vary from "strong" to "weak," as represented in the table by the length of the arrow.
- Forces in the diagram are either real or imagined. For example, a negative force in a particular situation might be "fear of facing retraining," which, in fact, is real—the change will require extensive retraining. But another negative force might be "fear of layoff," which, in fact, is mere rumor and thus imaginary; however, these negative forces remain in effect, whether real or imagined, so long as people perceive they might be true.

The conflicts of approach-avoidance that Lewin discusses are also prevalent in public health organizations. Typical questions pondered by employees facing a new system are, If I accept this new system, what will it mean to

TABLE **9.1.** Force field analysis of some of the typical change resistance comments

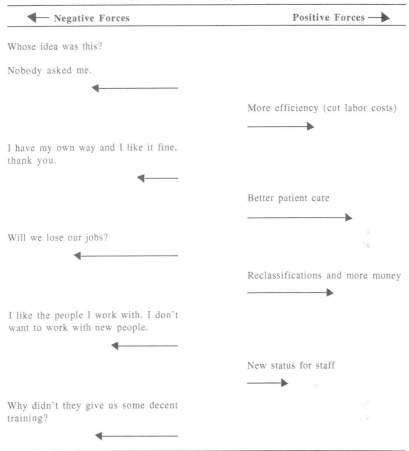

← Negative Forces	Positive Forces →
Whose idea was this?	
Nobody asked me.	
	More efficiency (cut labor costs)
I have my own way and I like it fine, thank you.	
	Better patient care
Will we lose our jobs?	
	Reclassifications and more money
I like the people I work with. I don't want to work with new people.	
	New status for staff
Why didn't they give us some decent training?	

me and my job? Will I have a job? How will it change my role? Will this new system lessen my role? The anxieties expressed by these questions are very clear and very real to the people within the system. It is important to remember that one person's microchanges are often another person's megachanges. As the system designers think they are making a minor change to enhance the total system, an individual end user may see the change as a megachange and resist it vehemently.

When a project implementer is designing the total "people" strategy for any system, it is important to involve the people from the very beginning and to understand clearly how groups function within the organization.

Practical Change Management Strategies

Change management is the process of assisting individuals and organizations to pass from an old way of doing things to a new way of doing things. A change process should both begin and end with a visible acknowledgment or celebration of the impending or just completed change.

Our culture is filled with empowering transitions. Our research indicates that there is not one change management strategy that can be used in every situation. Rather, it is essential for the change management leader to take the time to know the desired state (the vision or goal) and the particular organization and then to develop the appropriate strategies and plans to help facilitate the desired state.

Over the years, we have evolved a core model for the major process of change management. There are many options within this model, but we believe that it is helpful for leaders to have an overview map in mind as they begin to implement new information technology systems. The five-stage model that has proven effective for reducing barriers to technology change begins with an assessment and information-gathering phase.[6]

Assessment

The assessment phase of this model is the foundation for determining the organizational and user knowledge and ownership of the health informatics system that is under consideration. Ideally, this phase of the model begins even before the planning for the technological implementation of the new system. The longer the delay in beginning the assessment, the harder it will be to manage successfully the change and to gain ultimate user ownership.

There are two parts to the assessment phase. The first is to *inform* all potentially affected people, in writing, of the impending change. This written information need not be lengthy or elaborate, but it should alert everyone to the changes in process.

The second part involves *collecting information* from those involved in the change by the use of both surveys and interviews. The survey instrument should be sent to randomly selected members of the affected group. One person in 10 might be appropriate as a survey sample if the affected group is large. Five to 10 open-ended questions should assess the individuals' current perceptions of the potential changes, their issues of greatest concern about these changes, and their suggestions to reduce those concerns. Recording and analyzing the responders' demographics will allow more in-depth analysis of the concerns raised by these potentially affected people.

In the personal face-to-face interviews with randomly selected people at all levels throughout the affected portions of the organization, it is important to listen to the stories the people are telling and to assess their positive and negative feelings about the proposed health informatics system. These interviews should help in ascertaining the current levels of positive and negative feelings; what each person envisions the future will be, both with and without the new system; what each interviewee could contribute to making that vision a reality; and how the interviewee could contribute to the future success of the new system. These interviews provide critical insights for the actual implementation plan. Often, those people interviewed become advocates—and sometimes even champions—of the new system, thus easing the change process considerably.

An alternative or supplement to the one-on-one interviews is focus-group sessions. These sessions allow anywhere from five to seven people from across the organization to share their feelings and ideas about the current system and the new system.

Feedback and Options

The information obtained from surveys, interviews, and/or focus groups must now be analyzed, integrated, and packaged for presentation to both top management and to those directly responsible for the technical implementation. This is a key stage for understanding the strengths and weaknesses of the current plans, for identifying the major organizational areas of both excitement and resistance (positive and negative forces), for identifying the potential stumbling blocks, for understanding the vision the staff holds for the future, and for reviewing the options suggested by the staff for making the vision come true. If this stage occurs early enough in the process, data from the assessment stage can be given to the new system developers for review.

In the model, this phase is important in order to establish that the organization *learns* from the inputs of its staff and begins to act strategically in the decision and implementation processes.

Strategy Development

This phase of the model allows those responsible for the change to use the information collected to develop *effective change strategies* from an organizational perspective. These strategies must focus on a visible, effective process to "bring on board" the affected people within the organization. This process could include newsletters, focus groups, discussions, one-on-one training, and confidential "hand-holding." The latter can be especially important for professionals such as physicians who may not wish to admit ignorance and/or apprehension about the new system.

Implementation

This phase of our model refers to the implementation of the change management strategies determined to be needed for the organization, not to the implementation of the new system. The implementation of the change strategies developed must begin before the actual implementation of the new system. These behaviorally focused efforts consist of a series of steps, including informing and working with the people involved in a systematic and timely manner. This step-by-step progression toward the behavioral change desired and the future goals is important to each individual's acceptance of the new system. This is an effective mechanism for tying together the new technology implementation action plan with the behavioral strategies.

Reassessment

Six months after the new system is installed, the organization should conduct a behavioral-effects data-gathering process. This stage resembles the initial assessment stage—written surveys and one-on-one and/or focus-group interviews. Data gathered from this stage allow measurement of the acceptance of the new system, providing the basis for fine-tuning. This process also serves as input to the evaluation of the implementation process. It assures all the participants that their inputs and concerns are still valued and sought, even though the particular implementation has already occurred.

Conclusion

Change is difficult, but eventually it must occur. Successful stories of change continue to grow. Some of the change is smooth and some of the change is difficult, but nonetheless change is occurring in public health organizations.

It is not always easy to know exactly why a particular group resists change. However, experience shows that an intelligent application of our basic five-step change model—coupled with a sound technological implementation plan—leads to more rapid and more productive introductions of technology into organizations. The process can be expensive in terms of time and energy, but the cost is nowhere near the cost of an expensive technical system that never gains real user acceptance.

Perhaps most important, overall success in implementing change requires an emotional commitment to success on the part of all involved. The employees must believe that the project is being done for the right reasons—namely, to further the delivery of higher quality, more cost-effective health care. If employees generally perceive that a project is aimed at just "saving a quick buck" or at boosting someone's ego or status, that project is doomed to fail.

Questions for Review

Answer the questions that follow this short case:

The Department of Public Health in State X is in the process of installing a new system that will automate the collection of data related to stream pollution caused by runoff from coal mines. In the past, this data has been collected manually from handwritten reports submitted by public health assessors who sample streams, then entered manually into the minicomputer housing the department's public health data. Under the new system, the state's public health assessors will need to learn to use laptop computers housing programs that permit entry, collection, and transmission of data directly to the department's minicomputer. Personnel in the Data Assembly Unit of the department's Branch of Environmental Health will no longer enter data manually into the minicomputer, and department officers have not yet decided what duties those personnel will be assigned to, once the new system has been installed. The Chief of the Data Assembly Unit, Herman Wells, is a vocal opponent of the new system. He is well liked and well respected by his staff. Under the new system, Mr. Wells will no longer be responsible for assembling reports on stream pollution related to coal mines, a major part of his job under the old system; instead, these reports will be produced automatically under the new system. Mr. Wells has become embittered about the failure of the department to promote him after his many years of faithful service, and he holds a grudge against his boss and the department's officers; in fact, he wants the department to fail in its efforts to control stream pollution so that his arguments about how to effect the control will be justified. The Director, Branch of Environmental Health, is Homer Farren. Mr. Farren also is concerned about the new system; he fears that the automation will lessen his influence with Mary Rory, Head of the Bureau of Health Planning and Statistics, to whom he reports. Under the new system, Ms. Rory will no longer have to rely on Mr. Farren for compilation and distribution of stream pollution reports. Ms. Rory and other senior officers of the department view the new system as a much-needed improvement that will speed the reporting of stream pollution information and permit more effective action to prevent the pollution. They also see the new system as less expensive in the long run; it will permit eventual reductions in staffing levels and salary expense.

The director of the new information system project is Hank Greenberg. Mr. Greenberg has scheduled a meeting with all members of the Data Assembly Unit, including its chief, in an effort to explain the advantages of the new system and to gain employee buy-in. He fears that there will be strong resistance to the change brought about by the new system, and he is especially concerned about the influence that the unit's chief, Herman Wells, will have on the opinions of other members of the unit.

1. Identify the type(s) of change that the new system will create with respect to (a) the public health assessors, (b) the staff of the Data Assembly Unit, (c) Herman Wells, and (d) Homer Farren.
2. In which of these affected groups or individuals is resistance to the change likely to be strongest?
3. Which of the groups or individuals likely will be *least affected* by the change?

4. Should Homer Farren's resistance be classified as *resistance to a particular change* or as *resistance to the changer*?
5. Where would Hank Greenberg likely encounter the greatest intensity of resistance?
6. Describe the *organizational climate* into which the change will be introduced.
7. Describe the *magnitude of the change* for each player in this situation.
8. Explain how Hank Greenberg can use small-group theory in dealing with resistance to the change.
9. According to field theory, what are the positive and the negative forces in this situation?
10. According to field theory, what is the fundamental type of conflict that Hank Greenberg must deal with?
11. Explain how Mr. Greenberg can use the Practical Change Management Strategies model to smooth the transition to the new system? How can he use that model to address and minimize resistance he is likely to encounter in meeting with the Data Assembly Unit?

References

1. National Vaccine Advisory Committee. The measles epidemic: The problems, barriers, and recommendations. *JAMA* 1991;266:1547–1552.
2. Atkinson WL, Orenstein WA, Krugman S. The resurgence of measles in the United States, 1989–1994. *Annu Rev Med* 1992;43:451–463.
3. National, state, and urban area vaccination coverage levels among children aged 19–35 months—United States, April 1994–March 1995. *MMWR Morb Mortal Wkly Rep* 1996;45:145–150.
4. Vaccination coverage of 2-year-old children—United States, January–March, 1994. *MMWR Morb Mortal Wkly Rep* 1995;44:142–143, 149–150. Summarized in Gostin LO, Lazzarini P. Childhood immunization registries: A national review of public health information systems and the protection of privacy. *JAMA* 1995;274:1793–1799.
5. Satcher D. Keep up the progress on childhood immunization. *Public Health Rep* 1994;109:593.
6. Lorenzi NM, Riley RT. *Organizational Aspects of Health Informatics: Managing Technological Change.* New York: Springer-Verlag; 1994.
7. Bales RF. In conference. *Harvard Business Review.* 1954;32:44–50.
8. Deutsch M, Krauss RM. *Theories in Social Psychology.* New York: Basic Books; 1965.
9. Lorenzi NM, Mantel MI, Riley RT. Preparing your organization for technological change. *Healthc Inform* 1990;7(12):33–34.

10
Privacy, Confidentiality, and Security of Public Health Information

WILLIAM A. YASNOFF

Learning Objectives

After studying this chapter, you should be able to:

- Explain why it is important both practically and legally for public health organizations to maintain the confidentiality of information about individuals and to avoid releasing aggregate data that could identify an individual or a cohort.
- List and briefly describe the six principles of fair information practices.
- Describe a rule of thumb that can be used in determining the adequacy of a denominator in the release of aggregate public health data.
- List and describe the steps that a public health organization should take in establishing confidentiality agreements regarding health information.
- Describe at least four characteristics that a good password system should have.
- Describe the features of (1) smart cards, (2) biometrics, and (3) cryptography as computer security devices.
- Explain ways that public health organizations can prevent unauthorized access to their Internet-based systems and guard against attacks by intruders.
- List and describe two ways by which a public health organization can detect potential intruders of their systems.

Overview

Public health organizations need to protect the confidentiality of sensitive, identifying information about individuals to maintain the willingness of individuals to disclose such information and to adhere to laws affecting the handling of health information. Safeguarding the privacy, confidentiality, and security of such information is an important undertaking. A public health organization needs to adhere to the basic principles of fair information practices, as incorporated into the Privacy Act of 1974, and to develop and enforce confidentiality policies that govern the handling and release of public health data. Among security measures that an organization can institute to protect the integrity of information and guard against unauthorized access to it are passwords, smart cards, biometrics, and cryptography. In addition, a public health organization needs to be especially vigilant about potential intrusions into its computer systems, and particularly of those systems that rely or reside on the Internet. The use of proxy servers, session password mechanisms, and firewalls can help guard against mischievous attacks from the Internet, while intrusion detection measures can help an organization detect efforts to compromise systems.

Introduction

The practice of public health requires that we have access to very sensitive, identifying information about individuals. This type of information is essential if we are to perform our tasks of preventing and controlling the spread of disease. Access to this information, however, requires a careful balancing of the rights of individuals and the needs of the community. To date, public health practice has an excellent record of protecting the confidentiality of information obtained from and about individuals. This record helps maintain the confidence of the community and insures the continued willingness of individuals to disclose sensitive information to public health officials. Often, our ability to protect this information depends on statutory authority that prohibits any access or use of such information by individuals or groups who are outside the realm of public health.

We also have an obligation to disclose information about the health status of the community and trends of disease. In meeting this obligation, we must not compromise any individual's identity in releasing statistical information about the community. Avoiding indirect identification of individuals from the use of aggregate statistics is a continuing challenge.

Finally, as information systems are more widely applied in public health, the difficulties of protecting information increase. The public correctly perceives that all information systems that provide improved access to data for worthwhile and laudable purposes simultaneously increase opportunities for misuse of information. However, there are many tools and techniques available to insure that the electronic information is used only for appropriate purposes. Developers of public health information systems must be familiar with the application of these techniques.

In this chapter, we will define and discuss the concepts of privacy, confidentiality, and security as they relate to handling information about individuals in the practice of public health. We will briefly discuss the fair information practices that should be used by public health officials in the handling of such confidential information and the policies and procedures that public health organizations need to follow in this regard. We will conclude the chapter with a discussion of security arrangements that public health organizations need to make in order to prevent unauthorized access to the information.

Definitions

Terms such as *privacy*, *confidentiality*, and *security* often are subject to varying interpretations. In fact, they are often confused with one another. Before proceeding further, we will define these key terms.

Privacy may be defined as the right of individuals to hold information about themselves in secret, free from the knowledge of others. This definition implies that private information has not been disclosed to any third party.

Confidentiality is the assurance that information about identifiable persons, the release of which would constitute an invasion of privacy for any individual, will not be disclosed without consent (except as allowed by law). The exception for legal release of confidential data without an individual's consent may cause some concern until we realize that this exception implies "community" consent. Confidential data should never be released without consent—but community consent implies that the consent itself takes the form of legal requirements. In this context, *identifying information* represents any information, including but not limited to demographic information, that will identify or may reasonably lead to the identification of one or more specific individuals.

Security relates to the mechanisms by which confidentiality policies are implemented in computer systems, including provisions for access control, integrity of data, and availability of systems. Because security is, in this definition, dependent on and derived from confidentiality, it makes no sense to ask information technology personnel to develop a security plan until and unless the organization already has confidentiality policies in place.

A good analogy to the relationship between confidentiality and security is an access control system for a large building. A locksmith can provide security via excellent locks of various types to prevent and control entry to areas throughout the building. However, it is the confidentiality policy that tells the locksmith who gets the keys to which room. Without good confidentiality policies, security cannot be effective.

Fair Information Practices

The basis for confidentiality policy in public health is "fair information practices," a set of ideas defined in a 1973 study[1] and incorporated into the federal

Privacy Act of 1974, which has been discussed in Chapter 4. They represent a set of principles that define the responsibilities of an organization that holds confidential, identifying information about individuals. Although the Privacy Act applies only to federal agencies, the principles of fair information practices form an excellent basis for the confidentiality policy of any public health agency. The concept of fair information practices is built on the foundation that confidential, identifying information collected by a public health organization should possess the qualities of (1) relevance, (2) integrity, (3) a written purpose, (4) a need-to-know access, (5) the capacity for correction, and (6) consent of the individual or the community from whom the information was obtained.

Relevance

All information collected about individuals should be necessary and relevant to public health or be otherwise required by law. It is always tempting to collect whatever information that is easily collected under the assumption that it may be useful some day for something. However, the relevance principle requires us to avoid gathering information under such an assumption. The relevance principle recognizes that individuals are entitled to privacy: the benefits of information collection must therefore outweigh any individual privacy concerns. Another important aspect of information relevancy is that the collection of information should not be overly burdensome, intrusive, or coercive.

Integrity

Once information is collected, its integrity must be protected. The concept of integrity therefore means that we must take reasonable measures to prevent loss, interception, or misuse of the information. No unauthorized alteration or destruction of information may be permitted.

Written Purpose

All information collected should be consistent with written public health purposes and/or required by law. In practice, this concept means that every database must have a written purpose or purposes, and the usage of information in the database must be restricted to the stated purpose(s). A linkage of multiple databases should be considered a new database requiring a new written purpose.

Need-to-Know Access

All confidential Information should be accessible only on a need-to-know basis, both internally and externally. Public health organizations should require that all personnel sign confidentiality agreements at least annually. Moreover, an employee's access to confidential information should be terminated when duties change and the employee no longer has a job-related need to view the information. A public health organization should also prohibit an employee's disclosure of confidential information to someone who does not have the need to know it. Such a re-disclosure policy is essential to prevent loss of control of confidential information. After all, if such information is disclosed to an appropriate person who is allowed re-disclose it to someone else, it is no longer possible for the organization to enforce a confidentiality policy. Finally, a public health organization should submit any information it plans to disclose to an external entity for research purposes to an institutional review board (IRB)—for both practical and legal reasons. As John Christiansen points out in Chapter 4, the federal Health Insurance Portability and Accountability Act (HIPAA) permits disclosure of identifying information without an individual's consent for research purposes, but the law specifically recognizes the role of an IRB in such disclosures.

Opportunity to Correct Errors

Individuals should have access to information about themselves and the ability to correct this information to the extent allowed by law. As John Christiansen points out in Chapter 4, both the Privacy Act of 1974 and HIPAA make provisions for individuals to access information about them and to correct the information. Implicit in such provisions is the requirement that a public health organization maintain a public list of all databases so that individuals are aware that information about them may be in use. In fact, a key principle of fair information practice is that there must not be any secret databases. A public list of databases should contain the name of the database, a description of the information included, and a list of the information sources, excluding confidential sources. A system must be in place to respond to inquiries regarding information held about an individual, and this system must allow the individual to correct such information. As with credit reporting data, disputed data must be marked to indicate that the individual in question does not agree that the information is correct.

Consent

All information must be collected with the consent of the individual or else the community to whom it pertains. As we have indicated, community consent implies a legal basis that overrides the privacy interest of an individual. The consent must be informed. In the absence of community consent, a public health organization must disclose to an individual the purpose of the information collection, the data protections in place, and the consequences of withholding information, if any.

Organizational Policies and Procedures to Ensure Confidentiality of Information

It is essential for public health organizations to have appropriate confidentiality policies and procedures in place. These policies must be sufficiently comprehensive to encompass electronic information systems. Unfortunately, even today many public health agencies either do not have such policies or else have policies that do not fully conform to the principles of fair information practices.[2]

Confidentiality policies for restricting release of data are essential to prevent the inadvertent identification of individuals in the course of a release of data. All data releases by a public health organization should be reviewed, either manually or through use of an automatic computer-based approach. To control the potential for indirect identification, an organization should give special attention to the denominator of any count. For example, disclosing that one person in a population of 1 million has a particular health condition is not likely to result in the identification of that person. However, as the denominator decreases, the possibility that a released statistic will allow identification through the use of other available information increases. There is no absolutely secure cutoff for the size of the denominator. However, one rule of thumb that has proved to be useful is that the denominator must be greater than 50 in a population, or greater than 10 for a cohort. Table 10.1 provides examples of this rule of thumb in action.

Insuring that all personnel are familiar with confidentiality policies is essential. Confidentiality agreements signed upon employment and at least

TABLE 10.1. Examples of statistical denominators that are usually either adequate or inadequate to prevent inadvertent identification of an individual or a cohort: Rule of thumb method

Example	Adequate or Inadequate?
A public health assessment presents data showing that one person in a population of 50,000 has been diagnosed with metallic mercury poisoning.	Adequate
A study of eight families living in a remote Alaskan village presents data showing that one of the families has a head of household with a sexually transmitted disease.	Inadequate
A study presents data showing that one person in a population of 500,000 has a rare blood disorder.	Adequate
A table in a public health consultation presents data showing that of 30 different groups using water from 40 community wells, two groups have members with elevated levels of lead in their blood.	Adequate

· annually thereafter should include the definition of confidential information and indicate that such information is available on a need-to-know basis only and should not be re-disclosed. The agreement should direct the employee to ask his or her supervisor about any questions related to confidentiality. It should also indicate that confidentiality breaches will result in disciplinary action and that confidentiality must be maintained indefinitely.

Confidentiality agreements signed by data system administrators should contain special provisions, inasmuch as data system administrators have access to extensive confidential information because of their computer system responsibilities. Such provisions should indicate that information is to be used only as needed for administration of the computer systems and that access granted to others should only be in accordance with established policies and procedures. If possible, listed disciplinary actions for violations of the agreement by the data system administrators should include the possibility of termination on the first offense. If these individuals are not extremely sensitive to the issues of confidentiality, the entire organization will be at risk.

Security

Once appropriate confidentiality policies are in place, security mechanisms to ensure the enforcement of those policies must be established. These may be divided into authentication, insuring that the identity of the user is confirmed; data integrity, protecting information from of unauthorized alteration; and availability, preventing interference with system access for authorized users.

Authentication is at the heart of any security system. The choices regarding what access is provided or denied depend entirely on correct identification of the user. There are three basic methods to determine the identity of a computer user: (1) what the user knows (password); (2) what the user has (smart card); and (3) what the user is (biometrics).

Passwords

Passwords are by far the most common form of user authentication. Each user has a specific (usually self-chosen) combination of characters known to him or her and the system for use as a password. Entering this hopefully secret combination of characters identifies the user.

However, passwords have many practical drawbacks. First, most people choose very short dictionary words as passwords. A potential intruder may easily guess such passwords. The length of a password is important, because it determines the number of possible combinations. For example, a combination lock that opens with a single number is not nearly as secure as one with three numbers. Just so, a longer password is more secure from such guessing or the use of a trial and error method to determine a user's password. It is also very undesirable to use any dictionary words as a password, since many software packages exist that will simply try a dictionary's words in an attempt to gain unauthorized access.

Good passwords should be at least eight characters in length. They should also have more than one word connected with one or more digits or special characters. A good working model for passwords is "word1; word2." Passwords should not contain any familiar numbers, names, or words; for example, they should not consist of telephone numbers, birth dates, anniversary dates, Social Security or driver's license numbers, parts of a user's name or names of family members, or parts of a user's address, city, home town, etc. Passwords should never be written down anywhere—there is no security in an excellent password written on a Post-It™ note attached to a computer screen.

It is also important for a user to remember that if a password is entered over a network, particularly on the Internet, that password will travel "in the clear" unless it is entered on a secure page (such a page will have a closed lock or an unbroken key in the lower left corner of the browser). Passwords sent in the clear can easily be intercepted and used by hackers for unauthorized entry.

Finally, a password should have a short life. A user needs to change a password every two or three months. After all, the longer a password is in existence, the greater is the time frame by which a potential intruder can attempt to guess it or otherwise discover its nature.

Listed below are some of the password requirements imposed by the Centers for Disease Control and Prevention (CDC) on users of its systems:

1. A passcode is required to be created to gain access to all agency information technology systems.
2. The minimum allowable length for reusable passcodes is six characters.
3. Reusable passcodes must have a minimum effective life of at least one day, but no more than 90 days; identical or similar passcode reuse is prohibited for a minimum of 18 months.
4. Repeated unsuccessful attempts to login result in account suspension (this is the most effective means to prevent automated attacks at guessing passcodes for accounts).
5. Passcode sharing is prohibited.
6. Passcode content must be protected from disclosure to others and may not be displayed on the screen or displayed at the desk environment where it might be viewed.
7. Creating shortcuts for automatic entering of a passcode is prohibited.

Smart Cards

Smart cards are increasingly being used to improve the security of the authentication process. A smart card is a small device—the size of a credit card or even smaller—that displays a random number that changes periodically (usually every 60 seconds). The number displayed is included as part of the user password. Therefore, a user must not only provide a memorized password, but also must possess the smart card and enter a displayed number to gain access to a system.

Even if this combined password is intercepted, it is not helpful to a potential intruder, because its validity lasts no more than one minute. This type of improved authentication is strongly recommended for system administration personnel, because improper access to an account provides total access to both the system in question and perhaps the entire network.

The major disadvantages of smart cards are the possible inconvenience of having them always available, their cost (about $50 each), and the overhead of administration—keeping track of who has which smart card. Also, it is necessary for the clocks of the central computer and the smart cards to be synchronized to be sure both sides generate the same password. These challenges are not terribly difficult to overcome and, as a result, smart cards are rapidly increasing in popularity. Such cards are currently used at CDC to provide secure remote access to internal systems.

Biometrics

Probably the ultimate authentication is through biometrics: retinal scanning, fingerprint scanning, or voice identification. Fingerprint scanning in particular is now commercially available; it uses inexpensive devices (cost: approximately $100) and provides reliable and repeatable results. In Chapter 1, Patrick O'Carroll presents a scenario involving use of a thumbprint scanner now commercially available as an authentication device. Eventually, as such fingerprint scanning devices become built into computer keyboards, the use of this technique for authentication is likely to become much more widespread.

Cryptography

Protecting data integrity goes beyond authentication. Information must also be secure while in transit. Accomplishing this goal involves the use of *cryptography*—encoding messages so that they are intelligible only to the proper recipient. On a practical level, cryptography involves converting messages composed of "plain text" into new messages readable only with a key possessed by a user. Cryptography is a substantial discipline in its own right, and a complete description of it is beyond the scope of this text. Luckily, a working knowledge of very basic cryptography is more than adequate for its application in information systems.

The two basic elements of cryptography are the key and the algorithm. The *key*, analogous to a physical key used to open a lock, is a group of characters or numbers used to encode or transform a message into a form designed to be unreadable. The use of larger keys provides more security by making it difficult for a potential code breaker to test every possible combination of characters or numbers. At present, a key length of 128 bits is considered sufficient to provide a very high level of security. However, as computer power increases, key lengths will need to expand to ensure that a potential intruder's testing every possible combination remains impractical.

The *algorithm* is the method or steps used to apply the key to the message, producing an encoded result. Modern cryptography typically uses algorithms that have been fully disclosed and are well known. This use of algorithms allows standard devices and software to be available to perform encryption at very low cost.

One cryptographic technique growing in popularity is *public key cryptography*. With this technique, each user has both a public and private key. The *public key* is typically published in widely available directories, much like phone books. Anyone who desires to send a message to a person can encode it by use of the public key. Decoding the message, however, requires use of the *private key*, which is known only to the recipient. Therefore, anyone can send a message that can be read only by the desired receiver.

This technique is most widely used with the RSA cryptography algorithm. The RSA algorithm was invented in 1978 by Ron Rivest, Adi Shamir, and Leonard Adleman. This cryptographic method, which recently was placed in the public domain, requires a public key that is the product of multiplying two very large numbers, while the private key consists of the two factors. The security of the method depends on the difficulty of determining the factors of an extremely large number. A user may increase the security of an encrypted message by utilizing larger key sizes. Because the RSA algorithm is now in the public domain and can be used without payment of royalties, its popularity is likely to increase.

More recently, a more complex algorithm has been proposed for use as a federal standard. Called *Rijndael* (pronounced Rhine-doll), this data encryption formula was developed by Belgian cryptographers Joan Daemen of Proton World International and Vincent Rijmen of Katholieke Universiteit Leuven.

When transmitting information over a network, especially a public network like the Internet, a user should use encryption to prevent interception or alteration of the data.

Systems Availability and Computer Security

Availability of systems is another important aspect of computer security. Simply denying access to unauthorized users is not sufficient. Information systems must also be available to those users who need them. Making the systems available can be a difficult and challenging task, especially in the case of systems on the Internet.

Recently, there have been a number of high-profile attacks on Web sites; these attacks effectively paralyze affected sites by presenting an overwhelming number of requests for service. Known as "denial of service attacks," they are very difficult to defend against. Because even unauthorized users can attempt to gain access to a system, a large number of such attempts can effectively preclude usage by everyone.

In public health, this same type of scenario could occur in an emergency situation. A public health crisis might result in an overwhelming number of legitimate public requests for service to public health Web sites. Such crisis-level usage could effectively prevent use of the sites by public health officials and other emergency responders.

To address this problem, public health agencies must have a backup emergency Internet connection through an alternate Internet service provider. Such an arrangement allows emergency traffic to utilize this alternate channel. Only official personnel should be informed of this backup address.

The overall solution to "denial of service" attacks will require some changes to the Internet itself. Mechanisms will need to be developed to disconnect users who are rapidly generating huge numbers of repeated requests for service. Because these attacks represent a major problem for all Internet sites, it is highly likely that an effective preventive strategy will be developed soon. Meanwhile, designers of public health information systems must provide alternate access paths that can be activated in emergencies.

Internet Security

As Marion Ball indicates in Chapter 3, the Internet has been a boon to the development of public health information systems, because it provides a common user interface and a communications protocol accessible with Internet browser software. Information system developers, however, must understand the basic principles of Internet security to utilize this new tool properly.

The first of these principles is that a computer is not necessarily protected from malicious Web sites during the use of browser software. In particular, the Java language can run programs that may potentially have harmful consequences for a user's computer. To deal with this potential problem, some organizations have implemented "proxy servers" for Web browsing. The use of a proxy server means that the browser software does not run on a user's machine, but rather on another, "proxy" machine. The user's screen simply duplicates the view of the screen of the proxy machine. In this configuration, only the proxy machine is at risk from potentially harmful Java programs.

In the absence of a proxy server, the best strategy for gaining protection from potential damage from Web sites is to be sure that key files have been backed up. Of course, file backup is an essential part of computer usage in any case, and it should be a regular habit. If a file contains information that is important to a user or to an organization, then it is worth taking the time to create a backup regularly. Ideally, such backups should be done every day.

A second principle is that a user should employ one of two basic mechanisms currently in use to transmit and receive information in a secure fashion from a Web site. Both mechanisms involve the establishment of a "session password" used to encrypt information traveling back and forth between the user and the Web site. The first of these mechanisms, S-HTTP or "secure http," creates secure envelopes for messages that are then transmitted to and from the Web site. The other mechanism, "secure sockets layer" or SSL, creates a secure "pipe" between the user's machine and the Web server; SSL is transparent to any application, not just to a Web browser.

Either of these security mechanisms will result in a high level of resistance to message interception or alteration. Current Internet browsers have settings for the length of keys for secure applications. A user should be certain that key lengths are set to at least 128 bits. Browsers may initially be set for 40-bit keys that are inadequate to provide good security. After a user connects to a secure site, the security icon in the lower left-hand corner of the browser (either a key or a lock) will be closed or whole, indicating that security is in place. It is unwise to enter any sensitive information into a Web site unless the page into which the information will be entered is secure.

A third principle to follow in insuring the integrity of computer systems connected to the Internet is to use a firewall. In this context, firewalls have nothing to do with preventing the spread of flames or smoke, but rather with protecting computer systems from inappropriate access. A *firewall* is a separate, dedicated computer system that filters the packets of information from the Internet. Each packet of information has an indication of its source; therefore, a firewall can be programmed to intercept and discard packets from inappropriate sources. This filtering process provides substantial protection against access from inappropriate users. However, it is far from foolproof, because it is possible for a hacker to create Internet packets that appear to originate from a source other than the true sender.

A firewall can also limit the types of access provided to Internet users. It is possible, for example, to remotely log on to another system on the Internet and have access to some or all of the commands and information on that system. A firewall can prevent requests for log-on from reaching any of the systems inside the firewall. By configuring the firewall to allow only Web access, an organization can attain a significant degree of protection.

To minimize the potential for attack on the firewall system itself, an organization should take certain precautions. These precautions include mounting all disks as read only, so that a potential intruder cannot alter any information. Eliminating all unnecessary commands and services and allowing only a very small number of user accounts (that have very long and complex passwords) also is helpful. Although the percentage of Internet users trying to break into systems is quite small, the number of Internet users is so large (over 100 million people) that it is inevitable that attempts to inappropriately access your systems will be made.

Intrusion Detection

Another important element in the security plan is intrusion detection. After all, without a system in place to detect potential intruders, an organization will never find any. It is important to look for unusual access patterns or activities. There are two major types of evaluation techniques to permit an organization to detect unusual access patterns and activities: statistical and rule-based. *Statistical techniques* look at patterns of usage. For example, most systems have peaks of usage in mid-morning and mid-afternoon. A sudden surge of user activity in the middle of the night would therefore be highly suspicious and would require investigation.

Rule-based intrusion detection involves the assessment of certain conditions, the violation of which would indicate a possible problem. For example, if seven users try to log in simultaneously under the same user account, such an event would be highly likely to represent an organized attack. Most systems utilize the rule that a user account is locked after three failed attempts to enter a password. This is a good example of rule-based intrusion detection. Application of this rule makes it very difficult for a potential attacker to try thousands of passwords to gain illicit entry into a system.

In short, it is wise to assume that all systems are subject to attempted unauthorized use. An organization should plan accordingly. Above all, an organization should not make the mistake of thinking that its systems are too unimportant or uninteresting to potential hackers.

Conclusion

Computer security requires serious attention from knowledgeable personnel. It is important to back up key files on a daily basis and to use strong encryption for transmitting or receiving sensitive data. Users should be required to employ long passwords that are not dictionary words or other easy-to-guess information. Computer network security, in particular, requires expertise in authentication techniques, in encryption, and in deploying firewalls. Once comprehensive confidentiality policies are in place, it is possible to develop a security system to enforce those policies effectively.

Questions for Review

1. Briefly explain why community consent to release of public health information overrides individual consent.
2. Differentiate between *privacy, confidentiality*, and *security*, as those terms relate to public health information.
3. Assume that a public health employee has signed a confidentiality agreement that incorporates a need-to-know provision and prohibits re-disclosure of any information to which she gains access within her public health organization's systems. The agreement's term of enforcement is indefinite. Discuss the applicability of this agreement with regard to the following situations, assuming the information she has accessed is relevant to a project on which she is working:
   a. The employee discusses individual information she obtains with a colleague working on the same project.

   b. At lunch, the employee reveals the individual information to a friend
       working in a commercial enterprise not affiliated with the public health
       organization.
   c. During a weekend trip, the employee discusses the individual
       information with her husband.
   d. After the employee leaves this job, she begins self-employment and
       discusses the individual information with her best customers.
4. Robert Jameson, an epidemiologist for the Department of Public Health in
   State X, was born on May 5, 1965. His wife Mary works for the department
   as a sexually transmitted disease specialist. Mr. Jameson is about to change
   the password he uses to access the department's databases. Examine all
   the password possibilities below and determine whether each is suitable
   for use as a secure password. If the password is not suitable, explain why.
   a. Bob65
   b. Schlerx342
   c. 050565
   d. MarySTD
   e. Rjameson0565
   f. RJ1965
5. List the advantages and disadvantages of (1) smart cards and (2) biometrics
   as authentication devices for users of public health information systems.
6. Differentiate between a *key* and an *algorithm* in an encryption system,
   and explain the basic features of public key cryptography.
7. You are the principal data administrator in a public health department.
   Your department operates systems on the Internet. Explain how you can
   (1) guard against denial of service attacks, (2) protect computers from
   malicious Web sites while organization employees are browsing the Web,
   (3) ensure the integrity of your organization's information systems from
   external attack, and (4) detect efforts of intruders to gain access to your
   organization's systems.

References

1. Records, Computers and the Rights of Citizens: Report of the Secretary's Advisory
   Committee on Automated Personal Data Systems. Washington, DC: US Department of
   Health, Education and Welfare; 1973. Also available at: http://aspe.hhs.gov/datacncl/
   1973privacy/tocprefacemembers.htm.
2. O'Brien D, Yasnoff W. Privacy, confidentiality, and security in information systems of
   state health agencies. *Am J Prev Med* 1999;16:351–358.

11
Data Standards in Public Health Informatics

Daniel B. Jernigan, Jac Davies, and Alan Sim

Learning Objectives

After studying this chapter, you should be able to:

- Explain the detrimental effects and costs of having redundant, noncommunicating information systems in public health.
- Explain the nature of Health Level 7 as a major messaging standard for hospital information systems.
- List the advantages and disadvantages of a public health agency's using (1) a local vocabulary and (2) a universal vocabulary for a system.
- Briefly define the nature of (1) splitters and (2) lumpers as data vocabularies.
- Define (1) flat, (2) relational, and (3) object-oriented data formats in terms of the degree of complexity and usefulness of each.
- Explain what is meant by a *context* and an *information architecture* in the electronic exchange of information.
- Identify and describe the steps in the typical process by which a standard for data interchange is developed, and explain the roles of the American National Standards Institute and the International Organization for Standardization in standard setting.
- List at least three choices that a public health organization must make in trying to fit a national standard to a local project.
- Explain the differences between naming standards, transmission protocol standards, and software, and provide examples of each.
- Understand that many standards exist for different interrelated fields and know where to go to learn more if needed.

Overview

Public health organizations have lagged far behind hospitals and laboratories in adopting and implementing common data standards. Yet, public health in general must move to such common data standards if it is to fulfill its mission effectively. Without common data standards, public health organizations cannot share and otherwise maximize the use of health information. Such organizations must recognize, however, that replacing local vocabularies and grammar with universal codes provides both advantages and disadvantages. A number of forces are driving public health organizations to adopt and implement common data standards, including the provisions of the Health Insurance Portability and Accountability Act (HIPAA). Changes in these standards will require public health organizations to make many choices—in the nature of file formats, in the electronic exchange of data, and in the degree of complexity of the formats. Fortunately for public health organizations, a number of national standard-setting bodies have developed uniform standards that can be adopted and implemented, although choosing to adopt these standards is usually a balancing act involving some painful choices. The experience of the Washington State Department of Health in adopting and implementing common data standards illustrates some of these choices.

Introduction

Previous chapters have discussed the fundamentals of developing and installing effective and secure information systems in a public health environment. However, no matter how well designed and accepted an information system is, its usefulness will be severely limited if it cannot communicate in a meaningful way with other systems, both within and outside the organizational environment. Without standards for the data that is to be housed and processed by a system, the entire development and installation process will have been pointless.

Modern technological developments dictate that there be a common data language in public health. With advances in technology such as the computer and the Internet, the speed with which public health data can be collected, analyzed, and exchanged has increased dramatically. At the same time, as public health information activity gets faster and more complex, it becomes even more critically important that the data are being coded and communicated in a standard way. The development and use of *data standards*—a term that indicates uniform use of common terms and common methods for sharing data—will facilitate the efficient exchange of public health information.

The need for data standards in public health is not new. Even in the mid-19th century, William Farr recognized the importance of using common terms in developing a classification system for monitoring mortality in England. That list of terms led to the eventual development of the *International Classification of Diseases* (ICD),[1] now maintained by the World Health Organization (WHO). Farr noted in the Appendix to the First Annual Report of the Registrar General that

> The advantages of a uniform statistical nomenclature, however imperfect, are so obvious, that it is surprising that no attention has been paid to its enforcement in bills

of mortality. Each disease has in many instances been denoted by three of four terms, and each term has been applied to as many different diseases; vague, inconvenient names have been employed, or complications have been registered, instead of primary diseases. The nomenclature is of as much importance in this department of inquiry as weights and measures in the physical sciences, and should be settled without delay.[2]

The same need for uniform standards of nomenclature and classification exists today. Everyone benefits from a common approach to representing and exchanging public health data: those who collect it from outside sources, those who enter it into computer systems, those who analyze it, those who verify the findings, and those who communicate the information for use in public health interventions.

In this chapter, we discuss many of the issues associated with using uniform data standards for the exchange of public health information. We will begin with a short history of the challenges and developments in the exchange of health information. We will then define the context and meaning of common data standard terminology by the use of an analogy to a verbal conversation, including the use of a vocabulary and grammar. We will also discuss some of the efforts of major organizations to provide some level of standardization for data interchange between and among health organizations. Finally, by use of an actual short case history of one state health department's efforts to implement standards for data interchange, we will conclude the chapter by pointing out some of the complexities and challenges involved in adopting data standards.

The Historical Overview of Data Standards in Health: The Tower of Babel

Developing and using uniform data standards is a major challenge facing public health agencies as they move toward more electronic and automatic exchange of data. Fortunately, problems associated with collecting and communicating information are not unique to public health. The experiences of hospitals and healthcare providers can offer direction to public health departments and federal agencies making decisions about data standards. A brief history of efforts to integrate laboratory and hospital systems illustrates potential solutions to similar challenges in public health.

In the not too distant past, laboratory workers manually recorded the results of lab tests in logbooks and on paper reports that were sent to the patient's chart. Over time, laboratory devices were developed that performed routine tests automatically and provided the results on printed strips of paper. The printed result often was stapled into a logbook, with copies provided to the chart. These printouts were an improvement over handwritten results, but the management of data stored on paper is inefficient. Many of the laboratory devices eventually were configured to provide results electronically. Each device had its own unique format for communicating: The blood-testing machine spoke one language, the serum chemistry machine spoke another language, and the specimen-tracking computer spoke yet another. A number of laboratories took these electronic outputs and connected them to a central computer. The subsequent set of communicating computers and devices became known as a *laboratory information system* (LIS). The electronic connections for communicating between the instruments and the central computer, called *interfaces*, made it possible to access all the lab data from the various devices at a single computer terminal.

Interfaces greatly improved specimen tracking and the presentation of results; however, computer programmers had to undertake considerable work to translate the unique outputs of each of the machines into a format the LIS could understand. Laboratory directors were trying to build an integrated, intercommunicating laboratory, but they found themselves deafened by a cacophony of different languages. Adding a new device or purchasing a new LIS required that each of the disparate data formats be translated for the new device or system. This confusion in communication has been compared to the description of the Tower of Babel in the Book of Genesis.[3] During construction of that tower, the builders began to speak in different languages. The inability of the builders to communicate in a common language made building the great tower impossible. To overcome the Tower of Babel in laboratories by use of a common format for sharing the information, laboratories needed a *transmission protocol* recognizable to all participating systems.

Recognizing the costs and inflexibility of the old approach, the makers of lab devices and LIS developers came to agreement on standard electronic formats for communicating.[4,5,6] One common format was developed by a national developer of interfaces. Initially, interfaces were developed between each of the systems: billing–laboratory, laboratory–admissions, admissions–billing, and so on. Each interface was essentially unique; it could not be used with another system. These interfaces allowed for efficient data sharing, but they were time-consuming and expensive to develop and maintain, a fact that was especially evident as hospitals added new systems requiring even more interfaces. Programmers had to be brought back in to repeat the process of developing interfaces to connect each of the old systems to any new system.

In short, hospitals, especially those attempting mergers with other hospitals, found themselves in a similar situation as the laboratories, trying to connect more and more systems, each with a unique set of codes and electronic formats. These connections between systems were unique proprietary interfaces; they were not based on any common communication standard. Eventually, forces related to economy and effectiveness dictated that hospitals needed a common format for system interfaces, and these forces prevailed.

Working together, developers of *hospital information systems* (HISs) generated a common format for sharing data. The major messaging standard that developed for this purpose was *Health Level Seven* (HL7).[7] This standard has become the choice for interfacing of clinical data for most institutions. HL7 defines the data elements being exchanged, the timing of the interchange, and the format for multiple types of messages: orders, results, errors, services, and many others. By using a common message for communicating between disparate systems, hospitals can save a considerable amount of time and money when building interfaces.[8]

The Tower of Babel in Public Health

There are numerous noncommunicating systems in public health, just as there are such systems in hospitals and laboratory systems. City, county, and state health departments often use different and incompatible systems for collecting and analyzing data. Even different divisions within a single health department may have systems that cannot communicate with one another. In addition, state health departments use different systems provided by federal public health agencies. The reasons for the lack of compatibility vary. Computer systems may have a particular design because of *functional* requirements—for instance, clinical case management of patients in an immunization clinic. The systems may differ because of *policy* requirements within a health department—for example, requirements that allow only certain kinds of software to be installed and maintained by health department staff. The systems may also differ because of *external* requirements from federally funded programs for disease control. Although these reasons may be justifiable, they have contributed to a complex array of independent systems that have great difficulty sharing information and that impose a great burden on those entering and providing maintenance of data.[9] Some typical examples of the public health Tower of Babel are:

* an immunization clinic system that tracks measles vaccinations but cannot communicate with a public health lab system recording results from serum measles antibody tests;
* a prenatal clinic system that cannot communicate with a birth registry system; and
* a sexually transmitted disease monitoring system that cannot communicate with a communicable disease reporting system to identify patients with both hepatitis B and syphilis.

Even a casual examination of public health agencies will turn up other, similar examples of incompatible systems.[10] The net effect of relying on such systems is that opportunities for processing information more effectively are lost. For example, public health officials in charge of multiple public health information systems find themselves with an abundance of data. Unfortunately, these data cannot be easily combined. As a result, information of value to public health may be lost. This abundance of unusable data has been called "data smog" by the author David Schenk.[11] Schenk writes, "The character of information has changed: as we have accrued more and more of it, information has emerged not only as a currency, but also as a pollutant." The challenge to public health is to insure that, as more and more data are collected, these data generate more and more valuable information. Adhering to common data standards will help to meet that challenge.

Public health agencies have not fully capitalized on the value of common data standards to the extent that hospitals and laboratories have. But even while hospitals and laboratories have benefited from the implementation of data standards for communicating between information systems, they still need greater standardization. For public health as well as for such other institutions, the Health Insurance Portability and Accountability Act (HIPAA) holds promise of increasing the pace at which common data standards are implemented.[12,13] In Chapter 4, John Christiansen has discussed the impact that HIPAA will have on health information privacy. In addition, we need to point out that one of the goals of HIPAA is to improve the efficiency and effectiveness of health care through standardization of select shared electronic information. This law, once fully implemented, will certainly impact the business of health care by restructuring the way that health data are captured, transmitted, stored, secured, and managed. Likewise, it will impact public health by changes made to the source of most public health data. In turn, having a greater understanding of available data standards and their potential uses will allow public health to participate more fully in the information revolution occurring in health care and elsewhere.

Data Standards: A Figure of Speech

Public health agencies collect data in order to characterize, control, and prevent disease. Critical to this activity is the efficient *exchange* of unambiguous information. Such data become unambiguous by the use of a common language. In fact, one way to describe data standards in public health information exchange is to use the metaphor of a conversation. Like data standards, conversations use a *vocabulary* (i.e., a chosen set of words), require a *grammar* (i.e., a way of structuring the words), and take place in a certain *context* (i.e., a common setting for parties to exchange the words). Each of these three conversational components is useful for discussing available data standards and issues surrounding their implementation. Table 11.1 summarizes the analogy we will be using.

Vocabulary

Words are essentially representations of things and activities. Words that get used repeatedly are often coded, categorized, and cataloged in lists called

TABLE 11.1. The equivalence of the components of data standards to a conversation

Conversational Component	Data Standard Equivalent
Vocabulary: the words you choose for a conversation	Vocabulary: the coded terms to represent data that are being exchanged or stored
	Local vocabulary: a specific, proprietary set of terms that may limit data exchange
	Universal vocabulary: a nationally recognized set of terms maintained by others, which may have limited applicability to specific local uses
	Splitters: vocabularies that tease broad concepts into atomic elements
	Lumpers: vocabularies that gather several concepts into a single code
Grammar: the way you put the words together for a conversation	Format: the order and structure of data for storing or messaging
	Storage formats: use of spreadsheet or database files is a more static way to exchange data
	Electronic messaging format: a more dynamic way of exchanging data information using queries and acknowledgments
Context: the environment where you have a conversation	Information architecture: the designated infrastructure for supporting data exchange—software, hardware, resources, staff needed for communication, data security, confidentiality requirements, policy and regulatory requirements, etc.

vocabularies. In much the same way, health departments and hospitals maintain lists of codes that they use frequently—codes for counties, codes for reportable conditions, disease codes for death records, codes for identifying institutions, and reimbursement codes for common procedures that are performed. In general, these lists of codes or vocabularies can be described by how widely they are intended for use.

Local and Universal Vocabularies

Local vocabularies are usually defined for a specific purpose, often for a specific, proprietary application. *Universal* vocabularies are designed for broad use in disparate systems. For example, let's say that a health department needs a new system for recording information about licenses for water wells in the state. To maintain a current license, each well owner must provide the location of the well. The designers of the new licensing information system must choose how they will code the different data collected. As an example, let's take the data collected about the county where the well is located. Should the health department use the county codes from the old system (the local codes) or should it adopt *FIPS* (Federal Information Processing Standards) codes developed by the federal government (the universal codes)?[14] The old local codes are familiar to the data entry and data analysis staff and may make it easier to compare information collected in the new system to historical data. The new universal codes are not familiar to the staff, but having them in the database will allow adjoining states to combine data to develop regional statistics; they will also allow the water well information to be combined with other data sets at the health department that use the federal county codes.

There are always trade-offs in choosing between local and universal codes. For example, local codes are more easily updated or changed and can reflect specific local needs; however, local codes require maintenance by health department staff, and the use of local codes may impede rapid and efficient sharing of information. Universal codes do allow for better sharing of information, and the costs of maintaining them are borne by an outside agency. However, it may be difficult to get new codes when they are needed, and codes may not be available to represent all the information collected in a particular system. Choosing between a locally defined vocabulary and a universal vocabulary is essentially choosing the level of direct control one has over the codes in a system. In general, if the information is going to be compared or combined with other sources of information, then the use of universal codes is warranted. Table 11.2 summarizes the advantages and disadvantage of local and universal codes.

Splitters and Lumpers

Vocabularies can also be categorized by the degree to which the codes combine multiple concepts into single representations. In other words, vocabularies can be categorized as *splitters*, those that tend to tease concepts out into their more atomic elements, and *lumpers*, those that tend to gather concepts into a single code. Take, for example, the following narrative dictated by a pathologist evaluating a surgical biopsy: "The gallbladder was enlarged and red with pus easily expressed through the site of rupture." In addition to sounding truly repulsive, the narrative is also very difficult to represent with a single code. Translating that narrative into a single code like "enlarged gallbladder" would miss all the gory detail. Many newer anatomic pathology computer systems allow for these separate terms to be stored by use of codes from the *Systematized Nomenclature of Medicine* (SNOMED).[15] SNOMED is an example of a splitter vocabulary, because it permits storage of each concept in the sample narrative. (Vocabularies that function mainly to assign names to unique concepts, like SNOMED, are also known as *nomenclatures*.) A coding specialist using SNOMED for coding the gory gallbladder narrative into the computer system could choose separate codes for selected terms—for instance: T-63000 (Gallbladder), M-71000 (Enlarged), M-01780 (Erythematous), M-36880 (Purulent Discharge), and M-41611 (Rup-

TABLE 11.2. Advantages and disadvantages of using local and universal codes

Code Classification	Advantages	Disadvantages
Local	• Familiar to data entry and data analysis staff—no training required	• Requires maintenance by local health staff
	• More easily updated or changed than universal codes	• May impede sharing of information with other organizations not using the local code
	• Permits more readily comparisons of previously collected data to current data	
Universal	• Permits communication and sharing of data with other systems using universal codes	• May be unfamiliar to local staff—training may be required
	• Updating is the responsibility of the issuing organization and not the users	• Not as flexible or as subject to updating as local codes
		• May not be adaptable to represent all information of the local organization

tured Abscess). These separate codes can be used later as search terms for categorizing the data or for generating pathologic diagnoses. SNOMED version 3.5 contains 156,965 term codes in 12 separate lists of codes, or *axes*, containing names for different things. Axes of particular interest to public health include Living Organisms, Diseases and Diagnoses, Physiological Functions, and others. Newer versions of SNOMED (e.g., SNOMED RT and SNOMED CT) additionally contain relationships between the coded concepts as well as expanded clinical terminology.

Lumper vocabularies, on the other hand, do not attempt to provide names for all things and activities, but rather provide codes that combine multiple concepts into a single code. Let's take the following code for a laboratory test as an example: "Enzyme Immunoassay of Serum for Hepatitis A Virus Antibody." Here, the test code is actually a group of separate concepts that have been put together. Those separate concepts are "Enzyme Immunoassay," "Serum," "Hepatitis A Virus,", and "Antibody." A code to represent this collection of concepts can be found in the lumper vocabulary *Logical Observation Identifiers, Names, and Codes* (LOINC) as "13951-9."[16,17] Because LOINC codes are made up of known component concepts, the single code can be "exploded" to reveal the component parts. Thus, these lumper codes can serve as a single, unambiguous, representation of a complex set of concepts and, at the same time, the individual codes that make up the single code can be referenced and used for categorizing and routing the information. LOINC is an example of a vocabulary that takes separate component concepts, such as "serum" and "antibody," and connects them. The process of putting those components together is known as *coordination*. When codes are put together by use of defined component concepts prior to the release of the vocabulary, as is the case with LOINC, the codes are referred to as *pre-coordinated*. On the other hand, when users create new codes after the release of a vocabulary, the new codes are referred to as *post-coordinated*—that is, they have been put together after the fact. SNOMED codes, for example, can be post-coordinated. In general, if information is going to be compared or combined with other sources of information, vocabularies of pre-coordinated terms may provide for the most efficient and unambiguous movement of data. In contrast, the use of post-coordinated terms in such vocabularies may complicate the data movement.

Some vocabularies can be classified as both splitters and lumpers. An example of a vocabulary that has elements of both lumping and splitting is the *International Classification of Diseases—Clinical Modification* (ICD-CM).[18] Now in its ninth edition, this vocabulary has both atomic concepts like "fever" (780.6) and more lumped concepts like "Hepatitis A virus infection without mention of coma" (070.1). The ICD-CM differs from a nomenclature in that it is a *classification*, a vocabulary that has organized its codes into defined categories. In a classification, one can know that the code for "meningococcal encephalitis" (036.1) is a type of "meningococcal infection" (036.0), which itself is a type of "other bacterial diseases" (030–041). In other words, there is a *hierarchy* of relationships among the coded concepts. Newer releases of SNOMED will provide these kinds of relationships among its codes as well.

A number of additional "universal" vocabularies are available and useful for public health activities:

- *Current Procedural Terminology, Fourth Version (CPT4)*: codes and descriptors to represent health services (www.ama-assn.org/ama/pub/category/3113.html)
- *National Drug Codes (NDC)*: a set of universal product identifiers for human drugs (www.fda.gov/cder/ndc)
- *International Classification of Diseases for Oncology (ICD-O)*: an international coding tool for cancer registries maintained by WHO (www.who.int)
- *Unified Medical Language System (UMLS)*: an on-line tool analogous to a thesaurus for linking concepts common across different health care–related vocabularies (www.nlm.nih.gov/pubs/factsheets/umlskss.html)

Grammar

For any conversation to occur, two parties must choose a vocabulary that both parties can understand. However, it is not enough to have only the words: rather, both parties also must choose a way to put the words together so that the parties can understand each other. For instance, take the two following sentences:

"The disinfectant is contaminated by blood."

"The blood is contaminated by disinfectant."

Both sentences use the same words but mean very different things, depending on how they are arranged. To understand each other, both parties trying to communicate about blood and disinfectant must agree on the following order of words

"Thing being contaminated goes first; thing doing the contaminating is second."

For communicating information in public health in an efficient and unambiguous way, the order and structure of the data are as important as the vocabulary. A number of different formats (i.e., ways for structuring the data) allow data to be exchanged between parties.

Storage and Message

Storage Formats

Imagine two ways of having a conversation. One occurs through sharing more complete data collections such as written letters or diaries. Another is more like a face-to-face communication. The former is an exchange of relatively fixed information, whereas the latter is more dynamic—one question leading to another, with short bursts of information moving back and forth. The same alternatives can apply to the exchange of electronic information as well.

One alternative is that data can be stored in a structured, more fixed format, a *file*, and that file can be given to someone else for use. Files are usually formatted as either *flat* files (consisting of a table of rows and columns), or as a *database* file (a table, or set of tables, with columns, rows, and an accompanying description of the data with computer instructions for working with the data). There are many different "standard" file formats. Many of these formats are *de facto* standards—they have become standards through their frequent use, rather than through a formal consensus process. Standards that are developed through a formal consensus or regulated process are often referred to as *de jure* standards. Some common de facto standards in use as file formats are listed below:

- *Comma-delimited*: a flat file format with file extension *.csv, where commas are used to *delimit*, i.e., separate, the columns of a table; each row of the file represents a new record.
- *Tab-delimited*: a flat file format often with file extension *.txt, similar to comma-delimited, but tabs are used instead of commas.
- *Microsoft® Excel*: a proprietary database file format with file extension *.xls, known as a *spreadsheet*, i.e., a single table of rows and columns with some accompanying instructions for the computer to appropriately manipulate the data.

- *Lotus® 1-2-3*: a proprietary spreadsheet with file extension *.wk4.
- *Borland® dBASE*: a proprietary database format with file extension *.dbf.
- *Microsoft® Access*: a proprietary relational database format with file extension *.mdb.
- *SAS®*: a proprietary statistical analysis tool and file format with file extension *.ssd

If two parties are using the same file format to exchange information, they will be able to update their data easily by importing the files. If they are not using the same file format, then work will be required to change the format into something that can be imported.

Differences in file formats can lead to delays in public health interventions. For example, examine the following scenario: During an outbreak investigation, the Johnson County Health Department has chosen to store its data in the database Borland dBASE. Monroe County Health Department has started its own investigation as well, but has used the database Microsoft Access to store the data. Realizing that a statewide outbreak is occurring, the state health department begins coordinating the investigation and chooses to store the data in *Epi-Info*, a database provided by the Centers for Disease Control and Prevention (CDC), which uses a proprietary format different from either of the de facto standards used by the counties.[19] Each day, as new data are shared with the state health department, time and energy have to be devoted to translating and reformatting the data in order to combine them into a common, analyzable format.

In this situation, it is easy to see why use of a common file format would speed the sharing of data among the two counties and the CDC. In general, if data are to be exchanged in files, choosing a common file format for reporting, preferably a de facto standard, will lead to more efficient communication of public health information.

Electronic Messaging Formats

Data can be shared by exchanging files, but data can also be shared in a more dynamic way. A computer system can also "talk" with another, different kind of computer system through *electronic messaging*.[20] Such a more complex electronic conversation is most commonly employed in hospitals and businesses where the importance of sharing data efficiently and unambiguously may determine the life or death of a patient. Messaging, also called *electronic data interchange* (EDI), requires much more technological infrastructure than is needed for simply sharing data files; it requires a common set of questions and responses that both communicating systems understand. Take immunization registries as an example. The vaccine-preventable diseases section of the Washington State Department of Health has developed a large database to keep track of children's immunization status in the state. Oregon also has developed a health department registry database, but that database uses a different database design. When a child has moved from one state to another, is there a way that one database could automatically communicate with the other database to determine whether the child has any record of prior vaccinations? The answer is yes—through the use of HL7 messages.[21,22] By use of a structured format, the different messages being shared between the two computer systems simplistically might look like this:

Washington System:	This is the Washington State System, talking to the Oregon State System, requesting to know if you have any children with the last name "Munoz" and first name "Charlie"?
Oregon System:	This is the Oregon State System and I have 3 children with last name "Munoz" and first name "Charlie."
Washington System:	Do any of these children have a birth date of June 12, 1996?
Oregon System:	Yes, one child has the birth date of June 12, 1996.
Washington System:	Please provide the immunization records for this child.
Oregon System:	Hepatitis B vaccine at birth. Measles, Mumps, Rubella at 15 months, etc.

As you can imagine, this kind of automated query and response method requires a greater technological capability than does sharing files. However, messaging can provide much faster communication than can occur with periodic updating of databases. Additionally, the two-way conversation allows for dynamic transfer of information.

There are two major standards for messaging health information in public health: (1) HL7 and (2) *X12*, a national standard for exchanging business information.[23] HL7 standardizes the format and protocol for the electronic exchange of data among healthcare computer application systems. The standard, essentially a large document describing how to build specific electronic messages, provides formats for numerous types of information exchanges, such as requesting a new room for a patient, reporting ultrasound results, ordering intravenous fluids from the pharmacy, responding with an acknowledgment for further information, etc. HL7 not only defines the sequence in the message for certain data elements; it also defines the *data types*, the way certain kinds of data are structured, such as date/time (10/23/2000, 23/10/2000, etc.), name (Doe, John M., John M. Doe, etc.), phone (404-639-3311, +01(404) 639-3311), etc. HL7 currently can be used in public health for messaging between immunization registries[22] and cancer registries,[24] and for reporting results from emergency departments[25,26] and laboratories[27,28] to public health agencies.

The focus of X12 messages is on business-to-business operations. The *American National Standards Institute* (ANSI) has approved both HL7 and X12 for communicating clinical and administrative data, and it has approved X12 for healthcare business transactions. The ANSI Accredited Standards Committee X12

(ANSI ASC X12) has published more than 275 electronic message formats, called transaction sets, for ordering, shipping, and invoicing products, as well as for financial transactions for reimbursement and many other transaction types.[23]

One other important emerging standard for communicating health information is *XML*, or eXtensible Markup Language.[29] XML, and its cousin *HTML* (HyperText Markup Language), are maintained by the *World Wide Web Consortium* (W3C). Both XML and HTML use *tags* (e.g., <title>, <body>, <font>) to define the presentation/layout of a Web page on the Internet. You can get a good idea of what HTML looks like by choosing the "view source code" option on your Web browser. While HTML has predefined tags, XML provides the capability of defining tags for specific messages. XML has two major uses: (1) to provide structure and facilitate exchange of documents over the Internet, and (2) to facilitate the exchange and transmission of data between disparate applications and systems. Standard sets of XML tags have been defined for some disciplines like mathematics and chemistry, but there are no leading XML healthcare standards as yet. Version 3 of HL7 will be in XML, and that version may emerge as a national standard for clinical messages. There are many other XML-related standards that help define the grammar (*Document Type Definition*), interpretation of the data (*Resource Description Framework*), and content/semantics of the data (*Schemas*) for XML implementation. Further information about such developments can be found at the W3C Web site, www.w3c.org.

Flat, Relational, and Object-Oriented Data Structures

One way to look at the "grammar" or format of data being exchanged is to characterize it as either "storage" or "message," as previously described. Another way to characterize the format is by its degree of complexity in the way the data is structured. Generally, one can think of data as being formatted in at least three levels of increasing complexity: *flat*, *relational*, and *object-oriented*. Data can be both stored and messaged in any of these three hierarchies.

Flat Files

A *flat file* is basically a table for storing data. Columns are assigned for different data elements such as "Last Name," "Lab Test Name," and "Result". Rows represent individual records, such as the event of a patient's specimen being tested in the laboratory. The file might look like the following:

Johnson	RPR	Reactive
Doe	Culture	N. meningitidis
Smith	Hep A Virus	Positive
Munoz	Blood Lead	30

Some de facto standard flat files for messaging are the *UB92* (i.e., HCFA-1450) and the *HCFA 1500*, both used for Medicare insurance claims.[30] A format recognizable to communicable disease units in state health departments is *NETSS*, the National Electronic Telecommunications System for Surveillance: a flat file for sending reportable disease data to the CDC.[31] Data stored and messaged in a flat file may be easier to analyze and manipulate than when the data are in other formats; however, it does not easily represent the complex relationships and recurrences of data that are common in health care.

Relational Files

On the other hand, a *relational file* is designed to capture both repeating and related data elements. For instance, if patients are likely to have varying numbers of tests and results, then there could be separate, but linked, parts of the files for tests and results. Thus, a patient with several test results can be represented as easily as a patient with only one test. Using a relational database may be a more logical way to store public health data, because many findings in public health are likely to recur. While data can be stored in a relational database, relational structures can also be used for sending electronic messages. HL7 is an example of an electronic messaging format that uses a relational structure. For instance, when a laboratory result is sent by use of HL7, the message for a sexually transmitted disease screening panel (simplified for this example) looks as follows:

MSH|^~\&||LABMED-SOUTHWEST^68D0896766^CLIA|...

PID|1||78893565||JOHNSON^JACK|...

OBR|1||050994090000|220738^STD SCREEN^L|...

OBX|1|CE|5292-8^RPR-SYPHILIS^LN||REACTIVE|...

OBX|2|CE|6487-3^GONORRHOEAE ANTIGEN^LN||NEGATIVE|...

OBX|3|CE|14468-3^CHLAMYDIA ANTIGEN^LN||NEGATIVE|...

In this HL7 relational message example, the "|" is the delimiter separating the different data fields. The first segment, beginning with "MSH", indicates that a new message is being sent. For each message segment header (MSH), there can be one or more patient identification (PID) segments—here there is only one. For each PID, there can be one or more service request (OBR) segments—here there is only one. For each OBR, there can be one or more observation (OBX) segments—here there are three, one for each of the tests performed in the STD panel.

The relational structure of HL7 allows *electronic messaging* of more complex healthcare information more easily than does the use of flat files. In the same way, a relational database (e.g., Microsoft Access) allows data to be *stored* in a more complex way. In general, if you are going to be messaging or storing information that recurs—for instance, multiple lab tests per visit, multiple addresses per patient, or multiple contacts per case—the use of a relational structure for storage and messaging of data is warranted. Equally important, the use of a de facto or formal standard file format for storage or messaging will allow for more efficient and unambiguous communication of information.

The Object-Oriented Approach

Finally, the most complex of the formats for storage and message is the object-oriented approach. *Objects* are defined as independent, self-contained data packets that contain not only the data, but also the instructions for specific functions or procedures that can be performed with the data. Objects are developed by use of object-oriented programming languages such as JAVA and C++. Objects can be stored in an *object database management system* (ODBMS) and can be shared through a variety of transmission protocols. One architecture, in particular, the *Common Object Request Broker Architecture* (CORBA), has defined a protocol for sharing healthcare data by the use of objects; such data sharing is coordinated by CORBAmed.[32] At present, there are no widely implemented object-oriented standards directly applicable to public health activities.

Context

We have used the metaphor of a conversation to demonstrate the importance of standard vocabularies and formats in the electronic exchange of information. It is important also to consider the *context* in which a conversation occurs; some environments are simply better for communicating than others. While standards for vocabulary and format can lead to more efficient information exchange, additional steps can be taken to standardize other important information system elements. These might include common methods for sending data securely over the Internet, use of standard encryption algorithms for protecting patient confidentiality, agreements on use of a common web application for entry of various surveillance data, defining a set of interoperability requirements that all software purchases must meet, and others. A description of these different elements that together comprise the information system environment can be referred to as an *information architecture*. As with vocabularies and formats, use of standards throughout the architecture can improve the capture and communication of public health information.

Currently in the United States, surveillance data for various diseases is stored and communicated using disease-specific surveillance systems. For example, sexually transmitted disease cases are managed and communicated in a software tool that is unique and disconnected from other "stand-alone" systems in health departments for other diseases such as tuberculosis, HIV/AIDS, and childhood blood levels. As a part of efforts to integrate these disparate surveillance systems, CDC has developed the National Electronic Diseases Surveillance System (NEDSS). NEDSS, in one sense, is a response to the "Tower of Babel" that currently exists in public health reporting by providing the design of a common information architecture for sharing public health findings. NEDSS describes the "vocabulary" for public health information (i.e., the coded terms), the "grammar" for capturing and communicating the information (i.e., the format and structure of databases and electronic messages), and several other elements necessary for an integrated environment for public health surveillance information management. Standards are defined for various architectural elements including an integrated data repository, Web data entry, specific security methods, electronic messaging of health care information, data presentation and analysis, and more. Further information can be found at http://www.cdc.gov/.

It is important to remember that the choice of standards and elements in the information architecture may require additional resources or more complex software than older nonstandard systems. For example, the requirements in software, resources, and staff needed to support XML messaging over a secure internet connection with SNOMED codes and encrypted patient identifiers is very different from the requirements for using a flat file with no universal codes sent by mail on a floppy disk. As the complexity of the chosen standards within the information architecture increases, so will the complexity of the infrastructure and needed resources to support the data exchange increase. In general, when choosing data standards, public health agencies should account for the resources and infrastructure needed to support the full implementation of the standards in the information architecture so that the maximum benefit can be achieved. More on this issue is discussed in the section titled "Experience from the Field" later in this chapter.

Developing National Data Standards: Herding Cats

The development of data standards arises from a need to share data efficiently and unambiguously. However, the formal process for creating national data standards is not easy; it is much like trying to herd cats. Some organizations and corporations have come to agreement on acceptable solutions; others have not. The task of developing national data standards requires that academicians, software vendors, federal agencies, and others, each with their own agenda and investment of resources, must be brought together to develop a common specification. Such a task requires patience, creativity, and perseverance to bring the participants together.

Standardizing Standardization

Standards exist for paper sizes, just as standards exist for data interchange. We even have standards that define the thread width on a screw. However, navigating the plethora of standards and identifying the numerous, diverse areas requiring standardization can become a management nightmare unless a standards process is defined. The standards process helps determine how potential standards can be properly identified, balloted, changed, and retired in an iterative manner. Although the standards process may differ slightly from one *standards development organization* (SDO) to another, the functions of the standards process are similar. The steps that are typically involved in the standards setting process are listed below:

1. *Identify areas requiring standardization*: The first step is to identify the subject area of interest requiring standardization. For example, let us say that a previously unknown virus has been discovered that causes fever and abnormal movement in the arms and legs. Investigators have named this virus "Disco Fever Virus" (DFV). Soon after its discovery, state and local health departments identify the need to represent this concept in code sets for public health reporting. Clinics and hospitals, on the other hand, need this concept represented in code sets for reimbursement and billing purposes. In each case, standardized codes are desired to represent DFV infection, keeping in mind the different purposes, representations, and uses of these codes.

2. *Determine whether standards exist for the area of interest*: After querying the UMLS and researching standard code sets, many of which are accessible on the Internet, scientists determine that standard code sets such as ICD-9-CM and SNOMED do not have a code for DFV infection. They could generate a proprietary code to represent this concept in an internal application or database. However, given the fact that the clinic uses ICD-9-CM to represent a majority of infectious diseases, it would make sense to inform the standards development organization of the need to include and represent this concept in its coding classification scheme.

3. *Submit a proposal*: In most standards development organizations, a technical committee or working group is responsible for the development and submission of proposals for new or modified standards to the central governing board. In this example, a proposal justifying the need to develop a standard code for DFV infection would be submitted to the technical committee for consideration. The content and format of these proposals will vary from one standards development organization to another.

4. *Discussion/Debate*: Discussion and debate may occur at two levels. Discussion will first occur at the technical committee level. The merits of the submitted DFV infection proposal will be critiqued based on some form of evaluative criteria or guidelines used by the committee. At the second level, if the topic is of significant importance, the technical committee may recommend that the central governing board facilitate discussion and debate of the proposal. The central governing board, at the very least, will be involved in the final decision-making process to determine whether the proposal will be endorsed and incorporated into the standard.

5. *Review Process/Incorporate Changes*: Often, proposals are sent back to the submitter with changes, suggestions, and requests for further clarification. Submitters should expect each standards development organization to have some process to review and edit proposals. Submitters

should be prepared to make compromises and recommend alternative solutions in order to achieve consensus. When the changes have been agreed upon, the submitter incorporates these changes in the proposal.

6. *Consensus/Final Vote*: Once the technical committee has written up the specifications for the proposed additions or change to the standard, the proposal is described and balloted for approval by the central governing board. To gain approval, some specified majority of the central governing board must vote in favor of the items described in the proposal. Again, keep in mind that the balloting protocol may vary from one standards development organization to another.

In the example above, some negotiation has occurred between the submitters of the proposal and members of the technical committee. Once a consensus is reached, the governing board votes and approves the addition of a standard code representation for DFV infection.

Obviously, this example has been simplified. In reality, each step in the standards process requires significant effort, time, and understanding of the standardization needs. However, there are distinct advantages for the public health community to go through the standards process. Public health not only benefits from having influenced the development of a standard, but it also benefits from the experience and knowledge gained in the process. Equally important, the relationships forged with standards development organizations will prove invaluable, especially if other standards proposals are submitted in the future. Finally, the same approach on a less complex scale can be used to develop consensus solutions to communication problems in large health departments and public health agencies.

The Standard Bearers

Two organizations serve as the coordinator of standards development activities. Under the umbrella of these two organizations, standards are developed internally within technical committees and working groups or externally by accredited standards development organizations. Participants in these organizations represent diverse government and industry organizations:

* *American National Standards Institute* (ANSI): A voluntary standards organization that serves as the coordinator for national standards in the United States and as the US member body to the International Organization for Standards. ANSI accredits standards committees and provides an open forum for interested parties to identify, plan, and agree on standards; it does not itself develop standards. Standards are developed by SDOs. Some examples of ANSI-accredited SDOs are HL7 and X12.[33]
* *International Organization for Standardization* (ISO): Founded in 1946 as one of the two major international nontreaty standards organizations, ISO serves to coordinate and develop international voluntary consensus

standards that facilitate world trade and contribute to public safety and health. ANSI is the official US member body of ISO. There are numerous technical committees, including one on Healthcare Informatics.[34]

A Balancing Act

We have described the different kinds of data standards that are available and have attempted to show the benefits that standards can bring. It is also important to describe the potential problems that can arise in trying to fit a national standard to a local project. Choosing and implementing data standards is in some respects a balancing act. Public health agencies have to consider a number of possibly conflicting issues and determine how best to proceed. Some of the common concerns are listed below, each as a spectrum from one extreme to the other:

- *Free Versus Costly:* How much can you afford to spend on data standards? Some code sets must be purchased, such as SNOMED and CPT4. There are costs in purchasing the software or technical support to implement certain solutions, such as electronic data interchange, code translations, secure transmission over the Internet.
- *Local Versus Universal:* Are the codes you need in a standard vocabulary? No standard code set will meet all the needs of most public health activities. However, use of local codes will cause problems for data that will be shared and compared with other sources of data.
- *Home-Grown Versus Off-the-Shelf:* Where will you get the tools to use the data standards? As the complexity of the chosen data standards increases, software tools will be needed to use those standards. Home-grown solutions may save money but may be understood by only a single programmer. Off-the-shelf products may be advertised as "plug and play" but may cost more and may need to be "customized."
- *You Decide Now Versus All Decide Later:* How much input do you seek before choosing standards? Data standards allow for greater interoperability and ease of data exchange. In choosing standards, you should have a clear understanding of what data will need to be shared and with whom the data will be exchanged. Figuring these out first may avoid an uninformed choice as well as a delayed, "over-informed" committee decision.

Experience from the Field: The Washington State Department of Health

Implementing standards is like implementing good nutritional practices. Most American adults know what a healthy diet is, but most have not been able to change the way they eat. In the same manner, there is general agreement about the value of data standards, but individuals and organizations find it hard to change their daily practices to begin using them.

The Washington State Department of Health (WDOH) has been exploring integration of its notifiable condition information systems through standardization of data elements and data system architecture .The following are some of the experiences WDOH has had and the lessons learned in the process.

Electronic Laboratory-Based Reporting

Washington's initial foray into the world of standardization was the development of an Electronic Laboratory-Based Reporting system (ELR). This system allows clinical laboratories to submit mandatory notifiable condition reports electronically to WDOH, which in turn transmits the reports to the local health agency of the county where the patient resides.

Although simple in concept, ELR is impossible to implement without data and transmission standards. Early in the planning process, WDOH decided against mandating the use of proprietary standards and instead worked to understand emerging universal data vocabularies and electronic transmission standards. After extensive research, WDOH elected to implement ELR by using HL7 for the transmission format and LOINC and SNOMED as data vocabularies.[28] These decisions are consistent with general trends in the clinical laboratory industry. Ideally, they will allow automated, hands-off transmission of notifiable condition reports directly from laboratory information systems. This automated transmission of the reports will reduce the burden of notifiable condition reporting on the laboratories, decrease the amount of time necessary for public health agencies to get reports, and improve overall data quality.

However, the decision to use national standards did not lead to quick and easy implementation. WDOH soon learned that HL7, although considered a "standard," in fact is not used in the same way from one organization to the next. Each clinical laboratory participating in the ELR system spent time dissecting HL7 messages and reaching agreements about modifications needed to meet the public health HL7 message criteria. This meant that in-house information technology staff had to become very proficient in HL7. Althoug the staff's acquiring this proficiency was considered a good long-term investment, it added considerable time and cost to the ELR implementation.

Similarly, the decision to use LOINC and SNOMED required some serious discussion and consideration of trade-offs. As previously discussed, LOINC and SNOMED seem to be emerging national standards of choice for coding clinical laboratory data sets. Some commercial laboratories are beginning to move in this direction. The WDOH state public health laboratory has been adopting these code sets. However, LOINC and SNOMED are not yet widespread, and it will likely be a number of years before these standards are applied in the majority of clinical laboratory settings. Further, there will always be laboratories that do not use national standards, but instead continue to maintain their own internal code sets. Therefore, WDOH encourages the use of LOINC and SNOMED in notifiable condition reports. but recognizes the need to have mechanisms built into ELR that will allow the translation of proprietary standards into the accepted national standards. Ideally, that translation will occur at the originating laboratory, as the originating laboratory is in the best position to interpret its internal codes against the national code sets. As with HL7, this decision required the in-house epidemiology, information technology. and laboratory staff to become well versed in national vocabulary standards. again adding time and cost.

Disease Condition Database

Shortly after beginning work on ELR. WDOH began an effort to update the regulatory framework that supported the notifiable condition reporting system. As part of this effort. development began on an integrated database to serve as a repository for notifiable condition data. At the same time, a review of the existing paper-based reporting process was performed. All of these activities needed to happen at the same time because they are all related, and decisions affecting one part will affect the others. The rules dictate what information gets collected and in what format. The paper-based forms also dictate data format and therefore need to be consistent with the information system that the data will be entered into.

Between the various state and local programs that require reporting from laboratories. providers, or other entities, there were 51 different forms to be filled out. Each form had a different format and different data definitions. One form might ask for a patient's date of birth, while another asked for the patient's age at the time of the visit. This situation was difficult for the individuals who had to report information to public health; it also made it impossible to move toward an integrated information system. WDOH identified the data elements that were common to all reportable condition forms and sought agreement from the various state programs and local health agencies about how each data element will be defined and formatted. The data elements that proved to be the best candidates for initial standardization were those related to basic patient demographics (gender, race, address. age, etc.). WDOH was guided in selection of these elements by standardization efforts at CDC.

Although these discussions allowed WDOH to identify common data elements and to move to simplified, unified reporting forms, there were some difficult issues to overcome. Pragmatically speaking, data standards rarely provide an immediate benefit to the programs that must implement them. The benefits are more often seen in the long run, and they are generally accrued at the agency rather than at the individual program level. Individual public health programs find that their own proprietary standards work well for them. and they are reluctant to go through the pain of making a change when they will not see an immediate benefit.

Individual programs also often face the constraint of oversight from other state or federal agencies, which may impose specific data standards as a condition of providing funding to the programs. These constraints must be considered when an organization attempts to implement universal data standards. National efforts at the CDC to move to common data standards may help remove this historic obstacle.

Finally, it must be recognized that the brunt of implementing new data standards generally falls on people who will not see any real benefit from the change. Data entry clerks, laboratory analysts, and front-line program staff are the ones who will have to deal with the immediate drudgery of learning and implementing new codes sets. In general, these are not the people who will be running analyses and writing reports from this data; therefore, they may never come to understand the true value of implementing new, uniform data standards. Public health organizations developing such implementation plans must include these front-line staff in the planning as soon as possible and must allow adequate training time.

Conclusions

Much of current public health activity has been affected by the emergence of information technologies. Newer and faster ways to share data have impacted critical functions like the monitoring of infectious conditions and the identification of risk factors for disease. As the speed and availability of data increases, it becomes vitally important to use common methods for coding and exchanging data to assure that information being shared is translated into applied public health action. Public health practitioners must choose among different standard vocabularies, data exchange formats, and software tools for supporting implementation of data standards. Hospitals and laboratories have realized a number of benefits from standardized approaches to integrating information systems. Greater involvement at all levels of the public health community in the development and use of data standards should be equally beneficial to public health practice.

Questions for Review

Answer the questions at the end of the following short case:

The Office of Immunizations within the Bureau of Communicable Diseases in the Department of Public Health of State X operates a proprietary immunization registry. County public health agencies collect immunization data from private and public health care providers. These agencies then transmit the data to the Department of Public Health for entry to the state immunization registry.

There is no uniform data standard for use by the counties for collecting and reporting immunization data. A few counties have developed a shared immunization registry system. Most, however, operate home-grown systems. As a result, a school nurse wanting to verify the immunization records of a child who has moved into a county from another county usually must submit a paper form to the county in which the child received an immunization and wait several weeks for verification.

To permit automated entry of immunization data from some of the larger counties, information technology personnel within the state Office of Immunizations have developed interfaces between the systems of those counties and the state immunization registry system. However, most of the counties report immunization data to the Office of Immunizations on a monthly basis, using paper forms. Clerks within the Office of Immunization then enter the data manually into the state registry. Because of the sheer volume of monthly paper forms, there is usually a three-month backlog of immunization data, so that the state immunization registry is almost never current.

The Department of Public Health, in consultation with the state legislature, is considering a proposal to automate the collection and entry of immunization data statewide. This proposal would require both the Office of Immunizations and all state counties to adopt and implement HL7 as an electronic messaging system to speed data collection and immunization verification. Healthcare providers within each county would use the system to report immunizations to the county public health agency. The county health agency would then transmit the immunization data directly to the new immunization registry of the state Office of Immunization. The process would completely automate the collection and recording of immunization data. School nurses, in turn, could obtain automated verification of immunization from all county health departments via a relational database on a real-time basis.

1. What are the advantages of this proposed new system to (a) the Office of Immunizations, (b) counties, (c) health care providers, and (d) school nurses?
2. Explain the disadvantages to each of these entities of adopting and implementing the proposed HL7 system?
3. Which of the entities is *least likely* to observe a major benefit to be derived from implementation of the proposed HL7 system? Why?
4. Assuming that the new system is implemented, what are the implications for staff training by each of the entities in the system's operations?
5. If the counties and the Office of Immunization have been able to modify their current immunization systems to suit new applications, will this opportunity continue with the adoption and implementation of the HL7 system? Explain.
6. What factors should the Department of Public Health and state legislators consider in making a decision about mandating the adoption and implementation of the proposed new system?

References

1. World Health Organization. WHO Statistical Information System. Available at: http://www.who.int/whosis. Accessed September 1, 2000.

2. Farr W. *Vital Statistics: A Memorial Volume of Selections from the Reports and Writings of William Farr*. Metuchen, NJ: The Scarecrow Press; 1975:212.
3. *The Holy Bible*. King James version. Grand Rapids, MI: Zondervan Publishing House; 1995:Genesis 11:1–9.
4. Aller RD. Software standards and the laboratory information system. *Am J Clin Pathol* 1996;105(Suppl):S48–S53.
5. American Society for Testing and Materials. *Specification for Transferring Information Between Clinical Instruments and Computer Systems: ASTM E1394*. West Conshohocken, PA: American Society for Testing and Materials; 1992.
6. American Society for Testing and Materials. Technical Standards for Industries Worldwide. Available at: http://www.astm.org. Accessed September 1, 2000.
7. Health Level Seven. What is HL7? Available at: http://www.hl7.org. Accessed September 1, 2000.
8. Marotta DJ. HL7 in the 21st century: integrating medical information exchange. *Healthc Inform* 2000;17:46–48.
9. US General Accounting Office. *Emerging Infectious Diseases: National Surveillance System Could Be Strengthened*. GAO/T-HEHS-99-62. Washington, DC: US General Accounting Office; 1999.
10. Morris G, Snider D, Katz M. Integrating public health information and surveillance systems. *J Public Health Manag Pract* 1996;2:24–27.
11. Shenk D. *Data Smog: Surviving the Information Glut*. New York, NY: HarperCollins Publishers; 1997:30.
12. Office of the Secretary, Department of Health and Human Services. Health Insurance Reform: Standards for Electronic Transactions—Final Rule. *65 Federal Register*, no. 160 (2000):50312–72.
13. Department of Health and Human Services. The Administrative Simplification Provisions of the Health Insurance Portability and Accountability Act of 1996 (HIPAA). Available at: http://aspe.hhs.gov/admnsimp. Accessed September 1, 2000.
14. National Institute of Standards and Technology. Federal Information Processing Standards Publications. Available at: http://www.itl.nist.gov/fipspubs. Accessed September 1, 2000.
15. College of American Pathologists. Systematized Nomenclature of Medicine, International. Available at: http://www.snomed.org. Accessed September 1, 2000.
16. Regenstrief Institute. LOINC® and RELMA™. Available at: http://www.regenstrief.org/loinc/loinc.htm. Accessed September 1, 2000.
17. Huff SM, Rocha RA, McDonald CJ, et al. Development of the Logical Observation Identifier Names and Codes (LOINC) Vocabulary. *J Am Med Inform Assoc* 1998;5:276–292
18. National Center for Health Statistics, Centers for Disease Control and Prevention. *International Classification of Diseases, Ninth Revision, Clinical Modification (ICD-9-CM)*. Available at: http://www.cdc.gov/nchs/about/otheract/icd9/abticd9.htm. Accessed September 1, 2000.
19. Centers for Disease Control and Prevention. Epi Info. Available at: http://www.cdc.gov/epiinfo/. Accessed September 1, 2000.
20. Huff SM. Clinical Data Exchange Standards and Vocabularies for Messages. *Proc AMIA Symp* 1998:62–67.
21. Abernathy S. Immunization Registries to Exchange Data Using HL7. *HL7 News* July 1999. Available at: http://www.cdc.gov/nip/registry/hl7news.htm.
22. National Immunization Program, Centers for Disease Control and Prevention. Imple-

mentation Guide for Immunization Data Transactions using Version 2.3.1 of the Health Level Seven (HL7) Standard Protocol. Available at: http://www.cdc.gov/registry/hl7guide.pdf.

23. Accredited Standards Committee X12. Welcome to ASCX12. Available at: http://www.x12.org/. Accessed September 1, 2000.

24. National Center for Chronic Disease Prevention and Health Promotion, CDC. Working Toward Implementation of HL7 in NAACCR Information Technology Standards: Meeting Summary Report. Available at: http://www.cdc.gov/cancer/npcr/npcrpdfs/hl7mtg8.pdf. Accessed September 1, 2000.

25. National Center for Injury Prevention and Control, CDC. Data Elements for Emergency Department Systems (DEEDS) Release 1.0. Available at: http://www.cdc.gov/ncipc/pub-res/pdf/deeds.pdf. Accessed September 1, 2000.

26. Pollock DA, Adams DL, Bernardo LM, et al. Data Elements for Emergency Department Systems, Release 1.0 (DEEDS): A Summary Report. DEEDS Writing Committee. *J Emerg Nursing* 1998;24:35–44.

27. Pinner RW, Jernigan DB, Sutliff SM. Electronic laboratory-based reporting for public health. *Mil Med* 2000;165(Suppl 2):20–24.

28. Centers for Disease Control and Prevention. Health Level Seven Specifications for Electronic Laboratory-Based Reporting. Available at: http://www.cdc.gov/od/hissb/docs/HL7Spec.pdf. Accessed September 1, 2000.

29. World Wide Web Consortium (W3C). Extensible Markup Language (XML). Available at: http://www.w3.org/XML/. Accessed September 1, 2000.

30. Health Care Financing Administration (now Centers for Medicare and Medicaid Services). Medicare EDI Formats. Available at: http://www.hcfa.gov/medicare/edi/edi3.htm. Accessed September 1, 2000.

31. Centers for Disease Control and Prevention. National Electronic Telecommunications System for Surveillance. Available at: http://www.cdc.gov/epo/dphsi/netss.htm. Accessed September 1, 2000.

32. Object Management Group. CORBAmed. Available at: http://cgi.omg.org/homepages/corbamed/. Accessed September 1, 2000.

33. American National Standards Institute. ANSI Online. Available at: http://www.ansi.org/. Accessed September 1, 2000.

12
Evaluation for Public Health Informatics

Deborah Lewis

Learning Objectives

After studying this chapter, you should be able to:

- Explain the purposes of an evaluation of an information system.
- Describe the typical phases of an evaluation and their purposes.
- Differentiate between *formative* and *summative* characteristics of an evaluation, and explain why a sound evaluation needs to feature both characteristics.
- Explain why timeliness is important in an evaluation.
- Differentiate between subjectivist and objectivist evaluation methods, and describe the characteristics of each.
- List the characteristics of a well-developed evaluation report.
- Explain why evaluation of public health systems typically requires an evaluator to go beyond traditional evaluation models.

Overview

Both during development and after implementation of an information system, well-designed and timely evaluations are essential to help insure that the system accomplishes its intended purposes and is successful. In developing an evaluation, the evaluator needs to select an evaluation strategy and evaluation methods that are appropriate for analyzing the effectiveness of a system. Depending on the issues to be studied, an evaluator will select between subjectivist and objectivist methods or use a combination of both. Subjectivist strategies and methods focus on identifying the issues and the aspects of organizational culture that will impact system success. Objectivist strategies and methods, on the other hand, answer questions relative to specific and previously identified goals and objectives of a system. Regardless of the evaluation strategy and methods used, an evaluator's conclusions will be of little use if they are not communicated in a clear, focused, credible evaluation report that directly addresses the purpose of the evaluation.

Introduction

From planning, development, and implementation through determination of functionality, public health information systems rely on *evaluation*, the process of examining an information system to determine its effectiveness in meeting the needs of healthcare users. Well-designed evaluations provide the information that information system designers need to insure a system's functionality. Among other uses, evaluations are helpful in permitting system developers to develop and implement new public health information systems, to inform public policy decisions, and even to understand how the public can use health information on the Internet to make more informed healthcare decisions.

Evaluating health information systems often presents difficult challenges. In public health informatics, for example, an evaluation often deals with dynamic and ubiquitous data and with various information systems. Thus, system designers, implementers, and researchers must develop a comprehensive analysis that includes a broad range of evaluation methods. Moreover, the evaluation process is often complicated by the fact that many information applications, such as distributed electronic health record systems, are highly complex. In addition, the complexity of the evaluation task increases, in most instances, by virtue of the fact that systems implemented in field settings cannot be evaluated by use of traditional experimental methods. Finally, conventional analytic methods may be inadequate to describe the dynamic behavior of these systems over time. Although the set of evaluation tasks may be daunting, a properly designed evaluation can help to avoid the kind of costly failures discussed by Pete Kitch and William A. Yasnoff in Chapter 8.

This chapter will focus on the evaluation process as it applies to the wide range of information systems and programs that exist within the context of public health. We will begin by providing an overview of the phases of the typical evaluation and its purposes. After briefly examining development of evaluation strategies, we will review the nature and characteristics of the evaluation methods available. After discussing the desirable characteristics of an evaluation report, we will present a short case study that provides a reader the opportunity to apply the chapter's principles to an evaluation situation.

Phases of the Evaluation

A comprehensive evaluation of public health information systems includes multiple phases. It also requires an understanding of a range of methodologies. As the information resource being evaluated "matures" from development to deployment, the focus of the evaluation changes. We have adapted the phases of the evaluation process that we discuss here from Friedman and Wyatt[1]:

- Initially, it is important for an evaluator to understand the need for an information resource. At the initial phase, an evaluator studies the healthcare environment to identify the problem to be addressed and to focus the need for information resources. If the information system being evaluated is to be integrated into an organization, an evaluator will assess the organization's readiness for change and the attitudes of persons affected by the introduction of the system. This assessment phase will aid in the future success of a system's implementation. A more complete discussion of needs assessment can be found in Chapter 7.

- Early evaluation aids in the selection and development of a system because the results of the initial evaluation efforts often feed directly into the design phase. In the design phase, an evaluator studies the process of development. including the validation of the information system design.
- Early intervention and pilot studies then establish the usability and feasibility of an information resource. At this evaluation phase, an evaluation helps to confirm that the expected outcomes are consistent with the intended goals of the information resource. The feedback that is collected guides system redesign in preparation for deployment.
- The final phase includes deployment and integration of the information resource. The focus of the evaluation is on system performance and its impact on users and on the healthcare organization overall. Evaluation ideally becomes an ongoing process of evaluation and system redesign to meet the evolving needs of the healthcare enterprise.

Evaluation should begin as soon as system planning and development begins—while each phase may be perceived as equally important in supporting successful information system outcomes. Most evaluations, however, do not include all the phases we have described because, in reality, time constraints, limited funds, and organizational need generally dictate the evaluation focus.

Timing of the Evaluation

The timing of an evaluation is generally dictated by the purpose, scope, and maturity of the evolving system. Timing is important because evaluations generally contribute to the ongoing decision-making process in a system project; therefore, an evaluation is typically sought in a timely manner, and it is important that project staff allow enough time for an evaluation to be completed. After all, if an evaluation is conducted too rapidly, the quality and usefulness of the information obtained may suffer. On the other hand, an evaluation that takes too much time may be of little use, inasmuch as the system under development may undergo changes or become obsolete before it is implemented.

The challenge is to develop evaluations that are comprehensive enough to provide some support for effective system implementation and to offer rigorous evidence of outcomes. In this sense, evaluations are often a compromise.

They must balance the needs of the organization for timely information with the requirement of grounding the evaluation in data that genuinely reflect expected outcomes. The primary goal for evaluators is to provide the most rigorous and useful information possible to support the established goals of the information system.

Evaluation Strategies

Development of a comprehensive information system evaluation plan requires that an evaluator think broadly to include a variety of evaluation strategies that consider technical, economic, and organizational issues. An evaluation should be both formative and summative.[2] *Formative evaluation* produces information that can be fed back during the development and implementation to improve the likelihood of success of the project. A formative evaluation of information resources may seek to determine the answers to the following questions:

- Which information system should be selected and implemented?
- How much work redesign will be required to implement the system?
- How long will it take to implement the information system?
- What expectations does the staff have regarding the new system?
- How much will it cost to implement the system?

Summative evaluation, on the other hand, provides information about the effectiveness of the new information system.[3] Some questions that may be addressed by summative evaluation are as follows:

- Does the system work as designed?
- Is the system used as anticipated?
- Does the system produce the desired results?
- Is the system cost-effective?
- What are the effects of the system on the delivery of health services?

Formative evaluation, then, provides feedback to management and to system developers while a new system is under development, whereas summative evaluation occurs after a new system has been implemented.

Evaluation Methods

Evaluation in informatics employs a variety of methodologies. We will use the methodological framework described by Friedman and Wyatt[1] to categorize evaluation methods as either *subjectivist* or *objectivist* approaches. We will define these two approaches and provide examples from public health and medical informatics literature to help clarify their importance.

Subjectivist Evaluation

Subjectivist evaluation strategies focus on identifying the issues and the organizational culture that will impact system success. Subjectivist evaluation methods generally employ qualitative data collection. These methods are equally useful when the problem to be addressed by a system is still evolving and the system is early in its development or when the new system has been implemented. Subjectivist methods provide insight into the attitudes and opinions of potential system users and into the readiness of an organization/institution to accept the system. These methods provide an iterative process useful for securing a clarification of the issues, a clarification that is necessary to guide the direction, development, and implementation of the information system and to provide insight into users' acceptance of the system.[1] Figure 12.1 provides an overview of the process of subjectivist evaluation.

As Figure 12.1 indicates, subjective evaluation relies on such data collection processes as using focus groups, interviews and observations, retrospective data analysis, and systematic literature reviews. It obtains information from system users, system designers, and organizations. It uses this information to further develop research goals, to identify technical barriers to system success, to clarify organizational issues that may affect the success of the system, and to validate user issues and concerns.

Literature Reviews

Systematic literature reviews provide a historical perspective as well as a broad measure of the impact of information system evaluation within the research community. Because health informatics is a relatively new science, there are only a limited number of formal meta-analyses available to an evaluator. However, the use of systematic literature reviews offers system developers new insights by providing information about who is designing new systems or planning strategies for system deployment.[4]

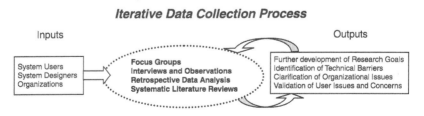

FIGURE 12.1. The process of subjectivist evaluation.

Retrospective Analysis of Data

A needs assessment may be a subjectivist approach when an evaluator identifies existing resources, services, and perceived need in order to provide a sense of the benefit of an information system for the organization. As an example in the literature, a study by Lange[5] examined 77 unique program-specific data systems existing within the Utah Department of Health in order to ascertain which databases contained identifiers representing "key program contacts"—persons who serve the mission of the health department. This needs assessment survey arose from a department-wide systems planning strategic plan that had the goal to create a resource that would implement standards and integrate data across programs within the Department of Health.

Focus Groups

In subjectivist evaluations, focus groups and interviews are important data collection strategies. An evaluator should use this methodology to assess users' perceptions and needs—both during system design and after system implementation. *Focus groups* bring together system users or program participants to discuss issues and concerns about the features of a system or program. The use of focus groups provides a forum for users' spontaneous reactions and ideas and often presents insights into organizational issues. An example of the use of focus groups in the literature appears in a study by Tang et al.[6] This study focused on gaining direct feedback from patients about their need for information regarding their individual health. Patients were asked to share their opinions about health education material they had received in the past. They were also asked to provide their reactions to new materials provided during focus group encounters and to describe what they perceived as desired attributes of patient education materials. The results of the focus group encounters were used to develop a set of criteria for the evaluation of computer-based patient education materials.

Interviews and Observational Studies

An example of the use of interviews and observational studies in subjectivist evaluation appears in Forsythe.[7] This body of ethnographic work spans multiple iterations of an evolving information system designed to assess health information needs and provide personalized explanation for patients with chronic migraine headaches. Patients and providers underwent both formal and informal interviews, and investigators conducted observational studies. During the course of the three-year project, investigators collected data used in the development of both the history-taking component and the explanation, or information provision, component of the system. Forsythe reflects that even with the extensive fieldwork that contributed to the development of the project, the design team still made personal assumptions that focused the ultimate system design. It was Forsythe's impression, in retrospect, that cultural assumptions held by systems designers may become embedded in a system, even though the designers did not intend for such assumptions to be incorporated. Forsythe's works highlights the importance of revisiting initial assumptions throughout the development of an information system. It provides an example of the iterative process that emerges as a new information system matures through the development and the implementation stages.

Objectivist Evaluation Methods

Whereas subjectivist evaluation methods are focused on identifying issues and evaluating the organizational culture into which a system will be introduced, objectivist methodologies answer questions related to specific, previously identified goals and objectives. Objectivist evaluations use empirical approaches and statistical analyses of quantitative data. Objectivist evaluations are focused more on a clinical event or an outcome under controlled conditions, rather than on the broader issues addressed by subjectivist evaluations. However, objectivist evaluations ideally are ongoing because of the ongoing changes occurring in healthcare delivery and the continual evolution of information systems. An objectivist evaluation, for example, might address the impact of a system on health care quality and costs; it might also address work flow redesign, the accuracy of data in public health databases, and/or evidence for new technology-based initiatives.[1]

In objectivist evaluation studies, participants or systems may be randomly assigned to the various treatment or control conditions in an experiment. In some cases, randomization may not be possible, in which case an objectivist evaluation may use quasi-experimental designs. An objectivist evaluation may use one group or multiple groups as subjects, and it may use post-test or, more often, both pre- and post-test evaluation components. Study designs that include two or more groups will usually have one group serving as the control. In crossover studies, participants will serve as their own controls. In objectivist evaluation studies, randomized clinical trials are generally considered the most scientifically rigorous design. Figure 12.2 provides an overview of the typical features of objectivist evaluations. The feedback loop from analysis to methodology represents the ongoing nature of systems evaluation. The lines are broken as a reminder that although evaluation and redesign are desirable, they are not always feasible due to time, funding, and other organizational constraints.

The literature on evaluations in health informatics provides numerous examples of objectivist evaluations. Here, we will present examples of different objectivist evaluation designs.

Experimental Designs

Cannon and Allen[8] evaluated the relative effectiveness of computer and paper-based reminder systems in the implementation of a clinical practice guide-

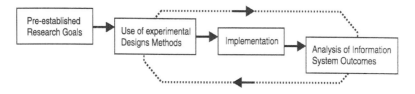

FIGURE 12.2. The process of objectivist evaluation.

line. In this study, 78 outpatient cases in a mental health clinic were randomly assigned, within clinician, to one of two reminder systems. One system was paper-based, and the other system was computer-based. The computer-based system, CaseWalker, reminded clinicians when guideline-recommended screening for mood disorder was due; it also insured conformity of the diagnosis of major depressive disorder to the criteria of the *Diagnostic and Statistical Manual of Mental Disorders*, Fourth Edition (DSM-IV), and it generated a progress note. The paper-based system consisted of a checklist inserted into the paper medical record. The study then compared screening rates for mood disorder and completeness of the documentation for the two systems. The computer-based system resulted in a higher screening rate for mood disorder (86.5% vs. 61% for the paper system, $P = 0.008$) and a higher rate of complete documentation of DSM-IV criteria (100% vs. 5.6%, $P < 0.001$).

In a randomized controlled trial, Overhage and colleagues[9] hypothesized that automated guideline-based reminders provided to physicians as they wrote orders could reduce errors of omission and improve health outcomes. This study randomly assigned to intervention and control groups faculty and house staff who used computer workstations to write orders. The study was conducted over 30 weeks. Three services were randomly assigned to be the intervention group and three services were controls. All physicians were provided with written versions of "corollary" orders based on accepted hospital guidelines. As physicians in the intervention group wrote orders, the computer suggested "corollary" order prompts. Physicians in the intervention group were found to have ordered the suggested corollary orders in 46.3% of instances in which they received a computerized reminder, whereas only 21.9% of physicians in the control group ordered the corollary orders ($P = 0.0001$). This study demonstrated that physician workstations linked to a comprehensive electronic medical record could be an efficient means of decreasing errors of omissions and of improving adherence to practice guidelines.

Cost-Benefit Analysis

An example of an objectivist evaluation involving cost-benefit analysis is a study of a teledentistry project within the US Department of Defense. The Total Dental Access (TDA) project enables referring dentists from the US Armed Forces worldwide to consult with specialists about the status of a patient.

TDA, used in over 50 dental clinics in Europe, focuses on three areas of dentistry: patient care, continuing education, and dentist–laboratory communications. One of the goals of TDA was to establish a cost-effective telemedicine system, while another goal was to increase patient access to quality dental care. An economic analysis of the teledentistry deployment was conducted to clarify the ongoing benefits of the program and to highlight its future potential. The results of the economic analysis demonstrated that the current teledentistry system generated a return on investment within one year of deployment and that future deployments would generate a return on investment within six months. This study demonstrated that providing dentists with easy, cost-effective access to specialists could improve the quality of care by facilitating better, more timely information for better decision-making by dentists and better communication between them and patients.[10]

Social Network Analysis

The literature also provides an example of the use of objectivist methodology for social network analysis in connection with a system. Aydin and others[11] evaluated the impact on patients and staff of the introduction of the CompuHx system into the Department of Preventive Medicine at the Kaiser-Permanente Medical Care Program in San Diego, California. CompuHx is a computer-based health appraisal system that assists nurse practitioners and physician assistants who work under the supervision of the medical staff to gather and record patient information for health appraisal and diagnosis. The purpose of the social network analysis was to determine how the new system affected work-related communication patterns among the staff. Nurse practitioners and physician assistants who used the system reported that they communicated more frequently with one another and with other staff and departments that could assist them in the performance of professional duties than did staff who did not use the information system. This frequent consultation and communication was found to have potential benefits for patient care.

Developing the Evaluation Report

Although every evaluator will use a different style for presenting an evaluation report, every report should meet basic standards for clarity, focus, and credibility. A good evaluation report meets the purpose of and objectives for the evaluation conducted. If the evaluation report does not address the purposes of the evaluation, it is a poor report, regardless of the quality of the report in terms of style and presentation method. Development of an evaluation report will depend on the original purpose, objectives, and evaluation approached used. An evaluation report writer also needs to consider the audience in developing the method of presentation. For example, technical language may appeal to system developers; on the other hand, a clear explanation of a system's impact on health outcomes will likely be of greater interest to healthcare providers. It may also be more effective to present the information in informal group meetings rather than as a written report.[1]

Conclusions

In this chapter, we have focused on basic evaluation models. It is important to recognize, however, that the complexities of public health problems and the disparate nature of public health settings sometimes require an evaluation approach beyond the approaches used in traditional evaluation studies. After all, system-wide informatics environments in public health will support data sharing across geographic distances and facilitate dissemination of health information to healthcare decision makers. Given the nature and use of public health informatics systems, their adoption may likely depend on the development of well-planned evaluations, evaluations that contribute evidence of benefit to the practice of public health and that are appropriately disseminated at professional meetings and in the literature of public health.

In the section titled "Questions for Review" that follows, we present a case study to assist the learner in synthesizing the information in this chapter.

Questions for Review

Read the following short case. Then answer the questions that are based on it.

A small rural clinic in State X has requested help from the state health department in addressing the healthcare needs of patients with diabetes. The clinic provides health care to patients through use of nurse practitioners and physician assistants who currently rely on telephone contact with physicians, who are 70 miles away in an urban medical center, for assistance with difficult cases. The director of the state public health department has asked you to lead a team to develop a technology-based strategy and initiatives that will support quality health outcomes for patients served by the clinic. You may select any four members of the state health department to serve on your team.

1. What expertise would you want on your team? Provide justification for your choices.
2. Assuming that you have assembled your team, what information will you need to begin planning your approach to the problem?
3. Because the focus of the problem solution to be developed is to be a technology-based initiative, you need to know about the existing infrastructure. State X has recently become a national demonstration site for new media, making any type of technology a possibility. You have also been given unlimited resources to carry out the project. It is important that your evaluation plan be well defined and documented, so

that you can show justification for the resources you propose and demonstrate outcomes for the patients that the technology-based initiative will serve.
    a. How will you begin?
    b. What evaluation approach would you consider to help you more clearly to identify the problems encountered by patients and providers of the clinic?
    c. Describe your initial evaluation plan, using formative methods.
4. On the basis of the initial evaluation, you have discovered that there has been an increase in the number of patients being treated for diabetic foot ulcers and other complications of diabetes. Chart reviews and discussion with the clinic's providers reveal that they do not always remember to incorporate clinical guideline recommendations in the care they provide. The providers have also stated that they are too busy to attend as many continuing education events as they would like, especially those events related to new medications for diabetes. Patients at the clinic state that they would like more information about diabetes care. Your team agrees that the following problems are important and would lend themselves to a technology solution:

- a need for the clinic's providers to have better access to consultants and specialists at the urban medical center;
- a need for patients to have access to diabetes care and diabetes management information;
- healthcare providers need support for clinical information and clinical decision making.

One idea that your team has is to develop a two-way video telecommunications system that will provide real-time visual and audio connectivity for professional consultations with specialists at the urban medical center.

A second idea is to develop a "virtual consumer health information center" that will provide diabetes care information for diabetic patients of the clinic. Patient access to this center is not an issue because funds are adequate to provide all clinic patients with connectivity via Web TV.

A third idea is to develop for the healthcare providers an electronic record system that will provide reminders regarding clinical guidelines and will include decision-support tools regarding medication selection and prescribing.

Your team believes that each of these initiatives is equally important in dealing with an identified problem. As a team leader, it is your responsibility to choose one of these initiatives and to describe the development of an objectivist evaluation plan.
    a. Describe your plan for the evaluation, and explain why you have chosen the particular methodology to be used.
    b. Create some mock data that results from your hypothetical evaluation and present it, along with a discussion of the results and outcomes for your proposed initiative. Assume that the audience for the evaluation is the healthcare providers at the clinic.

    c. Would your presentation method be different if the audience consisted of a system design team, rather than healthcare providers? How and why?

References

1. Friedman CP, Wyatt JC. *Evaluation Methods in Medical Informatics.* New York: Springer-Verlag; 1997.
2. Kaplan B. Addressing organizational issues into the evaluation of medical systems. *J Am Med Inform Assoc* 1997;4:94–101.
3. Anderson JG, Aydin CE. Overview: theoretical perspectives and methodologies for the evaluation of health care information systems. In: Anderson JG, Aydin CE, Jay SJ, eds. *Evaluating Health Care Information Systems: Methods and Applications.* Thousand Oaks, CA: Sage Publications; 1994:5–29.
4. Lewis DA. Computer-based approaches to patient education: A review of the literature. *J Am Med Inform Assoc* 1999;6:272–282.
5. Lange LL. Integrating public health data and information: A case example. In: Proceedings of the 1999 American Medical Informatics Association Symposium, Washington, DC, November 6–10, 1999:1104.6
6. Tang PC, et al. Meeting the information needs of patients: Results from a patient focus group. In: Proceedings of the 1997 American Medical Informatics Association Symposium, Nashville TN, October 25–29, 1997:672–676.
7. Forsythe DE. New bottles, old wine: Hidden cultural assumptions in a computerized explanation system for migraine sufferers. *Med Anthropol Q* 1996;10:551–574.
8. Cannon DS, Allen SN. Comparison of the effects of computer and manual reminders on compliance with a mental health clinical practice guideline. *J Am Med Inform Assoc* 2000;7:196–203.
9. Overhage JM, et al. A randomized trial of "corollary orders" to prevent errors of omission. *J Am Med Inform Assoc* 1997;4:364–375.
10. Rocca MA, et al. The evolution of a teledentistry system within the Department of Defense. In: Proceedings of the 1999 American Medical Informatics Association Symposium, Washington, DC, November 6–10, 1999:921–924.
11. Aydin CE, et al. Computers in the consulting room: A case study of clinician and patient perspectives. *Health Care Manage Sci* 1998;1:61–74.

Suggestion for Further Reading

Anderson JG. Evaluating clinical information systems: A step towards reducing medical errors. *MD Comput* 2000;17:21–23.

13
Ethics, Information Technology, and Public Health: Duties and Challenges in Computational Epidemiology

Kenneth W. Goodman

Learning Objectives

After studying this chapter, you should be able to:

- Differentiate between appropriate and inappropriate uses and users of information technology in public health under an electronic "standard of care."
- Explain why there is an ethical imperative to use appropriate information technology (IT) tools under an electronic "standard of care" in public health, and why failure to use appropriate IT tools can be as blameworthy as inappropriately using such tools.
- Explain the concept of "progressive caution" in the ethical application of information technology to public health.
- Explain the ethical tension inherent in attempting to maintain confidentiality of individual information while using modern IT tools to store group data.
- Explain why ethical considerations will not permit scientists to entrust decisions about public health interventions to computers alone.
- Identify *meta-analysis* and *data mining* as tools in public health research, and explain why such tools can themselves pose ethical challenges for scientists in making public health decisions.

Overview

The application of powerful information technology tools to the practice of public health poses ethical, in addition to practical, challenges. Under a modern, electronic standard of care, it can be as blameworthy to apply such tools inappropriately as it is not to apply them at all. Certain ethical guidelines can help public health scientists make sound decisions about what users and uses of information technology (IT) are appropriate in public health. Even with these guidelines, however, there remain some gray areas, particularly with respect to maintaining the privacy and confidentiality of public health information. The power of modern IT tools renders obsolete some previously sacrosanct guidelines about maintaining privacy and confidentiality. It is therefore necessary for public health practitioners to exercise "progressive caution" in applying information technology to the practice of public health. Developments such as bioinformatics pose acute challenges to maintaining privacy and confidentiality, as does the use of powerful computer technology as support for decisions about interventions. Finally, the interests of ethics and sound public health practice collide in the application of such modern tools as meta-analysis and data mining to public health problems. Even the time-honored practice of using and publishing case studies in public health research presents challenges to maintaining confidentiality of information, as the World Wide Web and other communication and education tools make it increasingly possible for readers to identify the individual(s) discussed in a case.

Introduction

At least as much as any other domains in the health professions and sciences, epidemiology and public health are information intensive. Public health is at ground, albeit not at heart, the collection, sharing. and analysis of data; and precious little of this effort uses 3-by-5 cards. The ancient, or at least traditional. thrust of public health informatics is best appreciated by picturing Aristotle, Paracelsus, John Graunt. and others building databases. sending e-mail, and surfing the Web in search of more and better information. We have digitized the Broad Street pump—along with its handle. its dirty water. and, in several respects, the very people who drink from it.

On balance, this is good news. The failure to use appropriate tools can be at least as blameworthy as using them carelessly or with ill intent. But attention to the intersection of ethics and public health informatics requires us to look more closely and with greater precision at the ways information technology (IT) is used and the issues it raises.

To begin, it is noteworthy that we are dealing with three broad. if not vast. areas of human inquiry: ethics, computing. and public health. This chapter addresses the intersection of computing (or IT) and public health. Previous work has explored the marriage of (1) ethics in epidemiology and public health[1-3] and. given our goals here, with somewhat greater specificity. (2) ethics, computing, and health care.[4]

So we have a number of tools (or at least predecessors) to guide us; this is good, given that the three-way intersection we are about to traverse is one formed by high stakes, the need for practical guidance. and the existence of principled disagreement.

Toward an Electronic "Standard of Care"

In science and the professions, standards evolve or are stipulated for a number of reasons. These include the need for a public evaluation metric, a system of professional goals and objectives, and a calculus for assigning blame. Contrary to what many people expect when ethics is given a seat at the health technology table, the result is not always nay-saying and hand-wringing; sometimes, perhaps often, ethics will *require* use of a new technology if it will promote or achieve independently scrutinized goals (e.g., better patient care, improved public health, etc.). This was clear at the dawn of interest in the intersection of ethics and health informatics, when it was noted that failure to use a computational tool might itself be blameworthy.[5]

The idea of a standard of care for public health informatics is motivated by these considerations. Such a standard will help make clear which uses and users of information systems are appropriate, why failure to use appropriate tools can be as blameworthy as inappropriate use, and why system evaluation is essential for an ethically optimized IT system. Throughout, we must attend to the fascinating tension between the need for science to progress and the demands of a reasoned and robust ethics; we call this "progressive caution."[6]

Appropriate Uses and Users of IT in Public Health

Nearly everyone would agree that a vital statistics database should be maintained and used for, say, reducing infant mortality and not, for instance, marketing infant formula. What's the difference? What makes the one use appropriate and the other inappropriate? While we consider these questions in some detail in what follows, we can lay out here some general strategies for answering them.

First and perhaps most obviously, not all uses and users are equal. We can begin to sort them out by looking at intentions, consequences, and values.

So, for instance, a database created with public funds to improve public health and promote public welfare is, well, a *public* database. This means that such a database is available for use by authorized public representatives for public purposes. A potentially inappropriate use of the database would therefore be for some sort of private gain or profit. This is not a comment on the free-market system. It is just an observation that the data in the database were collected by public representatives using public funds for the sake of public health. If the data were collected for proprietary purposes, it would have been necessary to disclose that in advance, if for no other reason than to allow the sources of the data to negotiate for their share of the profit. But then, of course, if a person is told that his or her personal information is going to be stored for proprietary purposes and an agreement over profit-sharing cannot be reached, and if that person then refuses to allow the information to be used, then the database would be less valuable, less useful, and less accurate as a *public health* resource.

So far, however, we have merely stipulated that the database is public, and tried to make a moral point out of it. More important and powerfully, we assign moral weight to the idea that the *intention* guiding the creation and maintenance of the database was to benefit the public. Intentions matter in ethics because they can aim for good or ill. In this case, the intention was a good one, and so hewing to it will constitute an appropriate use. This is emphatically not to say that proprietary uses are somehow inherently ill-intentioned—only that the use of public health information for public health should be regarded as more praiseworthy by virtue of the greater benefits that will accrue.

But suppose an evil database designer set about creating a computational resource for marketing untested home remedies, discriminating against minorities, or spreading panic. Surely this intention should not enjoy the same status as the other. Put differently, intentions (like IT uses and users) are not created equal. They are distinguished by, among other things, the consequences of their realization and the value we attach to the intention (whether realized or not). In part, because the evil database designer, if successful, will cause great harm, we judge her intentions to be morally inferior. Moreover, we value health over illness, stability over chaos, and so forth. Intentions and consequences, however, are not always so clear-cut.

Looking at matters in this way, we can also see why failure to use appropriate tools can be as blameworthy as inappropriate use—though this, of course, is true only when there is reason to believe the tools will have a positive or valued effect. Moreover, note that health IT tools require comprehensive and even systematic evaluation, and that this evaluation must occur in the context of actual use. Indeed, it has been convincingly argued that there is an ethical imperative to conduct such evaluation.[7] We can here explicitly extend this insight to public health informatics, at least provisionally, as we sort out the idea of an "electronic standard of care."

System evaluation also helps us make sense of particular uses and users of public health IT systems, at least to the extent that we need to determine for individual uses and users their efficacy and thereby part of their propriety.

We can now look at particular uses and users and see if our intentions-consequences-values metric does any good. For the sake of discussion, let's identify registry maintenance and querying, decision support and data analysis as uses; and government officials, students, and corporate investors as users. To be sure, there are many other actual and potential uses and users, and they might be combined in many ways. Indeed, with the lists just presented, we have nine possible scenarios, and we will not review them all. The idea is rather to give a sense of how the process might work.

We can do this with two easy (extreme) cases:

1. A government official wants to query (or build or maintain) a tumor or vaccine registry. If her *intent* is, say, identifying the incidence and prevalence of a certain neoplasm in a particular population, if the *consequence* of the query is closing a toxic waste site and reducing correlate morbidity and mortality.

and if we *value* reduced morbidity and mortality, then we should be seen to have identified an appropriate use and user.

2. Suppose now that the same registry is queried by an investor who is keen to predict for personal gain which anticancer agents will enjoy the greatest markets in coming years. Now the intent is commercial, the consequence is eroded public confidence in database security, and the value is entrepreneurship. The question of appropriate use and user should be easy to answer. (Again, the point is not to suggest that all commercial uses of public health data are inappropriate, only that proprietary and private uses cannot enjoy the same status as improved public health.)

Make no mistake: Many or most cases are vastly more complex than these. Rarely are data as unambiguous as implied in our little examples. In case 1, what about the problem of communicating health risks and the likelihood of engendering fear or even panic? What about people who lose their jobs if a factory is closed? In case 2, is there nothing to be said about the virtues of data sharing? On balance, though, we should say that ever more rigorous analyses of data that bear on the cases at hand will tend to point the way to ethically optimized solutions. Issues raised later in this chapter will give examples of this. In fact, ethical issues related to the use of IT should be seen as a subset of all ethical issues that arise in epidemiology and public health.

Such refinement, it is worth emphasizing, is precisely the task of applied ethics. The model is reasonably well evolved in clinical ethics and is applied with good results by many institutional ethics committees (as in hospitals). It is, if we may be forgiven the stipulation, the way to do ethics. The growing interest in codes of ethics is positive and noteworthy—but codes, guidelines, and lists of best practices are no substitute for robust and ongoing ethics education and analysis.

"Progressive Caution"

Ethics thrives on new science and technology. This is no less true in epidemiology and public health than in any other science. In the health professions, where the stakes are consistently high, the role of ethics is complex. When it comes to new technology, what role do we want ethical analysis to have? Should we be stomping our feet, shaking our heads, and clucking our tongues at the new technology, Luddites at the gates of progress? Or should we prefer facile boosterism, cheering each new gadget independent of its utility or consequences, cheerleaders at the edge of the abyss? The answer, of course, is straightforward: Neither. We want thoughtful analyses and practical guidance. We want science to progress, and we want to minimize risk. We want dispassionate reason and reasonable passion.

That is, we want a kind of "progressive caution" whereby we move forward, and that progress is tempered or leavened by attention to the kinds of details being scrutinized here. In a slightly different context, the idea of progressive caution was introduced thus: "Medical informatics is, happily, here to stay, but users and society have extensive responsibilities to ensure that we use our tools appropriately. This might cause us to move more deliberately or slowly than some would like. Ethically speaking, that is just too bad."[6(p9)]

Progressive caution captures the idea at the core of this chapter. It is perhaps best or most productive to put it in the form of a question: How should we arrange things so that we enjoy the benefits of new technology while reducing, minimizing, or mitigating the (potential) harms? Given that both the use and the failure to use IT raise ethical issues, the concept of progressive caution bids fair to help guide us as we consider the specific ethical issues that arise when IT is used in epidemiology and public health.

Privacy, Confidentiality, and Security

In Chapter 10, William A. Yasnoff discusses in some detail the technical issues associated with privacy, confidentiality, and security in health informatics. Here, we will discuss privacy, confidentiality, and security in an ethical context.

The intersection of ethics and health informatics almost immediately brings to mind questions of privacy and confidentiality. These issues are indeed what most people, scientists and laypeople included, worry about. But public health by its nature will require that we think about privacy and confidentiality in ways somewhat different than we might be accustomed to in clinical medicine, nursing, or psychology.

We might begin by recalling the difference between privacy and confidentiality. *Privacy* is best thought of as relating to *people* and their hope, goal, or right to be left alone and free of intrusion. You might, for instance, violate my privacy by peering in my window to study my behavior or by rounding up residual blood to analyze my genome. *Confidentiality* relates to *information*, the "holy secrets" of Hippocrates. You might violate my confidentiality by looking at my medical chart, or by querying the database that contains some or all of that information.

The core problem with confidentiality and electronic health media is this: We want simultaneously to make information easily accessible to appropriate users and inaccessible to inappropriate users. This is a problem, because the means for accomplishing the one are often in conflict with the means for accomplishing the other. But this air of dilemma is resolvable in a number of ways[8,9]:

- Technology, including security measures
- Institutional policies and procedures

- Education programs addressing the foundations and importance of confidentiality

These practical steps may be regarded as moral imperatives, measures to take as part of a comprehensive program to protect individuals' health information. But such protections cannot—and should not—be absolute. That is, there may be credible challenges to confidentiality, and many of the most interesting and important ones arise in public health.

Information, Consent, and Stigma

The most obvious way one might ethically set aside confidentiality is with the consent of those to whom the information pertains. This is often the case in research contexts: Investigators need to have access to personal health information, and subjects/participants agree to this access. Patients also routinely consent to release of information to third parties—e.g., insurers—for the sake of reimbursement of health professionals (though because they must provide such consent to be treated in the first place, one might plausibly wonder how voluntary such consent really is).

Public health IT poses special challenges to this model, in part because there are many cases in which it would be logistically or practically impossible for epidemiologists or public health officials to obtain consent from all those whose information they want to collect or analyze. In other contexts, too, society has set aside the notion of absolute confidentiality in exchange for the benefits of better health surveillance, monitoring, and analysis: information about transmission of various diseases, rates of vaccination, and so forth. Indeed, a great deal of personal health information is collected, stored, and processed by governments, universities, and other entities without any individual consent whatsoever. Institutional review boards oversee some of these efforts, but they do not oversee others. All represent, we might say, a price people are willing to pay in exchange for better public health.

But that willingness is not to be presumed come what may: It is, we might surmise, a gift from citizens in open societies. They trust health authorities to make sound decisions and recommendations based on the best available evidence, and they trust those authorities to acquire the evidence in the least intrusive ways possible. One of the ways to accomplish this is to render the data anonymous in salient respects. For instance, many public health surveillance efforts do not require the collection or storage of unique identifiers such as name, address, or Social Security number; all that is needed is case information, context, and so forth.

But the balance of the "special challenge" of public health IT is that health data achieve a distinctive synergy when they are stored in computers: It might not matter that you do not know my name if, for example, you know my disease, my race, my postal code, and my sexual orientation.[10,11] Either you will be able to identify me—to pick me out of the crowd—anyway, by virtue of these surrogate data ensembles, or your surveillance or research will come to associate my social, racial, ethnic, or other group with a malady or behavior in ways I would have objected to had I been given the opportunity to dissent.

Even in open societies, most people are ignorant of the ability of geographic information systems to characterize neighborhoods and draw inferences about ever-narrower social groups. Would people consent to these characterizations or inferences? Indeed, would they ever have agreed in the first place to allow their personal information to be digitized if they knew the kinds of inferences that might be drawn? What we have come to call "group confidentiality," or the idea that population subgroups have privacy and confidentiality interests,[12] has acquired recent currency, especially in genetics.

The Case of Bioinformatics

Completion of the project to map the human genome is ushering in what might come to be known as the golden age of molecular epidemiology. So, if there remain any doubts surrounding the importance of the tension here, we should be able to eliminate them with a brief excursus on computational genomics or bioinformatics.[13,14] For a variety of clinical and research purposes, including drug discovery, clinicians and scientists are increasingly able to digitize genetic information and store it in databases. Three key questions emerge from this effort, and they will continue to challenge our ability to get an ethical grip on all this new technology:

1. Does it make any real sense to talk about confidentiality when computers processing genomic data (perhaps in conjunction with other information) provide a high-powered way of identifying individuals whose idea of confidentiality might have been a piece of paper in a locked desk?
2. Consent to acquire information increasingly needs to take into account the idea that people might—or might not—want to learn the results of aggregate genetic analysis. In other words, if I agree to let you store and analyze my genetic data, does that mean you will later let me know what you learn? Will you have an unanticipated duty to disclose risks to people who might not want to hear of them?
3. What standards or assurances are available that error reduction is being addressed by the new technology? Complex databases and gene annotation protocols are ripe for both error and error-reduction strategies. With genomes as e-mail attachments and digitized genetic information being included in very large databases, the job of valid consent will be as difficult as required by any other aspect of biomedical research. There are several reasons for this. Some are independent of the role of information technology and some are greater because of computers.

Genetic information is not about one person; it is also information, in one degree or another, about a subject's relatives. These relatives might be identified in research (usually pedigree studies) without having consented to be subjects in the research. Genetic information is also to some extent also about members of one's racial or ethnic group, increasing the risk of bias and stigma—even as we might make use of the information for standard epidemiologic purposes. Genetic information increases in scientific (and other) value over time. This is due to the fact that, although we have sequenced the human genome, we are still mostly ignorant of the *function*s of most genes. As functional genomics progresses, we will have tomorrow the ability to conduct research that is not possible today. This increase in research potential is independent of the stored genetic information or tissue samples themselves. In other words, today's genetic database will increase in value tomorrow even if it is not changed or added to.

Can valid consent rise to these challenges? There is every reason to believe it can, especially as we ensure that the concept of valid consent as a process and not an event does not collapse into platitude and cliché. Indeed, the idea that consent is a process—which might, in fact, never end—might be precisely the way to ethically optimize the epidemiologic use of digitized genetic information. As has been commended in other contexts, there is potentially great value in special newsletters for subjects (and even communities) whose genetic information has been digitized and stored in an electronic database. Such newsletters would inform individuals, relatives, and communities of new and potential uses, including research, contemplated for the database. The database, if appropriately constructed, could provide the means for individual subjects to opt out of specific studies. For instance, suppose I am willing to consent to initial research in cancer genetics but not secondary research in neurogenetics. Once my genome is in your database, you will be able to let me know of the contemplated secondary use. And, if I dissent, you will be able to ensure that my genetic information is not included in your study.

Such a newsletter might also, it should be noted, provide a much better way of including subjects in the broad sweep of the research in general by informing them of study results, related research, and even ethical issues raised by the research! The positive potential for public health has not been adequately explored.

One way to think of these challenges is as challenges to our strategy of identifying intentions, consequences, and values. The strategy is not failsafe, but infallibility was never a promise of either science or ethics.

Decision Support

Our discussion of appropriate uses and users of IT systems will be of no small utility as we consider the issue of computational decision support in epidemiology and public health. In one sense, all computers used in epidemiology and public health are decision support systems—computers that help us navigate among the shoals of probabilistic data.

In clinical medicine and nursing, there are generally thought to be at least three kinds of decision support systems: reminder systems, consultation systems, and educational systems. Their functions are easily inferable from their names. It is not clear whether decision support in epidemiology and public health runs parallel to these three uses—what constitutes a reminder in clinical medicine, for instance, has no ready analog in the public health sciences. We can, however, identify two functions of ethical interest in decision support in epidemiology and public health; they are (1) interventions and (2) data synthesis, including meta-analysis and data mining.

Interventions

A decision support system might be used to help decide whether and when to begin an intervention program and what kind of intervention would be best or most efficacious. Why is there an ethical issue here? To answer this question, let's turn to clinical medicine.

What has come to be called the "standard view" of decision support in diagnosis suggests that humans are better than machines at functions as complicated as diagnosis.[15] Humans *understand* data better than machines (even if computers might be able to *process* it better and faster). The answers to questions about whether to close a well, commence an education program, or call for a quarantine are decisions that require more than digital firepower. They are decisions that require vast background knowledge, a scientific as well as an intuitive understanding of risk, and a more or less clear sense of how humans balance and trade off among competing goals. Computers cannot meet these criteria and likely will be unable to for some time.

It follows that although we might have a duty to use computers to help in making tough calls, we must not let the computers make the tough calls. This stance is appropriate whether we are contemplating needle exchange programs or foreign cattle bans, vaccination protocols or plague quarantines. Another way of putting this is that public health decisions are rarely if ever exclusively scientific, statistical, or what-have-you. Public health scientists and officials are faced with a difficult array of decision points such that the correct or best answer will rarely be arrived at with more information or more computing power. Rather, scientists and officials need to analyze their intentions or the goals they hope to achieve, the consequences of various decisions they might make or actions they might take, and the values that guide them.

The question of whether to intervene and which intervention to commend is, in part, an ethical one precisely for these reasons. It is perhaps not impossible that a decision-support system might one day be able to perform operations on human values as well as on data sets—but it is quite unlikely and, in any case, it will be quite a long time before that happens. The lesson in public health is the same as in clinical medicine and nursing: Computers should not be allowed to trump people.[15]

Data Synthesis and Computer-Based Research

Ever-increasing demands for data and evidence to inform guidelines and best practices have made it clear that we need computers to help us through all our information. Indeed, we now turn with increasing frequency to various forms of research synthesis to make sense of the data. The computational tools of research synthesis—meta-analysis and data mining will give us our best examples—are ways of eliciting conclusions, answers, or even mere suggestions from the apparent mess of data.

One way to think of this issue is by plotting ethical issues against scientific (un)certainty. That is, the most important and interesting ethical issues arise in cases of scientific uncertainty. Although it is true that even perfect knowledge will not answer all our ethical questions, it surely would make many of them easier!

The fledgling sciences (techniques, really) of meta-analysis and data mining provide us with many case studies about whether and when to use a computer in making scientific decisions. The debate over meta-analysis, which often turns on its methods and reliability, is important for any discussion of ethics in epidemiology, in general, and ethics, computing, and, epidemiology, in particular.[16]

Consider the case of meta-analytic studies of the effects of environmental tobacco smoke. In 1993, the US Environmental Protection Agency, relying on a meta-analysis of 11 studies of smokers' spouses, classified environmental or "second-hand" tobacco smoke as a Group A carcinogen, along with radon, asbestos, and benzene.[17] No problem so far—tobacco smoke is bad, people agree tobacco smoke is bad, a study shows that tobacco smoke is bad. The problem is that meta-analysis continues to engender intense debate about its accuracy and reliability. It might be, in other words and just for the sake of discussion, that we (in 1993) actually lacked adequate scientific warrant to rank environmental tobacco smoke as a Group A carcinogen. At any rate, the debate elicited the following remark[18]: "Yes, it's rotten science, but it's in a worthy cause. It will help us to get rid of cigarettes and to become a smoke-free society." We have described the ethics–computing–public health tension as follows:

> "In one respect, the very idea is incoherent: If one believes the science to be flawed, then how can it support a worthy cause? How even can the cause become worthy in the absence of credible evidence? (If environmental smoke does not harm children, then there is no reason to protect them from it, and so protecting them cannot be worthy.) But granting for the sake of discussion that the cause is worthy, it is nevertheless a severe form of ethical shortsightedness to suggest that the credibility of scientists, government institutions, and policy makers is a fair trade for a victory on one policy issue. Even the most craven utilitarian would recognize this to be a bad bet." [16(p160)]

Note that although the intention might be praiseworthy (to reduce environmental tobacco smoke) and the consequence a positive one (fewer people suffering the effects of second-hand smoke), the value we place on scientific method and credibility may sometimes outweigh the other considerations. It is also important to underscore that it can be very difficult to calculate future consequences—including future negative consequences.

Think of meta-analysis as a secondary or n-ary use of data. Such use matters, as it did with bioinformatics, because subjects or communities might have consented to the primary use but not necessarily the secondary or n-ary one. Now, this might matter little or not at all to subjects, especially if the risks of such research are minimal or absent and if (as is usually the case with meta-analysis) individuals cannot be identified from or in the data. Likewise, with data mining, also sometimes called "knowledge discovery" or "machine learning," we have the n-ary analysis of databases in search of patterns, trends, associations and the like. Used to great profit in science and business, data mining is emerging as a potentially valuable resource in health care.

Our concern is with valid consent in public health practice and research—specifically, the use of personal information for purposes other than originally intended. Data-mining technology promises public health trend-spotting, quality assessment, and outcomes research of depth and breadth unimagined a few years ago. Because this information is *personal* information, we need to ask whether those people the information is about would agree to such use. We need to look at three key considerations:

1. Is the database analysis something that was disclosed and consented to when the information was obtained?
2. Is the purpose of the data mining scientific, commercial, or both?
3. Are individuals identifiable in the database or as a result of the research?

The answer to question 1 is rarely "yes"; the use might be commercial; and the answer to question 3 will often be "generally" or "in principle." The feature of data mining that distinguishes it from more garden-variety forms of database research is the facility with which scientists (and others) can look through vast amounts of personal, identifiable information—again and again and again. (It is, therefore, a question at least of degree and perhaps of kind.) Each analysis is a further "experiment" for which we may generally presume that no consent has been obtained. Moreover, consent tools like newsletters are more useful for focused research programs where the goals of the research can be spelled out. In data mining, one might perform an analysis with all the effort and forethought that go into a MEDLINE search, for instance.

As with bioinformatics, more research is needed to clarify the ethical issues surrounding data mining. We include it here to give a sense of exciting new challenges to the standard model of valid consent. (How best, for instance, might one describe data mining in lay language to prospective subjects?) For now, the best consent for data mining research is likely to be obtained in advance, for noncommercial research, and for studies where individual identifiers are either not available or can be readily hidden.

Conclusion: The World Wide Web and Beyond

Case studies are an ancient and rightfully honored way to communicate, educate, and elucidate. The public health sentinel who learns about and shares information about an emerging malady does so, at least at the outset, by means of a case study. Clusters of cases capture our epidemiologic attention. That is just the way it works. But for the first time, news of rare, interesting, important, and otherwise noteworthy cases can be shared internationally and almost instantly. The problem is that the more distinctive a case is, the greater the likelihood that it will be possible to recognize or identify the individual(s) the case is about or to whom it pertains. What should we do about this?

It will not do to suggest that epidemiologists and public health scientists and officials should remain silent about such cases to protect the supposed confidentiality of heretofore-anonymous individuals.[19] But surely we need to do something to balance these two forces.

What should by now be clear is that people of good will have access to an ensemble of powerful conceptual tools, tools that have proven their worth in a broad variety of healthcare settings in which intelligent machines have been brought to bear. In the current instance, the best advice is that individuals and institutions that publish sensitive case reports need to adopt sound policies, acquire as much consent as possible, and, institutionally, ensure the availability of a robust ethics education program.[20]

What is in some domains a comfortable demarcation between practice and research becomes fraught and controversial in epidemiology and public health. This is unavoidable, but it presents us with splendid opportunities to apply and evaluate the tools of practical ethics. This will be especially true as ever-grander computers and data networks link scientists and officials from around the world. We will judge them by how well they use the networks in the service of public health, and by how well they attend to the concerns of individuals who, in a flash (or a click), may find themselves and their genes and maladies and behaviors out there for all to see.

Questions for Review

1. *Questions 1a–1d are based on the following scenario:* As a state public health executive, you have responsibility for maintaining and controlling a database containing data on all state residents who have been diagnosed with reportable diseases. Included in the database are certain identifiers, including names and addresses of individuals. In the course of performing your duties, you are approached by various individuals desiring access to the database. Using the ethical intent-consequences-value metric, determine your response to each of the following requests for access, assuming the access will be without the consent of individuals concerned:

    a. A pair of public health research scientists ask to access the database in order to conduct a study of an outbreak of measles in two public schools in a county, to determine whether a batch of vaccine may have been defective or whether certifications of vaccination may have been fraudulent.

    b. A prominent lawyer wants to obtain the names and addresses of individuals diagnosed with black lung disease in order to contact them to secure their agreement to participation in a law suit to be filed against coal mine operators.

    c. A major pharmaceutical company wants to obtain the names and addresses of individuals diagnosed with syphilis in order to secure their participation in a test of the effectiveness of a new drug that the company believes will seek out and kill latent spirochetes.

    d. A licensed physician specializing in treatment of sexually transmitted diseases wants to obtain the names and addresses of individuals diagnosed with STDs within the past two months in order to contact them for the purpose of building a practice.

2. Two epidemiologists have developed a computerized hair analysis system that detects the presence of unusual levels of arsenic in human subjects twice as fast as existing methods. Their extensive, private testing has proven the effectiveness of the system to their satisfaction, but the system has not been subjected to a formal testing process. The inventors have been assigned to study an outbreak of suspected arsenic poisoning in a community that relies on well water. Are they obligated to use the new system? Why or why not?

Questions 3 and 4 are based on the following case and are derived from DARPA 2001, Bio-Surveillance System, Proposer Information Pamphlet (Broad Agency Announcement [BAA] #01-17). Available on the Web at http://www.darpa.mil/ito/Solicitations.html. Accessed December 14, 2001, and Goodman, K.W. (2002). Ethics and Evidence-Based Medicine: Fallibility and Responsibility in Research and Practice. Cambridge and New York: Cambridge University Press.

A government in a democracy is worried about a bioterror attack. It seeks to support development of early warning technologies to reduce injury from such an attack, specifically to "develop, test, and demonstrate the technologies necessary to provide an early alert to appropriate emergency response elements about the release of biological agents, involving both natural and unnatural pathogens, against military or civilian personnel." The project will require using data from government and commercial health databases ("while maintaining patient privacy privileges"). These could include hospital emergency department records, 911 telephone calls, certain pharmacy and supermarket purchases, etc. (DARPA 2001, cited by Goodman 2002.) Such ubiquitous and automated surveillance would be impossible if consent were required from all people in a community.

3. What measures will make such surveillance ethically acceptable (or tolerable)?
4. How best should open societies balance public health and welfare against infringements of privacy and other rights and liberties?

References

1. Coughlin S, Beauchamp T, eds. *Ethics and Epidemiology*. New York: Oxford University Press: 1996.
2. Coughlin S, Soskolne C, Goodman K. *Case Studies in Public Health Ethics*. Washington, DC: American Public Health Association; 1997.
3. Geissman K. Goodman KW, et al. *Scientific Ethics: An Interactive, Multimedia, Computer-Based Training*. Atlanta: Centers for Disease Control and Prevention and Agency for Toxic Substances and Disease Registry: 1998.
4. Goodman KW, ed. *Ethics, Computing and Medicine: Informatics and the Transformation of Health Care*. New York: Cambridge University Press; 1998.
5. Miller RA, Schaffner KF, Meisel A. Ethical and legal issues related to the use of computer programs in clinical medicine. *Ann Intern Med* 1985;102:529–536.
6. Goodman KW. Bioethics and health informatics: an introduction. In: Goodman KW, ed. *Ethics, Computing and Medicine: Informatics and the Transformation of Health Care*. New York: Cambridge University Press: 1998:1–31.
7. Anderson JG, Aydin CE. Evaluating medical information systems: social contexts and ethical challenges. In: Goodman KW, ed. *Ethics, Computing and Medicine: Informatics and the Transformation of Health Care*. New York: Cambridge University Press; 1998:57–74.
8. National Research Council. *For the Record: Protecting Electronic Health Information*. Washington, DC: National Academy Press; 1997.
9. Alpert SA. Health care information: access, confidentiality, and good practice. In: Goodman KW, ed. *Ethics, Computing and Medicine: Informatics and the Transformation of Health Care*. New York: Cambridge University Press: 1998:75–101.
10. US General Accounting Office. *Record Linkage and Privacy: Issues in Creating New Federal Research and Statistical Information*. Washington, DC: U.S. General Accounting Office (GAO-01-126SP); 2001.
11. Sweeney LA. Guaranteeing anonymity when sharing medical data: the Datafly System. In: Masys DR, ed. *Proceedings of AMIA Annual Fall Symposium*. Philadelphia: Hanley & Belfus: 1997:51–55.
12. Alpert SA. Privacy and the analysis of stored tissues. In: *Research Involving Human Biological Materials: Ethical Issues and Policy Guidance*. Vol. II: Commissioned Papers. Rockville. MD: National Bioethics Advisory Commission; 2000.
13. Goodman KW. Ethics, genomics, and information retrieval. *Comput Biol Med* 1996;26:223–229.
14. Goodman KW. Bioinformatics: challenges revisited. *MD Comput* 1999;16:17–20.
15. Miller RA. Why the standard view is standard: people, not machines, understand patients' problems. *J Med Philos* 1990;15:581–591.
16. Goodman KW. Meta-analysis: Conceptual, ethical and policy issues. In: Goodman KW, ed. *Ethics, Computing and Medicine: Informatics and the Transformation of Health Care*. New York: Cambridge University Press; 1998:139–167.
17. Environmental Protection Agency. *Respiratory Health Effects of Passive Smoking:*

Lung Cancer and Other Disorders. Washington. DC: Government Printing Office (EPA/600/6-90/006F; GPO: 0555-000-00407-2); 1993.

18. Feinstein AR. Critique of review article. Environmental tobacco smoke: Current assessment and future directions. *Toxicol Pathol* 1992;20:303–305.

19. Snider DE. Patient consent for publication and the health of the public. *JAMA* 1997;278:624–626.

20. Markovitz BP, Goodman KW. Case reports on the Web: Is confidentiality being maintained? In Lorenzi NM. ed. *Proceedings of the Annual Symposium of the American Medical Informatics Association.* Philadelphia: Hanley & Belfus; 1999:1114.

Part III
Key Public Health
Information Systems

Introduction

In this part, we move to an examination of public health information systems that serve as major sources of data and information for public health practitioners and researchers.

In Chapter 14, Mary Anne Freedman and James A. Weed discuss the national vital statistics system. After briefly tracing the background of the development of this important source of information about births, deaths, and other events in the United States, they focus on the operation of the national vital statistics system, including the roles performed at the state and national levels and the nature of the vital statistics data files. The authors conclude the chapter with a discussion of innovations that enhance the system and its output and of the importance of vital statistics to the practice of public health.

In Chapter 15, Linda K. Demlo and Jane F. Gentleman provide coverage of systems that serve as sources of morbidity data. Using three major surveys operated by the National Center for Health Statistics (NCHS) as a basis of discussion, Demlo and Gentleman discuss the major challenges facing public health practitioners and researchers in securing timely, accurate, and reliable information about the incidence and prevalence of disease in the United States. After a discussion of concerns for the confidentiality, privacy, and security of morbidity data files and of the use of the NCHS's Research Data Center, the two authors provide an overview of present and future innovations in the computerization of survey data for retrieval, processing, editing, and dissemination. They conclude the chapter with a forward look at the continuing importance of morbidity data to the practice of public health.

In Chapter 16, Patrick W. O'Carroll, Eve Powell-Griner, Deborah Holtzman, and G. David Williamson discuss the importance and challenges of accessing and using risk factor data. After a discussion of the key risk factor systems in United States public health, the authors conclude the chapter with comments concerning the behavioral and other recognized risk factors that cause premature deaths, illnesses, injuries, and disability in the United States and a discussion of the importance of risk factor data as an element in the public health practitioner's tool kit.

In Chapter 17, Edwin M. Kilbourne discusses information system needs and resources in the area of toxicology and environmental health. After an introductory discussion of the scope and history of toxicologic and environmental health information, he discusses the nature and uses of types of major services and systems. He concludes the chapter with a discussion of bibliographic and factual databases available to the public health practitioner.

Neil Rambo and Christine Beahler conclude this part of the book with their discussion of knowledge-based information and systems in Chapter 18. After providing a definition of knowledge-based information, they discuss the challenges to the public health practitioner of locating useful public health information—on the Internet, in existing databases, in clearinghouses, and elsewhere. Rambo and Beahler provide useful guidelines for accessing useful knowledge-based information and conclude the chapter with a discussion of the importance of putting knowledge-based information to work in public health practice.

14
The National Vital Statistics System

MARY ANNE FREEDMAN AND JAMES A. WEED

Learning Objectives

After studying this chapter, you should be able to:

- Discuss the origins of the vital statistics system in the United States and explain the areas of responsibility of the states and federal agencies in maintaining the system.
- Explain the operation of the national vital statistics system with respect to the collection of data regarding births and deaths.
- Define the nature and the purpose of the Model State Vital Statistics Act.
- List the participants in and the provisions of the Vital Statistics Cooperative Program with respect to (1) training state and local personnel, (2) the Interstate Record Exchange Program, (3) vital statistics data files, and (4) classification of diseases.
- Explain the *International Classification of Diseases* as a tool for uniform standards in listing causes of death and explain how vital statisticians compensate for discontinuities caused by updates to this publication.
- Discuss recent innovations to enhance the vital statistics system, including (1) methods for automating classification of mortality cause-of-death data, (2) developments in electronic birth and death registration, (3) availability of data on CD-ROM and the World Wide Web, and (4) early release of preliminary data to facilitate surveillance.
- Explain why a comprehensive vital statistics system is important to the practice of public health.

Overview

The vital statistics system in the United States has always recognized the importance of collecting information about public health. Today, the national vital statistics system in the United States is a major cooperative effort between the states and federal agencies. The Vital Statistics Cooperative Program provides for collection of records of births. deaths, marriages. and other events on a national level. Moreover, increasing adoption of modern technology for record keeping and data exchange has resulted in faster and more accurate vital statistics reports. State data, supplemented by surveys administered by the National Center for Health Statistics within the Centers for Disease Control and Prevention, provide fundamental information for use in the arena of public policy and public health practice.

Introduction

The inception. development, and maintenance of a system to produce national vital statistics based on the local registration of vital events has been a major accomplishment of the United States during the 20th century. In this country, legal authority for the registration of births. deaths, marriages. divorces, fetal deaths, and induced terminations of pregnancy (abortions) resides individually with the states (as well as with cities in the case of New York City and Washington, D.C., and with territories in the case of Puerto Rico, the Virgin Islands, Guam. American Samoa. and the Commonwealth of the Northern Mariana Islands). In effect. the states are the full legal proprietors of the records and the information contained therein and are responsible for maintaining registries according to state law and for issuing copies of birth. marriage, divorce, and death certificates.

As a result of this state authority, the collection of registration-based vital statistics at the national level has come to depend on a cooperative relationship between the states and the federal government. This relationship has evolved over many decades, with its initial beginnings in the early development of the public health movement and the creation of the American federal system. In this chapter, a brief overview of this development will set the stage for a discussion of the components and uses of the present National Vital Statistics System.

Milestones in National Vital Statistics[1(p43–66)]

The registration of births, marriages, and deaths has a long history in the United States. beginning with a registration law enacted by the Grand Assembly of Virginia in 1632 and a modification of this law enacted by the General Court of the Massachusetts Bay Colony in 1639. In enacting this legislation. the early settlers. who were predominantly English. were following English customs in the new country. They were accustomed to the registration of christenings. marriages, and burials. In England, this kind of registration dated back to 1538, when the clergy in all parishes were first required to keep a weekly record of such events. In those early days, there was little or no statistical use made of such records, and certainly there was no thought of using them for health purposes. In the beginning, these records, along with wills and property inventories, were regarded primarily as statements of fact essential to the protection of individual rights, especially those relating to the ownership and distribution of property.

Although the Massachusetts law was based on English precedent, it differed in two important respects: (1) responsibility for registration of vital events was placed on government officers rather than on the clergy, and (2) the law called for the recording of vital events—births, deaths, and marriages—rather than church-related ceremonies. Connecticut and Plymouth, and eventually other colonies, followed a similar pattern.

Thus, at the basis of the vital registration system was the principle that the records are legal documents that help assure the rights of individuals. This principle was not sufficient, however, to create a fully effective registration system in the highly migratory American population during the 17th and 18th centuries, despite efforts to strengthen the registration laws. The impetus for a truly effective system came from the realization by some very astute statisticians and physicians, both here and abroad, that records of births and deaths, particularly records of deaths by cause, were needed for the control of epidemics and the conservation of human life through sanitary reform.

During the 17th century, parish lists of interments, usually including cause of death and age of deceased, were published in London as Bills of Mortality during epidemics of plague. The origin of vital statistics in the modern sense can be traced to an analysis of the English Bills of Mortality published by John Graunt (1620–1674) in 1662. Similarly, death records of some sort were apparently kept by American settlements from the earliest days. Disease ranked with starvation as a threat to the existence of many of the colonies; clergy compiled various lists of parish dead, and cemetery sextons made burial returns to town officers. For example, the clergyman Cotton Mather noted in 1721, during a severe smallpox epidemic in Boston, that more than one in six of the natural cases died, but only one in 60 of the inoculated cases did so. [1(p45)]

In the 18th and 19th centuries, the Industrial Revolution was associated not only with rapid urbanization and overcrowding of cities, but also with the deterioration of social and living conditions for large sectors of the population in Europe. Slums, crime, poverty, filth, polluted water, and epidemics of old and new diseases severely challenged the existing social order. As Dr. John R. Lumpkin has pointed out in Chapter 2, in England, as on the European and American continents, public health reformers became acutely conscious of the need for general sanitary reform as a means of controlling epidemics of disease—particularly cholera, but also typhoid, typhus, yellow fever, and smallpox. These early sanitarians used the crude death statistics of the time to arouse public awareness of the need for improved sanitation, and in the process they pressed for more precise statistics through effective registration practices and laws. The work of Edwin Chadwick (1800–1890) and Dr. William Farr (1807–1883) in England and of Lemuel Shattuck (1793–1859) in Massachusetts was instrumental in the development of public health organization and practice, including registration and vital statistics, during the 19th century. Thus, the history of public health is essentially the history of vital registration and statistics.

When the US Constitution was framed in the aftermath of the American Revolution, provision was made for a decennial census, but not for a national vital registration system. To obtain national data on births, marriages, and deaths, the decennial censuses in the latter half of the 19th century—1850 to 1900—included questions about vital events, such as: "Born within the year"; "Married within the year"; "Disease, if died within the year." These census items were introduced with the help of Lemuel Shattuck, against his better judgment. Indeed, the method came to be recognized as inefficient and the results as deficient, but the census questions were not abandoned until 1910, when the developing registration area was large enough to provide better national statistics.

The US Bureau of the Census was made a permanent agency of the federal government in 1902, and the enabling legislation authorized the Director of the Bureau to obtain annually copies of records filed in the vital statistics offices of those states and cities having adequate death registration systems and to publish data from these records. A few years earlier, the Bureau had issued a recommended death reporting form (the first "US Standard Certificate of Death") and requested each independent registration area to adopt it as of January 1, 1900. Those areas that adopted the form and whose death registration was 90% complete were to be included in a national death-registration area that had been established in 1880. In 1915, the national birth-registration area was established, and, by 1933, all states were registering live births and deaths with acceptable event coverage and providing the required data to the Bureau for the production of national birth and death statistics.

In 1946, responsibility for collecting and publishing vital statistics at the federal level was transferred from the Census Bureau to the US Public Health Service, first in the National Office of Vital Statistics and later (1960) in the National Center for Health Statistics (NCHS). In 1987, NCHS became part of the Centers for Disease Control and Prevention (CDC), US Department of Health and Human Services.

Operation of the National Vital Statistics System

Vital records and reports originate with private citizens—members of the families affected by the events, their physicians, funeral directors, and others. The responsibilities of these individuals are defined in states' laws. Birth registration is the direct responsibility of the hospital of birth or the attendant at the birth (generally a physician or midwife.) In the absence of an attendant, the parents of the child are responsible for registering the birth. Although procedures vary from hospital to hospital, usually the personal information is obtained from the mother; medical information may be obtained from the chart or from a worksheet filled out by the birth attendant.

Death registration is the direct responsibility of the funeral director or person acting as such. The funeral director obtains the data required, other than the cause of death, from the decedent's family or other informant. The attending physician provides the cause and manner of death. If no physician was in attendance or if the death was due to other than natural causes, the medical examiner or coroner will investigate the death and provide the cause and manner.

Reporting requirements vary from state to state. In general, the completed birth certificate must be filed with the state or local registrar within 10 days of the birth; death certificates must be filed within three to five days of the death.

Because the federal government has no constitutional authority to enact national vital statistics legislation, it depends upon the states to enact laws and regulations that provide for registration and data collection comparable from state to state. To achieve the needed uniformity for combining data from all states into national statistics, the federal agency responsible for national vital statistics recommends standards for use by state registration offices. The two primary standards are the Model State Vital Statistics Act and the US Standard Certificates and Reports.

The states are collectively represented in their dealings with the federal government by the National Association for Public Health Statistics and Information Systems (NAPHSIS), formerly (until May 1995) the Association for Vital Records and Health Statistics. NAPHSIS is a professional organization whose members include primarily, but not exclusively, the vital statistics executives and other employees of state registration offices. In addition to providing the states with a common point of contact with the federal government and numerous other professional organizations, NAPHSIS facilitates interstate exchange of ideas, methods, and technology for the registration of vital events and dissemination of vital and other public health statistics. NAPHSIS's progenitors date back to 1933, when it was organized as the American Association of Registration Executives.[2] Information about this important organization can be found on the NAPHSIS Web site at http://www.naphsis.org/.

US Standard Certificates and Reports

The standard certificates are the principal means of promoting uniformity in the data collected by the states. They are intended both to meet the legal needs of the system and to provide the data needed to be responsive to emerging public health issues. The standards are reviewed and revised approximately every 10 years through a process that includes broad input from data providers and users, including recognized experts in epidemiology and public health.

There have been 11 issues of the US Standard Certificates of Live Birth; 10 of the US Standard Certificate of Death (in 1915, the birth certificate but not the death certificate was revised); seven of the US Standard Report of Fetal Death (formerly stillbirth); four of the US Standard Certificate of Marriage and the US Standard Certificate of Divorce, Dissolution of Marriage, or Annulment; and two of the US Standard Report of Induced Termination of Pregnancy.[3]

The 1989 edition of the standard certificates is currently in use. In 1998, NCHS convened an Expert Panel to evaluate the 1989 version. The panel recommended revisions, which are currently under consideration by NCHS.[4] These revisions are expected to be implemented beginning in 2003. The panel's charge was to recommend the content, format, and item definitions of the new standard certificates, with the understanding that the certificates are no longer just paper documents, but a standard data set with an emphasis on electronic data collection. Thus, the 2003 revisions focus on data collection procedures in an electronic era.

Model State Vital Statistics Act and Regulations

A model act (or model bill) is proposed legislation drafted in a form that can be enacted into law by a state legislature. A model act is not a law itself.

The revision process for the Model State Vital Statistics Act and Regulations mirrors that of the standard certificates, although the model law is revised less frequently. The Bureau of the Census submitted the first model bill to the states in 1907, covering both birth and death registration. There have been several revisions over the century. The 1942 revision was the first to provide a statutory definition of vital statistics, defining them as "the registration, preparation, transcription, collection, compilation, and preservation of data pertaining to the dynamics of the population, in particular data pertaining to births, deaths, marital status, and the data and facts incidental thereto."[1(p5)]

The most recent full revision of the Model Act was in 1992.[5] Key provisions of the 1992 Model Act are shown in Table 14.1.

The 2003 standard certificate revision panel recommended that the Model Act be modified to accommodate the use of electronic signatures, standardized work sheets for data collection, and electronic transmission of source documents from the provider to the state registrar. These changes were adopted at the 2000 NAPHSIS annual meeting.[6]

The Vital Statistics Cooperative Program

In the early part of the 20th century, the Bureau of the Census and subsequent federal agencies responsible for the vital statistics system received unit record

TABLE **14.1.** Some key provisions in the 1992 Model State Vital Statistics Act

Act Category	Provisions
Authorization	• Provides for the establishment of an Office of Vital Statistics and a statewide system of vital statistics within a designated state agency and a naming of a state registrar with specified duties.
Birth registration	• Provides for the Office of Vital Statistics to register and certify each live birth in a specified manner and compels physicians and others to comply with the act. Other provisions specify the manner in which infants of unknown parentage, adopted children, and establishment of facts of a birth are to be handled.
Death registration	• Provides for filing of a certificate of death for each death occurring in the state, and places duties on funeral directors and physicians to comply with the act. Also requires a report on each fetal death if the fetus weighs 350 grams or more, or if weight is unknown and the fetus dies after 20 completed weeks of gestation or more. Establishes requirements for final disposition of a body.
Marriage registration	• Requires a record of each marriage performed in the state to be filed with the vital statistics office in a specified manner.
Divorce, marriage dissolution, annulment	• Establishes provisions for recording these events.
Amendment and disclosure of vital records	• Establishes procedures by which vital records may be amended and disclosed.
Enforcement	• Imposes duties on institutional heads, funeral directors, physicians, and others to comply with the act, and imposes penalties for failure to comply.
Technology	• The model legislation explicitly permits vital statistics offices to incorporate technological advances in records and information management.

Source: Centers for Disease Control and Prevention, National Center for Health Statistics, Model State Vital Statistics Act and Regulations, 1992 Revision.

data from the states in hard copy or microfilm. States were reimbursed for copying efforts at four cents per record. Data were transcribed (later key entered) at both the national and state levels as both states and federal government produced statistics. In 1971, NCHS began an experiment with the state of Florida to receive data on computer tape.[1] This effort expanded rapidly and evolved into the Vital Statistics Cooperative Program (VSCP). Under the VSCP,

NCHS partially supports state costs of producing vital statistics through a contract with each state. NCHS works with states to implement standards for data elements, editing and coding specifications, quality control procedures, and data transmission schedules.

Federal Activities in Training State and Local Personnel

The NCHS training and technical assistance program for state and local vital statistics staff incorporates a number of activities aimed at developing expertise in all aspects of vital registration and vital statistics. These include a complement of courses for registration staff, statisticians, and coding specialists; telephone and e-mail hotlines; periodic meetings; and on-site assistance. The on-site assistance program is designed to send a team of federal and state vital statistics specialists into states requesting assistance. In addition to focusing on the areas of most concern to the requesting state, the teams review the entire operation of the office and offer suggestions for improvements.

The Interstate Record Exchange Program

Prior to 1937, the federal government published birth and death statistics by place of occurrence. Starting in 1937, subnational statistics were published primarily by place of residence. Subsequently, states also began publishing their statistics by place of residence. Because residents of one state may be born or may die in a different state, a mechanism was needed to enable states to obtain records of vital events that occurred to their residents in other states. Thus, the Interstate Record Exchange Program was initiated. It is an agreement among the states to exchange records of out-of-state occurrences with the state of residence. The exchange agreements are negotiated and administered by NAPHSIS.[2] NCHS supports the arrangement by periodically providing states with lists of out-of-state occurrences.

Vital Statistics Data Files

One of the strengths of the vital statistics system is that it is a census rather than a survey. Thus, it includes a record of each vital event that occurs in the United States. Because all events are included, vital statistics can be used to examine data for small geographic areas, detailed demographic subgroups, specific causes of death, and rare events. The level of detail contained in each of the major vital statistics data files is described below.

The *natality* file contains demographic and health information recorded on certificates of all live births that occur in the United States. Demographic and health characteristics of the mother include age, race, Hispanic origin, education, birthplace, residence, marital status, medical risk factors of pregnancy, month that pregnancy prenatal care began, number of prenatal visits, tobacco use, alcohol use, weight gain during pregnancy, and obstetric procedures. Characteristics of the birth include birth weight, length of gestation, birth order, sex, plurality, method of delivery, Apgar score, complications of labor and delivery, abnormal conditions of the newborn, congenital anomalies, and attendant at delivery.

The *mortality* file includes demographic and medical information recorded on death certificates of all deaths that occur in the United States. Variables include residence, place of occurrence, month of death, age, race, Hispanic origin, birthplace, sex, educational attainment, occupation and industry of decedent (selected states), injury at work, marital status, type of place of death, and underlying and multiple causes of death.

The *fetal death* file includes demographic and health information recorded on reports of all fetal deaths of twenty weeks or more gestation that occur in the United States. The demographic and health characteristics of the mother and fetal death are similar to those for natality, but also include the fetal or maternal conditions causing death.

The *linked birth/infant death* data system contains records of all live births and infant deaths that occur in the United States. Three separate files are included in the system. One is a *numerator file* with linked birth-infant death records for each of the approximately 38,000 infants who die in the United States each year. The *denominator file* contains birth certificate information for each of the approximately four million live births. An additional file contains the relatively few infant death records that were not linked to birth certificates. The match rate is about 97–98%. Data are available for each of the birth cohorts from 1983 through 1991. Beginning with data year 1995, the data are organized by calendar year rather than by birth cohort to expedite data release.

Monthly counts of the number of *marriages* and *divorces* are obtained from each state. In addition, prior to 1996, states provided the total number of events by county of occurrence. Unlike the natality and mortality systems, detailed data for marriages and divorces have never covered the entire United States. NCHS obtained detailed data only from those states and territories with centralized registration systems. In addition, participating states provided a sample of records rather than their full marriage and/or divorce files. For data years prior to 1996, marriage data included demographic characteristics recorded on probability samples of records from up to 42 states and the District of Columbia (DC). Variables included bride's and groom's ages, race, marriage number, and previous marital status. Divorce data included demographic characteristics recorded on probability samples of records from up to 32 States and DC. Variables included husband's and wife's ages, race, and number of marriages. Other variables included marriage duration, number of children under 18, and physical custody of children. With data year 1996, NCHS ceased collecting detailed marriage and divorce data. Only the monthly counts are available.

International Classification of Diseases

Causes of death are classified for purposes of statistical tabulation according to the *International Classification of Diseases (ICD)* published by the World Health Organization (WHO).[7] The classification originated as the "Bertillon Classification of Causes of Death" prepared in the late 1800s by Dr. Jacques

Bertillon, chairman of the committee charged with development of a classification of causes of death for international use. In 1898, the American Public Health Association recommended that the classification be adopted by the United States and that it be revised every 10 years to keep abreast of advances in medicine.[1] The *ICD* is maintained collaboratively by WHO and 10 international centers, one of which is the WHO Collaborating Center for the Classification of Diseases in North America. To date, there have been 11 editions of the *ICD*, the most recent being the 10th revision (*ICD-10*), implemented in the United States in 1999.

Traditionally, a single cause of death has been selected for statistical tabulations. When the certifying physician indicates that more than one cause contributed to death, a procedure is required for selecting the cause to be tabulated. The *ICD* provides the basic ground rules used to code and classify causes of death, to identify the underlying cause of death, and to compensate for certifier errors in the cause of death statement. It also includes definitions of terms such as "underlying cause of death," "live birth," and "maternal death," as well as tabulation lists that define the cause of death groupings to be used for international comparisons. The *ICD* also delineates the format of the medical certification of death and specific regulations regarding the compilation and publication of statistics on diseases and causes of death.[7]

The introduction of a new *ICD* revision can create major discontinuities in statistical trend data. Discontinuities are measured through the use of "comparability ratios." These are obtained by coding a large sample of death records by both the previous and the current revisions and by calculating the ratio of deaths from a given cause as coded by the later revision to deaths from the same cause as classified by the earlier revision. As an example of the use of comparability ratios, Figure 14.1 shows age-adjusted death rates for selected causes of death from 1968 to 1997.

ICD-8 was in use during the period from 1968 to 1978. (In the United States, a modified version of *ICD-8* was adopted and published as *ICDA-8*.[8]) *ICD-9* was in use during the period from 1979 to 1998. In Figure 14.1, the nephritis comparability ratio of 1.74 indicates that 74% more deaths were classified to this cause in 1979 compared with 1978 solely because of the introduction of *ICD-9*. Similarly, the pneumonia death rate declined as a result of the change in revisions, whereas the suicide death rate remained unchanged. Preliminary estimates of *ICD-10* comparability ratios indicate that the change from *ICD-9* to *ICD-10* resulted in a large increase in deaths from Alzheimer disease, sizable increases in nephritis and septicemia deaths, a slight increase in deaths from stroke, HIV, and chronic lower respiratory disease, and a large decrease in pneumonia deaths.[9]

Mortality data for 1999 reflect the new cause-of-death classification system under *ICD-10*, including reorganized cause-of-death categories, and tabulation lists. The *ICD-10* list of 113 selected causes of death replaces the *ICD-9* list of 72 selected causes of death and is used to identify and rank the leading causes of death in the United States.[10]

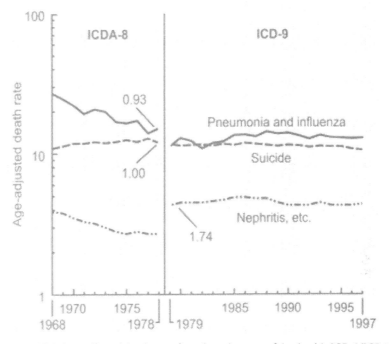

Figure 14.1. Age-adjusted death rates for selected causes of death with *ICD-9/ICDA-8* comparability ratios: United States, 1968–1997. (*Source:* Centers for Disease Control and Prevention, National Center for Health Statistics, National Vital Statistics System.)

Recent Innovations to Enhance the National Vital Statistics System and Its Output

Automated Classification for Mortality Cause-of-Death Data

In the late 1960s, NCHS began development of automated entry, classification, and retrieval of information reported on death certificates. The systems that automate the medical component of the death certificate have been continuously updated and refined. The major components of the automated mortality system are ACME, TRANSAX, MICAR, and SuperMICAR.

The *ACME (Automated Classification of Medical Entities)* program selects the underlying cause of death from the medical conditions reported on the death certificate. This system was developed to improve data consistency and facilitate the availability of multiple cause data. It has been used since

1968 and requires the manual coding of each entity (disease, accident, or injury) reported in the medical certification section of the death certificate. From those codes, which retain the location and order as reported by the certifier, the computer program automatically assigns the underlying cause of death by use of the selection and modification rules of the applicable revision of the *ICD*. Experienced *nosologists*—persons trained to classify diseases in accordance with an organized list of diseases and injuries—developed the computerized decision tables that drive the selection process, in consultation with medical specialists. These nosologists have achieved high levels of expertise in the practice of medical coding; in the interpretation and application of the *ICD* rules; in the training, apprenticeship, and qualification of new medical coders; and in the implementation of special projects on cause of death. The decision tables are updated periodically to reflect new information on the relationships among medical conditions and to convert the system to new revisions of the *ICD*.

TRANSAX (Translation of Axes) facilitates the tabulation and use of multiple cause-of-death data. The program translates the axis of classification from an entity to a record basis by accommodating linkages of entities provided by the *ICD*. For example, diabetes and acidosis both stated on the record become diabetes with acidosis.

MICAR (Mortality Medical Indexing, Classification, and Retrieval) was designed to replace the manual coding required by ACME. Data entry operators enter full text, abbreviations, or reference numbers for cause-of-death terms. After certificates are keyed, MICAR matches each entry to its dictionary and assigns the "entity reference number" that is the unique identifier in the dictionary for that cause. The records are then run through ACME to assign the underlying cause.

SuperMICAR takes the process one step further and allows the data entry operator to enter literal text as it appears on the death certificate. This information is processed in a similar manner to MICAR.

All US death records are coded through this system either in the state office or at NCHS. As of the year 2000, about six other countries were using the ACME component to select the underlying cause of death; an additional 19 countries have received copies of the software as part of their developmental work to implement automation for mortality.[10] Instruction manuals, which contain coding and data preparation procedures, short lists for tabulating mortality statistics, computer edits (consistency between age and cause of death, range edits, etc.), and procedures for querying cause-of-death statements, are available on the NCHS Web site (http://www.cdc.gov/nchs/).

Development of Electronic Birth and Death Registration

For most of the last century, the national vital statistics system was based primarily on paper recordings of over 6 million annual birth and death events

. by thousands of physicians, hospitals, funeral directors, and coroners. These records were typically transmitted through local registration officials, then keyed, queried, and edited as state offices received the records. The data were transmitted periodically to NCHS as files were completed. After labor-intensive processing in both state offices and NCHS, the data were released to the public on an annual basis as reports or electronic products.

Over the past 15 years, significant attempts to modernize the national vital statistics system have taken place. NCHS and the states have been working toward a vital statistics system in which birth and death certificates are created, edited, coded, queried, and corrected at the source point in electronic form; transmitted over high-speed lines to a central location in each state for any state processing and information management; and finally, electronically transmitted to NCHS on a frequent and regular basis.

This redesign, called the "current flow" system, shifts the data entry function from the state office to the source data provider who completes the original record; the original record would be electronic rather than paper. Data entry would employ standardized, automated editing systems to continually "clean up" the data by the states; changes and updates to the coded record would be transmitted to NCHS and entered in the data file on a continual basis.

Automation at the data source is a critical element of the new system. Electronic birth and death certificates (completed by hospitals, funeral directors, and physicians) facilitate record filing, reduce processing redundancies, increase timeliness, and can improve data quality. Experimentation with electronic birth certificates (EBC) began in the early 1980s. Currently, EBCs are in use in one or more hospitals in 48 states, and approximately 92% of all US births are registered electronically. However, most states operate a dual (electronic and paper) registration system, in part because state laws have often not kept pace with technology. The recent revision of the model law is intended to assist states in addressing these issues.[5]

Electronic death registration (EDR), however, has not progressed as rapidly, primarily because the death registration process is more complex than birth registration and involves many more data providers. In 1994, NCHS convened a steering committee to make recommendations for reengineering the death registration process. The group included representatives of federal agencies–NCHS, the Social Security Administration (SSA)–and professional organizations representing funeral directors, physicians, medical examiners, hospitals, medical records personnel, and state vital statistics offices (NAPHSIS). The committee's report provides recommendations and a framework for developing EDR systems in the United States.[12]

Recent advances in computer and network access technology have made the implementation of EDR systems feasible. Over the past several years, a number of states have begun developing systems. These efforts have been assisted by a NAPHSIS project, funded by SSA, to develop standards for EDR. This project, begun in October 1999, includes a survey of states to assess readiness for EDR, site visits to selected states, and two pilot projects. It is supported by an EDR Partnership Committee that includes representatives of major stakeholders. Standards developed through this project are available on the NAPHSIS Web site (http://www.naphsis.org).

State vital registration offices may need to refine their data processing systems to receive and process electronic records from source providers. Similarly, NCHS is reengineering its systems to receive, control, and process electronic data from the states. The internal NCHS system will provide staff with the capacity for on-line data retrieval for quality control, data tabulation, and report generation. The end result will be more timely vital statistics data at all levels of government.

Availability of Data on CD-ROM and the World Wide Web

Since 1996, NCHS has been releasing vital statistics files on CD-ROM. All data sets (birth, death, fetal death, linked birth/infant death, perinatal deaths) are now routinely distributed on CD-ROMs in ASCII and (for selected files) in SETS (Statistical Export and Tabulation System, a software package developed by NCHS to efficiently facilitate the use of data files on CD-ROM). The major vital statistics publications are available on the NCHS Internet home page, including the *National Vital Statistics Reports* and *Vital and Health Statistics* series reports. NCHS also put a number of (previously) unpublished statistical tables on the Internet and has begun to release *Vital Statistics of the United States* as an Internet report and as a CD-ROM.

Early Release of Preliminary Data to Facilitate Surveillance

As part of the current-flow system, in 1996 NCHS made a major addition to its product line with the development of the *preliminary files*. Starting with data year 1995, NCHS began releasing preliminary estimates of selected characteristics for 12-month periods based on the current-flow file without waiting for all records to be received and processed. The current-flow release includes detailed natality and mortality national data and preliminary state-level data.[13]

The preliminary data are published as *National Vital Statistics Reports*. The final natality and mortality files continue to be published, the schedule having been expedited by the current-flow process. Data from the current-flow file are treated as representative of complete data for the states and for the United States. This is accomplished by assigning a record weight to each vital record in the current flow file so that the sum of the records will equal independently obtained total counts of births, infant deaths, and deaths to persons over one year of age at the state and national level. Those counts represent the number of vital records filed each month in the state vital statistics offices.

The completeness of the preliminary files continues to increase. The 1996 preliminary file, published in October 1996, included 90% of births; the 1999 preliminary natality report, published in August 2000, included 97% of births.[14] In addition, publication of the final files has accelerated from 21 months after the end of the year for the 1995 natality file, to 15 months for the 1998 file.

Vital Statistics and the Practice of Public Health

Over several centuries of development, the nation's vital registration systems have evolved into the primary source of the most fundamental public health information. From the early beginnings of the movement to improve sanitation and to control disease, the data on deaths, especially causes of death, have been critical for identifying, tracking, and eventually understanding and controlling epidemics of communicable diseases. Today, mortality data are used more generally to study trends and differentials in all kinds of causes of death, both chronic and communicable, as well as those due to homicide, suicide, and unintentional injuries. In addition, infant mortality has traditionally served as a key indicator of general health conditions in a given population. The availability of mortality statistics for small geographic units, such as counties, has contributed uniquely to the value of these data for epidemiologic investigations and surveillance.

Statistics obtained from birth certificates, fetal death reports, and the linked birth/infant death file provide a wealth of information about infant health. Of current interest to the public health community are statistics on teenage and unmarried childbearing, birth weight, length of gestation, smoking during pregnancy, access to prenatal care, complications of labor and/or delivery, abnormal conditions of the newborn, and obstetric procedures. Healthcare providers and epidemiologists specializing in infant and child health monitor trends in these and other natality statistics.

Vital statistics also provide fundamental information in the arena of public policy. For example, out-of-wedlock childbearing is a topic of continuing high interest among national welfare policymakers. Similarly, national health policy is very much concerned with the problem of health disparities among various race and ethnic groups in the US population. In these and many other important policy issues, the vital statistics system constitutes a frontline source of information that leads to action programs, yields indicators of effectiveness, and generally guides the practice of public health.

Questions for Review

1. Explain why development and maintenance of a vital records system is a state responsibility, rather than a mandated federal responsibility.
2. Explain the role of the National Association for Public Health Statistics and Information Systems (NAPHSIS) in the relationship between state vital records systems and the federal government.

3. Under the existing vital records system, who is typically responsible for providing information for the registration of (1) deaths and (2) births?
4. What is the purpose of US standard certificates? How are they periodically revised?
5. Define a *model act* and explain the origin and purpose of the Model State Vital Statistics Act? List the provisions of the 1992 Model State Vital Statistics Act with regard to (1) authorization for a state Office of Vital Statistics, (2) provisions for birth registration, (3) provisions for death registration, and (4) provisions for marriage registration. Why is the Model Act not adopted in its entirety by all states?
6. Explain the purpose and the nature of the Vital Statistics Cooperative Program. What is the role of the National Center for Health Statistics (NCHS) in this program? Explain the federal role in (a) training state and local personnel and (b) the Interstate Record Exchange Program.
7. In what sense is the vital statistics system a census, rather than a survey? Explain the nature of (a) a natality file, (b) a mortality file, (c) a fetal death file, and (d) a linked birth/infant data system.
8. Why is the World Health Organization's *International Classification of Diseases* an important resource for use in the national vital records system?
9. Explain the importance and use of automated classification for mortality cause-of-death data in the NCHS system. Define the nature and purpose of (a) ACME (Automated Classification of Medical Entities). (b) TRANSAX (Translation of Axes), (c) MICAR (Mortality Medical Indexing, Classification. and Retrieval). and (d) SuperMICAR.
10. Why is the development of electronic birth and death registration a critical element in a redesigned national vital statistics system?
11. Explain the importance of a national vital registration system to the practice of public health. What public health-related uses are being made of vital statistics?

References

1. Hetzel AM. *History and Organization of the Vital Statistics System*. Hyattsville. MD: National Center for Health Statistics; 1997.
2. Association for Vital Records and Health Statistics. A History of the Association for Vital Records and Health Statistics. 50th anniversary 1933–83. Washington. DC: Association for Vital Records and Health Statistics: 1983.
3. Tolson GC, Barnes JM. Gay GA, Kowaleski JL. The 1989 revision of the U.S. Standard Certificates and Reports. *Vital Health Stat 4* 1991;(28):1–34.
4. National Center for Health Statistics. Report of the Panel to Evaluate the U.S. Standard Certificates and Reports. Hyattsville, MD: National Center for Health Statistics; April 2000.
5. National Center for Health Statistics. Model State Vital Statistics Act and Regulations: 1992 Revision. (PHS) 94-1115. Hyattsville. MD: National Center for Health Statistics; 1994.

6. National Association for Public Health Statistics and Information Systems. Resolution 2000-5: Amendments to the Model State Vital Statistics Act. June 28, 2000.

7. World Health Organization. *International Statistical Classification of Diseases and Related Health Problems: Tenth Revision.* Geneva: World Health Organization; 1992.

8. National Center for Health Statistics: *Eighth Revision International Classification of Diseases, Adapted for Use in the United States.* PHS Pub. No. 1963. Public Health Service. Washington, DC: US Government Printing Office; 1967.

9. Anderson RN, Minino AM, Hoyert DL, Rosenberg HM. Comparability of cause of death between ICD-9 and ICD-10: Preliminary estimates. *Natl Vital Stat Rep* 2001;49(2):1–32.

10. National Center for Health Statistics. ICD-10 cause-of-death lists for tabulating mortality statistics, effective 1999. *Instruction Manual Part 9.* Hyattsville, MD: National Center for Health Statistics; 1998.

11. Peters K. ed. *Proceedings of the International Collaborative Effort on Automating Mortality Statistics, Vol. I.* DHHS Pub. No. (PHS) 99-152. Hyattsville, MD: National Center for Health Statistics; 1999.

12. National Center for Health Statistics. Toward an electronic death registration system in the United States: Report of the steering committee to re-engineer the death registration process. Hyattsville, MD: National Center for Health Statistics; January 10, 1997.

13. Rosenberg HM, Ventura SJ, Maurer JD, et al. Births and deaths: United States, 1995. *Mon Vital Stat Rep* 1996;45(3, Suppl 2; 1–40).

14. Curtin SC, Martin JA. Births: Preliminary data for 1999. *Natl Vital Stat Rep* 2000;48(14):1–24.

15
Morbidity Data

Linda K. Demlo and Jane F. Gentleman

Learning Objectives

After studying this chapter, you should be able to:

- Differentiate between morbidity data used to measure prevalence and morbidity data used to measure incidence.
- Describe the National Health Interview Survey, including its basic survey methodology and its purpose.
- Describe the State and Local Area Integrated Telephone Survey, including its basic survey methodology and its purpose.
- Describe the National Health Care Survey, including its basic survey methodology, its components, and its purpose.
- List and explain at least five major challenges posed by current methods of collecting morbidity data with respect to data accuracy and data reliability.
- Explain why it is important for those collecting morbidity data to be able to insure respondents of confidentiality, and list the legislative and administrative requirements imposed on the National Center for Health Statistics (NCHS) with respect to data confidentiality.
- Explain the nature and the general purpose of research data centers, including the Research Data Center of the NCHS.
- Describe the current state of application of technology in NCHS surveys, and describe the nature of the challenges to survey administration posed by application of technology, including application of Internet approaches.

Overview

In the United States, the collection of accurate, representative morbidity data is important to public policy and public health practice. Three major surveys administered by the National Center for Health Statistics (NCHS) of the Centers for Disease Control and Prevention (CDC) illustrate some of the procedures in use and the challenges associated with this task. The National Health Interview Survey, the State and Local Area Integrated Telephone Survey, and the National Health Care Survey all serve as valuable sources of information about the state of public health in the United States, but at the same time they are beset with challenges in securing accurate and representative data. The NCHS Research Data Center and data centers operated by other agencies are important resources for public health researchers. In providing data that are crucial for studies. the NCHS must always maintain a concern for the confidentiality, privacy, and security of information it obtains. The continuing application of technology and of the science of informatics holds promise of improving the speed, validity, and reliability of data collection, but it also poses challenges to existing survey methods. In adapting to the use of such technological developments as the Internet and cellular telephones and in continuing to apply technological applications to data collection, the NCHS has the opportunity to address current and new data needs. At the same time, the task of coping with technological change comes with the danger of data error, offering a challenge in continuing to improve morbidity data collection and dissemination.

Introduction

At the most basic level, morbidity data reflect the level of sickness or disease, usually in a specified community or population group.[1(p1249)] Typically, two aspects of morbidity are of interest: *prevalence*, which measures the magnitude and burden of disease at a particular point or interval in time and is useful for diseases of long duration: and *incidence*, which reflects the new cases occurring over a defined time period and is useful as an indicator of the need for or success of preventive efforts. Information to document levels of morbidity may be obtained from a number of sources, such as special studies, disease registries, systems created for the mandatory reporting of notifiable diseases, etc.[2,3] Examples would include the Behavioral Risk Factor Surveillance System (BRFSS) administered by Centers for Disease Control and Prevention (CDC) and the states: population-based registries such as the Surveillance, Epidemiology and End Results program (SEER) supported by the National Cancer Institute; and various reporting systems such as the Vaccine Adverse Events Reporting System managed by CDC and the Food and Drug Administration. and the Drug Abuse Early Warning Network (DAWN), which focuses on tracking the magnitude of drug abuse problems and is supported by the Substance Abuse and Mental Health Services Administration.

This chapter describes current approaches to documenting levels of morbidity in the US population. It uses for illustrative purposes some of the population-based and provider-based surveys maintained by the National Center for Health Statistics (NCHS). Some of these surveys have been mentioned briefly in the previous chapter. In the course of this chapter's discussion, we will highlight the contributions of informatics in gathering. processing, analyzing. and disseminating such data.

Specifically, the focus here is on the following NCHS surveys: the National Health Interview Survey. the State and Local Area Integrated Telephone Survey, and components of the National Health Care Survey. Detailed information about NCHS surveys as well as numerous data files are available from the NCHS Web site at http://www.cdc.gov/nchs/.

The National Health Interview Survey (NHIS) collects information each year about approximately 107,000 people living in 41.000 households. The survey data, which pertain to health status, access to care and insurance. health services utilization, health behaviors, and other topics. are a principal source of information about the health of the civilian noninstitutionalized population in the United States.

The State and Local Area Integrated Telephone Survey (SLAITS) is a population-based survey mechanism for covering a wide range of health and health-related topics by utilizing the sampling frame of the ongoing National Immunization Survey (NIS).

The National Health Care Survey (NHCS) is a family of provider-based surveys with hospital, ambulatory, and long-term care components that provide information about the characteristics of patients seen in these settings and the services they receive, as well as characteristics of the healthcare providers.[4] These surveys. their characteristics, processes. and products, and the role of informatics in conducting them will be emphasized throughout this chapter, providing a framework for considering present and future accomplishments and challenges in the generation of morbidity data.

An Overview of Selected NCHS Surveys, Their Approaches to Collecting Morbidity Data, and Their Use of Informatics

The National Health Interview Survey (NHIS)

The NHIS is the principal source of information on the health of the civilian. noninstitutionalized household population of the United States. It has been conducted continuously since its beginning in 1957. Data are released on an annual basis. The US Bureau of the Census. under a contractual agreement, is the data collection agent for the NHIS. The data are collected through personal household interviews by Census interviewers. The sampling frame for the NHIS is redesigned every 10 years to better measure the changing US population and to meet new survey objectives. The new design is implemented five years after each decennial Census. Thus, the current design was implemented in 1995 and will be used through 2004. About 41.000 households containing about 107,000 persons are in the NHIS sample each year. The current sample was designed to oversample black and Hispanic subpopulations in order to increase the precision of estimates for those subpopulations. Plans for the next sample design, to be implemented in 2005, include oversampling these same two subpopulations, and perhaps others.

Households receive a letter in advance of the interview explaining the purpose of the survey, that participation is voluntary, and that confidentiality will be protected. The first contact made by the interviewer is at the home, and completing the interview may require more than one visit. The telephone is sometimes used to continue the interview at a later time.

The NHIS questionnaire underwent major changes in 1997. The redesigned questionnaire has a Basic Module (also called the Core), with questions that remain essentially unchanged from year to year, and more in-depth questions and/or questions on new topics added as supplements each year, as needed. The Basic Module contains three components: the Family Core, the Sample Adult Core, and the Sample Child Core. The Family Core component collects information on everyone in the family. Questions that can reasonably be answered by proxy are included in this section of the survey. The sample for the Family Core serves as a sampling frame for additional surveys (such as the Medical Expenditure Panel Survey, which is conducted by the Agency for Healthcare Research and Quality and collects additional data from some of the NHIS respondents about healthcare use, healthcare expenses, and health insurance coverage). Questions from the Sample Adult Core are administered to a randomly selected adult in each family, and a knowledgeable adult is asked questions from the Sample Child Core about a randomly selected child under 18. The random selection of a single adult and a single child was a new feature starting with the 1997 NHIS.

Many significant changes were made to the NHIS questions in 1997, including changes to the wording, recall period, context (surrounding questions), and positioning of questions, and the type and number of possible answers. One objective of the questionnaire redesign was to shorten the length of the survey, which now takes approximately 70 minutes on average to administer, including supplements. The previous major redesign of the NHIS questionnaire had been in 1982; by 1997, some substantial changes were needed to maintain relevance and adapt to changes. It was necessary and important to update the NHIS questionnaire because of demographic and societal changes, changes in the types of health problems occurring, changes in the healthcare delivery and health insurance systems, changes in knowledge about health risk factors, changes in treatments, new needs of health policy makers and other data users, and new regulations affecting government surveys. Table 15.1 indicates some of the changes made in the nature of survey questions asked.

The topics presently covered by the NHIS Family Core include health status and limitation of activity, injury, health care access and utilization, health insurance coverage, socio-demographic characteristics, income, and assets. The Sample Adult Core covers demographic characteristics, chronic conditions, health status and limitation of activity, health behaviors, and

TABLE **15.1.** A sample of health measures changed in or added to the redesigned 1997 National Health Interview Survey

Survey Area	Change(s)
Limitation of activity	New question to determine if anyone in the family is limited because of difficulty remembering or periods of confusion. Also, questions to determine if anyone in the family has difficulty walking without any special equipment and to identify children who receive special education or early intervention services.
Injuries	Questions in this redesigned section ask more specific questions about the external causes and circumstances of the injury event.
Medical expenditures	Question asking for an estimate of the annual household expenditure for medical care, including dental care.
Access to health care	Question asking whether reasons for changing usual source(s) of health care are related to health insurance only. Also, questions to identify persons who have delayed care for reasons other than costs and/or who have not gotten specific types of care that they needed.
Health conditions	Questions that used to cover 133 conditions in six condition lists are reduced to a single list consisting of several domains. Addition of a brief child behavior scale, or mental health indicator for selected children.
Immunizations	Addition of questions about chicken pox vaccination and adolescent immunizations.
AIDS	Addition of questions about self-perceived risk of infection and whether a list of risk items applies to the respondent.

Source: National Center for Health Statistics, Centers for Disease Control and Prevention. Availble at http://www.cdc.gov/nchs/about/major/nhis/hisdesgn.htm.

health care access and utilization. The Sample Child Core covers chronic conditions, limitation of activity, health status, health care access and utilization, and immunization.

Another major change in 1997 was the change from a paper-and-pencil questionnaire to a Computer Assisted Personal Interview (CAPI) instrument. Since then, interviewers have been using laptop computers to administer interviews.

The journey of interview data from their collection to their dissemination to the public is fraught with perils. The data pass through many hands and undergo numerous treatments before reaching the user. At each stage, errors may be introduced that reduce the quality of the data or delay their availability and therefore reduce their usefulness.[5] The journey is made less perilous by the application of modern informatics technology in the design and implementation of the survey, and in the processing, analysis, and dissemination of the data. Some examples follow.

The design of the NHIS sample is determined after years of research and analysis. Such work has been under way since 1999 for the next NHIS sample, to be implemented in 2005. Sophisticated survey methods and computerized algorithms are used in this research and/or in the ultimate implementation of the sample design—for example, to select primary sampling units (PSUs) and smaller geographical areas within PSUs to be surveyed. This provides sample adequacy, incorporates the desired oversampling of certain subpopulations, and ensures that sample sizes will be adequate to achieve desired levels of precision for certain critical estimates.

Interviewers receive computer-generated maps and lists to help them locate households to be surveyed. The management of interview case loads and deadlines in the 12 Census regional offices and between those offices and Census headquarters is facilitated by case management software. For example, interviewers receive the survey questionnaires and return the responses by connecting their laptop computers to their home or office telephones.

The use of CAPI software eliminates one step in the electronic capture of responses; instead of the responses being recorded by the interviewer during a paper-and-pencil interview and then later captured electronically, the data are electronically captured during the interview. The CAPI software automatically guides the interviewer through the maze of possible questions, displaying them on the computer screen for the interviewer to read aloud. The survey instrument ensures that the correct path, which depends not only on the sociodemographic characteristics of the respondent, but also on the responses to the health questions, is taken. The responses are typed in, and some responses are edited on the spot, during the interview. For example, the CAPI program can check that responses are within reasonable ranges and are consistent. Later, when the data reach the survey manager's headquarters, further editing is done by use of both computer programs and manual processing. Simple and elegant statistical computing techniques for outlier detection and statistical graphics can be used to edit the data. Software is available to apply complex statistical techniques for imputing missing values.

Nonresponse to survey items is a constant and insidious threat to the quality of interview data. Statistical analysis of nonresponse patterns by use of computing and modeling can permit nonresponse patterns and causes to be better understood.

The analytic usefulness of data files is enhanced by use of modern linkage software; matching and combining records from two or more data sets provides analysts with a richer set of variables at the microdata level. The use of software to test microdata files for the purpose of disclosure limitation enhances confidence in the ability to maintain confidentiality when microdata are released. See, for example, Zayatz and references cited therein.[6]

State-of-the-art dissemination technology permits data files and documentation to be delivered to users sooner, at less cost, and more compactly. NHIS data are now released via the Internet as well as on CD-ROMs, as discussed in the previous chapter. Release of the data on the Internet affords greater flexibility and ability to inform data users of updates and corrections.

Modern statistical computing methods and technology have enhanced the quality of analysis of survey data by statistical agency analysts and by outside data users. For example, software that takes into account the complex design of the survey is used to produce more accurate variance estimates. Multivariate models that perform lengthy iterative calculations on large files of survey data are fitted quickly, through use of personal computers. The use of statistical graphics enhances the ability of analysts to detect, perceive, and present patterns in the data. Exploratory, interactive data analysis and data mining techniques are widely used to analyze survey data.

Admittedly, the computer systems that alleviate some of the perils that affect data quality are themselves prone to errors. For example, a user of the current NHIS CAPI program sometimes has difficulty in backing up when it is determined by the interviewer that an incorrect path through the questions has been taken (e.g., because the respondent changes an answer or the interviewer entered an incorrect response). In addition, data linkage is prone to a not insignificant amount of error, usually because of inaccuracies or gaps in the data. Also, errors in the computer programs themselves can be a serious threat to the quality of data and data analysis. Such errors can occur at many different stages of data processing and analysis. Poor programmer training, poor programming habits, poor communication between programmers and their supervisors, and inadequate documentation of computer programs can cause errors that have significant impact on the ultimate usefulness of the data and the accuracy of analytic results.[7] Finally, poor communication between survey managers and survey sponsors can cause the writing of incorrect programs. A vigilant striving for data quality continues to be imperative as the NHIS and other surveys increasingly tap and enjoy the advantages of computer and communications technology.

The State and Local Area Integrated Telephone Survey

The State and Local Area Integrated Telephone Survey (SLAITS) is an NCHS survey mechanism that utilizes the sampling frame of the ongoing National Immunization Survey (NIS). The NIS is a telephone survey that was established in 1994 to meet the need for immunization coverage data for children 19–35 months of age for all 50 states and in 28 metropolitan areas. Fielding the NIS requires screening a very large sample of households in order to identify a sufficient number of households with children of an appropriate age for that study. The vast majority of the households initially contacted by telephone by the NIS do not contain such children. For example, in 1999, more than 2 million phone numbers were called in the search for households with age-eligible children, resulting in the identification of about 36,000 such households. SLAITS adds value to that effort by utilizing not just some of the families screened into the NIS sample, but also some of the families screened out of NIS, depending on the requirements of the particular SLAITS survey being conducted. SLAITS is termed a "mechanism" because it provides the capacity to field different surveys on a wide range of health- and welfare-related topics. For example, the SLAITS Survey of Children with Special Health Care Needs, sponsored by the Maternal and Child Health Bureau of the Health Resources and Services Administration, measures the prevalence and impact of special health care needs for all children. Table 15.2 provides an example of the kind of information that can be obtained using SLAITS.

The NIS, which is sponsored by the National Immunization Program (NIP) and NCHS, is based on a list-assisted random-digit-dialing (RDD) sample design. The NIS and SLAITS are therefore limited to households with telephones. NIP sponsors a set of immunization questions on NHIS, data from which can be used to adjust the NIS and SLAITS estimates to account for the fact that those surveys cover only households with telephones. For further discussion of adjustment for non-telephone coverage. see Battaglia et al.[8] and Frankel et al.[9]

The NIS and SLAITS also utilize modern informatics. For example, the NIS matches a long list of sample telephone numbers to a database of business telephone numbers to avoid calling business numbers, and a personal-computer-based autodialing system eliminates nonworking telephone numbers. The remaining telephone numbers are matched with a database of directory-listed residential telephone numbers to obtain as many household addresses as possible. This permits the NIS and SLAITS to mail introductory letters to these households before phoning them. Several on-line look-up topic-ori-

TABLE 15.2. Examples of the types of data available from SLAITS

Target Population	Subject
Children in low income families	• Public and private health insurance coverage and lack thereof
Children with special healthcare needs	• Utilization of and need for health and related services
Adults	• Barriers to health care for persons with chronic illness
Adults and children	• Asthma prevalence and treatment
Children between 4 and 35 months of age	• Satisfaction with pediatric care and pediatrician's advice

ented databases are integrated with the NIS Computer Assisted Telephone Interview (CATI) system. For example, NIS asks respondents to provide the names and addresses of their children's vaccination providers and to give consent for the providers to be contacted subsequently to obtain additional immunization history details. The CATI system looks up the vaccination provider's name and address information to confirm the information. Other automated edits are also built into the CATI system. These additional quality assurance procedures reduce the total cost of the data collection by reducing interviewer labor and respondent burden.

The National Health Care Survey

Components of the National Health Care Survey (NHCS) include the National Ambulatory Medical Care Survey, the National Hospital Ambulatory Medical Care Survey, the National Hospital Discharge Survey, the National Survey of Ambulatory Surgery, the National Nursing Home Survey, and the National Home and Hospice Care Survey. This family of surveys gathers data on the use of health services in the United States and the characteristics of both the patients and providers or facilities involved in the health care transaction. The resulting information is used by policy makers, planners, researchers, and others in the health community to monitor changes in the use of health care resources, the patterns of health conditions and diseases for which services are used, the impact of medical technologies, and the quality of care provided to a changing American population. Collectively, the surveys paint a picture of the evolving healthcare system and changes in morbidity and the content and source of care.[10] Table 15.3 provides an overview of the components of the National Health Care Survey.

All surveys are national probability sample surveys involving complex sample designs. Generally, data are collected by the US Bureau of the Census and processed by a private contractor. All surveys have historically had very high response rates (90% or higher), although, as with most surveys of physician practices, the National Ambulatory Medical Care Survey has experienced lower response rates in recent years. All surveys have evolved over time in response to changes in the healthcare delivery system and changing needs of data users.

The data are disseminated through a variety of mechanisms. Publications include NCHS Advance Data reports, Vital and Health Statistics Series 13 and 14 reports, journal articles, and various special reports. Microdata files are made available by tapes/cartridges, CD-ROMs, and downloadable files. Citation indices make evident the widespread use of NHCS data by researchers, public health professionals, and others.[11]

The National Hospital Discharge Survey (NHDS), the National Survey of Ambulatory Surgery (NSAS), and the National Hospital Ambulatory Medical Care Survey (NHAMCS) produce information about hospital utilization. The NHDS utilizes a three-stage sample design based initially on a subsample of

TABLE 15.3. The components of the National Health Care Survey

Component	Purpose
National Ambulatory Medical Care Survey	Samples physicians to obtain information about patients' symptoms, physicians' diagnoses, medications ordered or provided, and other services.
National Hospital Ambulatory Care Survey	Collects data on the utilization and provision of ambulatory care services in hospital emergency and outpatient departments, utilizing patient record forms for a systematic random sample of patient visits during a randomly assigned four-week reporting period.
National Hospital Discharge Survey	Provides information about characteristics of inpatients discharged from non-Federal short-stay hospitals in the United States, including diagnoses and procedures.
National Survey of Ambulatory Surgery	Collects data about surgical outpatient characteristics, expected method of payment, and diagnoses and procedures from both hospital-based and freestanding ambulatory surgery centers.
National Nursing Home Survey	Samples nursing homes and their residents to obtain information about the facilities and demographic characteristics, health status, and services received by current and discharged patients.
National Home and Hospice Care Survey	Secures information about agencies that provide home and hospice care and the services provided to current and discharged patients, using personal interviews with administrators and staff.

112 PSUs from the 1985–1994 NHIS. A subsequent sample is drawn of approximately 525 nonfederal, short-stay hospitals with probability proportional to size after stratification by hospital specialty/bed-size class and abstract service status. Some very large hospitals are included with certainty. Finally, a systematic sample of approximately 300,000 discharges is selected. Discharge data conforming to the Uniform Hospital Discharge Data Set (UHDDS) are collected by one of two methods: (1) manual abstraction of data from medical records by hospital staff or by Census field staff, or (2) the purchase of automated data from state data systems, commercial abstracting services, or directly from hospitals. Approximately 70% of the discharges are obtained in an automated form. Using a similar sample design and manual data gathering procedures, the NSAS collects data from a national sample of about 420 hospitals and 330 freestanding ambulatory surgery centers, which produce a sample of approximately 120,000 medical records.

The resulting data include patient demographics, expected source of payment, diagnoses, procedures, length of stay, hospital size, and geographic location. Because the NHDS has been fielded annually since 1965, it is a very rich source of trend data that have been used to track hospitalizations for specific diagnoses and procedures over time[12]; potentially avoidable hospitalizations[13]; and differences in hospital use for different population groups.[14] By combining NHDS and NSAS data, one can examine trends and trade-offs between inpatient and ambulatory surgery, although the NSAS has not been fielded since 1996. Recent NHDS data releases have highlighted a decrease in hospital admission rates and lengths of stay for patients with HIV/AIDS, presumably because of improved drug therapies.[15] An increase in lengths of stay for childbirth has also been observed.[16]

The sampling plan for the National Ambulatory Medical Care Survey (NAMCS) also begins with a subset of the NHIS PSUs. The second stage consists of a stratified sample of about 3,000 nonfederal physicians who are principally engaged in office-based patient care (excluding the specialties of radiology, pathology, and anesthesiology), drawn from the universe of about 300,000 physicians listed in the master files maintained by the American Medical Association and the American Osteopathic Association. Finally, the physician sample is divided into 52 random subsamples of approximately equal size. Each subsample is randomly assigned one of the 52 weeks in the survey year, and a systematic random sample of visits is selected from each physician's practice by use of a patient log or register for that week. Participating physicians, physicians' staffs, or occasionally Census field staff complete patient encounter forms for approximately 30 visits per physician. About 25,000 visits are sampled annually. To complement the NAMCS data, the National Hospital Ambulatory Medical Care Survey (NHAMCS) was fielded, using generally similar methods except for the use of a four-stage sample plan (PSUs, hospitals, emergency and outpatient departments, and patient encounters.) About 70,000 visits are sampled annually from about 440 hospitals.

NAMCS and NHAMCS data reflect visits to physicians, outpatient clinics, and emergency departments, including information on patient characteristics, expected source of payment, patients' complaints, physicians' diagnoses, diagnostic and/or screening procedures, medication therapy, planned future treatment, types of healthcare professionals seen, and causes of injury where applicable. NAMCS/NHAMCS data have been used to address such issues as office-based prevention, screening, diagnosis, and counseling practices[17,18]; prescribing practices[19]; visits for medical misadventure[20]; primary care referral patterns[21]; and sports-related injuries in children and young adults.[22]

The National Nursing Home Survey (NNHS) collects information from a stratified probability sample of about 1,500 nursing homes of the approximately 20,000 nursing homes in the coterminous United States. Within the homes, Census field staff collect information about the facilities through interviews with the nursing home administrators and staffs. In addition, data are collected on a sample of approximately 9,000 current residents and 9,000 discharged residents through a personal interview with the nurse or other person responsible for the resident's care, who consults the medical record to obtain the requested information.

Following similar procedures, the National Home and Hospice Care Survey (NHHCS) obtains information on about 10,800 current patients and 10,800 discharged patients. A two-stage stratified sample design is used, based on, first, a sample of approximately 1,800 hospices and home health agencies, and ultimately a systematic sample of current and discharged patients.

The NNHS and NHHCS patient-related information includes demographic data, caregiver and referral sources, length of service, patient charges, expected source of payment, diagnoses, types of services received, functional status/living arrangements, and reason for discharge. Facility-related information includes size, ownership, Medicare and/or Medicaid certification, occupancy rate if relevant, services provided, and expenses. NNHS and NHHCS data have been used to examine such issues as the quality of care provided to nursing home patients diagnosed with mental health conditions[23]; the relationship between infectious diseases among discharged nursing home patients and mortality[24]; and changes in utilization patterns indicating declining use of both nursing homes and home health services in recent years.[25,26]

The journey of the provider-based data from the original source or source document to publicly available published or electronic information is similar across all of the NHCS surveys. Each survey has a collection period of one year or less. However, survey operations typically span three or more calendar years, taking into consideration survey redesign, as appropriate, pilot testing, sample design, obtaining necessary approvals (such as from the Office of Management and Budget for response burden and an Institutional Review Board for human subjects protection), survey preparation, data collection, data processing, and dissemination. The time elapsed between the completion of data collection and public dissemination of data is typically somewhat less than one year.

As with the NHIS, the NHCS data pass through many hands and undergo numerous treatments, providing many opportunities for the introduction of error. All data collection instructions, concerns, or changes are communicated from NCHS through the Demographic Survey Division of the Bureau of the Census to the Census field staff. Most medical record abstractions are performed manually except for NHDS hospitals that submit automated discharge data to NCHS either directly or as part of a larger statewide database. Completed data collection forms are transmitted by Census staff to a contractor with responsibility for coding and keying. A variety of quality control activities occur. For example, a sample of records is re-coded to assure that error rates remain at acceptable levels; the error rates for the most recent NAMCS and NHAMCS surveys ranged from 0% to 1.8%. Raw data files and tapes are forwarded to the appropriate NCHS technical services staff for editing, cleaning, imputing, variance estimation, and conversion into a final, weighted data file, which provides the basis for analysis, report writing, and dissemination.

Also similar to NHIS procedures, the NHCS incorporates many sophisticated computerized algorithms and automated techniques for sample design and implementation, data processing and editing, detection of outliers, imputation of missing values, variance estimation, generation of statistical graphics, and dissemination techniques. A variety of data linkages strengthen the analytic potential of the surveys. For example, the NAMCS/NHAMCS and NHDS data can be linked to the Area Resource File, a database supported by the Health Resources and Services Administration and containing over 6,000 variables for each county in the United States; this file contains information about health facilities, health professions, measures of resource scarcity, health status, economic activity, health training programs, and socioeconomic and environmental characteristics.

NAMCS/NHAMCS data on medication therapy are enriched by data from a separate drug database containing information about therapeutic class, generic or brand name, Federal control schedule, and composition status. Future NHDS data releases will include hospital utilization data from the Department of Veterans Affairs and the Department of Defense, thereby broadening the range of national data on hospital utilization available for analysis. Similarly, an agreement has been reached with the American Hospital Association to link NHDS data with the AHA Annual Survey Database, which contains hospital-specific data items on utilization, organizational structure, facilities and services, finances, and personnel. This combined database will be available to researchers through the NCHS Research Data Center (see below). Unlike the NHIS, the NHCS currently does not incorporate computer-assisted techniques in the actual data collection process, although such approaches have been tested and are being considered.

The NHCS components have remained relatively unchanged over the past decade. However, they are currently being reexamined to assure that they reflect the many changes occurring within the health care delivery system and the experiences of patients as they utilize health care. Future modifications will go beyond a single, isolated healthcare encounter in order to better reflect an episode of care and to track functional status and health outcomes over time. More detailed clinical information will be obtained, particularly on drug therapies. In addition, provider and facility induction questionnaires will be expanded to gather more information about the characteristics of the delivery setting and the interrelationships among components of the healthcare system. This will enable better understanding the influence of the delivery system on morbidity, quality, and outcomes of care.

Challenges in Measuring Morbidity

A number of interrelated issues pose special challenges in the generation and use of morbidity data. Table 15.4 provides an overview of some of the challenges to be discussed.

Producing nationally generalizable information on morbidity is often a by-product of a survey or other data gathering effort that was designed to serve multiple needs—not merely the need to generate morbidity data. One major issue is the inclusiveness of the data obtained. In the case of a specific disease or health condition, does the information available capture all the cases needed (and avoid double counting) in order to make a national estimate? Different data sources, such as personal interviews, physical exams, or administrative data, have associated strengths and limitations that affect the quality of morbidity data.

A recent *Morbidity and Mortality Weekly Report (MMWR)* focused on surveillance for asthma by drawing upon data from the National Hospital Discharge Survey, the National Hospital Ambulatory Medical Care Survey (emergency department data only), the National Health Interview Survey, and mortality data from the vital statistics system.[27] The authors documented up-

TABLE 15.4. Some challenges in measuring morbidity

Challenge	Nature of the Issues
Survey sample	• Issues related to the inclusiveness of the data collected and whether information available captures all cases needed and avoids double-counting
Medical coding	• May not reflect emerging diseases and related conditions
	• Differences in specifications of codes may influence comparability of data from different sources
Data reliability	• Provider-based morbidity often taken from truncated administrative sources
	• Limits imposed on the number of diagnostic codes captured for further analysis, resulting in undercounts
	• Bias in coding created by incentives inherent in the Medicare payment plan
	• Nonreporting of undiagnosed morbid conditions by self- and proxy reports
	• Need to obtain data on certain conditions from two or more surveys of different sources
	• Selection bias in personal interview surveys
Survey instrument design	• Interviews may be subject to more inaccuracies than other survey design modes
	• Tradeoffs in long recall vs. short recall periods in securing care recipient reports of illnesses
Disease-related problems	• Difficulty in securing accurate data on incidence and prevalence of certain diseases (e.g., cancer)

ward trends in self-reported asthma and use of services for asthma treatment. However, it was not possible to ensure that all cases were included (e.g., hospital outpatient clinic use was omitted), or that there was no double counting (e.g., the same person could have had multiple office visits during the course of a year or could have been hospitalized in addition to seeing an office-based physician). Thus, it was not possible to come up with a single national figure reflecting morbidity due to asthma.

Another *MMWR* examined the impact of arthritis and other rheumatic conditions on the US healthcare system. Using data from the NHCS, the authors concluded that "arthritis and other rheumatic conditions have a large impact on hospitalizations, ambulatory-care visits, and home health care, with women accounting for most of this impact and all persons aged less than 65 years accounting for a substantial portion."[28(p349)] Again, a national estimate of morbidity due to these conditions could not be generated because some persons may have experienced multiple discharges or encounters, and some care was missed, because data were not gathered from settings such as chiropractors' offices and rehabilitation, physical, and occupational therapy services.

There are also a number of issues associated with the specification of diagnostic codes and the processes by which they are assigned; these issues have implications for morbidity data. Typically, information on morbidity is reported by use of the categories and codes of the *International Classification of Diseases* (*ICD*), now in its tenth revision,[29] although the ninth revision continues to be used for morbidity coding in the United States. (There is no standard classification currently in use for coding functional status.) Provisions exist for modifying the *ICD* between formal revisions. Nevertheless, as new diseases emerge and epidemiologists and other researchers focus their efforts on better understanding and tracking those diseases, existing coding systems may not accurately reflect emerging diseases, such as HIV/AIDS. Care must be taken to examine codes for related conditions that may have been used in the absence of codes for the condition of interest and to review the underlying medical records documentation to assure that the diagnostic information is accurate and relevant.

Differences in the specification of codes used to define a condition of interest may influence the comparability of data from different sources. For example, in the *MMWR* analysis of arthritis and other rheumatic conditions cited above, the codes used to define the conditions were specified by the National Arthritis Data Workgroup and are much more inclusive than they would typically be in the case of more routine reporting of healthcare utilization.

Another problem is that provider-based morbidity data frequently are taken from administrative data, the reliability of which remains a concern. One source of error in morbidity data derived from hospital discharge records is the limit imposed on the number of diagnostic codes that are taken from hospital records and captured for further analysis. For example, if a maximum of five diagnostic codes can be recorded, any further diagnoses that were made during a hospital stay will be omitted from the record. The result will be an undercount of diagnoses. The limit on the number of codes will also cause bias: minor illnesses will be undercounted more than major illnesses, and the longer the hospital stay, the more diagnostic codes will be uncounted.

In the mid-1970s, the Institute of Medicine (IOM) conducted three national studies that looked at the reliability of three sources of hospital discharge data: (1) discharge abstracts processed by private abstract services reflecting care provided to Medicare and Medicaid patients in 1974; (2) records generated by the Centers for Medicare and Medicaid Services (formerly Health Care Financing Administration) from claims submitted by participating hospitals to receive Medicare reimbursement for patients discharged during 1974; and (3) hospital discharge data from NCHS's National Hospital Discharge Survey based on data abstracted from hospital medical records and reflecting discharges for the entire noninstitutionalized US population in 1977.[30] In a comparison of the original data with the data re-abstracted by the IOM field team for all diagnoses combined, levels of agreement were 63.4%, 58.4%, and 65.2% for the NHDS data, Medicare records, and private abstract service records, respectively, using 4-digit comparisons of *ICD-8* codes.

In the IOM studies, levels of reliability for individual diagnoses varied considerably, ranging from 79.6% for bronchopneumonia to 37.5% for chronic ischemic heart disease for the NHDS data and 4-digit comparisons. Reliability increased with more inclusive diagnostic groupings and decreased for records with multiple diagnoses and co-morbidities. For some cases, particularly when the patient had many medical problems, it was impossible for the field team to determine which diagnosis should be regarded as "principal" and which data source (the IOM or original data) should be viewed as "correct." In the NHDS study, these indeterminate cases ranged from 6.5% with 4-digit coding to 2.0% with the broader NCHS categories typically used for reporting. For almost every diagnosis, the likelihood that it would be correctly included among the list of diagnoses appearing on the NHDS abstract was greater than the likelihood that it would be correctly designated as "principal" (for diabetes the figures were 99.8% and 65.7%). The degree to which these discrepancies present a problem obviously depends on the purpose for which the data are used. Improvements could be attained if the discharge summary were routinely used to abstract information on principal diagnosis, rather than the face sheet of the medical record, and if the operative report were routinely used to abstract information on principal procedure.[30]

The 1983 advent of prospective payment of hospitals by the Medicare program introduced new problems regarding the reliability of morbidity data. Under the prospective payment system, a hospital provides up to five diagnostic codes and three procedure codes to the Centers for Medicare and Medicaid Services, which processes the codes through the GROUPER computer program to designate a diagnosis-related group (DRG), which is multiplied by various weights to determine the amount of payment. The Office of the Inspector General for the Department of Health and Human Services conducted a study to determine the amount of incorrect coding and whether DRG "creep" was occurring. In a national sample of hospitals (minus the states of New York, New Jersey, Massachusetts, and Maryland, which were "waivered" out of the prospective payment system at that time) and a sample of Medicare discharges from those hospitals between October 1, 1984, and March 31, 1985, the investigators found an error rate of 20.8% in DRG coding. A statistically significant 61.7% of those errors benefited the hospital financially, whereas the rest penalized the hospital.[31] The error rate is consistent with the IOM study conducted a decade earlier. Although the IOM found discrepancies between the Medicare record and the IOM abstract for 41.6% of all cases combined and coded to 4 digits, when investigators compared the cases by DRGs, 19.2% of the cases were discrepant.[30] To the degree that such errors persist and such data are released by hospitals for purposes other than Medicare payment, they will likely influence the accuracy of morbidity data.

More recent studies of the reliability and validity of diagnostic information on hospital discharges tend to be state- or institution-specific, rather than national in scope. Nevertheless, they continue to reveal problems. For example, as part of a larger validation study of the Complications Screening Program (CSP), a quality assurance tool that identifies in-hospital complications potentially indicative of problems with the quality of care, McCarthy et al.[32] examined whether medical records contained clinical evidence supporting the *ICD-9-CM* discharge diagnosis and procedure codes used to identify the complications. The study design involved a retrospective record review of 485 randomly sampled 1994 hospitalizations of Medicare beneficiaries in Connecticut and California. Objective, explicit chart review instruments were developed that itemized key clinical criteria to confirm the diagnosis and procedure codes. Findings were presented for 11 surgical and 2 medical screens. For all surgical cases, 68.8% of case records included objective clinical evidence, 11.8% contained only a physician note, and 19.4% contained no evidence. The corresponding numbers for medical cases were 43.7%, 26.4%, and 29.9%, respectively. The rates of confirmatory clinical evidence varied by complication screen, ranging from 86.7% for reopening of surgical site to 50.0% for postoperative pneumonia. The study did not include the full range of *ICD-9-CM* codes, and the review criteria were very specific. Regardless, to the degree that morbidity analyses are based on the types of cases examined here, the validity of the reported diagnoses may be questioned.

Morbidity data may also be obtained from interview surveys and physical exams. Morbidity data from interview surveys such as NHIS are subject to more inaccuracies than data obtained by physical examination. An obvious flaw in morbidity data gathered by either self or proxy report is the nonreporting of undiagnosed morbid conditions. In addition, terminological variations, wishful thinking, and a respondent's reluctance to divulge what is very private information may contribute to the inaccuracy of morbidity data gathered by personal interview. Interview data gathered by proxy are generally less accurate than data obtained directly from the subject, and they also yield higher item nonresponse rates. Either a proxy or a nonproxy respondent may lack medically precise knowledge about a condition. Recognizing that inherent difficulty, the managers of the NHIS discontinued the practice of coding chronic health conditions through use of *ICD* codes when the revised NHIS questionnaire was introduced in 1997. It was felt that the use of *ICD* codes appeared to confer a higher degree of precision to the data than was appropriate.

The NHIS has traditionally collected information on health conditions in two ways: (1) by asking directly whether the respondent had been diagnosed with specific conditions, and (2) by ascertaining indirectly which conditions were the causes of behaviors related to ill health, such as contacting a physician's office, staying in bed, and/or cutting down on normal activities. The latter approach yields lower rates for a condition, because the respondent will mention the condition only if it triggered contact with the healthcare system or caused a reduction in the individual's ability to function. Thus, the latter rates tend to exclude conditions with negligible impact. Also, results from the latter approach are confounded by differences in socioeconomic status, because persons of lower socioeconomic status are less able to stay home from work, to limit their activities, or to seek medical care; thus when such respondents do not demonstrate those behaviors, their health conditions are not counted. For further discussion of this issue, see Madans.[33]

The two types of rates have their respective valid uses. For example, NCHS regularly publishes prevalence rates derived from direct questions about the presence of chronic conditions—see, for example, Collins,[34,35] Adams et al.,[36] and Benson and Marano.[37] In addition, Hing and Bloom[38] published rates of chronic conditions for persons with functional dependency. The two types of rates can differ considerably. For example, the diabetes prevalence rate was estimated to be 9.7% for persons aged 45 and older, based on the following question asked of sample adults in the 1997 NHIS: "Have you EVER been told by a doctor or other health professional that you had diabetes or sugar diabetes?" On the other hand, the proportion of people who have diabetes that is the cause of a functional limitation was estimated to be only 2.5%, based on asking the *same* sample adults the following questions if they indicated that they had a functional limitation: "What conditions or health problems cause you to have difficulty with these activities?"[39]

The 1997 NHIS designers also introduced a new practice of requiring nonproxy responses to a large section of the survey containing questions that are much more accurately answered by self-report. For example, a proxy cannot with certainty answer a question such as "Has a doctor or other health professional ever told you that you had [a particular chronic condition]."

A related problem arises with conditions for which afflicted persons might live either in the community or in an institution. Alzheimer disease and other dementias provide a relevant example. Using NCHS data, one would need to obtain and combine estimates from the NHIS (a population-based survey) and the NNHS (a facility-based survey) in order to capture data representing (almost) the entire population of the United States. Within NCHS, an internal workgroup is analyzing the technical issues associated with making such combined estimates.

Another problem in measuring morbidity via personal interview is the selection bias caused by the fact that ill people may be less able to report accurately and completely, or they may not report at all. For example, data for a person who is in the hospital temporarily will normally be obtainable only by proxy from other family members. In the case of the NHIS, if a hospitalized person is selected as the sample adult, it is unlikely that the interviewer will be able to administer that portion of the survey. And a hospitalized person who lives alone will probably not be contacted at all, so that household will be counted as a noninterview.

Cancer is an example of a chronic disease for which it is difficult to measure both incidence and prevalence. In the gathering of cancer incidence data, it is common to assign the date of diagnosis as the date of commencement of the disease, but clearly the disease began earlier than the date of diagnosis. Furthermore, the stage of the disease at the time of diagnosis varies greatly and is not always known or recorded. Prevalence of cancer is difficult to measure because of as-yet-undiagnosed cases and because it is not generally straightforward to assign a date after which a cancer patient may be considered to no longer have cancer. The natural histories of certain common cancers (e.g., breast and prostate) are such that people surviving longer than five or even ten years cannot necessarily be considered cured.[40]

Finally, in the questioning of a respondent about morbidity history, there are trade-offs between using a long recall period and using a short one. If a respondent is asked about illnesses occurring over the last year, some incidents are likely to be forgotten, especially less severe ones, whereas if a short recall period is used, the resulting counts and rates will be lower and subject to higher statistical variation. Also, annualization of counts and rates based on a shorter (less than one-year) recall period requires strong assumptions to be satisfied. For example, if it is known that 100 individuals responded that they had a cold during a three-month recall period, that count can be multiplied by four (under certain assumptions) to obtain an annualized count of 400 colds per year, but it cannot be concluded that 400 *individuals* would have had a cold during a 12-month period, because some people have multiple colds in a year, whereas others have none or only one cold.

Concerns for Confidentiality, Privacy, and Security

Because health information, including morbidity data, is among the more personal types of data, such data are especially vulnerable or susceptible to invasion of privacy. There are also more tangible risks, such as loss of employment or insurance coverage if such information is divulged. The potential for unauthorized or accidental transmission of confidential information is increased by the rapid growth of electronic information exchange. At the same time, mechanisms to guard against unauthorized release and to build in controls and systems checks are enhanced by greater reliance on informatics.

The ability to guarantee the confidential treatment of data received from respondents to all NCHS surveys is fundamental to the conduct of the NCHS mission. The quality and quantity of information NCHS collects and disseminates would suffer severely without such assurances, and the consequences (both legal and professional) would be crippling. In the absence of any other constraint, NCHS would seek all means at its disposal to treat data with the utmost security and respect for privacy of individuals and establishments. However, a set of laws exists that provides a strong legal basis for doing so.

Legislative and Administrative Requirements

The legal underpinnings for NCHS's confidentiality policies derive from the Public Health Service Act, the Privacy Act of 1974, Title 18 of the United States Code, and the Health Insurance Portability and Accountability Act (HIPPA). Section 308(d) of the Public Health Service Act (42 USC 242m) requires that whenever NCHS requests information, it must inform the person or establishment providing the information about the uses to be made of it, which are usually limited to statistical research and reporting. Thereafter, the NCHS is limited to those specified uses, and only NCHS staff or its qualified agents may use the information. The NCHS may never release identifiable information without the advance, explicit approval of those providing the information or described in it. The Privacy Act of 1974 (5 USC 552a) provides for the confidential treatment of individual records maintained by a Federal agency according to either the individual's name or some other identifier. The law also prohibits any use of those records for purposes other than those for which they were collected. Among the law's other provisions is the requirement to establish appropriate administrative, technical, and physical safeguards to protect records. Under Title 18 of the US Code 1905, the Federal Law Governing Federal Employees' Behavior, federal employees are subject to severe penalties for disclosing confidential information.[41] Collectively, these statutes provide for fines of up to $5,000 and/or imprisonment and removal from public office for failure to adhere to their provisions. Finally, as discussed by John Christiansen in Chapter 4, HIPPA imposes responsibilities on those who handle individual health information.

The NCHS Research Data Center

The coterie of people who produce a survey have a genuine desire for the data to be used by the public. At the same time, it is ethically, practically, and legally necessary that confidentiality of the individuals or organizations that provided the data be preserved. After all, nonresponse rates will rightfully go up if respondents are not confident about the confidentiality of their personal information. But analysts whose projects are beneficial to society may require information at levels of detail that cannot be provided in publicly released data. In response to the need for more detailed data than can be released, NCHS and other agencies have created research data centers that provide analysts with controlled access to microdata.

NCHS provides two modes of special access via its Research Data Center (RDC)—on-site access and remote access. In both cases, potential RDC users submit a detailed proposal to the RDC, indicating the purpose of the analysis to be undertaken, specifying the software, methods, and data to be used, and describing the output files. If the proposed analysis is generally sound and can be undertaken without breaching confidentiality, the proposal is approved, and the analyst arranges either to visit the RDC or to electronically submit an analytical computer program using SAS as the programming language. The remote access software system returns the program's output to the analyst's registered e-mail address. Restrictions are different for remote access than for on-site access. A fee is charged for use of the RDC, and users sign a confidentiality agreement. Identifiers such as names and social security numbers are removed from NCHS data used in the RDC, and strict disclosure limits are enforced. User-written computer programs and their output are scanned and screened by RDC staff, both manually and by use of special software. Complex systems are required to permit this screening process to be highly automated. For more details, see the RDC Web site at www.cdc.gov/nchs/r&d/rdc.htm. The guidelines for operations applying to users of the NCHS Research Data Center are listed below:

Guest researcher (on site)

- RDC staff constructs necessary data files including merged user data
- PC SAS, SUDAAN, STATA, FORTRAN, and HLM available
- Other statistical packages available with sufficient lead time
- Output subject to disclosure review
- Disclosure review guidelines published in NCHS Staff Manual on Confidentiality
- [a] Analyses (paper output and computer discs) passing disclosure review can be taken off site
- Center requires staff oversight
- Open only during normal working hours

Remote access

- RDC staff constructs necessary data files including merged user data
- Ability to submit analytical computer programs via e-mail
- Output returned by e-mail to user's registered address
- SAS programs only, certain procedures and functions not allowed:
  - PROC TABULATE and PROC IML not allowed
  - LIST and PRINT not allowed—no listing of individual cases

- R_, FIRST., LAST., not allowed—no selection of individual cases
- No cell fewer than five observations; if found, other cells also suppressed
- Job log scanned for conditions that spawn case listings
- Manual disclosure limitation review where necessary

The Continuing Potential to Computerize Survey Data Retrieval, Processing, Editing, and Dissemination

For current surveys, and certainly for surveys of the future, there is a potential for greatly increased reliance on informatics and the electronic retrieval, processing, editing, and dissemination of morbidity data. However, the degree to which this occurs may depend on the complexity of the survey, the nature of the data items of interest, the data source, the state of technological development, and the further evolution of standardized data definitions and formats.

Currently available software packages offer a variety of options, including point-and-click survey instrument design vs. programming; a variety of data editing capabilities (data editor, built-in logical checks, and routing capabilities); multiple data export features (ASCII, statistical package, and relational files); different data structures (central, meta, hierarchical, and rostering); documentation options (edit log, word processing version of the survey instrument); and a variety of special features including case management, multilingual capabilities, and multimedia and software help desks.[42] Tailoring these and other options to specific applications requires careful consideration of advantages and disadvantages.

The 1997 change to CAPI by the National Health Interview Survey offered a number of improvements. Interviewers now read the questions to the respondent from the screen of a laptop computer, and the responses are entered electronically on the spot, instead of being written down on paper during the interview and captured electronically later. The use of CAPI permits some immediate editing to be performed by the computer program, and it permits corroboration by the respondent, who is still present at the time of such editing. The computer also ensures that correct skip patterns are followed as the interviewer and respondent take what can be a complex path through the questions. When the time comes during the interview for an adult respondent to be selected from among the family members, the computer program selects an adult, ensuring randomness and adherence to the survey protocol. A randomly selected child is similarly identified. The questionnaire can be displayed on the computer screen in either English or Spanish, changing languages on command by the interviewer. On-line help is available for the interviewer and/or the respondent. Notes made by the interviewer can be captured in the file and attended to later, at Census or at NCHS. The path of the interview, including the time spent on each question, backups, corrections, etc., can be recorded for future research and analysis. For example, this tracking allows trouble spots in the questionnaire to be identified and studied.

Plans are under way to upgrade the software used in the NHIS instrument from CASES software in a DOS environment to Blaise software in a Windows environment. This upgrade will provide enhanced data editing capability and will generally be more interviewer-friendly. When respondents' signatures are needed, it will also enable NHIS to use devices to collect them electronically, doing away with the present cumbersome and expensive system of using paper forms, tracking the forms if they are not submitted on time by the interviewer to the Census Bureau, and storing the forms. The new instrument will also be able to use audio-CASI (audio computer-assisted self-interviewing) technology to afford more privacy to respondents when especially personal questions are asked. With audio-CASI, the respondent self-administers the survey using a laptop computer, listening to questions on audio headphones and entering responses into the computer. The response categories are usually displayed on the screen; the questions may or may not be.[43]

Also in the NHIS future are relational databases to store in-house and public use data files, and a metadata repository to organize the multiple and complex versions of NHIS documentation. These will facilitate editing, imputing, dissemination, and access to NHIS data.

The Internet offers new, much faster, and much less expensive ways to collect interview survey data. The ability to ensure security of transmitted data over the Internet has improved. Households with Internet access are far from representative of all households, but the proportion of households with Internet access is increasing, and such access is now provided in public places such as libraries.[44] The use of mixed-mode survey designs (combining, say, an Internet survey with an in-person or a telephone survey) could compensate for the bias in an Internet-only survey, and statistical methods could be developed to adjust for this bias, just as NIS and SLAITS adjust for nontelephone bias, as previously described.

The use of the Internet to gather data would fundamentally alter the nature of surveys like the NHIS, replacing a face-to-face encounter with a live interviewer with an impersonal computer interaction. Indeed, the name of the survey—the National Health *Interview* Survey—would no longer be appropriate: Webster's Dictionary[45(p765)] defines the verb *interview* as "to meet, visit" and the noun *interview* as "a meeting of people face to face to confer about something." Dillman predicted that, just as computer-assisted interviewing by telephone has increasingly been used as a replacement for in-person interviewing, "self-administered surveys, which leave interviewers out of the data collection process entirely, will become the dominant method of surveying early in the 21st century."[46] (Self-administered surveys are administered by regular mail, courier, fax, e-mail, and touch-tone telephone entry, as well as by the Internet.) For further discussion of these issues, see also Dillman.[47,48]

Also, if the present version of the NHIS were administered via the Internet, methods would have to be developed to ensure that a specific person—e.g., the sample adult—was actually the one providing responses over the Internet.

SLAITS has already used privacy-enhancing technology. A New Jersey survey on HIV testing and HIV risk behaviors was used to test the effectiveness of Digit-Grabber® dialed digit meters. This technology permits respondents to answer telephone questions in a relatively anonymous way and without other people in the room hearing the answers. Half of the respondents were offered the Digit-Grabber, and half were not. The SLAITS results suggested that those not offered the relative privacy of the Digit-Grabber technology were less likely to report engaging in behaviors that may carry a social stigma, such as same-sex sexual behavior. Previous research by Turner et al. led to similar conclusions.[49]

Cellular telephone exchanges are currently excluded from the NIS Random Digit Dialing sampling frame, but at some time in the future, the NIS and SLAITS will have to modify their data collection procedures to deal with the increasing prevalence of cellular telephones in the United States. At present, it is not desirable to call cell phone users and ask them to participate in a survey if the receivers of the calls are required to pay for the call. If charging arrangements for cell phone use evolve into a flat fee system, however, respondents will not have to bear an extra cost for participating in phone surveys. Other issues will also have to be dealt with, such as how to sample households when residents have their own individual phone numbers as well as or instead of a household phone number.

As previously noted, the National Health Care Survey utilizes computerized algorithms and automated approaches in sample design and implementation and in a variety of data processing, editing, and analytic activities. Much less reliance on informatics and electronic assistance has occurred with respect to the actual data gathering. In considering whether to introduce CAPI techniques into the NAMCS, survey administrators concluded that CAPI would lend itself well to the interview of physicians to determine whether they were in scope for the survey and to obtain information about their practice characteristics. However, that is a very small portion of the overall data collection effort. Because of the absence of computers or appropriate software in many physicians' offices and the lack of resources for survey administrators to leave a computer in the office to be used for data input (most of the patient data are recorded by office personnel), it was decided that CAPI would not be cost-effective at this time. Various scanning and imaging techniques are viewed as promising for obtaining patient information from medical records and are still under consideration.

CAPI continues to hold a great appeal for the nursing home and home and hospice care surveys as a means of reducing edit requirements, aiding in data storage, and facilitating the drawing of patient samples through electronic lists. An additional advantage is the ability to build in as many data quality and consistency checks as possible so that problems are discovered and corrected during the interview or at the time of data abstraction while it is still possible to obtain the correct information. Developmental work has been initiated with the expectation that long-term care surveys after 2002 will be computerized.

The majority of patient records (from a minority of hospitals) are obtained electronically for the NHDS. Since the 1988 redesign, automated discharge data have been received from roughly 170 facilities. Manual data collection occurs in a core sample of hospitals and in all other facilities not providing automated data. The automated data come from individual facilities (some of which provide a complete census of their discharges, which are then sampled), private vendors, or state governmental and professional entities. The schedule for data receipt ranges from monthly, to quarterly, to semi-annually, to yearly. The automated data files are not standardized. They arrive in different formats, including reel-to-reel tapes, diskettes, c-tapes, and e-mail and Internet files. Formats vary and may be ASCII, EPSDIC, blocked, variable, or fixed. These data cannot be used without the investment of considerable staff time and effort in data conversion and verification because of the multiple formats.[50]

With respect to NCHS facility-based surveys, because the surveys focus on different settings of health care with different types of data collection, a single electronic approach may not be appropriate. Instead, these surveys may use different software that could feed data into a data warehouse for storage, manipulation, and linkage across surveys. There are many potential options, with a variety of advantages and challenges. Nevertheless, significant progress in obtaining automated morbidity data would seem to rest at least partially on further standardization of data definitions, codes, formats, and modes of transmission, requiring a concerted, collaborative effort on the part of state and federal governments, healthcare professional and provider organizations, and industry groups. Progress could be facilitated by wider use of standardized, computerized medical records. Progress may be complicated by the transition to the use of *ICD-10-CD*, which is currently used for mortality data but not for morbidity data.

Some improvement in the consistency of diagnostic codes may be attained by the use of computer products called "encoders," of which there are basically two types. One type uses a branching logic system, in which the coder first enters the main term from a diagnosis or procedure and then follows a series of questions resulting in a code assignment. The other resembles an automated code book, encompassing a screen that resembles the alphabetical index and tabular list of the *ICD-9-CM*. Some automated systems incorporate the GROUPER algorithm, which results in the assignment of a DRG for payment purposes.[51] These systems may improve the reliability of coding by the inclusion of prompts to consider related codes and look for co-morbidities and complications that could influence the code assignment. They may also lessen the accuracy of coding by optimizing coding in order to increase reimbursement. Regardless, automated systems should improve the reliability of coding in the sense of "repeatability," such that the same code would be obtained in repeat examinations of a record. However, the issue of validity (whether the medical record and the code accurately capture the clinical nuances of the patient's condition and care) remains an open question—at least for some cases.

Another policy initiative with the potential to increase the consistency and quality of morbidity information is HIPAA. Section 263 of the HIPAA provisions for administrative simplification requires the National Committee on Vital and Health Statistics (NCVHS) to "study the issues related to the adoption of uniform data standards for patient medical record information and the electronic exchange of such information."[52] After receiving input from a variety of private and public sector groups, the Committee identified three major barriers to electronic interchange: (1) limited interoperability of health information systems, (2) limited comparability of data exchanged among providers, and (3) the need for better quality, accountability, and integrity of data. The Committee's report will include recommendations for addressing these issues.

A Look Forward

The need for morbidity data is permanent and enduring. What will change are the things we measure and the way we measure them. New public health challenges will emerge, generating new data needs. Advances in informatics will provide new opportunities for gathering, processing, and disseminating data. These new technologies offer significant improvements in the quality and timeliness of data. However, they also offer new ways to make mistakes, including bigger mistakes. As always, we must develop coping mechanisms to deal with the potential for error. To keep our surveys relevant, we must be willing to change and, when appropriate, to adopt new methods and technology. We must contend with the uncertainties caused by the plethora of alternatives that are offered to us and do our best to move forward. Sharing information and experiences, by means such as this book, will facilitate such progress.

Questions for Review

1. You are a researcher interested in obtaining information about the current state of the public's health in the United States. For each of the information items listed below, indicate the best source of information, choosing among (1) the National Health Insurance Interview Survey, (2) the State and Local Integrated Telephone Survey, and (3) any components of the National Health Care Survey.
   a. Information about hospital utilization by family members
   b. Information about how many children have special needs for health care
   c. Information about families' health care access and healthcare utilization

    d. Information about morbidity due to injuries

    e. Information about the number of persons covered by health insurance plans

2. *Questions 2a and b are based on the following short case:* In a research project to estimate the incidence and prevalence of a certain disease, a public health scientist can obtain data from three sources: (1) a study conducted by interviewing a random sample of the noninstitutionalized population, in which the questions used a short recall period of three months to obtain information from healthcare recipients, with no proxy responses permitted; (2) a study conducted by interviewing a random sample of the noninstitutionalized population. in which the questions used a long recall period of one year to obtain information about health care recipients; with proxy responses permitted; (3) complete administrative records furnished by hospitals, with one record per hospital stay, in which at most three diagnostic codes describing the reasons for the hospital stay were captured; and (4) complete mortality records, each identifying the underlying cause of death and multiple contributing causes of death. as well as specifying the age and sex of the deceased.

    a. What are the limitations of each of the four data sources in terms of likely data accuracy. completeness, and reliability?

    b. What are the strengths of each of the three data sources in terms of data accuracy, completeness. and reliability?

3. The NCHS Research Data Center does not permit remote users to use cells containing fewer than five observations in the application of SAS programs. If such a cell is discovered in a user's computer output, all other cells are suppressed, regardless of the number of observations included in the other cells. Explain why such a policy is necessary to protect the confidentiality of individuals represented in the data.

4. List at least three reasons that administering the present version of the National Health Interview Survey via the Internet would be problematic.

5. Explain the impact of using "encoders" in an effort to improve the consistency of diagnostic codes. Are there any disadvantages?

References

1. *Webster's Encyclopedic Unabridged Dictionary of the English Language.* New York: Gramercy Books: 1996.
2. MacMahon B, Pugh T. *Epidemiology: Principles and Methods.* Boston: Little. Brown and Company; 1970.
3. Fox J, Hall C, Elveback L. *Epidemiology: Man and Disease.* London: The MacMillan Company; 1970.
4. US Department of Health and Human Services. *National Center for Health Statistics Programs and Activities: Monitoring the Nation's Health.* Hyattsville, MD: US Department of Health and Human Services: 1999.
5. Gentleman JF. Health information analysis: potentials and impediments. In *Health*

Information for Canada. Report of the National Task Force on Health Information Statistics. Ottawa, Canada; 1991; Statistics Canada.

6. Zayatz L. Data masking for disclosure limitation. In *Proceedings of the National Conference on Health Statistics*. Washington, DC: National Center for Health Statistics; 1999. Proceedings available on CD-ROM from National Center for Health Statistics, Aug 2–4, 1999.

7. Kernighan BW, Plauger PJ. *The Elements of Programming Style*. Second Edition. New York: McGraw Hill; 1978.

8. Battaglia M, Malec D, Spencer B, Hoaglin D, Sedransk J. Adjusting for noncoverage of nontelephone households in the National Immunization Survey. In *Proceedings of the Section on Survey Research Methods*. Alexandria, VA: American Statistical Association; 1995:678–683. Aug 13–17, 1995. Orlando, Florida.

9. Frankel M, Srinath KP, Battaglia M, Hoaglin DC. Reducing nontelephone bias in RDD surveys. In *Proceedings of the Section on Survey Research Methods*. Alexandria, VA: American Statistical Association; May 13–16, 1999. St. Petersburg Beach, FL, pp. 934–939.

10. Bernstein AB, Hing E, Burt C, Hall MJ. Trend data on medical encounters: tracking a moving target. *Health Aff (Millwood)* 2001;20:58–72.

11. McLemore T, Bacon WE. Establishment surveys of the National Center for Health Statistics. In *Proceedings of the International Conference on Establishment Surveys*. Buffalo, NY; June 27–30, 1993: American Statistical Association, Alexandria, VA.

12. Feinglass J, Brown JL, LoSasso A, et al. Rates of lower-extremity amputation and arterial reconstruction in the United States. 1979 to 1996. *Am J Public Health* 1999;89:1222–1227.

13. Pappas G, Hadden W, Kozak LJ, Fisher G. Potentially avoidable hospitalizations: inequalities in rates between US socioeconomic groups. *Am J Public Health* 1997;87:811–816.

14. Kozak LJ, McCarthy E, Moien M. Patterns of hospital use by patients with diagnoses related to HIV infection. *Public Health Rep* 1993;108:571–581.

15. National Center for Health Statistics. Decreasing hospital use for HIV. Health E-Stats. Available at: http://www.cdc.gov/nchs/products/pubs/pubd/hestats/hivchart.htm. Accessed March 29, 2002.

16. National Center for Health Statistics. Longer hospital stays for childbirth. Health E-Stats. Available at: http://www.cdc.gov/nchs/products/pubs/pubd/hestats/birthchart.htm. Accessed March 29, 2002.

17. Salive M, Guralnik J, Brock D. Preventive services for breast and cervical cancer in U.S. office-based practices. *Prev Med* 1996;25:561–568.

18. Thorndike A, Rigotti N, Stafford R, Singer D. National patterns in the treatment of smokers by physicians. *JAMA* 1998;279:604–608.

19. Aparasu R, Fliginger S. Inappropriate medication prescribing for the elderly by office-based physicians. *Ann Pharmacother* 1997;31:823–829.

20. Burt C, Arispe I. Emergency department visits for medical misadventure. Poster session at the Academy for Health Services Research and Health Policy Annual Meeting, Los Angeles, CA, June 25–27, 2000.

21. Franks P, Clancy C. Referrals of adult patients from primary care: demographic disparities and their relationship to HMO insurance. *J Fam Pract* 1997;45:47–53.

22. Burt C, Overpeck M. Emergency visits for sports-related injuries. *Ann Emerg Med* 2001;37:301–308.

23. Castle NG, Shea DG. Mental health services and the mortality of nursing home residents. *J Aging Health* 1997;9:498–513.

24. Beck-Sague C, Banergee S, Jarvis WR. Infectious diseases and mortality among US nursing home residents. *Am J Public Health* 1993;83:1739–1742.

25. Bishop CE. Where are the missing elders? The decline in nursing home use, 1985 and 1995. *Health Aff (Millwood)* 1999;18:146–155.

26. Health, United States, 2001 with Urban and Rural Health Chartbook. Hyattsville, MD: US Department of Health and Human Services; 2001, 289.

27. Mannino D, Homa D, Pertowski C, et al. Surveillance for asthma—United States, 1960–1995. *Mor Mortal Wkly Rep CDC Surveill Summ* 1998;47:1–27.

28. Impact of arthritis and other rheumatic conditions on the health-care system—United States, 1997. *MMWR Morb Mortal Wkly Rep* 1999;48:349–353.

29. World Health Organization. *International Statistical Classification of Diseases and Related Health Problems, 10th Revision.* Volume 2. Geneva: World Health Organization; 1993.

30. Demlo L, Campbell P. Improving hospital discharge data: lessons from the National Hospital Discharge Survey. *Med Care* 1981;19:1030–1040.

31. Hsia D, Krushat WM, Fagan A, Tebbutt J, Kusserow R. Accuracy of diagnostic coding for Medicare patients under the prospective-payment system. *New Engl J Med* 1988;318:352–355.

32. McCarthy E, Iezzoni L, Davis R, et al Does clinical evidence support *ICD-9-CM* diagnosis coding of complications? *Med Care* 2000;38:868–876.

33. Madans J. The measurement of health status in the United States. In Proceedings of the Symposium on Health and Mortality. November 1997, Brussels, Belgium. 19–22. Available at: www.un.org/esa/population/pubsarchive/healthmort/c.pdf.

34. Collins JG. Prevalence of selected chronic conditions: United States, 1990–1992. *Vital Health Stat 10* 1997;(194):1–89.

35. Collins JG. Prevalence of selected chronic conditions: United States, 19931995. National Center for Health Statistics. *Vital Health Stat 10* 2001:Forthcoming.

36. Adams PF, Hendershot GE, Marano MA. Current estimates from the National Health Interview Survey, 1996. National Center for Health Statistics. *Vital Health Stat 10 (200)* 1999(212 pg).

37. Benson V, Marano MS. Current estimates from the National Health Interview Survey, 1995. National Center for Health Statistics. *Vital Health Stat 10 (199)* 1998.

38. Hing E, Bloom B. Long-term care for the functionally dependent elderly. National Center for Health Statistics. *Vital Health Stat 13 (104)* 1990.

39. Schenker N, Gentleman JF, Rose D, Hing E, Shimizu I. Combining Estimates from Complementary Surveys: A Case Study Using Prevalence Estimates from National Health Surveys of Households and Nursing Homes. To appear in Public Health Reports, 2002, Vol. 117.

40. National Cancer Institute of Canada. *Canadian Cancer Statistics 1995.* Toronto, Canada: National Cancer Institute of Canada; 1995.

41. US Department of Health and Human Services. *National Center for Health Statistics Staff Manual on Confidentiality.* Hyattsville, MD: US Department of Health and Human Services; 1997.

42. Dorn-Havlik S, Mulrow J, White G. Final Report. *NCHS Activity 2: CAPI Benchmarking.* Washington, D.C.: Ernst & Young, LLP; 2000.

43. Couper MP, Baker RP, Bethlehem J, et al. *Computer Assisted Survey Information Collection.* New York: Wiley; 1998.

44. Taylor H. Does Internet research work? Comparing online survey results with telephone survey. *International Journal of Market Research* 2000;42:51–63

45. *Webster's New Universal Unabridged Dictionary*, Second Edition. New York: Simon and Schuster; 1983.

46. Dillman DA. Mail and other self-administered surveys in the 21st century: the beginning of a new era. Available at: http://survey.sesrc.wsu.edu/dillman/. Accessed March 29, 2002.

47. Dillman DA. *Mail and Telephone Surveys: The Total Design Method.* New York: Wiley; 1978.

48. Dillman DA, Bowker DK. The Web questionnaire challenge to survey methodologists. Available at: http://survey.sesrc.wsu.edu/dillman/. Accessed March 29, 2002.

49. Turner CF, Ku L, Sonenstein FL, Pleck JH. Impact of ACASI on reporting of male-male sexual contacts: Preliminary results from the 1995 National Survey of Adolescent Males. In: Warnecke R. ed. *Proceedings of the Conference on Health Survey Research Methods.* Breckenridge, Colorado; 1995. Proceedings available at: www.cdc.gov/nchs/data/proceed.pdf. Accessed March 29, 2002.

50. Mulrow J, White G. Final Report. NCHS *Activity 1: Gain a Clear Understanding of Division of Health Care Statistics Current Process, Needs, and Requirements.* Washington, DC: Ernst & Young, LLP; 1999.

51. Abdelhak M, Grostick S, Hanken M, Jacobs E. *Health Information: Management of a Strategic Resource.* Philadelphia: WB Saunders Company; 1996.

52. National Committee on Vital and Health Statistics. *Report to the Secretary of the U.S. Department of Health and Human Services on Uniform Data Standards for Patient Medical Record Information.* Washington, DC: National Committee on Vital and Health Statistics; 2000.

16
Risk Factor Information Systems

PATRICK W. O'CARROLL, EVE POWELL-GRINER,
DEBORAH HOLTZMAN, AND G. DAVID WILLIAMSON

Learning Objectives

After studying this chapter, you should be able to:

- Define a risk factor data system and discuss how such systems complement morbidity and mortality data systems.
- Explain how risk factor data systems help public health officials to focus on the primary prevention side of the "prevention paradigm."
- Describe in detail the history, nature, uses, maintenance, and limitations of at least one important national-level risk factor data system.

Overview

Risk factor data systems are a relatively recent addition to the information systems arsenal of public health professionals. These systems complement vital statistics data systems and many morbidity data systems by providing information on factors that lie earlier in the causal chain leading to serious illness, injury, or death. There is a great variety of risk factor systems in use at the present time: some are designed to produce estimates for use at the national or regional level, whereas others are state- or local-level systems. Some focus on "pure" (predisease) risk factors (e.g., risk-taking behavior), whereas others focus on early disease states that represent risk factors for subsequently more serious disease or death. Some systems are designed to give cross-cutting estimates of many risk factors for a given population and time period (e.g., the Youth Risk Behavior Surveillance System), whereas others focus on particular risk factors or conditions (e.g., the Drug Abuse Warning Network). The Behavioral Risk Factor Surveillance System is a very rich data system that has been in use for some years. In this chapter, it is discussed in detail to illustrate the breadth, depth, complexity, and myriad uses of risk factor data systems.

Introduction

Vital statistics systems were the first widely used, institutionalized data sources for public health. These systems made it possible to track major trends in natality and mortality on a large scale. Health officials have been using these familiar vital statistics systems for centuries.[1] Indeed, the phrase "leading cause of death," which is based on simple comparative counts of deaths by various causes, has become almost a euphemism for "high-priority public health problem." More advanced uses of mortality data have been developed to better measure preventable (or at least premature) loss of life, such as the years of potential life lost index.[2] Such basic and advanced uses of vital statistics data remain a staple of public health assessment to this day.

However, over time, public health officials increasingly recognized the limitations of an over-reliance on vital events for monitoring population health status, prioritizing public health threats, and targeting research and prevention programs. From this recognition has sprung a variety of newly institutionalized data systems, based not on health events but on *risk factors* for health events. These risk factor data systems, although relatively recent in vintage, have become some of our most powerful tools for assessing community health and monitoring progress toward prevention.

In this chapter, we will discuss the nature of risk factor data systems, focusing in particular on the Behavioral Risk Factor Surveillance System (BRFSS) as illustrative of the risk factor data systems currently in use. We will begin with the reasons for the existence of such systems, then move to a discussion of the disease prevention paradigm that underlies them. After providing an overview of some of the major risk factor surveillance systems currently in use, we will examine the nature, history, participation patterns, and data uses of BRFSS to illustrate the importance of such systems to maintaining and improving public health.

Why Develop Risk Factor Data Systems?

Several trends led to the need for better data for prevention. One such trend, at least in the United States, was demographic. During the latter half of the 20th century, the population pyramid shifted toward the older age groups. For example, the proportion of the US population 65 years of age and older increased from 8.1% in 1950 to 12.7% in 1998—an increase of 57%.[3] Chronic diseases are an important cause of death in older age groups, but opportunities to reduce chronic disease mortality generally precede death by many years and even decades. As such, chronic disease death counts *per se* primarily indicate what the public health community should have been focusing on years or decades ago. This suggests the need for data more proximally related in time to the underlying causes of chronic disease deaths. In addition to the prevention of chronic disease mortality, the public health community also began during this period to focus on other new challenges, such as the prevention of deaths from environmental exposures, occupational hazards, injuries, and even violence. As with chronic diseases, salient points of preventive intervention for mortality from these causes often precede death by many years.

Scientific research in the past century has clearly elucidated the underlying causes of and antecedents to many causes of premature death. For example, the role of smoking,[4] hypertension,[5] and certain blood lipoproteins[6] as causal factors for heart disease mortality were thoroughly explored and documented in the latter half of the 20th century. The potential role of exercise and proper diet in preventing heart disease mortality was likewise explored during this period.[7] As the importance of these risk and protective factors became clear, the focus of many public health programs shifted from preventing mortality *per se* to reducing or mitigating the population prevalence of known risk factors (e.g., smoking) and increasing the prevalence of protective factors. This shift also contributed to the need for better means to monitor the incidence and prevalence of risk factors (including risk behaviors) among the population.

The 20th century witnessed unprecedented progress in preventing premature mortality and in lengthening the human lifespan, particularly among Western nations. With this progress, the public health community began to focus on the *quality* as well as the quantity (longevity) of life. For example, the prevention of chronic disease itself became a practical goal, in addition to the prevention of *mortality* from chronic diseases. Likewise, the prevention of disabilities from injuries and, whenever possible, the prevention of injuries *per se* were added to the prevention of injury mortality as a public health goal. In this context, means other than vital statistics systems were obviously needed to measure the incidence and prevalence of morbidity (e.g., diabetes), disability, and indicators of risk factors and social problems with long-term or multiple impacts on health and well being (e.g., alcohol abuse, smoking, and teenage pregnancy). Risk factor data systems were developed in light of all of these trends and needs.

The Prevention Paradigm

Risk factor data systems allow the public health community to monitor the fundamental causal factors that lead to death, disease, or disability. From the public health perspective, a focus on the incidence and prevalence of these risk factors moves the "prevention paradigm" in the right direction, away from tertiary prevention (e.g., emergency therapy to prevent death from a myocardial infarction) toward secondary prevention (e.g., treating hyperlipidemia and hypertension) and primary prevention (e.g., promoting healthy lifestyles, preventing smoking). Figure 16.1 illustrates this shift from disease treatment toward identification of risk factors for purposes of primary and secondary prevention. Note that certain diseases may be considered "risk factors" for other more serious diseases. Clinical depression, for example, is both a treatable disease in its own right as well as a key risk factor for suicide.[8]

Primary Prevention ←	←	←	Secondary Prevention	←	←	← Tertiary Prevention
			(intervention to prevent more serious disease)			(treatment)
		RISK FACTORS				OUTCOMES
Risk Factors → → (pre-disease/injury)		→ → Disease & Disability → → (minor→serious)				Serious and untreatable disease; death
Smoking		Increased upper respiratory infections, hypertension, COPD, emphysema; pre-cancerous lesions				Myocardial infarction, cancer
Social isolation; family history of depression or suicide		Clinical depression; suicidal thoughts, suicide threats, attempted suicide				Suicide
Unsafe sexual behavior		Gonorrhea. syphilis. genital herpes. HIV+				AIDS
Sedentary lifestyle, poor dietary habits		Obesity, hypertension, Type II diabetes				Heart disease, complications of diabetes

FIGURE 16.1. Risk factor data systems and the prevention paradigm.

Uses of Risk Factor Data Systems

Risk factor data systems support public health practice in several key dimensions. First, determining the prevalence of various risk factors in a community is a key part of community health assessment, one of the core functions of public health.[9] This assessment gives community leaders and health officials the data they need to set priorities for prevention programming. Nationally standardized risk factor data systems also allow comparisons across states and geographic regions as well as comparisons in particular states and regions over time. Such comparisons give additional information for targeting prevention programming and resources for research.

Risk factor data systems are also a very powerful means of monitoring the impact of prevention programs. Consider, for example, a statewide campaign to reduce the prevalence of smoking, the ultimate goal of which is to prevent smoking-related diseases. It would be nearly impossible to attribute reductions in heart disease or cancer mortality 30 or 40 years hence to such an intervention. However, monitoring the prevalence of smoking as a risk behavior is comparatively straightforward, using standard risk factor survey instruments. Data on risk factor trends are also very useful at the national level, where such data are used to predict the health problems that our country will face years into the future and to target new prevention resources toward the reduction of the prevalence of key population risk factors.

Key Risk Factor Data Systems

A variety of important risk factor systems are in place throughout the country. Some data systems are national in scope, and they allow only national and regional estimates. Others are developed or modified locally and applied to purposes such as community planning for health. Some risk factor systems focus on behavioral risk factors, others on environmental risk factors, others on health conditions (such as hypertension) that are precursors or markers for subsequent serious disease; a variety of others focus on specific conditions or concerns (e.g., youth suicide attempt surveillance in Oregon,[10] and the incidence of emergency department visits consequent to drug abuse as monitored by the Drug Abuse Warning Network[11,12]). Several key national data systems are presented in Table 16.1. Other national systems can be accessed from Web sites at the Centers for Disease Control and Prevention (CDC) (http://www.cdc.gov), at the Agency for Toxic Substances and Disease Registry (http://www.atsdr.cdc.gov/), and at many state departments of health (e.g., Georgia's State-level BRFSS, at http://www.ph.dhr.state.ga.us/epi/brfss/index.shtml).

Before discussing BRFSS in some detail, we will provide an overview of the other systems presented in Table 16.1.

The National Health and Nutrition Examination Survey (NHANES)

The National Health and Nutrition Examination Survey (NHANES) is treated extensively in Chapter 33, and it will therefore be covered only briefly here. First authorized by the National Health Survey Act of 1956, NHANES collects information about the health and diet of people in the United States. The data collected have been used to influence policy and improve the health of the US population in many ways. For example, data from NHANES have been used for such purposes as determining the prevalence of iron deficiency, osteoporosis, and overweight, thus providing a basis for public health strategies. As a whole, NHANES focuses on a variety of behaviors that put individuals at risk, including the prevalence of smoking and of practices associated with HIV. In addition, of course, the survey provides a rich source of sample data about the state of public health.

The current NHANES that began in 1999 is the eighth in a series of national examination studies conducted in the United States since 1960. The current NHANES emphasizes a detailed personal interview, a health examination, and a nutrition interview. The primary objective is to collect high-quality health and nutrition data and to release it in a timely manner. The goals associated with this objective include providing an estimate of the number and percent of persons in the US population and in designated subgroups with selected health conditions and risk factors; to monitor trends in the prevalence, awareness, treatment, and control of selected diseases; to monitor trends in risk behaviors and environmental exposures; to analyze risk factors for selected diseases; to study the relationship between diet, nutrition, and health; to explore emerging public health issues and new technologies; and to establish national probability samples, including a sample of genetic material for future genetic research. For more information, see http://www.cdc.gov/nchs/nhanes.htm.

TABLE 16.1. Some national-level risk factor surveillance systems

Data System	Subjects	Contact Information (Organization: Telephone No., Web address[¶])
Behavioral Risk Factor Surveillance System (BRFSS)	≥18 years old	Behavioral Surveillance Branch, Division of Adult and Community Health, National Center for Chronic Disease Prevention and Health Promotion, CDC; (770) 488-2455. http://www.cdc.gov/nccdphp/brfss/about.htm
National Health and Nutrition Examination Survey (NHANES)	1–74 years olds	Division of Health Examination Statistics, NCHS, CDC; (301) 458-4096. http://wonder.cdc.gov/wonder/sci_data/surveys/hanes/hanes.asp
The Mortality Followback Survey Program (NMFS)	≥ 15 years old	Division of Vital Statistics, NCHS, CDC; (301) 458-4561. http://wonder.cdc.gov/wonder/sci_data/mort/followbk/followbk.asp
National Vital Statistics System: Linked Birth/Infant Death Files	Infants (< 1 year old)	Division of Vital Statistics, NCHS, CDC; (301) 458-4034. http://wonder.cdc.gov/wonder/sci_data/natal/linked/linked.asp
Youth Risk Behavior Surveillance System (YRBSS)	Youth (grades 9–12)	Division of Adolescent and School Health, NCCDPHP, CDC; (770) 488-3259. http://www.cdc.gov/nccdphp/dash/yrbs/

¶ The Web addresses (URLs) in this table for NHANES, NMFS, and the Linked Birth/Infant Death Files allow direct query of these data systems via the CDC WONDER query engine. General purpose URLs for these risk factor systems are provided in the related text below.

The National Mortality Followback Survey Program

The National Mortality Followback Survey Program (NMFS), begun in the early 1960s by the National Center for Health Statistics (NCHS), uses a sample of US residents who die in a given year to supplement the death certificate with information from the next of kin or another person familiar with the decedent's history. This information can then be used for study of the etiology of disease, of demographic trends in mortality, and other health issues. The 1993 NMFS, the most recent completed survey, drew a sample of 22,957 death certificates and used measures to ensure adequate representation of persons under age 35, women, and the black population.

The focus of the 1993 NMFS was on five subject areas:

- Socioeconomic differentials in mortality
- Associations between risk factors and cause of death
- Disability
- Access to and utilization of healthcare facilities in the last year of life
- Reliability of certain items reported on the death certificate

Designed in collaboration with other agencies of the Public Health Service, the Department of Health and Human Services, and the National Highway Traffic Safety Administration, the 1993 NMFS has provided a rich source of data on deaths due to homicide, suicide, and unintentional injury and on risk factors associated with deaths in the US population. Although each NMFS includes new survey items and emphases, many items are the same from one NMFS to the next in order to facilitate trend analysis. For more information, see http://www.cdc.gov/nchs/about/major/nmfs/nmfs.htm.

National Vital Statistics System: Linked Birth/Infant Death Files

The Linked Birth/Infant Death files provide a data set that is a very valuable tool for monitoring and exploring the interrelationships between infant death and risk factors that are present at birth. This data set links information from the death certificate to information from the birth certificate for each infant under one year of age who dies in the United States, Puerto Rico, the Virgin Islands, and Guam. This linkage permits use of many additional variables available from the birth certificate for the purpose of conducting more detailed analyses of infant mortality patterns. Included in the linked files is information from the birth certificate about:

- age;
- race;
- Hispanic origin of the parents;
- birth weight;
- period of gestation;
- prenatal care usage;
- maternal education level; and
- marital status of the mother.

This information is linked to information from the death certificate such as:

- age at death, and
- underlying and multiple cause of death.

This linkage permits detailed study and analysis of the relationships between risk factors and infant mortality. For more information, see http://www.cdc.gov/nchs/datawh/nchsdefs/urban.htm.

The Youth Risk Behavior Surveillance System (YRBSS)

The Youth Risk Behavior Surveillance System (YRBSS) monitors priority health-risk behaviors that contribute to the leading causes of mortality, morbidity, and social problems among youths and adults in the United States. It monitors six different categories of behaviors:

- behaviors that contribute to unintentional and intentional injuries;
- tobacco use;
- alcohol and other drug use;
- sexual behaviors that contribute to unintended pregnancy and sexually transmitted disease, including HIV infection;
- dietary behaviors; and
- physical activity.

The YRBSS consists of national, state, and local school-based surveys of representative samples of 9th through 12th grade students and a national household-based survey of 12- through 21-year-olds. The national surveys are conducted by the CDC. State and local education agencies administer the state and local surveys, with technical assistance from the Division of Adolescent School Health, National Center for Chronic Disease Prevention and Health Promotion, CDC. A principal purpose of YRBSS is to promote health personal behaviors and address the prevention of priority health risks among adolescents and youth. The YRBSS is administered every two years during odd-numbered years.

Among the data limitations of YRBSS is the fact that most state and local surveys do not gather enough data from minority populations in their jurisdictions to allow for accurate separate analyses of subgroups. Moreover, the specific categories sampled vary by jurisdiction. It is also important to recognize that no personal identifiers are collected for participants at the state and local level and that permission to use data from state and local surveys must be obtained from the state and local education agencies conducting such surveys. For more information, see http://www.cdc.gov/nccdphp/dash/yrbs/.

The Behavioral Risk Factor Surveillance System (BRFSS)

To illustrate the rich and complex nature and uses of risk factor data systems, as well as the challenges and limitations inherent in such systems, it is instructive to examine in detail a particular and important example: the Behavioral Risk Factor Surveillance System.

The BRFSS is a collaborative project of the CDC and the U.S. states and territories. The BRFSS, administered and supported by the Behavioral Surveillance Branch (BSB) of the National Center for Chronic Disease Prevention and Health Promotion, is an on-going data collection program designed to measure behavioral risks, clinical preventive health practices, and healthcare access among adults 18 years of age or older. The objective of the BRFSS is to collect uniform, state-specific data on preventive health practices and risk behaviors that are linked to chronic diseases, injuries, and preventable infectious diseases in the adult population. Data are collected from a random sample of adults (one per household) in each state through a monthly telephone survey. Currently, all 50 states, the District of Columbia, and the territories of Puerto Rico, Guam, and the Virgin Islands participate in the BRFSS. By 2000, over 180,000 adult interviews were completed annually. The BRFSS is the foundation upon which many successful state and health agency programs are built. It is recognized throughout the healthcare and disease prevention communities as an important and powerful tool in the development, implementation, and evaluation of healthcare programs. The system is a data-tracking source for federal and state programs. It supports CDC-wide disease prevention efforts, defines disease burden, identifies high-risk populations, assists in decision making and the allocation of resources, and can be used to evaluate disease prevention efforts at the national, state, and local levels.

History of BRFSS

The impact of personal behaviors such as smoking, physical inactivity, weight control, and alcohol abuse on disease risk received wide recognition in the United States during the 1960s and 1970s.[13] Information on such personal behaviors was sometimes available from national surveys, but state-specific data were not available on a regular basis. The lack of timely, accessible state-level data impeded the efforts of many state health departments to develop and implement health education and risk reduction programs or to track health risks for their residents.[14] At the same time, use of telephone surveys showed that they were a reliable and affordable alternative to in-person household surveys for some purposes. By 1980, telephone surveys were accepted as a mechanism for states to collect information on the prevalence of behavioral risk factors in their populations.[15] In response to the new opportunities offered by telephone surveys, the CDC began working with state health departments in 1981 to develop a system for estimating the prevalence of behavioral risk factors in state adult populations, using random digit-dialed telephone surveys.[16,17] Cross-sectional surveys were conducted during 1981–1983 by CDC in collaboration with 29 state health departments to develop standardized survey methods for obtaining population-based estimates of the prevalence of personal health practices and behaviors among adults. In 1984, 15 states collected data continuously throughout the year, completing an average of 100 interviews per month. Data were collected on six individual-level risk factors associated with the leading causes of premature mortality among adults: cigarette smoking, alcohol use, physical inactivity, diet, hypertension, and safety belt use. A standard core questionnaire was developed by CDC for states to provide data that could be compared across states. Except for physical activity, for which there were no standard questions available, the initial survey included existing questions from national surveys such as the National Health Interview Survey and the National Heart, Lung, and Blood Institute surveys on hypertension. The initial questionnaire was designed to last no more than 10 minutes, so that states could include their own questions after the core. Although the surveys were designed to collect state-level data, a number of states from the outset stratified their samples to allow them to estimate prevalence for regions within their respective states.

Data collection was a state-directed activity; however, CDC had primary responsibility for developing the survey instrument, providing protocols and guidelines on collection activities, processing and weighting the data, and disseminating summary surveillance reports. The CDC developed survey protocols to assist states and to promote comparability among states, although from the beginning there was state variability in sampling methodology and collection activities. For example, states were initially encouraged to use cluster designs based on the Waskberg method, but some states used simple random samples.

The number of states participating in the surveillance system grew annually, and by 1994 the BRFSS had become a nationwide system. Changes in the design of the survey also occurred during the first decade of the survey. Beginning in 1988, optional, standardized sets of questions on specific topics (optional modules) were made available to the states to allow comparable data on an expanded number of topics. Selection of new subject areas for the BRFSS was based on input from states and CDC about priority topics, as well as on the willingness of other divisions and centers at CDC to provide additional financial support for the BRFSS. Development of the questionnaire became a more cooperative federal-state effort. The partnership was formalized with the creation of the BRFSS Working Group, comprised of selected BRFSS state representatives and CDC staff. The working group participates in establishing BRFSS policies and procedures, including changes to the survey instrument, modifications of protocol, and other matters related to data collection and dissemination. Over the years, there was general agreement among states and CDC that the BRFSS core would not exceed 80 questions, so that states could continue to add their own questions. By the early 1990s, there was no room for additional expansion of the BRFSS core. In 1992, the survey was redesigned to allow some questions to be asked annually (fixed core) and others to be asked every other year (rotating core). In addition, five core spaces were reserved for newly arising topics of public health importance (emerging core). The BRFSS core questionnaire now contains questions on HIV/AIDS; cancer screening and other clinical preventive services; diabetes; and additional tobacco-related questions. Table 16.2 provides an overview of the BRFSS questionnaire plan for the years 1993–2000.

TABLE **16.2.** The BRFSS Questionnaire Plan, 1993–2000

Fixed Core		Rotating Core I (Odd Years)		Rotating Core II (Even Years)	
Topic	Number of Questions	Topic	Number of Questions	Topic	Number of Questions
Health status	4	Hypertension	3	Physical activity	10
Health insurance	3	Injury	5	Fruits and vegetables	6
Routine check-up	1	Alcohol	5	Weight control	6
Diabetes	5	Vaccinations	2		
Smoking	1	Colorectal screening	4		
Pregnancy	1	Cholesterol	3		
Women's health	10				
HIV/AIDS	14				
Demographics	14				
Total: Women	53	Total:	22	Total:	22
Men	42[§]				

[§] The total number of questions for men does not include 11 questions on pregnancy and women's health.

Federal and State Roles

The state BRFSS programs, located within the state health departments, oversee all aspects of data collection, including hiring appropriate staff, ensuring that interviews are conducted according to the interview schedule each month, and training and evaluating interviewers. Data are forwarded to the CDC for processing and weighting. The responsibility for the BRFSS at CDC lies with the BSB, which is located in the Division of Adult and Community Health in the National Center for Chronic Disease Prevention and Health Promotion. The BSB is responsible for purchasing randomly generated telephone number samples for use in the survey, programming the states' questionnaires for computer-assisted telephone interviewing, editing monthly data files, reformatting data to adhere to a common CDC standard, generating quality control reports to facilitate monitoring activities, and computing annual weighting factors. The BSB is also responsible for producing data sets for analysis, preparing annual tabular summaries of BRFSS data for each state, and preparing annual summary prevalence reports reflecting estimates across states for selected variables. Additionally, the BSB collaborates with and provides assistance to the states for data collection, analysis, interpretation, and utilization. It also coordinates and facilitates the exchange of technical information among the states.

The costs of completing a BRFSS interview vary by state, but they currently average about $100–$150 per interview. The CDC and the states share the cost of the survey. CDC provides approximately half of the cost of the interviews to the states through an annual cooperative agreement award. The states provide the remainder of the costs, either through funds obtained from specific federal programs, from state programs, or from other mechanisms.

Uses of the BRFSS

An important aspect of the BRFSS is how data are disseminated and utilized within states. The greatest and most beneficial impact of analysis and use of the data is at the state and local levels. BRFSS data are used to conduct trend analysis, support program decisions, target resources, facilitate program evaluation, and make comparisons among states and regions, and, in some cases, counties or cities. States also use the data to educate the public and make public officials aware of health risks and disease prevalence. Most data from the BRFSS are linked to specific objectives, such as the Healthy People 2010 initiative.[18] Such use of the BRFSS provides state policy makers with informed options for public health policy decisions. Although use of the BRFSS for decision making is central, it is not the exclusive function. Nearly all states prepare reports or fact sheets to educate the public, the health professional community, and legislators about the current status and trends in lifestyle patterns in their states.

How BRFSS data are used to address specific health issues varies by state. BRFSS data have been used to support tobacco control legislation in most states. For example, in California the data were influential in supporting the passage of Proposition 99 Tobacco Tax legislation, which generated millions of dollars in state funds to support health education and chronic disease prevention programs. In Oregon, the state health department used BRFSS state-added questions to evaluate the effect of the bicycle helmet legislation on safely helmet use. With passage of the National Breast and Cervical Cancer Mortality Prevention Act by Congress in 1990, funds became available to state health departments to establish breast and cervical cancer programs. Surveillance data on use of mammography and Pap tests from the BRFSS produce critical information to states about baseline cancer screening levels and provide a means to monitor breast and cervical cancer control program impact. There are other specific examples of state use of BRFSS data:

* Alabama used BRFSS data to support legislation restricting indoor smoking and mandating seat belt use.
* Alaska assessed the health risks of special populations such as Alaska natives and American Indians.
* Connecticut identified population and age groups at increased cancer risk on the basis of their behaviors.
* The District of Columbia used data to support project "WISH" (Women Into Staying Healthy), a breast and cervical cancer prevention program.

- Michigan used BRFSS data to develop, implement, and evaluate statewide programs to reduce the risk of cardiovascular diseases.

Disseminating BRFSS findings within states is an important part of the surveillance system. As part of the cooperative agreement funding mechanism, CDC requires states to demonstrate how they have analyzed and disseminated BRFSS data. State-specific BRFSS data are also published in state medical journals[19] and in peer-reviewed scientific journals.[20]

The task of analyzing data from the BRFSS and encouraging and promoting analysis of the data elsewhere rests primarily with researchers within CDC's BSB; however, researchers throughout CDC frequently analyze and publish findings from the BRFSS. A few examples can be used to illustrate the analytic role and responsibilities at CDC. One common approach is to analyze health risk behavior prevalence patterns across states—e.g., drinking and driving.[21] Another analytic approach is to examine aggregated data. This approach is exemplified by an examination of the prevalence of walking for physical activity.[22] A collaborative effort was undertaken by staff in the Epidemiology and Analysis Section, another center at CDC, and the Oregon Health Division to analyze BRFSS data from state-added questions.[23]

Some of the work conducted by researchers outside CDC has been on measurement properties of the BRFSS. Currently, more than 30 scientific publications on properties of selected BRFSS measures have been identified. Examples of recent studies of this type include comparison of BRFSS estimates for safety belt use with state observational surveys of safety belt use[23]; comparison of BRFSS state estimates for current smoking with estimates from the Census Bureau's Current Population Surveys[24]; a South Carolina comparison of BRFSS estimates for hypertension with physiologic measures from the same population[25]; and a comparison of estimates of self-perceived health status and chronic disease risk factors from a managed care member survey with those from the BRFSS.[26] Most of these studies reported very high reliability and validity for BRFSS data.

Recently, several new studies have been initiated, including one focusing on the use of the BRFSS as a source for national estimates of selected health risk behaviors. This study compares estimates from BRFSS data with data from the National Health Interview Survey, an in-person household survey (see Chapter 15).

Analysis of BRFSS data has heightened the visibility of the system, and dissemination of the data has increased. The average number of publications in professional journals using BRFSS data increased from about 8 per year in the 1980s to about 18 per year during the 1990s. A bibliography maintained by BSB contains over 500 references for articles and reports using BRFSS data and published between 1982 and July 2000. These publications represent a mixture of aggregate and state-specific data analyses, epidemiologic studies focusing on the distribution of risk factors at a point in time, changes and trends over time, and area comparisons.

Caveats in Using BRFSS Data

The BRFSS employs a complex survey design, and analysis of the data requires the use of analytic software that takes the characteristics of the design into account. Those characteristics, including unequal probability of selection, clustering of observations, stratification, and non-response, may result in incorrect standard errors and confidence intervals. These characteristics may further result in misleading tests of significance when one is using standard statistical software packages that do not take these factors into account. Use of standard statistical packages with a weighting variable should yield the same point estimates as sample survey software packages, but the standard error of the estimated prevalence and other measures of variability are often underestimated. The extent of underestimation is related to the degree of intra-cluster correlation for variables being analyzed: The higher the intra-cluster correlation, the greater the underestimation of variability.

Other Design Characteristics Affecting BRFSS Data Use

Users of BRFSS data should keep several other characteristics of the BRFSS in mind.

Coverage

Not all US households have telephones. Currently, it is estimated that, overall, about 5% of the population cannot be reached by telephone.[27] The percentage of households with telephones varies by region, state, and populations within a state. For example, telephone coverage is lower in the South (92%) than in other regions of the United States. Coverage by states ranges from 87% to 98%. However, there is also variation by geographic areas within states and by population subgroups. For example, about 17% of Native American households are without telephones, compared with 15% of black households and 5% of white households. Because the BRFSS relies solely on telephone interviews, the potential exists for response bias due to undersampling of populations most likely to lack telephones. Although no direct adjustment is made for telephone coverage, poststratification weighting adjusts for some of the effects of noncoverage. Studies comparing estimated prevalence for persons with telephones versus persons without telephones have been reported to be similar.[28]

Other protocol characteristics may exclude small portions of the total adult population. For example, the BRFSS excludes institutionalized individuals. Although this is a relatively small proportion overall, this exclusion may introduce more bias in some groups than in others (i.e., the elderly, where an estimated 5% are institutionalized). The survey does not conduct proxy interviews, so that noninstitutionalized individuals who are unable to respond to a telephone interviewer are also excluded. Finally, the BRFSS is administered in Spanish as well as in English in many of the states that have large Hispanic populations, but people who speak only languages other than English and Spanish are excluded.

Self-Reporting

There may also be some limitations on the reliability and validity of self-reported behaviors, with some behaviors overreported and others underreported. However, in general, studies that have looked at this issue with BRFSS data have generally reported high reliability and validity.[29,30] A related issue shared by all anonymous telephone surveys is that self-reported data cannot be verified by physical measurement or visual means.

Response Rates

Telephone surveys such as the BRFSS generally have higher refusal rates than those conducted in-person.[31] Further, response rates may vary by demographic characteristics such as age and education, with elderly persons and those with lower educational attainment disproportionately refusing to be interviewed in telephone surveys.[32]

Current and Future Directions of BRFSS

Among the directions taken by BRFSS either currently or in the future are substate analysis of data and improvements in the technology used to secure, analyze, and deliver survey results.

Substate Analysis

The BRFSS has a long history of local-level use. Currently, 40% of states geographically stratify samples to enable them to produce substate prevalence estimates. County of residence is the most common strata selected, but others include state health regions, health districts, town of residence, or census tract. States that geographically stratify their samples generally have higher numbers of completed interviews than other areas, but most also combine the data for the strata over several years to increase the total number of respondent interviews available for analysis. In addition to stratification to obtain smaller area estimates, some states conduct independent local surveys. Such surveys may use the BRFSS questionnaire as is; others use selected questions and add their own topics of interest. Examples include King and Snohomish counties (Washington), Harlem (New York), El Paso (Texas), San Francisco Bay Area (California), SPARC project (region in three Northeastern states), and Fulton County (Georgia).

Recognizing the growing need for more local data, the BSB is conducting a pilot project for producing city-level data. The purpose of the project is to develop the capacity to provide BRFSS data sets for larger metropolitan areas, using existing data. The pilot project combines data for 1997–1999, uses county codes to identify the appropriate primary metropolitan statistical area or metropolitan statistical area, and then reweights the data, using intercensal estimates for these metropolitan areas. Estimates from this new data file are currently being assessed, and a release of the data as a public use data file is expected within the next year. There are many benefits of using BRFSS for local estimates. Among these benefits is the fact that the surveillance system is well established in all states, it is relatively inexpensive to operate, it provides flexibility that allows for adding locally relevant questions, and it provides very timely and readily available data.

Information Technology and BRFSS

Traditionally, dissemination and communication of BRFSS results were limited to summary reports of descriptive data made available on request and through CDC's Morbidity and Mortality Weekly Report Surveillance Summaries. Although these reports provide useful information, they represent only a small proportion of the potential uses of BRFSS data. An overall strategy for maximizing the communication and dissemination of BRFSS data in a variety of formats to different audiences was devised and implemented. As a result, BRFSS now capitalizes on information technology by providing annual data files on CD-ROM and, via the Web site—http://www.cdc.gov/brfss/ —downloadable data files, survey instruments and other documentation materials, sets of trend analysis tables for the states and the nation, and sets of demographic-specific tables of estimates of risks and conditions, including bar charts for comparison of areas or survey years. In addition, Web-based training modules for interviewers and training for analysts are being developed. Additional projects now being completed include a searchable index allowing identification of question text, response categories, and type of question for items included in the BRFSS from 1984 to 2000; a searchable index of publications using BRFSS data from 1982 to 2000; and Webcast projects to provide training, survey protocol changes, and a forum for a series of lectures on analysis of BRFSS data. CD-ROMs containing historical data for 1984–1990 are also available, as is a CD-ROM containing a PowerPoint overview of BRFSS.

Conclusion

Although we have focused largely on national risk factor data systems, with primary emphasis on BRFSS as an example, it is important to note that such systems exist at the state and local levels as well. Taken together, these systems are crucial resources for disease control and prevention. Risk factor data systems have become important tools for monitoring fundamental behaviors and exposures that put people at risk for death, disease, or disability. Such monitoring allows preventive intervention early in the chain of causation. Risk factor-oriented intervention is extraordinarily powerful, in that the reduction of the exposure to certain risk factors (e.g., tobacco use) can decrease the risk for a great host of untoward outcomes. Risk factor data systems not only support public health practices at the community and state levels, but they also are invaluable aids in the establishment and support of the national agenda for public health policy.

Questions for Review

1. Explain why vital statistic and morbidity data systems alone are inadequate to support modern public health practice and policy. How do risk factor data systems complement vital statistics and morbidity data systems? List and explain the key uses and dimensions of risk factor data systems.
2. Explain the mechanisms by which (a) the National Health and Nutrition Examination Survey (NHANES), (b) the Mortality Followback Survey Program, (c) the Linked Birth/Infant Death Files, and (d) Youth Risk Behavior Surveillance System (YRBSS) collect risk factor data. How do these surveys differ in their focus and their target survey audiences?
3. Under what circumstances might a public health researcher interested in risk factor data at the state level look for a risk factor data source other than the Behavioral Risk Factor Surveillance System (BRFSS)?
4. Explain the roles of federal and state public health organizations in the operation of BRFSS. How is BRFSS funded? How are states held accountable for disseminating the data?
5. List the uses to which data from the BRFSS are put at (a) the national and (b) the state level. To what extent have BRFSS data been used in scientific research?
6. Explain the limitations of BRFSS data in terms of (a) survey coverage, (b) survey reporting, and (c) response rates. How do these limitations affect the reliability of BRFSS data?
7. What benefits accrue to states that choose to stratify BRFSS data?
8. Explain how information technology is improving the dissemination and communication of BRFSS results.

References

1. Tyler CW, Last JM. Epidemiology. In: Wallace RB, Doebbeling BN, eds. *Public Health and Preventive Medicine*. Norwalk, CT: Appleton & Lange; 1988:5–33.
2. Trends in years of potential life lost before age 65 among whites and blacks—United States, 1979–1989. *MMWR Morb Mortal Wkly Rep* 1992;41:889–891.
3. National Center for Health Statistics. *Health, United States, 2000*. Hyattsville, MD: Centers for Disease Control and Prevention; 2000:123.

4. Centers for Disease Control and Prevention. Office on Smoking and Health. *The Health Benefits of Smoking Cessation: A Report of the Surgeon General.* DHHS Publication No. (CDC)90-8416. Washington, DC: Public Health Service; 1990.

5. Kannel WB. Fifty years of Framingham Study contributions to understanding hypertension. *J Hum Hypertens.* 2000;14:83–90.

6. Wallace RB, Anderson RA. Blood lipids, lipid-related measures, and the risk of atherosclerotic cardiovascular disease. *Epidemiol Rev* 1987;9:95–119.

7. Luepker RV. Heart disease. In: Wallace RB, Doebbeling BN, eds. *Public Health and Preventive Medicine.* Norwalk, CT: Appleton & Lange; 1988:927–948.

8. Wulsin LR, Vaillant GE, Wells VE. A systematic review of the mortality of depression. *Psychosom Med* 1999;61:6–17.

9. Institute of Medicine. *The Future of Public Health.* Washington, DC: National Academy Press; 1988.

10. Fatal and nonfatal suicide attempts among adolescents—Oregon, 1988-1993. *MMWR Morb Mortal Wkly Rep* 1995:44:312–315, 321–323.

11. Roberts CD. Data quality of the Drug Abuse Warning Network. *Am J Drug Alcohol Abuse.* 1996;22:389–401.

12. Swisher JD, Hu TW. A review of the reliability and validity of the Drug Abuse Warning Network. *Int J Addict* 1984:19:57–77.

13. Somer AR, Weisfeld VD. Individual behavior and health. In: *Public Health and Preventive Medicine.* Norwalk, CT: Appleton-Century-Crofts; 1986.

14. Remington PL, Smith MY, Williamson DF, Anda RF, Gentry EM, Hogelin GC. Design, characteristics and usefulness of state-based behavioral risk factor surveillance: 1981–1986. *Public Health Rep* 1988;103:366–375.

15. Dillman DA. Which is best: The advantages and disadvantages of mail, telephone and face-to-face surveys. In: *Mail and Telephone Surveys: The Total Design Method.* New York: John Wiley and Sons; 1978:39–78.

16. Gentry EM, Remington PL. Hogelin GC, et al. The behavioral risk factor surveys: II. Design, methods and estimates from combined state data. *Am J Prev Med.* 1985; 6:9–14.

17. Marks JS, Hogelin GC, Jones J, Gaines K, Forman M, Trowbridge MF. The behavioral risk factor surveys: I. State-specific prevalence estimates of behavioral risk factors. *Am J Prev Med.* 1985;6:1–8.

18. US Department of Health and Human Services. *Healthy People 2010* (Conference Edition in Two Volumes). Washington, DC: US Department of Health and Human Services; January 2000.

19. Heath GW, Smith JD. Physical activity patterns of Georgia adults: Results from the 1990 behavioral risk factor surveillance system. *South Med J.* 1994;87:435439.

20. Wingard DL, Cohn BA. DES awareness and exposure: The 1994 California behavioral risk factor survey. *Am J Prev Med.* 1996:12:437–441.

21. Liu S, Siegel PZ, Brewer RD, Mokdad AH, Sleet DA, Serdula M. Prevalence of alcohol-impaired driving. Results from a national self-reported survey of health behaviors. *JAMA.* 1997:35:1069–1078.

22. Siegel PZ, Brackbill RM. Heath GW. The epidemiology of walking: Implications for promoting physical activity among sedentary demographic groups. *Am J Public Health.* 1995:85:706–710.

23. Nelson DE, Grant-Worley JA, Powell K. Mercy J, Holtzman D. Population estimates of household firearm storage practices and firearm carrying in Oregon. *JAMA.* 1996:275:1744–1748.

24. Arday DR, Tomar SL, Nelson DE, Merritt RK, Schooley MW, Mower P. State smoking prevalence estimates: A comparison between the Behavioral Risk Factor Surveillance System and Current Population Surveys. *Am J Public Health* 1997;87:1665–1669.
25. Giles WH, Croft JB, Keenan NL, Lane MJ, Wheeler FC. The validity of self-reported hypertension and correlates of hypertension awareness among blacks and whites within the stroke belt. *Am J Prev Med* 1995;11:163–169.
26. Cogswell ME, Nelson DE, Koplan JP. A comparison of health status in a large managed care organization to the general population. *Health Aff (Millwood)*. 1997:16:219–227.
27. GENESYS Sampling System, unpublished document. 1996.
28. Anderson JA, Nelson DE, Wilson RW. Telephone coverage and measurement of health risk indicators: Data from the National Health Interview Survey. *Am J Public Health* 1998:88:1392–1395.
29. Jackson C, Jatulis DE, Fortmann SP. The Behavioral Risk Factor Survey and the Stanford Five-City Project Survey: A comparison of cardiovascular risk behavior estimates. *Am J Public Health* 1992;82:412–416.
30. Bowlin SJ, Morrill BD, Nafziger AN, Lewis C, Pearson TA. Reliability and changes in validity of self-reported cardiovascular disease risk factors using dual response: The Behavioral Risk Factor Survey. *J Clin Epidemiol* 1996;49:511–517.
31. Groves RM, Lyberg LE. An overview of nonresponse issues in telephone surveys. In: Groves RM, et al. eds. *Telephone Survey Methodology*. New York: John Wiley; 1988:191–212.
32. Groves RM, Kahn RL. *Surveys by Telephone: A National Comparison with Personal Interviews*. New York: Academic Press; 1979.

17
Informatics in Toxicology and Environmental Public Health

EDWIN M. KILBOURNE

Learning Objectives

After studying this chapter, you should be able to:

- Understand the particular importance of large, searchable databases in the practice of toxicology and environmental public health.
- Be aware of the history underlying the development of databases used in both clinical practice and public health.
- Be familiar with some of the major sources of information concerning toxicology and environmental public health.
- Understand the ways (other than information searching) in which information systems facilitate the practice of toxicology and environmental health and be aware of how multiple systems work together to enable health workers in different roles to interact effectively.

Overview

The use of information systems to support the areas of toxicology and environmental public health is necessarily extensive because of the large numbers of potentially toxic substances with which environmental health specialists and toxicologists must deal. In this chapter, the author presents a brief history of informatics in these areas and then proceeds to discuss in some detail the various categories of information systems that support environmental public health and medical toxicology. The author's focus is on services available for unambiguous chemical identification, on bibliographic search and retrieval systems, on authoritative "factual" databases, on threat-identification databases, on diagnostic tools, on systems to support case management, and on surveillance systems. The chapter concludes with the presentation of an imaginary scenario in which many of the information tools discussed are brought to bear on an emergency posing a threat to public health.

Introduction: The Scope of Information Needs in Toxicology and Environmental Public Health

Of all disciplines in public health, environmental health and toxicology are among those that benefit most from computerized information systems. These systems enable practitioners to cope with the extraordinarily large number of potential etiological (toxic) agents that pose potential health threats to the public. As of this writing, Chemical Abstracts Service (CAS), a service operated by the American Chemical Society that registers all known chemical compounds, has well over 18 million organic and inorganic chemical substances registered.[1] Although the numbers of chemicals with significant potential for human exposure are far fewer, they nevertheless number at least in the tens of thousands.[2] There are thousands of compounds approved for use as medicines, and there are hundreds to thousands more in quasi-medicinal use (health foods, herbal tonics and remedies, vitamins, and nutritional supplements). To all these must be added the frequent interactions among chemicals to which humans may be exposed. Indeed, diet itself may substantially influence the response to chemical exposures.[3]

Such a large body of knowledge challenges the ability of even the most learned and experienced specialist's ability to practice without the support of some sort of information system. Of the information systems available, computerized systems are the most comprehensive and the easiest to manage. There are specific challenges in environmental public health and toxicology that can be more easily met with the assistance of computerized information systems. These include:

- Definitive identification of substances to which people are exposed or potentially exposed
- Facilitating access to literature on the expected or possible health effects of specific agents
- Providing quick and easy access to expert consensus on difficult clinical and public health questions regarding specific chemicals
- Providing information to interested parties and the public on the location(s) of possible sources of chemical contamination in the environment
- Providing assistance in diagnosis of difficult cases of illness with a possible toxic cause
- Supporting poison centers in provision of advice and collection of data on poisoned patients[4]
- Quantifying the extent to which people are exposed to toxicants and the resulting morbidity and mortality

The goal of this chapter is to describe the ways in which the available health information services and technology assist in facilitating both the workflow and the interactions among diverse parties involved in environmental health and in clinical and preventive toxicology. Although there is purposeful emphasis on the systems and services most used in the United States, many international readers will find the information relevant to environmental public health in their own countries.

History

The information services and systems currently available to toxicology and environmental public health arise out of two distinct movements affecting US medicine and public health. These are the poison control movement of the early 1950s and the environmental protection movement that began to exert a substantial effect on US public policy in the late 1960s and the early 1970s. Interestingly, the systems that have their roots in these two movements are still somewhat separable and distinct. However, such distinctions have begun to blur with increasing recognition of the common aims of clinical (medical) toxicology and environmental public health.

Information to Support the Clinical Encounter

During World War II and the post-war period, chemical technology improved greatly, and an increasing number of new and diverse drugs and chemical products became widely available for use in the home. In 1952, a study done by the American Academy of Pediatrics showed that over half of unintentional injuries to children were due to the ingestion of potential poisons.[5] The first poison control center in the United States opened in 1953 in Chicago under the leadership of Dr. Edward Press.[6] At that time and ever since, the principal goal of US poison control centers has been to provide information helpful in the acute care of individuals exposed to potentially harmful chemical substances.

As the number of poison centers grew, the need for comprehensive and authoritative information on potential toxicants grew in importance. The US Public Health Service (USPHS) became involved in the collection, dissemination, and updating of information on toxicants. States were asked to designate poison control centers, and the USPHS National Clearinghouse for Poison Control Centers provided them with periodically updated sets of 5-by-8-inch index cards with information useful in the acute care of patients affected by specific toxicants (Figure 17.1).

This system served the country from the late 1950s through the early 1970s. Speaking with physicians who practiced during this era, the author learned of problems with the index card system. For example, prior to official updates, cards were frequently updated locally with handwritten information of unclear quality. In addition, because of the emergent nature of many poisonings, cards often made their way out of the card set, were taken to the bedside, and were frequently lost. These aspects of the system made it unreliable.

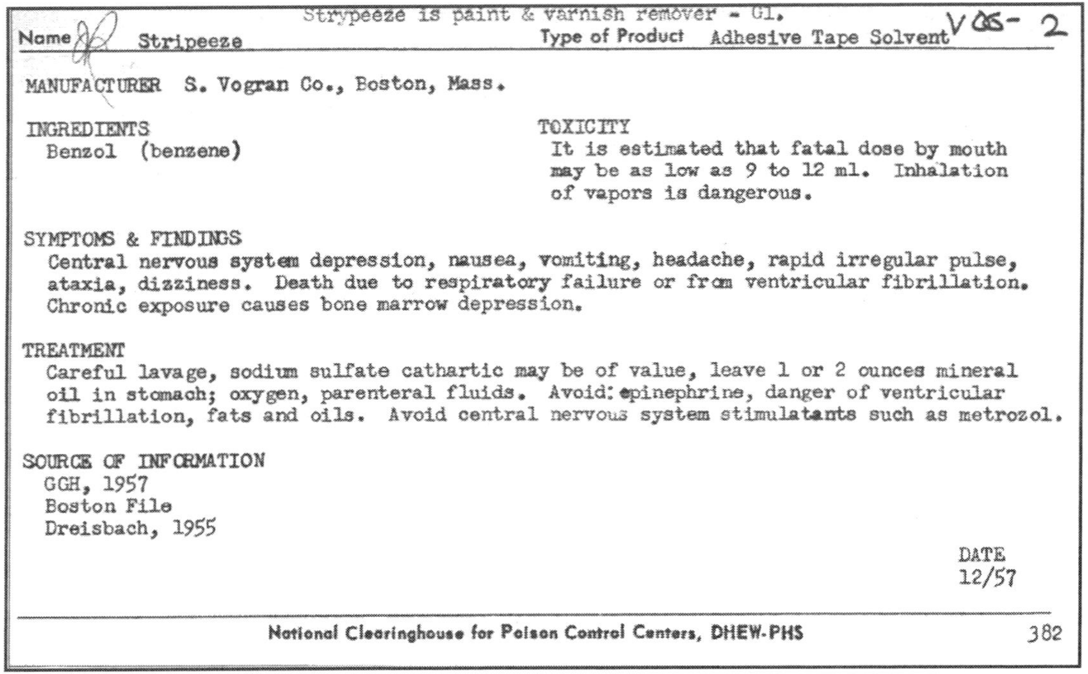

Name   Stripeeze   Stripeeze is paint & varnish remover – GL,   V   OG – 2

Type of Product   Adhesive Tape Solvent

MANUFACTURER   S. Vogran Co., Boston, Mass.

INGREDIENTS
Benzol (benzene)

TOXICITY
It is estimated that fatal dose by mouth may be as low as 9 to 12 ml. Inhalation of vapors is dangerous.

SYMPTOMS & FINDINGS
Central nervous system depression, nausea, vomiting, headache, rapid irregular pulse, ataxia, dizziness. Death due to respiratory failure or from ventricular fibrillation. Chronic exposure causes bone marrow depression.

TREATMENT
Careful lavage, sodium sulfate cathartic may be of value, leave 1 or 2 ounces mineral oil in stomach; oxygen, parenteral fluids. Avoid: epinephrine, danger of ventricular fibrillation, fats and oils. Avoid central nervous system stimulants such as metrozol.

SOURCE OF INFORMATION
GGH, 1957
Boston File
Dreisbach, 1955

     DATE
     12/57

National Clearinghouse for Poison Control Centers, DHEW-PHS   382

FIGURE 17.1. Example of a 5 x 8-inch card from one of the sets supplied to poison centers by the USPHS National Clearinghouse for Poison Control Centers. Although this particular card provides information about the composition of a specific commercial product, comparable information was not available for the great majority of such products until the 1970s.

Another weakness was the fact that the system addressed principally the toxicity and treatment of generic chemical substances. But understandably, patients frequently reported exposure to brand-name commercial products rather than generic chemical substances. There was no comprehensive, centralized source of information on the precise chemical formulations of the nonpharmaceutical commercial products.

The old system took a quantum leap forward in the early 1970s, when Dr. Barry Rumack undertook a comprehensive survey of companies marketing commercial products, asking for information on their precise chemical formulations. The response rate to this survey was overwhelmingly high, and the study effort required so much time, effort, and space that Dr. Rumack was forced to move it out of the hospital and continue it independently. He formed a company (the predecessor of Micromedex®) that produced a microfiche product including both (1) clinical information on specific toxicants and (2) precisely which commercial products contained those toxicants and in what concentrations.

This combination of these two types of information had tremendous clinical utility, and the microfiche product was an instant hit. This was the original Poisindex®, which rapidly became the principal information source for most US and Canadian poison centers. In the late 1980s, the product was made available in CD-ROM format for computers and computer networks, further facilitating rapid access to the most clinically relevant parts of the database.

Information to Support Environmental Public Health

The National Library of Medicine (NLM) has had a central role in providing access to information supporting environmental public health activities. NLM traces its origins back to the US Army Surgeon General's office, which, in 1836, budgeted $150 for "medical books" for officers.[7] The Library expanded greatly within the Department of the Army during the 19th century. In 1956, Congress passed Public Law 84-941, which gave the NLM its current name and placed it within the USPHS. NLM was charged by Congress with improving health in the United States by facilitating access to the world's biomedical literature.[8] NLM began computerizing data in earnest in 1965 with the creation of the Medical Literature Analysis and Retrieval System (MEDLARS). MEDLARS was initially developed primarily for the purpose of managing data required to produce and publish the Index Medicus. However, it ultimately evolved to support literature searches for health professionals.[9]

In 1966, in the context of increasing public concern regarding the potential adverse health consequences of chemicals in the environment, the President's Science Advisory Committee evaluated the availability of toxicologic data and concluded that "there exists an urgent need for a much more

coordinated and more complete computer based file of toxicological information than any currently available and, further, that access to this file must
be more generally available to all those legitimately needing such information." This finding led to the creation in 1967 of NLM's Toxicology Information Program (TIP). The objectives of TIP were to create automated toxicology
data banks and to provide toxicology information and data services.

TIP antedated even the creation of the US Environmental Protection Agency
(EPA) in 1970. During the remainder of the 1970s, awareness of environmental issues increased in the United States. Concern about the environment grew
as a result of the extensive publicity received by such shocking examples of
environmental contamination as the Love Canal. In 1980, Congress passed
the Comprehensive Environmental Response, Compensation, and Liability
Act (CERCLA, also known as "Superfund"). Although the lion's share of
Superfund monies was directed to the EPA to deal with the problem of abandoned sites with hazardous wastes, significant new funding was made available to NLM to continue and intensify its programs to organize toxicologic
data and enhance access to them.

In 1994, TIP was renamed TEHIP (Toxicology and Environmental Health
Information Program), a name that more accurately reflects the mission and
content of the databases offered. TEHIP is overseen by NLM's Division of
Specialized Information Services (SIS). Although SIS covers other specialized areas, the bulk of the databases offered cover toxicology and environmental health. TEHIP currently offers a broad array of databases containing a
wide range of toxicologic and environmental health information. TEHIP is
now a major function of SIS. The mission of TEHIP is broader than TIP in that
TEHIP (1) provides selected core information resources and services; (2) facilitates access to national and international information resources; and (3)
strengthens the information network of toxicology and environmental health.[10]

Types of Services and Systems in Toxicology and Environmental Public Health

The workflow in environmental public health and medical toxicology is supported by numerous different categories of information systems, including:

- Services for unambiguous chemical identification
- Bibliographic search and retrieval systems
- Authoritative "factual" databases
- Threat identification databases
- Diagnostic tools
- Systems to support case management
- Surveillance systems

The remainder of this chapter is devoted to a survey of these systems.

Unambiguous Chemical Identification

The number of known chemical substances is extremely large and growing at an astonishing rate. By 1984, some five million chemical substances had been synthesized. As of this writing in May 2001, that number exceeds 18 million. Many of these are complex chemical molecules, which can only be fully and unambiguously identified with reference to their three-dimensional molecular structure. Although there are internationally accepted conventions for naming complex molecules, the use of alternative schemes, including systematic, "generic," proprietary, incomplete, or trivial names, is frequent, even in the peer-reviewed scientific literature. Thus, the unambiguous identification of the precise chemicals to which toxicologic information refers is problematic.

The Chemical Abstracts Service (CAS), a division of the American Chemical Society, has developed the CAS registry, a comprehensive database identifying specific chemical structures and associating them with a CAS registry number (CAS RN or "CAS number").

The NLM and other sources of toxicologic information make use of CAS numbers for unambiguous identification of the chemicals discussed in literature citation and factual databases (see below). NLM's ChemIDplus service (available over the Web) has an extensive list of synonyms that can be related to the basic compounds.[11] For almost 100,000 entries, each compound is displayed graphically, showing its two- or three-dimensional structure and facilitating the comparison of compounds' pharmacological or toxicological structure-activity relationships. ChemIDplus has the additional useful feature of directing the user to other databases with information about the compound. Such databases include not only databases maintained by NLM but also those of selected regulatory or scientific organizations maintained by state, national, or international agencies or organizations. NLM frequently provides hyperlinks to these databases.

Other NLM databases support the identification-by-synonym feature. For example, the Hazardous Substance Data Bank (HSDB) contains an extensive list of synonyms and is capable of resolving synonyms into unique (CAS-identified) chemicals in many instances, independently of the ChemIDplus service. However, the synonym function cannot be depended upon to be as comprehensive as that of ChemIDplus.

The ChemIDplus synonym resolution feature is quite extensive and impressive. For example, it is capable of resolving the street names "horse," "smack," and "junk" to "diacetylmorphine" (CAS number 561-27-3), a chemical synonym for the drug heroin. Common chemicals frequently have large numbers of obscure synonyms. For example, HSDB's synonyms for isopropyl (rubbing) alcohol are: AI3-01636, ALCOOL ISOPROPILICO (ITALIAN), ALCOOL ISOPROPYLIQUE (FRENCH), AVANTINE, Caswell No 507, (Component of) Hibistat, DIMETHYLCARBINOL, EPA Pesticide Chemical Code 047501, FEMA NUMBER 2929, IMSOL A, IPA, ISOHOL, ISOPROPYL AL-

COHOL, ISO-PROPYLALKOHOL (GERMAN), LUTOSOL, PETROHOL, PRO,
n-Propan-2-ol, PROPAN-2-OL, I-PROPANOL (GERMAN), i-Propyl alcohol,
SEC-PROPYLALCOHOL, I-PROPYLALKOHOL (GERMAN), SECONDARY
PROPYL ALCOHOL, and Visco 1152. Moreover, there are some 60 names for
this compound in ChemIDplus.

Finally, it is impossible for any chemical identification service unambiguously to link one term to another if that term is itself used ambiguously—that
is, if the term is used to refer to more than one compound. For example, the
acronym "MDA" is linked in ChemIDplus both to the industrial curing agent
and azo dye intermediate methylenedianiline and to the altogether chemi-
cally dissimilar 3,4-methylenedioxyamphetamine or "ecstasy," a drug of abuse.
The user would have to interpret from the context of his/her query which
compound was meant.

Bibliographic Databases

Because of its pioneering and longstanding investment in computerizing the
citations to the literature of health and medicine, NLM dominates the area of
bibliographic databases that are relevant to toxicology and environmental
health. Derivative products exist and are marketed commercially; they may
have added-value features related to advanced methods of indexing and retrieval. Nevertheless, the initial data source is NLM.

NLM has two named bibliographic databases of substantial importance for
toxicology. These are TOXLINE and MEDLINE (both available over the Web).
Both databases have evolved greatly over the years. TOXLINE's usefulness has
historically centered on its coverage of publications and technical and governmental reports not covered in MEDLINE and is therefore complementary to
MEDLINE. In the past, there has been substantial overlap between literature
accessible through TOXLINE and MEDLINE. However, these problems are being
resolved as of the writing of this chapter and will be gone or greatly diminished
soon. For now, TOXLINE information in the MEDLINE-indexed journals
("TOXLINE core") can be pursued most easily directly within MEDLINE. The
current Web interface is called PubMed, which is available at http://
www.ncbi.nlm.nih.gov/entrez/query.fcgi. Using PubMed provides toxicology
information seekers with the advantages of PubMed searching, with related
records, MeSH term selection, document delivery, and linking out features.[12]

Bibliographic searching is a particularly useful exercise when one is involved in toxicological research or toxicological or environmental health
practice in situations that are not urgent or emergent. Putting together a co-
gent search strategy may take time, as does the selection and finding of the
individual articles to which MEDLINE or another source has guided one. To
this must be added the time required to digest the literature and arrive at
useful conclusions.

Factual Databases

Databases containing facts or authoritative opinions can be particularly useful in situations in which rapid action is required. In environmental public health emergencies (e.g., significant chemical spills and releases) and in medical toxicologic emergencies (e.g., overdoses), authoritative facts and predeveloped peer-reviewed conclusions have great utility, because they can form the basis for rapid rational action at a time of emergency. In these situations, bibliographic databases are less useful because of the time and effort required to locate, review, and draw conclusions from appropriate literature citations.

The Hazardous Substances Data Bank

Because of its broad and comprehensive coverage, the Hazardous Substances Data Bank (HSDB; available via the Web at http://toxnet.nlm.nih.gov/ was labeled by an Institute of Medicine committee as the "default" database among NLM's group of on-line factual databases. HSDB is tremendously useful, particularly in the sphere of public health, as a source of quick and authoritative information on subject chemicals. Like all of NLM's toxicological factual databases, it is organized into records, each covering an individual chemical substance and associated with a specific CAS number. Some 4,500 of the most commonly encountered chemical substances are covered.[13]

HSDB is of potential use to a wide array of health professionals because of the comprehensive nature of its coverage of individual substances. Each chemical record contains a large number of standardized fields, and these fields cover a number of different categories of information (see category names, below) required by the broad array of health professionals likely to be involved in an exposure situation. For example, public health and emergency medical personnel can be guided by the *human health effects* and *emergency medical treatment* sections of the record. Additional data helpful to both clinical and research personnel may be found in the *animal toxicity studies*, *metabolism/pharmacokinetics*, and *pharmacology* field groups. Personnel charged with clean-up and prevention of further exposure will be interested in the *environmental fate and exposure* and the *environmental standards and regulations* sections. Those entrusted with prevention planning and the safety of occupationally exposed persons will likely use the *chemical safety and handling, manufacturing/use information,* and *occupational exposure standards* information categories. Chemists and analytical toxicologists will benefit from both the *chemical/physical properties* and *laboratory methods* sections. All will benefit from the *special references* section, a list of review documents particularly relevant to the specific chemical. An *administrative information* section lists changes and updates made to the record.

Poisindex

The Poisindex system is a widely used factual database that is a proprietary product available on CD-ROM from Micromedex, Inc., a company that is a major developer of toxicologic and pharmacologic information. Poisindex is particularly focused toward providing the information needed by providers of clinical care, particularly in emergency circumstances. It serves two important functions: (1) linking the common or trade names of products with their constituent generic substance or substances and (2) identifying the toxicity of the individual generic component or components and discussing appropriate treatment. Hundreds of thousands of industrial, commercial, pharmaceutical, and biological substances are covered, and each of these is linked to one or more of over 900 management documents providing information on clinical effects, range of toxicity, and treatment protocols for exposures involving the substances. Table 17.1 provides the classes of substances covered in Poisindex®.

Specific types of information available from Poisindex include substance identification and pseudonyms, clinical effects, lab tests for monitoring and diagnosis, therapeutic maneuvers, pharmaceutical treatment, antidotes, complications, and prognosis. Poisindex has made great use of hypertext linking to enhance mobility around the database. Moreover, patient management

TABLE 17.1. Categories of substances covered in Poisindex®

Common household products	• Cleaners
	• Personal care products
	• Insect and pest protection
Industrial chemicals	• Manufacturing agents
	• Industrial cleaners and solvents
	• Protective agents
Pharmaceutical products (generic and trade names)	• Prescription
	• Over-the-counter
	• Veterinary
	• Street drugs
Biological entities	• Plants and plant products
	• Animal venoms and toxic products
	• Microbial toxins

Source: Adapted from information provided on the Micromedex Web site (http://www.micromedex.com).

systems used by poison centers to document and record patient information smoothly integrate access to Poisindex so that the center personnel can easily alternate between giving and receiving information, thus facilitating the work flow in what can be a very high-pressure, busy environment.

HazDat

The Agency for Toxic Substances and Disease Registry (ATSDR) has a number of factual databases regarding environmental toxicants. They are largely part of the HazDat family of data systems. HazDat is ATSDR's exposure and health effects Web database. It is the scientific and administrative database developed to provide access to information on possible human exposure to hazardous substances from Superfund sites or from emergency events and on the health effects of hazardous substances.

HazDat contains information on contaminated sites, including data that identify the contaminants, their concentrations, and the media in which they were found. Other information provided includes the impact on the population, community health concerns, ATSDR public health threat categorization, and ATSDR recommendations. HazDat contains substance-specific information such as the ATSDR Priority List of Hazardous Substances, health effects by route and duration of exposure, metabolites, interactions of substances, susceptible populations, and biomarkers of exposure and effects. Moreover, HazDat contains data from the US EPA Comprehensive Environmental Response, Compensation, and Liability Information System (CERCLIS) database, including site CERCLIS number, site description, latitude/longitude, operable units, and additional site information.

ToxFAQs

In the Web interface for HazDat, there are call-outs for other useful information sources on environmental toxicants. The ToxFAQs (short for toxicological frequently asked questions) is particularly suitable for supporting communication with the lay public regarding environmental health hazards. It is a series of summaries about hazardous substances. These are excerpted from the ATSDR Toxicological Profiles and Public Health Statements. Each fact sheet serves as a quick and easy-to-understand guide written so as to be understandable by a toxicologically unsophisticated reader. Answers are provided to the most common questions about exposure to hazardous substances found around hazardous waste sites and the effects of exposure on human health.

ATSDR Toxicology Profiles

Mandated by Congress under CERCLA, ATSDR produces "toxicological profiles" for hazardous substances found at National Priorities List (NPL or "Superfund") sites. These hazardous substances are ranked according to frequency of occurrence at NPL sites, toxicity, and potential for human exposure. Toxicological profiles are developed from a priority list of 275 substances. ATSDR also prepares toxicological profiles for the Department of Defense (DOD) and the Department of Energy (DOE) on substances related to federal sites. As of March 2001, the profiles covered more than 250 substances.

These documents are most notable for being extremely comprehensive. For this reason, they can be extremely useful to professionals whose work requires in-depth knowledge of toxicological properties of a particular substance. The documents are quite large and therefore have not, so far, been made available over the Internet. They are published on paper. However, they have recently become available commercially as products on CD-ROM.

Information on Health Threats and Environmental Monitoring

In response to proponents of the community's "right to know" about toxic hazards to which they may be exposed, a number of data sources have been developed. These data represent the findings from required reporting by industries that may pollute, from monitoring of the environment, and from the results of specific environmental investigations. The governmental agencies principally involved in providing these data are the US EPA and ATSDR. ATSDR's information on specific instances of health threats is included in HazDat, as are the public health assessments of Superfund sites.

Toxics Release Inventory

The Toxics Release Inventory (TRI), published by the US EPA, informs citizens regarding toxic chemicals that are being used, manufactured, treated, transported, or released into the environment. It contains information concerning waste management activities and the release of toxic chemicals by facilities that manufacture, process, or otherwise use these substances. The list of currently reportable substances includes over 600 individual chemicals and chemical categories.

The data are compiled by EPA and made available to the public. Access to the information was initially quite cumbersome. However, EPA's current interface operates over the Web (http://www.epa.gov/tri/) and is user-friendly. Users may indicate their geographic area of interest or may focus the output in other ways (e.g., all sites dealing with a particular substance). They are able to see the amounts of environmental releases, by chemical, in the area of interest. "Drilling down" into the data permits the identification of specific source-enterprises, identifying them by name and street address. Thus, one may identify the reported environmental chemical releases of any particular company itemized by year, by chemical substance, by quantity emitted, and even by the environmental route of pollution (i.e., to air, surface water, injection well, or land).

Such information is of great help to those trying to identify the types of pollution problems in a community and to identify the sources. Moreover, because remedies may differ substantially by chemical type, these data may help identify solutions to environmental contamination problems.

Diagnostic Aids

One of the most challenging tasks faced by consulting clinical practitioners (and sometimes public health officials) is diagnosing the problem. Diagnosis may be problematic in toxicology and environmental health because of the great number of possible causative agents. It is difficult for even very expert personnel to keep track of and mentally evaluate all possible causes for a given clinical picture.

Texts (whether paper or electronic) and the scientific literature constitute the ultimate references supporting the diagnosis of a specific toxicant-mediated syndrome. Unfortunately, current bibliographic retrieval systems do not necessarily present information in the way a diagnostician needs to receive it.

One product is worthy of mention as an important step forward toward solving this problem. The SymIdx (symptom identification) module of the Lexi-Comp™ CD-ROM Clinical Reference Library can be very helpful in cases (or public health problems) in which a toxic cause is suspected but the agent is not clear. This module takes multiple symptoms and signs as input. The user receives lists of pharmaceuticals, other chemicals, and biologically produced compounds (e.g., animal venoms, toxic plants) associated with the selected symptoms. Each list is ranked in descending order by the number of symptoms attributed to each agent. Such a list can be an important start for further diagnostic investigation and ultimate identification of the causal agent.

Poisoning Case Management

Patients, their friends and family members, or their healthcare providers seek expert advice about the evaluation and treatment of toxic or potentially toxic human exposures to chemical substances over two million times per year. Despite their number, the cases are distributed throughout the population. It is infeasible to have substantive clinical toxicologic expertise at every healthcare facility to which poisoned patients might come for evaluation and treatment. Accordingly, approximately 70 regional poison control centers (poison centers) located around the country share their toxicologic expertise with callers who may be healthcare providers or members of the public.

Because of the many potential clients of poison centers, the call volume may be high. At any given moment, the specialists in poison information (SPIs) may have several active cases, all of which need further follow-up. While dealing with these cases, they intermittently need to access computerized sources of data. Moreover, SPIs pass on active cases to others at the end of a shift.

A type of computer-based patient record system specific to poison centers has been developed and deployed at most poison centers around the country. There are currently four companies that produce this type of software, and these systems perform the following ideal functions to varying degrees:

- Record and display information on:
  - Patient identification and demographics
  - Exposure: toxicant, dose, context
  - Symptoms, signs, laboratory findings
  - Follow-up calls
  - Eventual outcome
- Operate with sufficient efficiency and ease to allow the SPI to record and read information while continuing to carry on the telephone conversation
- Change rapidly between patients
- Provide a legible and easily understandable account of the case to an SPI who takes over at shift change
- Allow (or facilitate) consultation of computerized data sources (especially Poisindex) during a call
- Hold data and produce reports providing data for:
  - Improved case management
  - Administrative reports
  - Regular reports of summary call information to the American Association of Poison Control Centers for its Toxic Exposure Surveillance System (required for poison center accreditation)

Surveillance

In general, surveillance in toxicology and environmental health is not as well developed as in the infectious disease arena. Nevertheless, two outstanding systems are worthy of mention.

ATSDR maintains an active, state-based Hazardous Substances Emergency Events Surveillance (HSEES) system to describe the public health consequences associated with the release of hazardous substances. Systems cataloging chemical spills and releases prior to HSEES had little public health utility. The HSEES system has four goals:

1. Describe the distribution and characteristics of hazardous substances emergencies
2. Quantify morbidity and mortality experienced by employees, responders, and the general public as a result of hazardous substances releases
3. Identify risk factors associated with the morbidity and mortality
4. Provide data on which to base strategies to reduce morbidity and mortality from hazardous substance releases

The American Association of Poison Control Centers (AAPCC) collects summary information from each call to accredited poison centers as part of the Toxic Exposure Surveillance System (TESS). TESS currently acquires over two million records per year. Summary findings are published annually and serve to direct attention to the poisoning problems with which poison centers most frequently deal and to those that are most frequently fatal.

An Imaginary Scenario Involving Multiple Systems

The distinct systems and databases described in this chapter all serve complementary purposes. An imaginary scenario involving events with health consequences may best make this point.

A tractor-trailer truck carrying cylinders of an industrial gas jackknifes and turns over near a populated area of County X. A cloud of visible fumes is emitted from cylinders that are damaged in the wreck. The cylinders are labeled as carrying liquid fluorine. The director of county emergency services connects with the Internet and accesses HSDB. Within five minutes she is able to radio important information to firefighters, police, and EMTs who have not even reached the area yet.

She warns them that inhalation of even very small quantities of concentrated fluorine gas may cause death, and she describes the required protective equipment for dealing with fluorine liquid and gas at close range. She also warns that fluorine gas may be heavier than air and may collect in low-lying areas and may not dissipate promptly. She advises firefighters of special techniques for fighting fires associated with fluorine (which is not itself flammable but supports combustion). She advises police and firefighters of the US Department of Transportation's official recommendation for an initial evacuation radius. She describes the acute symptoms and signs of fluorine exposure to EMTs to let them know what to expect and advises them regarding treatment that can be administered in the field (oxygen, possibly bronchodilators), and maneuvers to avoid (mouth-to-mouth respiration).

Following a protocol set forth in the local emergency management plan for chemical spills and releases, she contacts the county health officer, and together their departments contact local health care facilities and the regional poison center to advise them of the situation and to allow them to prepare for possible casualties.

The Medical Director of the poison center accesses his CD-ROM copy of the ATSDR toxicological profile on fluorides, hydrogen fluoride, and fluorine to prepare himself to answer any in-depth specialized clinical questions that arise. He also downloads the ATSDR ToxFaqs sheet on the same subject. He distributes it to the SPIs answering the phones to aid them in responding to queries from the public about the release.

The county health officer downloads the same document and gives it to his media relations specialist to use in preparing a press release about the incident. He also informs the state officer, since environmental measurements beyond local capacity to conduct will be required before the area can be declared safe. The state health officer will also see that the incident is reported to HSEES.

Unfortunately, it turns out that some people have been exposed to the gas. As patients begin to arrive in his Emergency Department, one resident physician, doubting whether the cause is really fluorine, enters his patients' primary symptoms into a computerized diagnostic program. He is reassured when fluorine comes up as a strong possibility.

The SPIs have been reviewing the Poisindex management protocol for fluorine, available over their poison center's CD-ROM server and local area network. They are now fully prepared to advise healthcare providers on management of exposed persons. Their medical director will back them up on difficult or atypical problems. Cases that come to the attention of the poison center will be reported to TESS.

The Future

This situation represents an idealized scenario of the ways in which public health, healthcare, and first responder personnel could work together effectively to deal with a chemical emergency. Note that persons in each role require knowledge of and access to information tailored to his or her responsibilities. Further progress in toxicology and environmental public health requires both the ongoing enhancement of the information systems we use and the proper training of public health and healthcare personnel in how to use them.

Questions for Review

1. List and explain the key reason(s) that access to searchable databases may be more important for environmental public health than for other fields.
2. What factors led to the emergence of the poison control movement in the 1950s? Why were paper-based information files unsatisfactory for poison control? What key information was not provided by paper-based information sources regarding the treatment of poisoning with particular chemical substances?
3. Review the evolution of the National Library of Medicine (NLM) and its projects to support the practice of environmental health. Whose history of work in the environmental arena is longer, that of the US EPA or of the NLM?
4. What are the relative advantages and disadvantages of (a) bibliographic information systems and (b) information systems containing authoritative peer-reviewed data in addressing environmental health problems?
5. Why is unambiguous chemical identification important? How is this identification enhanced by current technology?
6. What is the usefulness of having technical databases written for the lay public?
7. In what ways is a poisoning case management system different from the prototypical computer-based patient record? In what ways is it the same?
8. What are the potential ultimate benefits of on-line reporting of chemical spills and releases and their health consequences?

Acknowledgments

The author owes a debt of thanks to Barry H. Rumack, MD, William O. Robertson, MD, Jeanne Goshorn, and Philip Wexler, all of whom provided much background information, advice, and helpful comments.

References

1. Chemical Abstracts Service. CAS registry number and substance counts. Available at http://www.cas.org/cgi-bin/regreport.pl. Accessed May 20, 2001.
2. National Research Council (U.S.) Steering committee on Identification of Toxic and Potentially Toxic Chemicals for Consideration by the National Toxicology Program. *Toxicity Testing: Strategies to Determine Needs and Priorities.* Washington, DC: National Academy Press; 1984.
3. Evans AM. Influence of dietary components on the gastrointestinal metabolism and transport of drugs. *Ther Drug Monit* 2000;22:131–136.
4. Litovitz TL, Klein-Schwartz W, Caravati EM, Youniss J, Crouch B, Lee S. 1998 Annual Report of the American Association of Poison Control Centers Toxic Exposure Surveillance System. *Am J Emerg Med* 1999:17:435–487.
5. Grayson R. The poison control movement in the United States. *Industrial Medicine and Surgery.* 1962;31:296-297 as cited in: Wax PM. Historical principles and perspectives. In: Goldfrank LR, Flomenbaum NE, Lewin NA, Weisman RS, Howland MA, Hoffman RS, eds. *Toxicologic Emergencies.* 5th Ed. Norwalk, CT: Appleton and Lange; 1994:7.
6. Press E, Mellins RB. A poisoning control program. *Am J Pub Health.* 1954;44:1515–1525.
7. National Library of Medicine. NLM long-range plan. Available at http://www.nlm.nih.gov/pubs/plan/lrp/contents.html. Accessed March 29, 2002.
8. Committee on Toxicology and Environmental Health Information Resources for Health Professionals, Institute of Medicine. *Toxicology and Environmental Health Information Resources: The Role of the National Library of Medicine.* Washington: National Academy Press; 1997.
9. Miles WD. *A History of the National Library of Medicine.* NIH Publication No. 85-1904. Bethesda MD: National Institutes of Health; 1982.
10. National Library of Medicine. Fact Sheet. Toxicology and Environmental Health Information Program. Available at http://www.nlm.nih.gov/pubs/factsheets/tehipfs.html. Accessed March 29, 2002.
11. National Library of Medicine. ChemIDplus. Available at http://chem.sis.nlm.nih.gov/chemidplus/. Accessed October 27, 2000.
12. Goshorn J. Next Generation TOXLINE. NLM Technical Bulletin. Available at http://www.nlm.nih.gov/pubs/techbull/jf01/jf01_toxline.html Accessed May 18, 2001.
13. National Library of Medicine. Fact Sheet. Hazardous Substances Data Bank. Available at http://www.nlm.nih.gov/pubs/factsheets/hsdbfs.html. Accessed October 27, 2000.

18
Knowledge-Based Information and Systems

Neil Rambo and Christine C. Beahler

Learning Objectives

After studying this chapter, you should be able to:

- Define primary, secondary, and tertiary knowledge-based information.
- Explain the challenge to public health workers of using the abundance of so-called gray literature now available on the Internet, and both the challenge and the benefits of the conversion of traditional health-based publications to the Internet.
- Explain why, despite the appearance to the contrary, that knowledge-based information on the Web is not all easily accessible and why public health information is more difficult to locate than clinical information.
- Explain the principles of a keyword search of a database that is not highly structured and well indexed.
- Describe the nature of such information search tools as MEDLINE, CDC Wonder, the National Guideline Clearinghouse, Sociological Abstracts, PsyINFO, the National Technical Information Service, TOXNET, and the Hazardous Substances Data Bank.
- Describe options available to a public health worker for obtaining full-text documents that do not appear in full on the Internet, along with the trade-offs involved.
- Explain why both knowledge-based and evidence-based resources are being increasingly applied to the public health field, and explain their usefulness in policy formulation.

Overview

Knowledge-based information has become increasingly important to the practice of public health. As technological developments have made such information more readily available, the challenge to the public health worker, ironically, is learning to access it, including learning to access and use the so-called gray literature. Fortunately, a number of databases are readily available to public health workers, but a searcher must know how to use keyword searches and other tools to access and use them. Such sources as CDC Wonder, PubMed, the National Guideline Clearinghouse, Sociological Abstracts, and TOXNET furnish a cornucopia of information to public health workers, but it is crucial to know how to use them and to understand the nature of the information they contain. It is also important for public health practitioners to know how to obtain copies of articles, because full-text documents are not usually available via the Internet, and the trade-offs involved in selecting a delivery source. The greater availability of both knowledge-based and evidence-based information sources has significant implications for the development of public health policy.

Introduction: Toward a Definition of Knowledge-Based Information

Many of the preceding chapters in this part of the textbook—indeed, of the text itself—demonstrate that data are the foundation of public health practice. For example, numbers related to birth, deaths, and the incidence of disease and injury provide critical data that give a snapshot of what is occurring in a population at a given time. Combined with other such snapshots, such data can provide evidence of trends or confirmation of the effect of interventions.

In this chapter, however, we are concerned with knowledge-based information rather than data. In its simplest sense, *knowledge-based information* is that information derived from the professional literature of a field of knowledge. Knowledge-based information is part of a class of information used to support *evidence-based practice*, derived from work done in the development of an approach to clinical practice known as *evidence-based medicine*. One article defines evidence-based medicine as "the conscientious, explicit and judicious use of current evidence in making decisions about the care of individual patients."[1] The relationship between knowledge- and evidence-based information will be considered at the end of this chapter.

In the field of health care, Hersh distinguishes between patient-specific and knowledge-based information.[2] According to Hersh, *patient-specific information* is information collected on an individual patient, as in a patient's medical record. In contrast, knowledge-based information in health care is information that is derived from observations or research concerning many patients. The purpose of knowledge-based information is to create new knowledge regarding the effectiveness of clinical interventions, knowledge that can then be applied in the treatment of individual patients.

In the same way, data from public health information systems can be thought of as population-specific information. Knowledge-based information in public health is derived from many observations, from perhaps an intervention involving many populations or many interventions concerning a single population. For example, knowledge-based information might consist of data systematically gathered from tuberculosis control interventions among Native Americans in several communities. Such information is no longer a snapshot. Rather, it is a summary of observations carried out in the field. It is a research report, and thus leads to new knowledge.

Knowledge-based information is not simply text-based. Some text—news and announcements, for example—are essentially ephemeral. But *knowledge-based information* cumulates and contributes to a growing body of knowledge, in contrast to data. A Web site containing public health news and related information is a text-based system. But that same Web site may also be a knowledge-based system if it provides access to research findings. For instance, agency and organization Web sites, such as those hosted by state health departments, the Centers for Disease Control and Prevention (CDC), the Health Resources and Services Administration (HRSA), the National Association of County and City Health Officials (NACCHO), and the Association of State and Territorial Health Officials (ASTHO), are likely to be hybrids. They contain news and announcements—"text"—and also guidelines based on research findings—"knowledge." In the same way, journals in the field, such as the *American Journal of Public Health* and the *Journal of Public Health Management and Practice*, may be hybrids containing a mixture of textual and knowledge-based information.

Hersh also identifies the following three categories of knowledge-based information:

1. *Primary* knowledge-based information consists of the primary literature, broadly defined, such as original research reports in journals, books, proceedings, and other venues.
2. *Secondary* knowledge-based information is information that indexes the primary literature. For example, MEDLINE is a secondary resource. It and similar indexes provide access to and organize primary resources. Similarly, a bibliography is a secondary knowledge-based information resource.
3. *Tertiary* knowledge-based information provides reviews of, summarizes, or synthesizes the primary literature. Review articles in journals are tertiary resources, as are textbooks and monographs that synthesize whole areas of knowledge. A less familiar form of tertiary resources are compilations of secondary resources—they gather *metadata* (or descriptions of data about) secondary resources.

The focus of this chapter is on secondary and tertiary resources, as defined by Hersh. Practitioners, after all, usually consult these resources for an obvious reason: Although a practitioner will typically scan a few journals in his or her specialty on a regular basis, there usually isn't time for more comprehensive direct use. The reason is that the primary literature is not cumulated or synthesized. Mining the contents of primary literature takes both time and skill. Another barrier to the direct use of primary resources is that results—that is, the contribution that such literature makes to decision making—are never certain: there is no way to predict whether the investment of time will pay off in one instance or not. Tertiary resources, on the other hand, add value to the primary literature by summarizing and synthesizing the findings, thus distilling primary research and making it more directly applicable to decision making, and increasing the likelihood of potential value to decision making. Secondary resources organize primary literature and make it more accessible. Organization and synthesis—adding value—meets the needs of the practitioner by limiting the time necessary to acquire useful knowledge.[3]

Issues Related to Access and Reliability of Knowledge-Based Information

Professional journal articles, textbooks, and conference proceedings are the most organized and controlled sources of research information—"controlled" in the sense that these standard publication channels involve forms of professional review for quality and scientific rigorousness. Such sources involve a formal peer review process, and the production and distribution channels are understood and predictable.

Other formats—including printed technical reports and, increasingly, Web sites—are less well controlled and reliable. For these formats, review processes may not be in place. The author or producer of a Web site may be an individual, with no organization backing the veracity of the site's content, either explicitly or implicitly. In a bibliographic sense at least, such *gray literature* is also less accessible because there are traditionally no secondary resources to describe and organize it.

An irony of gray literature is that while the literature is considered inaccessible because of the lack of a centralized publication and distribution process and the lack of organization by secondary resources, it is far from inaccessible in the ordinary sense of the term. On the contrary, we may be deluged by it. Technical reports from federal, state, and local agencies pile up on desks, while Web sites—possibly relevant and perhaps useful—proliferate. Such resources are inaccessible in a bibliographic sense. They are inaccessible in the sense that they are not controlled and organized, and cannot be accessed from an index. The lack of bibliographic access to gray literature means the reader has no guide to its use—no terminology control, no relationship mapping, and no sense of comprehensiveness—things a secondary resource should provide.

However, because of the proximity and convenience of the Web, the irony of gray literature is that public health practitioners will increasingly find that it is *more* accessible—as the term is more generally understood—than the standard professional organs. For example, journals are likely to be confined to special or academic libraries; they may therefore be more difficult to access for those not affiliated with the host institutions than are the Web sites housing gray literature.

Even the professional organs that have appeared as traditional print publications are in transition to electronic formats. An access-related benefit of this movement is that the contents of a journal, once directly accessible to only one user at a time as it is pulled from a library shelf, can now be accessed from any location providing the opportunity to log on to the Internet. Of course, the issue of who is authorized to access Internet-based resources is complex. It involves a mix of licensing agreements, affiliation or memberships, and subscription and use fees. Nevertheless, the fact that such material is available on the Internet and thus not restricted to a single location is a great boon to access. The technical complications, however, actually limit access more severely than the location. If a would-be user is not part of an academic institution or an agency that subscribes to an electronic publication, for example, access will be denied or at least restricted without the direct payment of a fee to the publisher for each article.

It is clear that the convergence of strong technologic and economic forces is changing publication practices, patterns, and formats. It is also clear that more print publications will move to various forms of online availability, either exclusively or in conjunction with print analogues. What is less clear is who will have more access and who will have less, and who will pay for what level of access at what point in the process.

The developments are changing the way that scientific information is disseminated. A case in point is PubMed Central, which is based on the idea that scientific research, especially research that is funded by public dollars, should be freely accessible to all who need it.[4] Such a resource requires fundamental changes in the ownership of information and in the roles of authors and publishers. At the same time, it takes advantage of the promise of networking technology to increase access to knowledge for all.

Searching Knowledge Resources

Imagine that you are responsible for community health assessment in a local public health agency. You attend a community meeting at which participants express considerable concern that several children have recently been hit by cars while crossing the streets or playing near driveways. Someone raises a question about what has been done or could be done to prevent the incidents. You are not sure, and you decide to locate information about such incidents.

But where do you look? For an increasing number of public health professionals—those with access to a computer and an Internet connection—the easiest approach is probably a "quick and dirty" Web search. By the use of

Google, a general Web search engine (http://www.google.com), you could
type "child pedestrian injuries" and retrieve over 21,000 Web pages of information about such injuries. Results will vary according to the Web search
engine used because of differences in indexing methods and search algorithms. How does a searcher, even a casual searcher, make sense of the retrieval of thousands of pages? An obvious technique is to ignore the large
number of sites retrieved, to assume that those listed first are likely to be most
relevant, and to scan the first few pages for the best of the limited lot. Such a
technique makes sense.

Although such general Web searching is both undeniably convenient and
instructive about what is "out there," it has many limitations that make it
unreliable for a serious search. The major drawback is that the information
content of the Web pages retrieved may not be vetted by anyone. The onus of
evaluating the quality of the information provided is on the searcher: *caveat
lector*. In the area of public health practice and policy, this burden is not
trivial. It follows that sticking to known and trusted resources is a good way
to limit exposure to bad information. Fortunately, the Web sites of familiar
state and federal agencies—including the CDC, HRSA, and the Environmental Protection Agency (EPA)—relieve the public health researcher of the burden of determining what information to trust.

Another way that a public health researcher can save time in an information search to is use a site containing a *Web portal*—a selected and organized
compilation of links to other sites. For example, portals like those offered by
HealthWeb from the University of Michigan and HealthLinks from the University of Washington provide links to numerous health-related sites. If, as
another example, you needed to access information about child pedestrian
injuries, the CDC Web site provides an "injury" portal to the National Center
for Injury Prevention and Control (NCIPC).[5]

Although the Web provides access to a super-abundance of information,
there is a risk in over-relying on it. The danger is that casual searchers will be
lulled into a sense that if information cannot be located by use of a general
search engine on the Web, it must not exist. Of course, such is not the case.
Most science research reports and most of the public health knowledge base
are contained within special databases—special databases that may be accessible on the Web but are not accessible through use of a general Web search
engine. Rather, a searcher needs to use search interfaces that are usually specific to a particular database to extract information from these databases.

In this section, we examine a number of these more specialized resources.
Many of them require little more than some time to learn the search syntax
and the other peculiarities of the interface to the database. In fact, there are
few barriers to a typical public health practitioner's use of these resources. We
describe a comprehensive search approach and show how to use many of
these resources. The approach we describe, however, is one that a professional
librarian might use to conduct a fairly comprehensive search for the highest

quality of information available; it is unlikely to be used by a public health worker. Nevertheless, the search process illustrates the use of key knowledge resources in public health and demonstrates the activities involved in conducting a serious search.

Finally, it is necessary to point out that, by its nature, public health information is more difficult to locate than clinical information. Clinical information, after all, is most often found in relatively few, peer-reviewed databases. Public health information, on the other hand, spans a number of disciplines—including biomedicine, the social sciences, law, and business—and it therefore necessitates broad-ranging searches in databases that are highly structured (MEDLINE, from the National Library of Medicine, is an example) or else largely unstructured. Moreover, public health information does not appear in the form of the randomized controlled trials that form the gold standard for clinical literature; in fact, such controlled trials are almost nonexistent in public health.

Using Tools for a Search on the Topic of "Child Pedestrian Injuries"

For illustrative purposes, we will use the topic "child pedestrian injuries" to illustrate the complexities of a search for public health information. The key databases for this topic are

- *Biomedicine*: MEDLINE, EMBASE, CINAHL (Cumulated Index to Nursing and Allied Health Literature)
- *Social Science*: Sociological Abstracts, ERIC (Educational Resources Information Center), PsycINFO
- *Government*: NTIS (National Technical Information Service), PAIS (Public Affairs Information Service, NIOSHTIC (National Institute for Occupational Safety and Health Technical Information Center)
- *Transportation*: TRIS (Transportation Research Information Service)
- *Business*: ABI Inform
- *General*: Dissertation Abstracts, Expanded Academic Index, full-text newspaper databases

Access to such databases varies. Some are available at no charge on the Web, such as MEDLINE from the National Library of Medicine. Others are available to those who have an affiliation—for example, with a university—or else privileges to use an academic library to conduct research. Still others, such as EMBASE, are available only for a fee through a commercial search service such as Dialog. The latter are usually accessed with assistance from a librarian at a university or at a government agency.

Of course, the need to search numerous databases affects both the accuracy and the reliability of the search. The problem is ameliorated somewhat by the use of highly organized and indexed databases, in which professional index-ers assign subject headings from a controlled vocabulary after analyzing all entries. Such headings make it unnecessary to include synonyms, spelling variations, or equivalent conceptual terms in the search. For example, a search of PubMed for articles that discuss the effectiveness of seat belts in preventing motor vehicle injuries can be accomplished by virtue of the fact that PubMed provides "seat belts" as a subject heading. On the other hand, a search in a database that does not provide subject headings might entail considering such terms as "safety belt(s)," "seatbelt(s)," "booster seat(s)," "lap belt(s)," "shoulder belt(s)," "seat restraint(s)," "car seat(s)," "restraining device(s)," "safety harness(es)," and more.

It is often useful to conduct a keyword search of databases with no single controlled language or of databases with little indexing. Such a search retrieves any citation, abstract, or full-text document that includes the keyword(s). It is important to recognize, however, that keyword searching is literal in that retrieval is based on word occurrence only and not on meaning. Getting around this drawback requires a searcher to use synonyms, spelling variations, and equivalent conceptual terms. A pleasing exception to this requirement is a keyword search in PubMed (http://www.ncbi.nlm.nih.gov/entrez/query.fcgi), which provides automatic linking of keywords to appropriate indexing terms. Still, the advantages of keyword searching include the ability to search numerous databases with one search strategy. A disadvantage is the impossibility of including every conceptual and textual variation in a search—and losing search precision as a result.

It is important to remember that keyword searching is the only searching available in databases that are not indexed and that the nature of a keyword's precision of meaning helps establish the difficulty of the search. For example, the keyword "pedestrian" is relatively precise and singular: It has one very precise meaning—a person on foot in a motor vehicle environment. There are no significant synonyms and no second meanings of the term. Using this keyword therefore makes the search relatively easy. On the other hand, a search on a more difficult topic, such as effective interventions into injuries from speeding, might include the use of multiple keywords, such as "speed(ing)" and "speed limit(s)." Moreover, in many articles the terminology is implicit—for example, an excessive speed such as 75 mph is mentioned in the article, and it is assumed that the reader will recognize the velocity rate as an issue of speed. Finally, the terminology itself might differ from one country to another: for example, in the United Kingdom and in other European countries, speeding intervention is referred to as "traffic calming."

Another problem in locating public health information is the lack of specificity in the conceptual "location" of the material. The concepts employed in database searching were developed by the military in the 1940s. The search terminology still reflects this history. A "hit" is the retrieval of relevant information, and a "direct hit" refers to the retrieval of information that is an exact match to the information need. The terms originally referred to the use of radar to locate a target, and a hit is most possible when there is a discrete point in space where the target resides (i.e., a meeting of coordinates). It is much more difficult to locate information when you are unable to find an exact location, or when the information resides in more than one discrete place. For example, in the field of clinical medicine, it is relatively easy to locate articles concerning drug treatment options for tuberculosis. This information can be found in a discrete space, grouped into a coherent category. The search in PubMed would be "tuberculosis/dt" or tuberculosis with the subheading of drug therapy. This search targets the appropriate set of information, which can be further limited by language, publication year, randomized controlled trials only, etc. In public health, most topics occur on a continuum rather than defining a discrete space.

For example, an effort to retrieve relevant information about effective interventions in child pedestrian injury must address the following location issues, or else information retrieval becomes increasingly difficult:

- End points to be measured or prevented might include death, broken bones, head injuries, or any injury, regardless of the seriousness.
- Should the information retrieved focus on the drivers or the children? If children, what age? Should it be preschool age, elementary school age, or teenagers?
- What types of intervention should be examined? Should it be legal interventions, educational interventions, or environmental modification interventions, or all three?
- What research methodology is stringent enough for this study? Assuming that there will be few, if any, randomized controlled trials, will case-control studies be acceptable? Is there any room for qualitative methods in the study? Are reports from newspapers and magazine articles acceptable?

In addition to the complications caused by the spread of public health topics over many disciplines, yet another complication is that many of these topics are couched in social science terminology rather than in a more sharply defined clinical vocabulary. The terminology is, therefore, less specific and more difficult to pinpoint. Of special concern in conducting database searches is the use of "implicit" versus "explicit" information. For example, in the topic of "injuries to child pedestrians," the scenario is most often that a traffic accident occurred. However, in many studies, this information is assumed, rather than stated. Including the concepts of "crash" and/or "accident" will therefore not retrieve all relevant information.

A Search Example: Data Sources for Child Pedestrian Injuries

In this section, we will present an example of the use of certain knowledge-based resources to locate information about the topic of child pedestrian injuries. We will discuss the nature of each resource used and the information the resource can provide.

CDC Wonder

CDC Wonder (http://wonder.cdc.gov) provides a single point of access to a variety of CDC reports, guidelines, and numeric public health data. Users may log on either as anonymous users or as registered regular users. Being a registered regular user entitles a searcher to save searches and to receive e-mail from the system that provides notification of the search results that are available. Figure 18.1 provides a view of the screen that a user would encounter in a search for information about child pedestrian injuries. Clicking on the *Injury Mortality Data* link would provide the searcher with pedestrian death statistics by state, by age, and by gender. For children ages 5–9, for example, a searcher would learn that the death rate for pedestrians throughout the country was 1.21 per 100,000 in 1999.

PubMed

PubMed is the National Library of Medicine's search service. It provides access to MEDLINE and other NLM databases. MEDLINE is NLM's premier bibliographic database, covering a broad swath of biomedical and healthcare topics. It contains bibliographic citations and author abstracts for more than 4,300 journals from the United States and 70 other countries, although the emphasis of MEDLINE is on English-language journals. MEDLINE contains more than 11 million citations, some as recent as the previous week and others dating as far back as 1966. Conducting a search of PubMed on the topic of child pedestrians could start with the entry of keywords, as follows:

> pedestrian* AND children* AND (motor vehicles OR automobiles OR traffic accidents OR accident prevention)

Note that the keywords *pedestrian* and *children* are both truncated, as indicated by the use of the asterisk as a truncation symbol. The entry indicates that *pedestrian* and *children* are root words. *AND* and *OR* are Boolean operators. The *AND* is exclusive, limiting the search to only those documents in which all the words connected by *and* in the search statement occur. The *OR* is inclusive; it retrieves documents that contain any of the words linked by *or* in the search statement. The parentheses indicate that all terms within must be searched first. Figure 18.2 shows a screen obtained from the use of this search.

Motor vehicles, automobiles, traffic accidents, and accident prevention are all subject headings in MEDLINE. By constructing a search statement in the manner we have shown, a searcher could retrieve all documents that contain any of these terms first; then, the entire set will be joined by *pedestrian* and *children*.

This search strategy retrieves 241 documents. A searcher may reduce the number of documents retrieved by setting limits on the publication year or

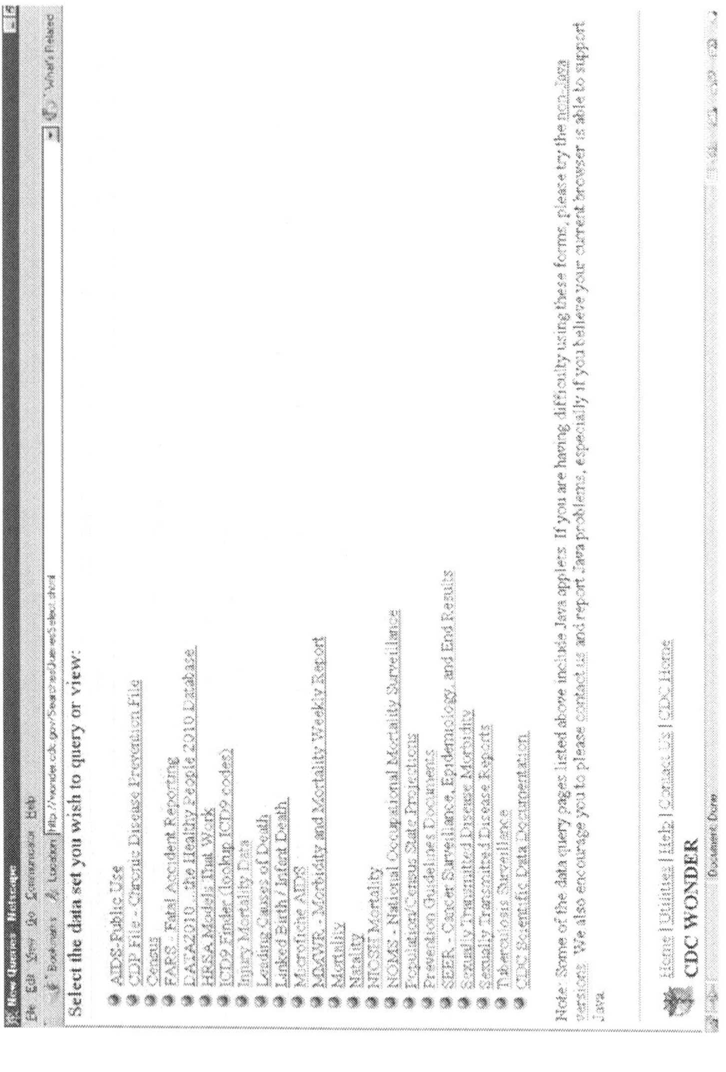

New Queries – Netscape

File   Edit   View   Go   Communicator   Help

Bookmarks   Location [http://wonder.cdc.gov/SearchSelect/select.shtml]   What's Related

Select the data set you wish to query or view:

- AIDS Public Use
- CDP File – Chronic Disease Prevention File
- Census
- FARS – Fatal Accident Reporting
- DATA2010 – the Healthy People 2010 Database
- HRSA Model That Work
- ICD9 Finder (lookup ICD9 codes)
- Injury Mortality Data
- Leading Causes of Death
- Linked Birth / Infant Death
- Mortuche AIDS
- MCMR – Morbidity and Mortality Weekly Report
- Mortality
- Natality
- NHOST Mortality
- NOMS – National Occupational Mortality Surveillance
- Population/Census State Projections
- Prevention Guidelines Documents
- SEER – Cancer Surveillance, Epidemiology, and End Results
- Sexually Transmitted Disease Morbidity
- Sexually Transmitted Disease Reports
- Tuberculosis Surveillance
- CDC Scientific Data Documentation

Note: Some of the data query pages listed above include Java applets. If you are having difficulty using these forms, please try the non-Java versions. We also encourage you to please contact us and report Java problems, especially if you believe your current browser is able to support Java.

Home | Utilities | Help | Contact Us | CDC Home

CDC WONDER

Document: Done

FIGURE 18.1. A view of a CDC Wonder screen in a search. (*Source:* Centers for Disease Control and Prevention. Department of Health and Human Services.)

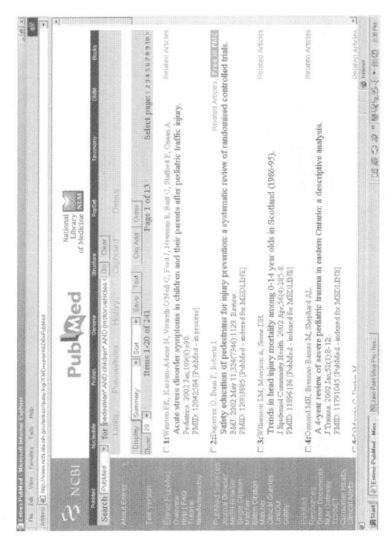

FIGURE 18.2. A screen in a search of PubMed using the search statement. (*Source:* PubMed, National Library of Medicine.)

the publication type. Clicking on *Limits* at the top of the screen and then choosing "randomized controlled trial" as a publication type reduces the set to only four articles.

The National Guideline Clearinghouse

The National Guideline Clearinghouse (http://www.guideline.gov) is a public resource for evidence-based clinical practice guidelines sponsored by the Agency for Healthcare Research and Quality, the American Medical Association, and the American Association of Health Plans. These guidelines are defined as systematically developed statements designed to assist practitioners and patients make appropriate decisions. Searching may be conducted in three different files—disease/condition, treatment/intervention, and organization. All guidelines are available with a full summary, but many are also available in full-text on-line. A search in this database for "pedestrian" retrieves three guidelines, one of which is available full-text from the database. Figure 18.4 shows the search.

Sociological Abstracts

Sociological Abstracts provides access to sociology literature and related disciplines. It includes abstracts of articles selected from over 2500 journals, conference papers, dissertations, and sociology book abstracts. The database is published by Cambridge Scientific Abstracts. Because it is not primarily a health-related database, the search strategy for a health topic can be broad without fear of returning too many irrelevant hits. Searching with the terms "pedestrian* and child" returns just six articles. One is entitled "The urban environment and child pedestrian and bicycle injuries: Interaction of ecological and personality characteristics." This article, by Christopher Bagley, appears in the *Journal of Community and Applied Social Psychology* (1999;2:281–289). From the title alone, it appears that this article is highly relevant to our search. But note that the journal is not indexed in MEDLINE; therefore, limiting the search to MEDLINE would not have turned up this information. Sociological Abstracts is provided at no charge at many universities; it is also available commercially through such database vendors as Dialog.

PsycINFO

PsycINFO, published by the American Psychological Association, provides bibliographic coverage of 1,300 psychology journals in addition to bibliographic coverage of a variety of books, dissertations, and technical reports. It is especially relevant for injury prevention materials because of its emphasis on psychological skills and effective safety training. PsycINFO uses "pedestrian accidents" as a subject heading. The following search, performed in PsycINFO, retrieved 50 relevant documents published in the 1998–2000 time period:

pedestrian accidents (subject) and child* (keyword)

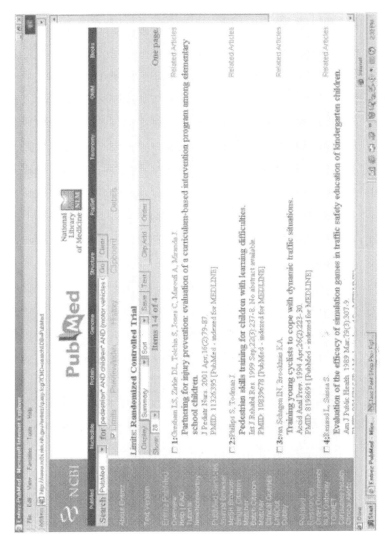

FIGURE 18.3. A search in PubMed setting limits of "randomized controlled trial." (*Source:* PubMed, National Library of Medicine.)

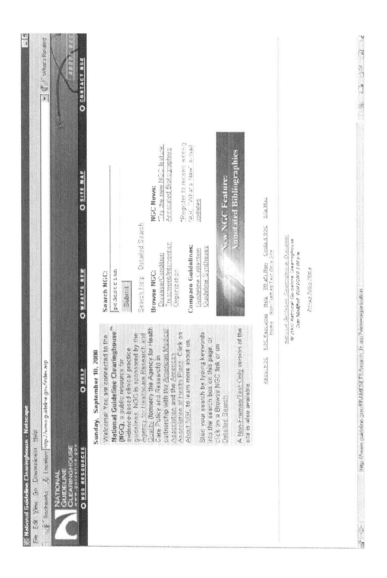

FIGURE 18.4. A screen from a search of the National Guideline Clearinghouse. (*Source:* The National Guideline Clearinghouse).

A number of the articles retrieved by this search strategy are in journals not indexed by MEDLINE—for example, "Characterization and prevention of child pedestrian accidents: An overview," authored by J.P. Assailly and appearing in the *Journal of Applied Developmental Psychology* (1997;18:257–262).

National Technical Information Service

National Technical Information Service (NTIS) provides bibliographic coverage of government documents, research reports, journal articles, and data files for sale by NTIS. It provides many unique documents not available in other databases. Each record may be found on microfiche at depository libraries or may be purchased directly from NTIS. A search in this database using keywords "child" and "pedestrian" retrieved numerous relevant documents not available in other databases. One example is "Epidemiology of injuries in Hispanic children; phase two," by P. Agran and D. Winn. The study was performed by the University of California at Irvine and sponsored by the National Center for Injury Prevention and Control. A case-control study of pedestrian injuries was utilized to identify risk factors for pedestrian injury among Hispanic children, resulting in development, implementation, and evaluation of a research-driven community pediatric pedestrian intervention.

A Second Search Example: Locating Chemical/ Environmental Health Information

A second example of a search will focus on chemical/environmental health information, which is of interest to consumers as well as to public health practitioners. A major source of information about this subject is TOXNET (http://toxnet.nlm.nih.gov), a cluster of databases covering a range of toxicology, hazardous substances, and environmental health topics. All of these databases are available via the Internet from the National Library of Medicine at no charge. This source provides full-text information—a document in its entirety rather than a citation and an abstract that refers to a specific document that may be available only in print.

The following search example will illustrate one possible use of these databases:

Assume that an environmental health specialist in Los Angeles has heard about the dangers of 1,1,1–trichloroethane and needs to know more about the chemical in order to determine whether it is present to the community at dangerous levels.

Once on the Internet, the specialist connects to TOXNET and selects the Toxic Release Inventory database for the reporting year 1999 (the most recent available.) The TRI is a database that provides information about estimated releases in the environment of many of the toxic chemicals. TRI is searchable by chemical name or by CAS (Chemical Abstracts Service) registry number, facility name(s), facility location (by state, city, county, or zip code), or amount of release. Figure 18.5 shows the TRI search screen.

Searching TRI for 1,1,1–trichloroethane in Los Angeles retrieves two records. It is also possible for our specialist to restrict the geographic area of concern further through a search of Los Angeles by zip code. On the page listing the records, an icon permits a searcher to perform calculations on the records in order to derive total calculations for environmental releases and off-site waste transfer. According to this information, all the environmental release is air release, rather than water, land, or underground injection. Figure 18.6 shows the screen containing the calculations.

The Hazardous Substances Data Bank

Having located information about the industrial release of 1,1,1–trichloroethane via TOXNET, our specialist now consults the Hazardous Substances Data Bank (HSDB), a scientifically peer-reviewed database containing full-text information on human and animal toxicity, safety and handling, environmental fate, and governmental regulation. HSDB is an excellent source of information about the chemical of interest. A search of HSDB provides the screen shown in Figure 18.7.

It is always easier to search HSDB by CAS number, a unique identifier that obviates a search through myriad records.

The HSDB record for 1,1,1–trichloroethane describes two major forms of exposure: (1) industrial solvent exposure and (2) exposure of adolescents from sniffing glue. The record indicates that there is no conclusive evidence of carcinogenicity from exposure to the chemical; however, exposure does cause central nervous system depression that ranges from headaches and lightheadedness to coma and death. The estimated daily intake of the chemical from air is 0.110 parts per billion (ppb)—0.420 ppb in urban/suburban areas and 1.20 ppb in source-dominated areas. The "Human Health Effects" section of the record details the expected symptoms at various exposure levels. The regulations regarding exposure limits appear in the "Environmental Standards and Regulations" section as well as in "Occupational Exposure Standards."

Our search for information about 1,1,1–trichloroethane is over.

Document Delivery and Library Services

Prior to the mid-1990s, all of the resources we have identified were more difficult to access and use. Searchers often had to have specialized, client-side software to search the databases and master arcane search languages. In addition, it was necessary for searchers to establish accounts, dial, and pay for modem-mediated, dedicated communication networks. Obviously, a searcher of these databases had to be highly motivated.

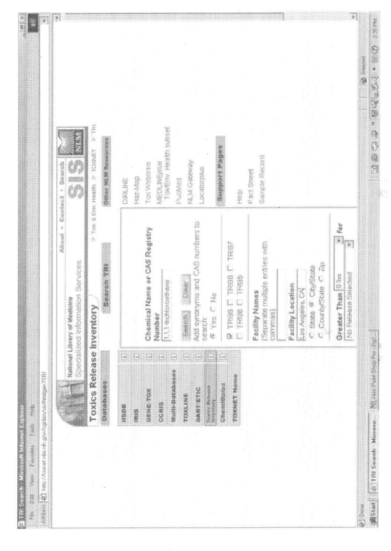

FIGURE **18.5.** Screen showing the Toxic Release Inventory search screen. (*Source:* TOXNET, National Library of Medicine. Available at: http://toxnet.nlm.nih.gov.)

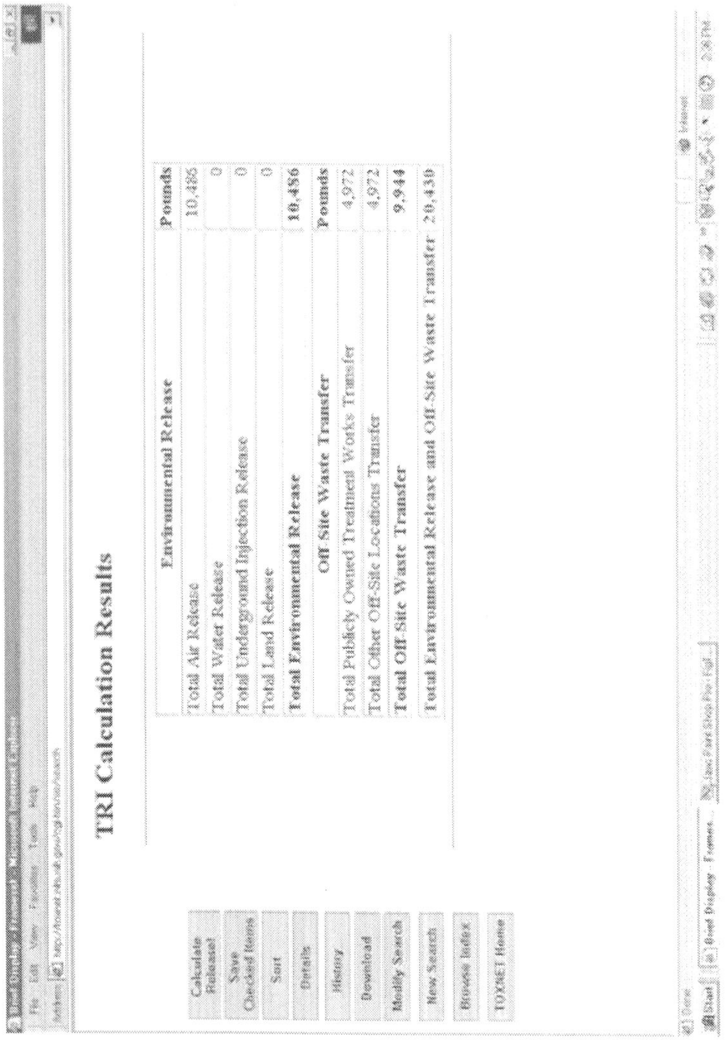

TRI Calculation Results

Environmental Release	Pounds
Total Air Release	10,485
Total Water Release	0
Total Underground Injection Release	0
Total Land Release	0
Total Environmental Release	10,486

Off Site Waste Transfer	Pounds
Total Publicly Owned Treatment Works Transfer	4,972
Total Other Off-Site Locations Transfer	4,972
Total Off-Site Waste Transfer	9,944
Total Environmental Release and Off-Site Waste Transfer	20,430

Calculate Release!

Save Checked Items

Sort

Details

History

Download

Modify Search

New Search

Browse Index

TOXNET Home

FIGURE 18.6. A view of the TRI screen showing calculations. (*Source:* TOXNET, National Library of Medicine. Available at: http://toxnet.nlm.nih.gov.)

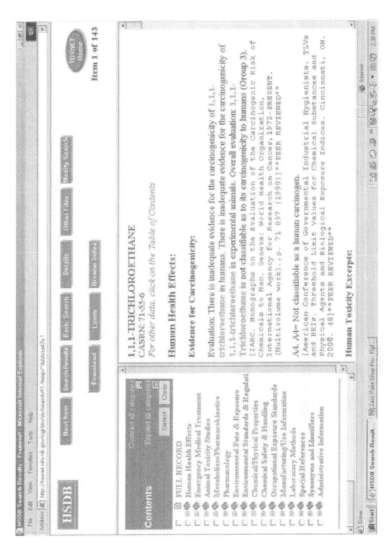

FIGURE **18.7.** Results of a search for 1,1,1–trichloroethane in the Hazardous Substances Data Bank. (*Source:* Hazardous Substances Data Bank.)

Since then, the rapid spread of the Internet has fueled a transition of these resources to easily accessible Web-based tools. Now, with a computer and an Internet connection, a user can access these resources at any time from any location, often without having to establish accounts and pay access charges.

This technological advance has had profound implications for access and use. Using these resources prior to the Internet required overcoming barriers of time, skill, and cost, effectively limiting use to librarians and some researchers and educators who either did not have librarian support or needed to search directly. The point is that very few practitioners were searchers of these resources. Now, the barriers to practitioners have been greatly lowered.

Still, the result of a database search today may be a set of citations and abstracts. The search phase may be complete, but finding answers to questions may not be. In fact, finding those answers may require obtaining copies of the identified articles, chapters, or reports. How does a searcher obtain those copies? Unfortunately, there is no single, simple answer. For one thing, it depends on the source of the information.

For example, the National Library of Medicine's PubMed offers an integrated document-ordering feature. The feature is known as Loansome Doc. Following the Loansome Doc screens, a searcher is instructed to contact a Regional Medical Library (1-800-338-7657 or http://www.nnlm.gov) for a referral to a library that will provide this document delivery service. Fees and other terms of service will vary by provider. The Regional Medical Library (contact information given above) can provide more details.

However, there are no services similar to Loansome Doc available through the other databases referred to in this chapter. The ready availability of documents from the National Library of Medicine (NLM) is a result of NLM's dedication to ensuring that these information services are available to health professionals throughout the country. As part of this effort, NLM has fostered the development of a national network of libraries that together provide the Loansome Doc service.

However, there are many document suppliers that can deliver copies of articles identified from searches of multiple databases in many different disciplines, usually for a fee. A directory of suppliers with links to their Web sites can be found at http://www.library.vcu.edu/docsup. In addition, state and local public libraries can usually obtain copies of journal articles and books through interlibrary loan. This service is usually free for registered users of the library system. There is a trade-off between using commercial suppliers and using public libraries: The commercial supplier will cost in dollars but not in time to deliver the item; the public library may not cost in dollars but will most likely take more time to deliver a document.

Services other than document delivery that may be of interest to a public health worker are database searching, search consulting, and search training. Asking a librarian about the availability of these services can be useful. Public health practitioners can contact the area Regional Medical Library for a referral to libraries that provide these services.

From Research to Practice: Putting Knowledge-Based Information to Work

Knowledge-based information has been defined as "information derived from the professional literature of the field." Technically, evidence-based medicine (from which evidence-based public health practice has evolved) includes clinical expertise and information about a particular patient as well as the pertinent professional literature. However, this comprehensive view of evidence-based medicine is not usually reflected in practice. In most discussions and/or literature about evidence-based medicine, clinical expertise and patient information are largely ignored, leaving the professional literature as the primary component of evidence-based medicine. In such a typical situation, knowledge-based information and evidence-based medicine become largely synonymous.

Systematic reviews and meta-analyses are research methods at the high end of the knowledge-based resources. Systematic reviews in clinical medicine were originally summaries of relevant randomized controlled trials (RCTs) performed in a systematic way so that other researchers could duplicate the results. However, because there is a paucity of RCTs available in many clinical areas and almost none available in public health areas, systematic reviews employ the best external evidence available: RCTs when possible, and comparative studies or primary studies when no RCTs exist. Meta-analyses are systematic reviews that employ a quantitative method to summarize results. Both originate with population-based studies. The application of population-based studies to individual patient care seems less appropriate than their application to the health of society at large, or the public health arena.[7]

Both knowledge-based and evidence-based resources are being increasingly applied to the public health field. Their usefulness in maintaining and improving the health of populations is intuitive but difficult to demonstrate, given the fuzziness and complexity of relevant information. Policy formulation is an area where this type of information support could be essential. For example, in a systematic review exploring the effectiveness of driver education as an intervention in motor vehicle crashes, the review's authors found that there is no evidence that this education is effective in reducing crash involvement.[8] They recommend that schools and communities consider other options, such as graduated licensing. In another article in the same supplement, a comparable review found graduated licensing to have some effectiveness as an intervention in adolescent driving.[9] Driver education has been a mainstay in high schools in this country for many years, reflecting a huge financial and philosophical investment, but in this example of the application of knowledge-based and evidence-based information, the investment appears to have provided little payback.

There are many other examples of public health policies that are rooted in belief rather than evidence. As budgets tighten, and pressure for increased accountability mount, it becomes more important to put into practice those policies that show strong evidence of their effectiveness. Applying the evidence to policy and practice—using knowledge-based information—is a necessary step toward accomplishing this goal.

Questions for Review

Questions 1–10 are based on the following short case:

You are a public health specialist interested in securing information about the incidence of AIDS in children ages 0–6 in the United States and how these children receive treatment. You have access to the Web at your workplace.

1. List some of the end points, focus issues, and types of intervention you might want to guide your search.
2. Explain how you would conduct a search of gray literature on the Internet and why this literature is not always inclusive, accurate, and reliable. What is the central paradox relating to the accessibility of this literature?
3. Your general search engine search of the Internet turns up more than 800 hits on the topic of children with AIDS and the treatments used. What technique would you use to limit the number of hits you need to review?
4. Assume that you find a Web portal regarding AIDS in children on one of the Internet sites you locate by use of a general Internet search engine. Explain what this portal is and why it might provide access to information relevant to your search topic.
5. Explain how you might use CDC Wonder to obtain relevant information. How could you limit your search to obtain relevant information only on children?
6. Explain how you would frame a keyword search to limit your search of databases with no controlled indexing terms.
7. Explain the advantage of using PubMed in your search.
8. How would you conduct a search of the National Guideline Clearinghouse, a search of Sociological Abstracts, a search of PsycINFO, and a search of the National Information Technical Service?
9. In your search of the Internet by use of a general search engine, you find references to several articles whose titles seem relevant to the purpose of your search, but the articles themselves are not available in full text on the Internet. Your public health organization does not currently have a membership in or an affiliation with an organization that can provide you with these copies.
   a. Explain your options for obtaining hard copies of these articles.
   b. What are the trade-offs involved in making your choice?
10. You decide that you need help in database searching, search consulting, and search training in order to conduct your search. How would you go about identifying the availability of these services?

References and Notes

1. Sackett DL, Rosenberg WM, Gray TA, Haynes RB, Richardson WS. Evidence based medicine: What it is and what it isn't. *BMJ*. 1996;312:71–72.
2. Hersh, WR. *Information Retrieval: A Health Care Perspective*. New York: Springer-Verlag; 1996.
3. Information needs and uses of the public health workforce—Washington, 1997–1998. *MMWR Morb Mortal Wkly Rep* 2000;49(6):118–120.
4. PubMed Central is located at http://PubMedCentral.nih.gov. Background information on this development can be found elsewhere on the National Institutes of Health Web site at http://www.nih.gov/about/director/pubmedcentral/pubmedcentral.htm.
5. The general HealthWeb site is located at http://www.healthweb.org. The public health area is at http://healthweb.org/browse.cfm?subjectid=80. The HealthLinks site is located at http://healthlinks.washington.edu. The public health portal section is at http://healthlinks.washington.edu/inpho. The Injury-Related Web sites portal is located at http://www.cdc.gov/ncipc/injweb/websites.htm.
6. Beahler CC, Sundheim JJ, Trapp NI. Information retrieval in systematic reviews: Challenges in the public health arena. *Am J Prev Med*. 2000;18:6–10.
7. Tonelli MR. The philosophical limits of evidence-based medicine. *Acad Med* 1998;73:1234–1240.
8. Vernick JS, Li G, Ogaitis S, MacKenzie EJ, Baker SP, Gielen AC. Effects of high school driver education on motor vehicle crashes, violations, and licensure. *Am J Prev Med*. 1999;16:40–46.
9. Foss RD, Evenson KR. Effectiveness of graduated driver licensing in reducing motor vehicle crashes. *Am J Prev Med*. 1999;16:47–56.

Part IV
New Challenges, Emerging Systems

Introduction

In Part IV, we examine many of the challenges that public health informatics specialists and, indeed, all public health practitioners face. We also take a look at several of the systems that are emerging to provide public health practitioners with fast access to critical information.

In Chapter 19, Denise Koo, Meade Morgan, and Claire Broome explore one of the new challenges facing public health: collecting data in such a way as to accommodate the needs of users within a variety of systems. After a discussion of the need for data in public health, the authors explore the current situation in data collection with regard to public health surveillance. They proceed to discuss several motivators for change in data collection, including the unsatisfactory nature of the ubiquitous stovepipe categorical systems, the deficiencies of current systems, mounting concerns about security and confidentiality, and the opportunity to transform the practice of public health. After a discussion of enablers of change in data collection, including the Internet, the authors conclude with a discussion of the National Electronic Disease Surveillance System (NEDSS) as an example of the new directions that public health data collection must follow.

In Chapter 20, Robb Chapman discusses another challenge facing public health—finding means to access data quickly and easily. First tracing the forms and the history of data access, Mr. Chapman focuses on present-day considerations for building public health data access systems, including choosing a suitable architecture and capitalizing on the promise of the data web as an access mechanism. He also cautions against over-reliance on the Internet as a data access tool.

In Chapter 21, Carol L. Hanchette provides an introduction to geographic information systems (GIS) as tools for organizing and displaying data. Using numerous examples of the utility and versatility of GIS, she discusses GIS functionality in the public health setting. She also provides an extensive discussion of implementing and using GIS systems—on small, departmental, and enterprise-wide scales. Dr. Hanchette addresses many of the issues associated with GIS—personnel and training issues as well as social/institutional issues such as confidentiality, security, agency coordination, and organizational politics. After a discussion of both the limitations and the lessons to be learned from GIS experience, she concludes the chapter with a discussion of the implications of emerging technologies, including the Internet, for GIS development and use.

In Chapter 22, Robert W. Linkins focuses on immunization registries as tools for increasing immunization rates in the United States and for effecting a reduction in the rates of morbidity and mortality attributable to vaccine-presentable disease. After providing a definition and a developmental history of such registries, Dr. Linkins focuses attention on the national Initiative on Immunization Registries and its purposes. In particular, he discusses the recommendations of the National Vaccine Advisory Committee with regard to several registry issues: protecting the privacy of individuals and the confidentiality of information, overcoming technical and operational challenges, ensuring recipient and provider participation, and determining the resources needed to develop and maintain immunization registries. Dr. Linkins cites statistics that demonstrate the efficacy of immunization registries and points out their dependence on the development of integrated health information systems.

In Chapter 23, William A. Yasnoff and Perry L. Miller discuss yet another kind of emerging systems, decision-support and expert systems. To illustrate both the complexity and the utility of such systems in public health practice, they provide an example of the use of decision-support systems in childhood immunization forecasting. Through coverage of IMM/Serve, they discuss such design issues as encoding in various forms of knowledge and knowledge representation; the system development process; testing such a system both manually and through automated tools; implementation; local customization; and maintenance. They conclude the chapter with a discussion of system development strategies, including criteria that can be used to determine the desirability of decision support and expert systems.

Part IV ends with Chapter 24, in which Larry L. Dickey and John D. Piette focus on the delivery of preventive medicine in primary care through information technology. Among the tools that they discuss are the electronic medical record, the comprehensive risk assessment, and interactive voice response systems for preventive care assessment. The authors also discuss the use of information technology for preventive care service delivery, for preventive care reminders, and for preventive care auditing. They point out that, although information technology is unlikely to replace the health-promoting relationships of primary care clinicians with their patients, it holds promise of promoting public health and preventing disease much more effectively and efficiently than ever before.

19
New Means of Data Collection

Denise Koo, Meade Morgan, and Claire V. Broome

Learning Objectives

After studying this chapter, you should be able to:

- Describe the current situation in public health with respect to data collection and data sharing, as indicated by public health surveillance systems.
- List and discuss the factors that are providing the motivation and the opportunity for public health practitioners to move to developing and using systems that provide for integration of public health systems and healthcare systems and that permit efficient, effective sharing of data across system boundaries.
- Discuss the characteristics of the data collection and surveillance systems of the long-term future in public health.
- List some of the barriers and requirements that public health must address in developing the ideal health information systems of the long-term future.
- Describe the Centers for Disease Control and Prevention's National Electronic Disease Surveillance System as a model for future public health systems, including its short-term and long-term objectives.

Overview

The current challenges to public health in collecting, analyzing, and sharing data necessary to promote the health of the population is exemplified by the current inefficient systems used for public health surveillance. Current data collection systems lack interoperability, speed, and comprehensiveness, among other deficiencies. In part, these inadequacies are products of distinct funding streams and a compartmentalized approach. Yet, many forces now at work are motivating public health and the healthcare system in general to move toward an integrated, efficient, and comprehensive approach to the collection of data important to public health. These forces include recognition of the deficiencies of current data collection and data sharing systems, interest in acquiring new data, the continuing proliferation of systems at all levels, concerns about security and confidentiality, and the opportunity to transform the practice of public health. Such enablers of change as public policy and the multiple developments in information technology are also driving the effort. A new public health initiative, the National Electronic Disease Surveillance System (NEDSS), is a primary example of the long-term vision of data collection and data sharing in public health. NEDSS's long-term vision is of complementary, interoperable electronic information systems that permit automatic gathering of health data from a variety of sources on a real-time basis, facilitating the monitoring of the health of communities, assisting in ongoing analyses of trends in and detection of emerging health problems, and providing information for setting public health policy. Although that long-term vision faces numerous barriers to and requirements for its realization, the comprehensive, as opposed to disease-based, approach used by NEDSS exemplifies the electronic capture and sharing of information between the healthcare system and public health that will move the United States toward data collection systems that will support public health practice in the 21st century.

Introduction: The Need for Data in Public Health

The mission of public health is to promote the health of the population. The emphasis of this mission is often on prevention, especially primary prevention, rather than on treatment. Public health practitioners are interested in intervening as early as possible in the causal pathway of disease or disability, preferably before the manifestation of disease. Thus, for the public health professional, areas of interest or study include factors in the pre-exposure environment (including air quality, poverty, access to health care, education status) and the presence of hazardous agents (whether chemical or biological), behaviors, and exposures. In addition to collecting data on these determinants or risk factors for disease, public health officials monitor the occurrence of health events/conditions and deaths, as well as the activities of the healthcare and public health systems and their effects on health. Together, these data enable public health officials—in collaboration with policy makers—to arrive at informed decisions about the most effective mechanisms for intervention. Because the most appropriate data sources vary for a given problem or disease, public health professionals frequently must combine information from multiple, usually incompatible systems and sources to obtain a more inclusive and accurate depiction of the problem—for example, to arrive at an accurate estimate of incidence, to determine the prevalence of behavioral or environmental risk factors, and to ascertain the availability and use of preventive services related to the disease or condition. Usually, the various systems from which public health professionals derive the necessary information do not communicate with one another, nor do they connect with systems operated in the healthcare industry.

Yet, if public health is to address such continuing future problems as disease prevention and control, and if it is to deal with future public health crises in a fast and effective way, it must have quick and comprehensive access to data across system boundaries—access that ties together public health systems at the federal, state, and local level, and access that integrates public health and healthcare industry systems. The vision of public health systems of the future is very different from the reality of public health systems of today. This chapter will discuss the forces that are driving public health to develop and implement integrated systems that will enable practitioners to acquire and share information quickly. It will also present a vision of the future of public health information systems, including the new directions, as exemplified by the NEDSS and the barriers to and requirements of such systems, as well as some strategies for attaining this vision.

The Current State of Public Health Surveillance

Public health surveillance is defined generally as the ongoing systematic collection, analysis, and interpretation of health-related data for use in the planning, implementation, and evaluation of public health practice.[1,2] Surveillance is a key data-driven activity of public health. The Centers for Disease Control and Prevention (CDC) recently conducted an inventory of all its public health information systems, identifying 120 surveillance systems in use at CDC, of which 71 were used by or exchanged data with partners in state and local health departments (unpublished data). These systems use data from various sources, some of which are collected from healthcare providers, laboratories, individuals, or directly from medical records and birth and death certificates explicitly for surveillance purposes. Other systems make secondary use of existing administrative data, such as hospital discharge data or workers' compensation or other insurance data, for surveillance. Methods of data collection vary, but traditionally they have consisted largely of paper reports that are either mailed or faxed or of telephone reports. Figure 19.1 presents a sample state case report form that is characteristic of the paper reports existing today.

In some instances, public health officials conduct resource-intensive chart review with an abstraction form, and attempting to use administrative data frequently requires them to wait for the availability of unwieldy, difficult-to-use data tapes from the primary source.

This current situation is exemplified by the schematic in Figure 19.2, which depicts several of the existing surveillance information systems, their data sources, and information flows. As is clear from CDC inventory results and from this figure, CDC programs provided with funding by Congress for the surveillance, study, and control of specific diseases—for instance, for tuberculosis (TB), sexually transmitted diseases (STDs), acquired immunodeficiency syndrome (AIDS), and lead exposure—employ independently

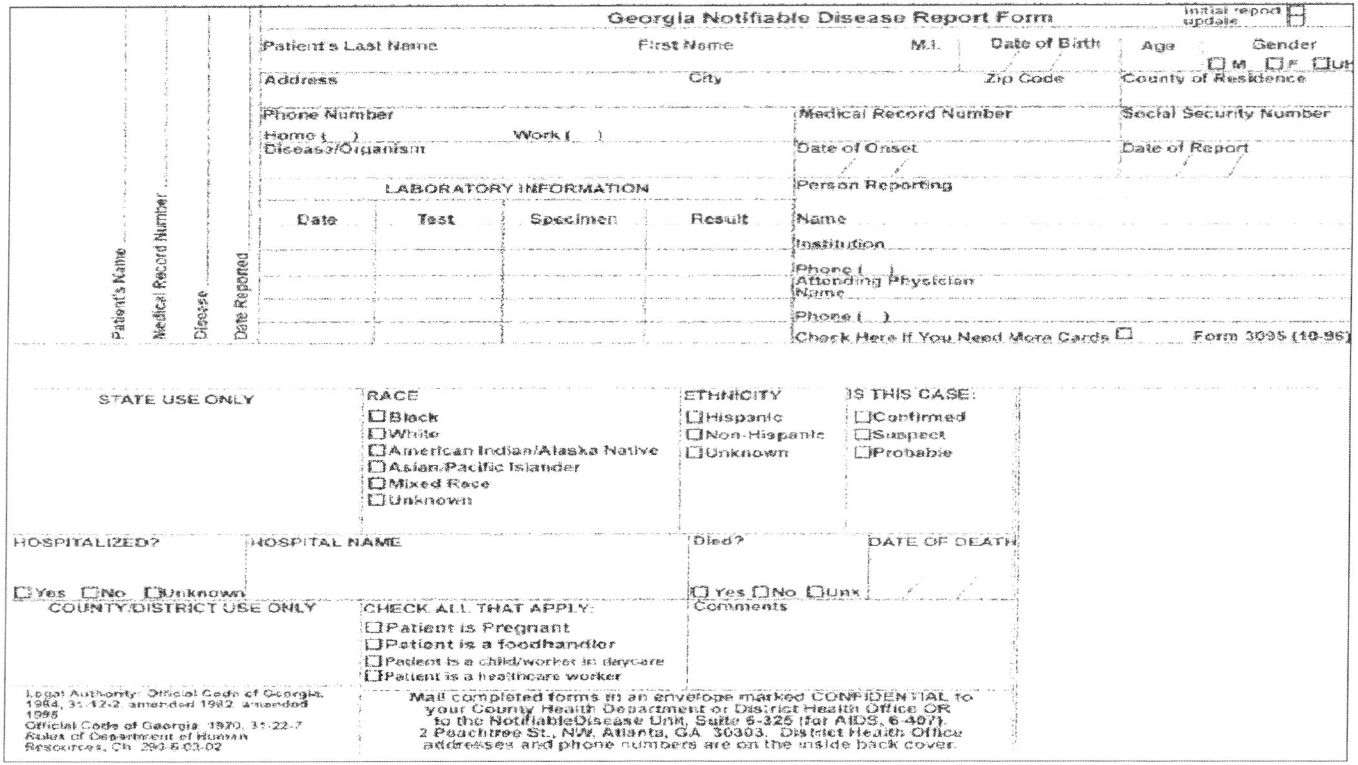

Georgia Notifiable Disease Report Form

Initial report ☐ update ☐

Patient's Name
Medical Record Number
Disease
Date Reported

Patient's Last Name | First Name | M.I. | Date of Birth / / | Age | Gender ☐M ☐F ☐U

Address | City | Zip Code | County of Residence

Phone Number
Home ( ) Work ( )
Medical Record Number | Social Security Number

Disease/Organism | Date of Onset / / | Date of Report / /

LABORATORY INFORMATION

Date	Test	Specimen	Result

Person Reporting
Name
Institution
Phone ( )
Attending Physician
Name
Phone ( )
Check Here If You Need More Cards ☐ Form 3095 (10-96)

STATE USE ONLY

RACE
☐Black
☐White
☐American Indian/Alaska Native
☐Asian/Pacific Islander
☐Mixed Race
☐Unknown

ETHNICITY
☐Hispanic
☐Non-Hispanic
☐Unknown

IS THIS CASE:
☐Confirmed
☐Suspect
☐Probable

HOSPITALIZED?
☐Yes ☐No ☐Unknown

HOSPITAL NAME

Died?
☐Yes ☐No ☐Unk

DATE OF DEATH / /

COUNTY/DISTRICT USE ONLY

CHECK ALL THAT APPLY:
☐Patient is Pregnant
☐Patient is a foodhandler
☐Patient is a child/worker in daycare
☐Patient is a healthcare worker

Comments

Legal Authority: Official Code of Georgia, 1984, 31-12-2, amended 1992, amended 1995
Official Code of Georgia 1970, 31-22-7
Rules of Department of Human Resources, Ch. 290-5-03-02

Mail completed forms in an envelope marked CONFIDENTIAL to your County Health Department or District Health Office OR to the NotifiableDisease Unit, Suite 6-325 (for AIDS, 6-407), 2 Peachtree St., NW, Atlanta, GA 30303. District Health Office addresses and phone numbers are on the inside back cover.

FIGURE 19.1. A sample state case report form. (*Source:* Georgia Department of Public Health. Available at: http://www.ph.dhr.state.ga.us/epi/disease/art/epiform.gif. Accessed April 2, 2002.)

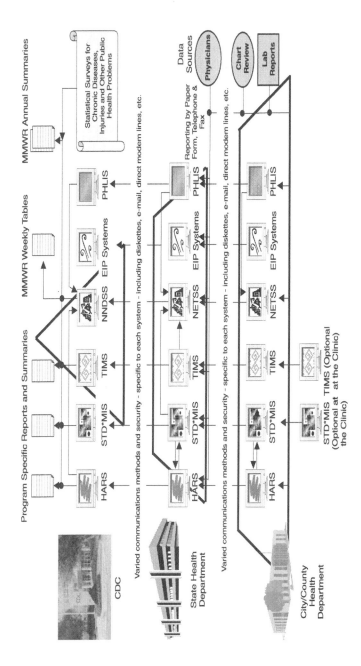

FIGURE 19.2. Existing surveillance information systems, data sources, and information flows. CDC, Centers for Disease Control and Prevention; EIP, Emerging Infections Program; HARS, Human Immunodeficiency Virus/Acquired Immunodeficiency Syndrome Reporting System; NNDSS, National Notifiable Diseases Surveillance System; NETSS, National Electronic Telecommunications System for Surveillance; PHLIS, Public Health Laboratory Information System; STD*MIS, Sexually Transmitted Disease Management Information System; TIMS, Tuberculosis Information Management System.

developed disease-specific computer applications for use at the state (and sometimes local) level for the collection, entry, and analysis of surveillance data, and for transmission of data to CDC. The distinct funding streams, the mechanisms for delivering clinical care and health services, the partners and data sources (e.g., STD program managers and clinics for STDs, TB program managers and clinics for TB, and clinical laboratories for blood lead levels)—all promote such independence. Some examples of these systems for infectious diseases, depicted in the figure, include the human immunodeficiency virus/AIDS reporting system (HARS), the Sexually Transmitted Disease Management Information System (STD-MIS), and the Surveillance System for Tuberculosis (SURVS-TB), now replaced by the Tuberculosis Information Management System (TIMS). Examples of such systems for other conditions include the Adult Blood Lead Epidemiology and Surveillance program (ABLES) and the Childhood Blood Lead Surveillance System.

These systems have played an important role in standardizing data collection and reporting across the nation for their respective diseases. As such, they provided, and continue to provide, information that is crucial to public health practice. However, a crucial shortcoming of these systems is that they are not horizontally integrated. The variables common to multiple systems, classification and coding schemes, user interfaces, database formats, and methods for transmitting or analyzing data are not standardized and/or cannot be reused. Most of these applications do not allow the import or export of data. Personnel at local and state health departments are required to use multiple, incompatible applications to enter and analyze data; data cannot easily be exchanged, linked, or merged by different programs (e.g., notifiable disease reports and laboratory reports of isolates) or be used to evaluate problems by person (e.g., co-morbid conditions or later occurrence of a second disease) over time and geographic area. As the sophistication of local and state health departments in computing and information management and the need to exchange and use electronic data have increased, the shortcomings of the initial uncoordinated and unstandardized efforts to computerize surveillance have become apparent.

Motivators for Change

Yet there are forces at work that are compelling the public health system to make changes in the approaches and systems for collecting data. These forces include the inefficiencies of current stovepipe categorical systems, the deficiencies of current systems in general, a growing interest in acquiring data from new sources, the proliferation of information systems in the public health industry, concerns about the security and confidentiality of health information, and the opportunity to transform the practice of public health in general. In addition, certain enablers of change, including federal law and developments in information technology, are driving public health toward making changes in data collection systems.

Stovepipe Categorical Systems

This disease-based approach to prevention and control, with its accompanying disease-specific surveillance information systems, has made it more difficult for state and local health departments to assess the diseases and health problems in their communities efficiently. In order to evaluate the overall health of their jurisdictions, local and state health officials must use and access multiple information systems. For example, maternal and child health programs cannot easily access data in the independent surveillance information systems for monitoring childhood lead poisoning, asthma, and vaccine-preventable diseases. It was clear by the mid-1990s that a more efficient, nonduplicative change in the approach to conducting public health surveillance and to building information systems to support these activities was needed.[3,4]

Deficiencies of Current Systems

In addition to the need for efficiency, there are other key motivators for a change in approach. Current surveillance systems generally capture only a fraction of cases, in a delayed and labor-intensive fashion. Underreporting to public health, particularly from physicians, has been well documented.[5-10] Many providers do not know how or to whom to report diseases, or else they believe that disease reporting is a burden that detracts from their clinical responsibilities. Few healthcare providers understand the importance of public health surveillance, the role of the provider as a source of data, and the role of the health department in response. As well, some of these surveillance systems are more targeted at specific sites, such as STD clinics, thus limiting the completeness of data when patients are not seen and treated at such specialized clinics.[11] Data in these systems are also frequently delayed,[12-14] in part because of the burdens of reporting and duplicative data entry on participants either in the healthcare system or at the local or state health department. There are also substantial delays and challenges in obtaining and using final hospital discharge data or data from other sources for secondary use for surveillance.[15-17]

Interest in Acquiring New Data

Interest in acquiring new data is also driving public health toward the development of more efficient and effective data collection systems. Public health, after all, will benefit by collecting more timely and complete data not only from current data sources, but also from new sources. Highly critical is the need for more information for public health—for example, data useful for detecting bioterrorist events and emerging infectious diseases. In the past, public health has designated specific conditions or syndromes as important for notification to public health. However, concerns about bioterrorism and the relative uncertainty about the exact biological or chemical agent that a terrorist will choose to use as a weapon give rise to an interest in capturing somewhat *less* specific data in a *more* timely fashion, such as collecting "real-time" data on the occurrence of suspicious respiratory syndromes (i.e., possible early anthrax, plague, smallpox, or tularemia) in order to generate a more rapid and effective public health response.[18] Early access to these data in electronic format, *as they are entered*, is highly desirable. For a more effective public health response to bioterrorism or to other, less urgent problems, it is also anticipated that new data sources, such as emergency room or prescription or over-the-counter pharmacy data—or even, potentially, school absentee or 911 call data—may supply useful information. Many of these data may not provide detailed information about the persons involved, but their timely availability may signify important trends that lead to earlier detection and response to a public health problem.

The Proliferation of Information Systems

The increasingly widespread use of information systems, both at the state and local health department as well as in medical and other information systems, provides another motivator for a change in approach to collecting data for public health. Many state and local health departments have developed systems to meet a range of internal data needs. These departments wish to simplify reporting to CDC programs by using a single electronic approach—for example, by secure Internet transmission—and without re-entry of data into CDC systems. This problem is even more pressing at the most common primary data sources, the information systems of the healthcare provider or the laboratory. It would be unrealistic to expect that the healthcare system would use, in addition to its own information systems, multiple freestanding public health information systems built to meet the needs of a particular federal program. Thus, the increasing sophistication of both the healthcare system and the public health system underscore the need for an integrated approach to gathering public health data from key primary data sources, an approach that facilitates capture and use of data that are already in electronic form. Such an approach will, of necessity, also acknowledge the interdependence of the public health and the healthcare systems and improve the efficiency of systems to support both.

Concerns about Security and Confidentiality

Even a discussion of direct electronic access to clinical data and of integration of public health systems with healthcare systems heightens the concerns of consumers about the security and confidentiality of their personal data. In reality, the use of electronic information systems actually provides an opportunity to *improve* the security and confidentiality of medical data.[19] After all, a definition of *security* includes the technological, organizational, and administrative processes designed to insure that only authorized persons access data systems. It is widely acknowledged that the technology exists for markedly improved security and protection of electronic health information, and the National Research Council (NRC) has made recommendations for how to insure such security.[20] Several institutions have collaborated to demonstrate the feasibility and efficacy of an approach that incorporates these recommendations.[21] Nationally, security standards for health information systems that closely follow the NRC recommendations are under development as part of the Health Insurance Portability and Accountability Act. In addition, given the general public's concerns about privacy and confidentiality, CDC has developed agency-wide Internet security standards and a secure Internet pipeline for transmission of data (described further below) that are consistent with the NRC recommendations for security of health-related data. It is hoped that these standards will eventually facilitate secure electronic exchange of appropriate data between public health and the healthcare system.

The Opportunity to Transform the Practice of Public Health

The closer integration of public health and the healthcare system and the timely capture of data at its origin will provide unprecedented opportunity to transform the nature and practice of public health. Elimination of repeat data entry or manual data transcription reduces the opportunities for mistakes, thus hopefully leading to improved data quality, or at least the ability to determine the specificity and quality of the data directly. And direct capture of clinical or other data for public health purposes means that public health will not simply conduct surveillance as it always has, only a bit faster and with slightly more data; rather, this new, integrated approach will provide public health with the opportunity to use new methods of detecting public health problems sooner than before, facilitating earlier identification of persons at risk and more timely interventions.

Enablers of Change

Accompanying the motivators of change that we have discussed are certain developments that enable that change. These developments include shifts in public policy and innovations in technology.

Policy: The Health Insurance Portability and Accountability Act (HIPAA)

Standards for exchanging electronic data are the critical glue for improving the sharing and use of health information among systems. In 1996, the US Congress passed the Health Insurance Portability and Accountability Act (HIPAA) (P.L. 104-191), which—at the request of healthcare providers and the industry that finances health care— contained provisions for administrative simplification. It mandated the development, implementation, and use of standards for exchanging financial and administrative data related to health care. These provisions required the Secretary of the Department of Health and Human Services (DHHS) to adopt national uniform standards for electronic transactions related to:

* health insurance enrollment and eligibility, healthcare encounters, and health insurance claims;
* the establishment of identifiers for healthcare providers, payers and individuals, as well as code sets and classification systems used in these transactions; and
* security of these transactions.

Rules for all of these have been published (except the rule for the individual identifier, which has been delayed until appropriate privacy protections are in place), and HHS has adopted final rules for transaction standards and code sets. (For up-to-date information about the status of these standards, see the Administrative Simplification page on the DHHS Web site, available at: http://aspe.os.dhhs.gov/admnsimp.) Anyone who conducts these transactions electronically will be required to use these national standards, which are largely based on existing private sector data standards and include input from standards development organizations, the healthcare industry, and state and local government.

Agreement on standards is particularly challenging because of the diverse needs of the groups who record and use health information, including providers, payers, administrators, researchers, and public health officials. Most of the coding systems or standards proposed for HIPAA have been designed for business purposes, not to facilitate the assessment of the quality of health care or other data needs of public health.[22] However, HIPAA has provided the impetus for various standards development organizations (SDOs) and terminology and coding groups to work collaboratively to harmonize their separate systems[23] (see also http://www.hipaa-dsmo.org). For example, two American National Standards Institute (ANSI)-accredited SDOs, the Accredited Standards Committee X12N (http://www.x12.org)—which has dealt in the past principally with standards for health insurance transactions—and Health Level Seven (HL7, http://www.hl7.org)—which has dealt with standards for clinical messaging and exchange of clinical information within healthcare institutions (e.g., hospitals)—have collaborated on a standardized approach for providing supplementary information to support healthcare claims. The payer, billing, and clinical arenas had traditionally remained separate from their respective standards organizations.

Until recently, public health agencies had not worked closely with SDOs such as X12 or HL7, nor with clinical coding systems. Thus, neither healthcare information systems nor public health information systems took into account approaches that would facilitate public health surveillance, such as electronic transmission of laboratory data directly to public health agencies, use of medical codes designated by public health as relevant, capture and coding of behavioral or environmental risk factors in the medical record, or the recording of race and ethnicity or educational background with the enrollment of a patient.

But such approaches are necessary to the development of integrated data systems for public health. Such systems require a clear definition of public health data needs and the sources for these data, consensus on data, and communications standards—to facilitate comparability and exchange of data—and policies to support data sharing while preserving data security, along with generation of mechanisms and tools for accessing and disseminating data in a useful manner. Public health practitioners, through the activities of the NEDSS initiative (described below) and the Public Health Data Standards Consortium—which includes public health and health services research interests (http://www.cdc.gov/nchs/otheract/phdsc/phdsc.htm)—are attempting to improve the utility and re-usability of data captured in clinical systems for population-based health. It is also expected that the re-usability of clinical data will facilitate the ability to measure and improve the quality of care, patient safety, and clinical cost-effectiveness, and address other issues of concern to those involved in health care as well as in public health.

Information Technology

Another enabler of change in data collection appears in the form of recent changes in technology. These changes provide new opportunities for data collection and analysis and will facilitate the transformation of public health surveillance in this country. The innovative technologies will (1) allow more timely and secure reporting of public health data; (2) reduce the burden of reporting on healthcare providers; (3) facilitate receipt of easily utilized data at already overworked public health agencies; and (4) provide access to data across governmental and political boundaries—while at the same time enforcing appropriate privacy and confidentiality restrictions on the sharing of information. Table 19.1 summarizes the changes in information technology that we will discuss.

The Internet

The first and most important of these new technologies is the Internet. The Internet will affect both the collection and dissemination of data. First, it will enable more rapid collection of data from healthcare providers and infection control professionals, allowing them to report data directly to local and state-based public health computer systems by use of only an Internet-connected computer with a Web browser, rather than filling out a piece of paper and

TABLE 19.1. Changes in information technology enabling changes in data collection

Changes in Information Technology	Expected Impact
The Internet	• Will enable more rapid data collection and analysis by use of only an Internet-connected computer with a Web browser; will also enable comparisons across systems and levels.
Extensible Markup Language (XML)	• Will provide standardization for transferring data from system to system and from the healthcare setting to the public health setting.
Industry standards for information systems design and development	• Will enable state and local systems to tailor their systems to use technologies that are consistent across systems, enabling the development of such tools as virtual databases.

faxing or mailing it. Second, public health decision makers will also be able to access and analyze data through the Internet and a browser, in turn providing these decision makers access to more timely information about emerging public health problems. Also, as laws regarding confidentiality and the use of health-related data are refined at the state and local levels, Internet access to these systems will allow staff to retrieve data at appropriate levels of detail from their own jurisdictions *and* to compare and monitor data regarding public health problems in neighboring areas as well. In anticipation of increased use of the Internet for public health surveillance (as well as for other activities), state and local health departments are being equipped with secure Internet access as part of the US national Health Alert Network (HAN).[18]

Extensible Markup Language (XML)

A new technology closely tied to the Internet is the Extensible Markup Language (XML, see http://www.w3.org/XML/). XML will provide a more flexible method of transferring data from information system to information system. Properly constructed and standardized XML documents will provide not only public health data, but also the information that permits these data to be used in the appropriate context. For example, XML documents could contain, in addition to raw disease indicators and rates, standardized descriptions of the sources of the data, how they were collected, and their reliability. Such information will allow public health professionals to better interpret the information and make appropriate policy decisions. However, although XML does show considerable promise in facilitating the transfer of raw data and the exchange of processed information, it alone is not sufficient. Detailed specifications for the application of generic XML standards will be needed to insure that public health information needs are met. These efforts must be coordinated across the entire public health enterprise if the potential of XML is to be realized.

The standards development organization HL7 is among the leaders in adopting XML technology for the transfer of information within the healthcare setting, with the necessary additional specification[24,25] (see also HL7 Web site). The new version 3 of HL7 will provide standard definitions for XML markup of document structure and content. This new version will remove much of the optionality and lack of true standardization associated with older versions of HL7. Through version 3's more rigorous adherence to rules for markup and the use of standard vocabularies for coding data elements, healthcare professionals will expend less effort to retool existing systems and transform data from "HL7-compliant" applications, thus allowing healthcare systems to send and accept the information needed for public health surveillance.

Standards for Information Systems Design and Development

A related advance, of which HL7 is simply one example of many, is the increased use of industry standards for information systems design and development. Historically, many systems relied on particular software packages and hardware vendors. As interoperable standards for software become more widely disseminated, state and local health departments will be able to tailor their systems to use technologies that are consistent with the information technology standards (hardware and software) within their state governments; at the same time, these departments will still be able to plug in solutions developed for the public health community at large. As a hypothetical example, software written in the Java programming language to detect outbreaks of infectious disease could be used on virtually any computer that a state or local health department might have, whether the computer is Intel and Microsoft, Sun and UNIX, or an Apple Mac.

An example of the advantages of these types of standards is the ability to create distributed "virtual" databases. Currently, many of the disease-specific programs have data systems that either cannot share data or that must significantly transform those data before they can be transferred into and out of other systems. Although standards such as HL7 can assist in this transformation and transfer process, sending messages back and forth still requires many steps. By the combination of the Internet and XML with appropriate security protocols, it will be possible to create virtual databases that physically exist in different places but that, to an information system user, appear as though they are all a single, local database. The advantages of such an approach are evidenced by a pilot effort already under way. The CDC, in collaboration with the US Bureau of the Census, has developed a prototype application known as Data Web (see Chapter 20). By using formally structured metadata to describe the content of various databases, the Data Web system can dynamically link notifiable disease reports (numerators) with the most current population data (denominators) maintained by the Bureau of the Census to create maps showing rates of disease by state and county. Future versions will allow even more databases to be linked in a fashion consistent with privacy laws and confidentiality guidelines.

New Directions: NEDSS

Vision for the Future

An example of the kind of integrated data collection and surveillance system we have discussed as a desirable development in public health is a new public health initiative spearheaded by CDC, the NEDSS. The *long-term vision* for NEDSS is that of complementary, interoperable electronic information systems that:

- gather health data automatically from a variety of sources on a real-time basis;
- facilitate the monitoring of the health of communities;
- assist in ongoing analyses of trends and detection of emerging public health problems; and
- provide information for setting public health policy.

This vision incorporates some key implications. First is the assumption of ongoing, automated capture and analysis of data, including automated algorithms for detecting aberrations of potential importance. Second is the point that these data are already electronic, and that there will be no need for re-entry of data. Third is that this more comprehensive approach would support efficient data collection via access to multiple critical sources—such as computerized medical and laboratory records as well as sources of data outside the health arena (e.g., environmental monitoring systems, highway traffic crash data)—for multiple programmatic uses, and *not* through the building of myriad independent systems for single diseases or programs. Finally, at the core of this vision is the closer integration of the public health and the healthcare systems, an integration that should lead to improved provision of health care as well as public health.

In a scenario from this future, suppose a patient sees a physician with respiratory symptoms. As the physician enters the symptoms in the patient's electronic medical record, the differential diagnosis pops up on the screen.

Because a public health agency would have worked with those developing the computerized patient record, diagnoses such as plague or anthrax might be included, depending on the geographic location or epidemiologic characteristics of the patient. Data could be available from public health computers about the prevalence of or concern regarding various conditions that month or that season. The computer would recommend diagnostic tests, some of which are more relevant for public or community health than for the care of the individual patient, such as measles immunoglobulin M for a fever and rash, or a stool culture for *Salmonella* for diarrhea. When these test results become available and a diagnosis is made, these data are automatically shared with the public health agency. Such sharing insures that the public health authority is made aware of all individual cases in a timely fashion—facilitating early public health intervention if the numbers or trends appear to reflect more than the random occurrence of sporadic cases. Although it is a more complex application, one could also imagine a collaboration with clinical laboratories to retrieve specimens if further testing such as molecular fingerprinting were indicated.

In a simpler scenario, the computer might track the rate of drug resistance among isolates of various bacteria and flag increasing resistance to antibiotic *P*. Suppose that, through a query of pharmaceutical databases across the country, a public health official notes an increase in utilization/sales of this antibiotic in the same annual period over the last several years, prior to and concurrent with the increase in resistance. Regardless of whether this is cause or effect, the official sends an electronic notice to healthcare providers for these areas of the country, pointing out the likely decreased effectiveness of drug *P*. In addition, the official makes plans to step up the campaign for the judicious use of antibiotics, including insuring that a warning automatically appears whenever a provider writes an electronic prescription for this antibiotic for a patient whose clinical status is consistent with infection by resistant bacteria.

Barriers and Requirements for the Future

This exciting vision remains a vision for the future, not for tomorrow. The 1995 report of the US Public Health Service, entitled *Making a Powerful Connection: the Health of the Public and the National Information Infrastructure*, highlighted in a similar fashion the opportunity to integrate public health and healthcare delivery and argued that in order to move in this direction, "health-care organizations and the public health community will need to coordinate not only their roles and responsibilities, but also their information systems."[26] The report described several requirements for the development of "logically integrated health information systems, in which information collected once can serve multiple purposes." The authors cited the need for nationally uniform policies for data standards, privacy and security, unique identifiers, and data sharing. They also mentioned organizational and financial barriers as well as a lack of informatics training in public health as impediments to the development of such policies. An additional requirement for achieving this long-term vision, presumably subsumed under the category of data standards, includes a standardized electronic medical record, although recommendations for the eventual adoption of standards for the electronic exchange of medical record data were also presented to the Secretary of HHS by the National Committee on Vital and Health Statistics in July 2000, as required by HIPAA (available at http://ncvhs.hhs.gov). Public health officials will need to ensure that evolving standards for a computer-based patient record[27] facilitate its use by public health—for example, for the purpose of the exchange of clinically relevant data for public health surveillance, with appropriate and secure protection of privacy and confidentiality.

Privacy of Health Information

Having similar standards and coding for data will not be useful if it is not permissible to share the data. Maintaining the privacy of a person's health information is a key requirement for allowing the sharing of data with others. Health information privacy refers to "an individual's claim to control the circumstances in which personally identifiable health information is collected, used, and disclosed."[28] Much of the current privacy protection of health information is based on a patchwork of state laws and regulations that predate the electronic age and do not provide adequate protection for either paper or electronic health information.[29,30] Consumers have many understandable concerns about the potential for misuse of electronic health records in this dawning era of computerized medical records. Health information privacy is, therefore, a hotly debated topic.

However, public health officials have generally protected the privacy of health information and constrained its use for public health purposes. CDC and the Council of State and Territorial Epidemiologists (CSTE) have recently attempted to clarify the existing myriad of federal and state privacy laws affecting public health departments by developing a "Model State Public Health Privacy Act" (http://www.critpath.org/msphpa/privacy.htm). This Model Act states that public health departments may justifiably acquire, use, and store personally identifiable health information for public health purposes provided they respect the privacy and security of the information. In addition, because no federal statute currently exists that protects the confidentiality of all personally identifiable health data, HIPAA requires that the US Secretary of HHS promulgate privacy standards by regulatory authority for transactions covered by HIPAA. As John Christiansen has discussed in Chapter 4, HHS recently published a rule for Standards for Privacy of Individually Identifiable Health Information that includes a definition of protected health information and descriptions of disclosures that may occur only with consent and disclosures that may occur without consent, such as disclosures to public health for surveillance purposes.[31]

Unique Health Identifier

Related to the issue of privacy is the issue of unique health identifiers, especially for individuals. One of the standards mandated by HIPAA is that of establishing a unique health identifier for individuals, one that would allow for longitudinal and geographic links among a patient's healthcare records. Unique health identifiers for individuals (in addition to those for providers, health plans, and employers) would not only increase the availability and quality of information for improved clinical care of the patient, but would also facilitate the exchange and linkage of health data for population-based functions like public health surveillance. However, in part because of fears about privacy, and because there is as yet no overarching federal law protecting health information privacy, the United States still has not defined a mechanism for assigning unique health identifiers to individuals. In fact, current US appropriations laws prohibit any further movement on this matter until such a unique health identifier is legislatively approved.[32]

Organizational Issues

Although this chapter describes many technical advances as facilitators for new approaches to data collection, integration of public health and healthcare delivery systems is not primarily a technical problem, but rather a political, as well as an organizational, problem. The programmatic orientation and organization within public health, described earlier in this chapter and seen at local, state, and CDC levels, is also reflected within the DHHS. HHS is organized into 11 operating divisions, of which CDC/ATSDR is only one. Clearly, other HHS agencies have responsibilities for and collect data from the public and various parts of the healthcare delivery system. Some of these data are also useful for public health. However, each of these agencies operates independently and develops partnerships with its own programmatic contacts, not unlike the partnerships developed by CDC's disease-specific programs with their state-based counterparts (e.g., Centers for Medicare and Medicaid Services [CMS] with state Medicaid or Medicare directors; Food and Drug Administration with state food agencies).

Acknowledging the need for increased coordination around data issues, HHS formed the HHS Data Council in August 1995. The Data Council coordinates all health and human service data collection and analysis activities of HHS. These activities include developing an integrated health data collection strategy, coordinating health data standards, and dealing with health information and privacy issues. The Data Council is also the focal point for HHS interactions with the National Committee on Vital and Health Statistics (NCVHS), an external advisory committee to the Secretary of HHS in the areas of health data policy, data standards, privacy concerns related to health information, and population-based data (see Chapter 14.) It is hoped that the Data Council and its related activities will facilitate a more comprehensive approach to health and the healthcare system. However, the challenges of coordinating the efforts of these agencies and their partners at local, state, and federal levels cannot be understated; similar organizational challenges have already been recognized in the medical informatics field.[33-35]

NEDSS Activities

Although there is much work ahead to attain the vision we have described, CDC, together with its public health partners, has initiated various activities directed toward realizing it (for more detail, see http://www.cdc.gov/nedss). The vision for NEDSS is depicted schematically in a public health-centric view in Figure 19.3.

Note that, compared with the activities in Figure 19.2, data collection and analysis are conducted with shared rather than independent facilities and tools. In addition, data interchange takes place by use of standardized electronic formats. Figure 19.3 also depicts standardized electronic data interchange (EDI) with regard to some of the myriad data sources outside public health. It should be clear from this description and the figure that NEDSS will rely on cross-cutting standards. CDC and its partners are building a common standards-based framework for surveillance information systems, one that consists of a common data architecture, a consistent user interface, open systems architecture standards, and standardized, secure Internet transmission of data to public health.

The common data architecture consists of several components—a public health conceptual data model, data definitions, and coding. These components provide a foundation for standardization of public health data collection, management, transmission, analysis, and dissemination. The public health conceptual data model (PHCDM) documents the categories and properties of data needed for surveillance (e.g., about persons or populations, health-related activities, case definitions, risk factors), and the relationships between them (e.g., a person can have many episodes of illness but each episode can have only one date of onset, with many dates for multiple specimens.) A supplement to the data model will also provide detailed standards for certain core data elements, including variable definition, with valid values for possible responses, and standards for how to collect, code, calculate, store, and present a data element.

Together, these elements of the data architecture provide a framework for organizing data standards and guidelines and facilitating data comparability and exchange with other systems. The PHCDM is intended to serve as a vehicle for communicating and reconciling the information needs of public health at all levels. And by providing a common starting point in terms of data constructs for database design, it will also reduce development efforts for computerized information systems used in public health. Logical data models from which database design models and physical models are subsequently derived may all be different in their implementation in a given state or public health program, but their mappings back to the PHCDM will be

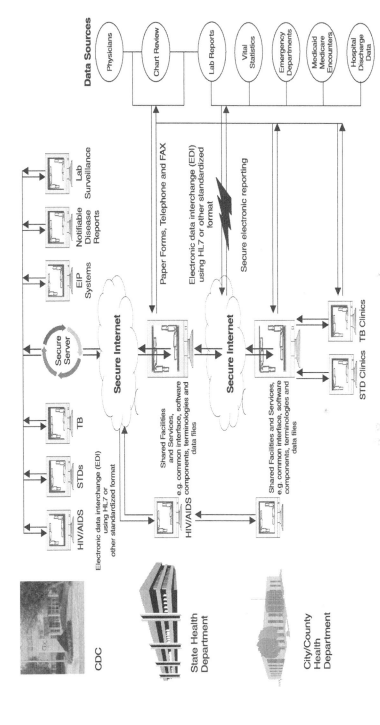

FIGURE 19.3. Proposed integrated surveillance systems solution. CDC, Centers for Disease Control and Prevention; EIP, Emerging Infections Program; HIV/AIDS, Human Immunodeficiency Virus/Acquired Immunodeficiency Syndrome; STDs, Sexually Transmitted Diseases; TB, Tuberculosis.

maintained, facilitating sharing of information among information systems. The data model also is critical to the development of standards for the exchange of information among public health and healthcare providers. The PHCDM facilitates communication of public health data needs to national standards-setting bodies such as HL7. Many classes and attributes in the PHCDM originated with HL7's Reference Information Model (RIM), given its comprehensive representation of the clinical world. However, use cases and concepts in the PHCDM have also been proposed to HL7, to broaden the scope of the RIM from the care of the individual patient to the care of populations, whether these are populations in an intensive care unit of a hospital, persons enrolled in a specific health plan or working in a given industry, or persons at high risk for a specific disease. CDC is spearheading efforts to harmonize the PHCDM with the RIM, to (it is hoped) mutual benefit. Table 19.2 provides an overview of the goals and objectives of the Public Health Conceptual Data Model:

Through NEDSS development activities, separate surveillance information systems will no longer have a different look and feel, and CDC programs

TABLE 19.2. Stated goals of the public health conceptual data model

PHCDM Goal	Purpose
Provide a framework for organizing data standards and guidelines	• Provide a context for data standards guidelines and permit persons working on data standards to determine areas for which data standards and guidelines are required.
Reduce development effort for computerized information systems used for public health	• Provide reusable analysis and database design; develop a common starting platform that can be used or modified, all reducing systems development time and cost.
Enhance data sharing through consistency	• Minimize the need for complex data mapping and transformation processes prior to sharing or reusing data.
Represent public health data needs to national standards-setting bodies	• Provide the ability to collaborate with national health informatics standards-setting bodies to define standards for the exchange of information among public health agencies and healthcare providers.
Facilitate collaboration between CDC and its state and local partners in public health	• PHCDM to serve as a vehicle for collecting and reconciling information that meets the needs of public health at all levels.

Source: Public Health Conceptual Data Model, Centers for Disease Control and Prevention. Available at: http://www.cdc.gov/nedss/Data models/phcdm.pdf. Accessed April 2, 2002.

will not develop tools separately for functions that are shared across systems, such as automated electronic capture of data from the healthcare system and data analysis or dissemination. In addition, NEDSS will use commercial off-the-shelf products when appropriate. NEDSS also includes or will include standards for items such as the user interface of the system and components such as registry matching or XML messaging. The user interface standards provide guidelines for consistent graphical user interfaces, whether for Windows or for browser-based systems.

These CDC constituents and any other information systems tools used at state and local health departments are intended for employment in the context of an information systems architecture containing elements that can be implemented in a modular fashion. Consistent with the rest of NEDSS activities, the information systems architecture also incorporates standards-based, open systems, thus providing a structure around which public health information systems can be integrated. This approach permits development, pilot testing, and implementation of NEDSS in phases at various sites in state and local health departments, using commercial industry standards. State and local health department partners will not be required to use CDC-developed software or components. This standards-based approach and the modular architectural framework should facilitate the sharing of data and reports among public health organizations at all levels.

In addition, given the need for a single, secure mechanism for transmitting data to CDC, NEDSS will make use of CDC's Secure Data Network (SDN), which protects Internet-based systems that involve the transmission and processing of sensitive or critical data. The SDN is a security subsystem based on standard security technology that:

- verifies client identity;
- controls access to protected Internet-based activities—file uploads, file downloads, sensitive Web pages, Web-based programs;
- encrypts data during transmission across the public Internet;
- certifies that information must have originated from a particular individual; and
- certifies that access to information is accessible only to a particular individual or group.

This network meets standards recommended by the National Research Council and is consistent with those that will be recommended as part of HIPAA security standards. It is hoped that the SDN lays the groundwork for direct, secure electronic exchange of data between public health and the healthcare system.

Related CDC Infrastructure Activities

NEDSS will rely on a public health workforce that has robust access to the Internet, the capacity to make secure connections, and the ability to use its data and information systems. The Health Alert Network (HAN) is a related activity that is designed to insure that all full-function local and state public health agencies have Internet access and training as well as access to distance-based learning technologies. HAN provides a vital infrastructure for NEDSS. In addition, public health has recognized the need for new skills among the public health workforce. These skills require an understanding of the role of data modeling and standards and the use of increasingly sophisticated information technology. Public health informatics, after all, is the "systematic application of information and computer science to public health practice, research, and learning".[36] For the promotion of the development of integrated systems for sharing data electronically with the health care information infrastructure, it will be essential for *all* public health workers to have a basic understanding of public health informatics, and for some workers to develop a deeper understanding of the application of informatics to gathering data for public health. CDC has made some initial efforts to develop the needed educational programs through a one-week general overview course in public health informatics for public health program managers[37] and a two-year public health informatics fellowship for training persons interested in careers in public health informatics (see http://www.cdc.gov/epo/dphsi/informat.htm). It is hoped that through expansion of these programs and through partnerships with the National Library of Medicine, which sponsors training programs in medical informatics at academic medical centers across the country, the numbers of public health workers trained in informatics will steadily increase. These efforts are critical for assembling the pool of workers that will build and maintain our public health information systems in the future.

Current Pilot Efforts

The NEDSS approach incorporates both long-term and short-term objectives. It is important to begin to capture electronically and use data from the healthcare system *now* if the long-term objectives are to be accomplished. Many of the activities we have described, especially those related to the data model and interactions with health informatics standards organizations, are geared toward influencing, in the future, how and what data are collected *a priori*. However, CDC and its public health partners are also conducting various pilot projects designed to capture data directly from providers, or to exchange data electronically as it presently exists and use it. In this process, public health is learning about the technical and policy implications and challenges of direct electronic sharing of data from outside public health.

These pilot efforts are aimed at capturing data that already exists in the private healthcare sector. Often, these are data that public health currently uses and that usually require paper-based reporting and re-entry of data. In Hawaii, for example, the State Health Department established a partnership with several laboratories.[38] Electronic capture of private sector laboratory data more than doubled the number of notifiable disease reports, reports that were also more complete and timely than those in the usual paper-based notifiable disease system. This particular effort did not rely on the use of national data standards. CDC and its public health partners, on the other hand, are exploring the electronic capture of key laboratory data through the use of standard HL7 messages containing data coded in LOINC and SNOMED clinical vocabularies.[39,40] CDC has also developed HL7 messages for use by immunization registries[41] and is piloting the use of HL7 messaging for cancer registries.[42] For further information, see Chapter 22.

Other pilot projects are geared more toward capturing data that exists in the healthcare system but are currently not widely available or used by public health. The Data Elements for Emergency Department Systems (DEEDS) project attempts to standardize information capture in emergency departments.[43,44] These standards are being pilot-tested, with sharing of emergency department data directly with the state health departments in Oregon[45] and North Carolina. The ultimate goal is routine electronic public health reporting for trauma, infectious disease, etc., triggered automatically by data entries in clinical emergency department records. Pharmacy data are another type of data underutilized by public health. A project in Massachusetts demonstrated the utility of electronically available health maintenance organization pharmacy data for detecting 18% more cases of active tuberculosis than were reported to the State Health Department.[46] In addition to hospital discharge databases, large data repositories, such as that of a large national clinical laboratory, have also been shown to contain data useful for public health purposes.[47] And, given the strong interest in early detection of a bioterrorist event, many state or local health departments are attempting to capture and use nonspecific healthcare system data such as 911 calls, Emergency Management System responses, emergency department and other acute care visits, and intensive care unit beds or admissions, in addition to hospital clinical data on diseases or syndromes and medical examiner or death certificate data, by cause of death or syndrome.[18,48] CDC's National Center for Health Statistics is working with partners, including the National Association for Public Health Statistics and Information Systems (NAPHSIS), to develop standardized electronic birth and death certificates that should improve the timeliness, completeness, and utility of vital statistics reporting (see http://www.naphsis.org and Chapter 14.)

In recognition of the complexities and longer-term nature of the goal of capturing and using data from already existing electronic information systems, some state health departments and CDC programs have designed their systems so that providers can enter data in a protected fashion directly over the Internet. These notifiable disease systems in the states of Colorado, Kansas, and New York, the CDC unexplained deaths surveillance project, and the Hazardous Substances Emergency Event Surveillance System not only allow direct data entry by participants in the system, but also are designed to permit

direct queries of the data and feedback of reports. CDC also worked with state
and local health departments to set up similar, temporary surveillance systems in emergency departments during events such as the World Trade Organization meeting in Seattle in December 1999, as well as the 2000 Democratic
and Republican national conventions. The experiences with these systems
underscore the value of supplying immediate feedback and analytic capacity
to data providers and other participants in the system. However, to the extent
that these systems require data entry activities distinct from those undertaken
during routine provision of care, they may unduly increase the burden of
reporting for healthcare providers and may not be sustainable in the long run.

Conclusions

The continuing changes in the healthcare system in the United States, the
increased emphasis on standardization of healthcare transactions, and the
advent of the Internet and other advances in information technology are con-
verging with a strong and growing interest in capturing an increasing amount
of health-related data electronically. Public health organizations, therefore,
are attempting to take advantage of these opportunities by moving away from
independent disease-based or programmatic systems to collect data through a
more comprehensive approach that involves capture of data that are already
electronic, especially from (although not limited to) the healthcare system.
The development of integrated and comprehensive public health information
systems requires the ongoing cooperation, collaboration, and contributions
of public and private organizations. These organizations include but are not
limited to state and local health department epidemiologists, public and private medical and public health laboratories, state and federal vital statistics
programs, federal agencies (e.g., in addition to the DHHS agencies, the Department of Transportation, the Environmental Protection Agency, and the
Department of Labor), managed care organizations, professional organizations, and national standards development organizations.

Indeed, the efforts of CDC and its public health partners, as exemplified by
NEDSS, fit within a larger framework of activities at the federal level. Together with the National Center for Health Statistics (part of CDC) and the
HHS Data Council, the NCVHS is developing a vision for health statistics for
the 21st century, one that is supportive of the concept of integration of public
health and healthcare delivery systems (http://ncvhs.hhs.gov/). It is intended
that the vision reflect all manifestations of health and healthcare delivery,
while also encompassing population health, healthcare delivery systems, and
the interactions between the two. This vision will integrate and coordinate
public and private data sets, as well as data collected and maintained at the
national, state, and local levels. NCVHS also recommends building and integrating the health information infrastructure through a set of technologies,

standards, and applications that support communication and information to develop a national health information infrastructure.[49] NCVHS has described three types of presumably integrated computer-based health records—(1) personal (consumer), (2) healthcare provider (clinical care), and (3) community— for monitoring the health of the public and outcomes. NCVHS has recommended that this infrastructure be driven by patient care and health status, and not by reimbursement. This comprehensive view is consistent with the long-term direction in which public health needs to go.

Exciting opportunities exist today to transform many of public health's monitoring functions and to integrate them more closely with the health care information infrastructure. To be most effective, the public health community must be able to use data from many different sources both within and outside of public health, with rapid dissemination of data to those who need to take action to protect the health of the public. In deciding to develop such integrated systems, the United States is joining such countries as Australia,[50] Great Britain,[51] and Canada,[52] in all of which efforts are well under way to integrate public health and health information systems and activities.

Questions for Review

1. *Questions 1a-c are based on the following short case:* Governmental authorities have alerted the CDC that reliable information establishes the strong possibility that a terrorist group plans to expose the populations of five major cities to deadly anthrax. The CDC has been asked to coordinate efforts to detect early diagnoses of anthrax with the healthcare providers of the five cities, with the local public health organizations, and with state health departments of the states in which the five major cities exist. At present, the overburdened healthcare providers and laboratories in these five cities use a hodge-podge of slow and incomplete paper-based systems to report the existence of notifiable conditions to local public health departments. Local public health departments manually enter the data from paper-based forms into their computer systems, none of which communicate directly with other local systems or with the various state systems. Local public health departments then send the captured data to their respective state health departments in the form of data tapes or on diskettes, which are loaded into computerized state health department surveillance systems. The state health departments in the five states in which the cities are located must manipulate the data in order to make it available to the CDC.
   a. List at least five reasons that the existing systems will likely be too slow, inefficient, and ineffective in alerting the CDC to the occurrence and magnitude of outbreaks of anthrax poisoning.
   b. Explain the factors that have led to the situation depicted, in which a

    variety of health authorities have developed independent and incompatible systems for reporting morbidity.

  c. Explain how the NEDSS system, if fully deployed at this time, would permit the CDC to collect more complete data on anthrax outbreaks rapidly. Identify the reasons that NEDSS would likely be a more effective means of capturing data, analyzing the data, and comparing the data across the five cities.

2. Identify at least four factors that serve as motivators for change in the way that healthcare providers and public health organizations are collecting, sharing, and analyzing data needed to protect public health. Explain the contribution that each of these factors is making.

3. In what sense do (1) public health policy and (2) recent changes in information technology serve as enablers of change in the way that healthcare providers and public health organizations collect and exchange data?

4. Explain how Extensible Markup Language (XML) functions in enabling changes in public health data collection and transfer.

5. Explain why the increased use of industry standards for information systems design and development is important to the change that must occur in the way that public health collects and shares data.

6. In what sense are (1) privacy of health information and (2) unique health identifiers requirements for future public health data collection systems? Why are unique health identifiers so controversial that Congress has reserved the right to approve their implementation?

7. In what sense is integration of public health and healthcare delivery systems a political and an organizational problem, rather than merely a technical problem?

Acknowledgments

We would like to thank Dan Friedman, PhD., and John P. Fanning, for their helpful comments.

References

1. Thacker SB, Berkelman RL. Public health surveillance in the United States. *Epidemiol Rev* 1988;10:164–190.

2. Teutsch SM, Churchill RE, eds. *Principles and Practice of Public Health Surveillance.* New York: Oxford University Press; 2000.

3. Thacker SB, Stroup DF. Future directions for comprehensive public health surveillance and health information systems in the United States. *Am J Epidemiol* 1994;140:383–397.

4. Morris G, Snider D, Katz M. Integrating public health information and surveillance systems. *J Public Health Manag Pract* 1996;2:24–27.

5. Marier R. The reporting of communicable diseases. *Am J Epidemiol* 1977;105:587–590.

6. Kirsch T, Shesser R. A survey of emergency department communicable disease reporting practices. *J Emerg Med.* 1991:9:211–214.

7. Konowitz PM, Petrossian GA, Rose DN. The underreporting of disease and physicians' knowledge of reporting requirements. *Public Health Rep* 1984;99:31–35.

8. Simpson DM. Improving the reporting of notifiable diseases in Texas: Suggestions from an ad hoc committee of providers. *J Public Health Manag Pract* 1996:2:37–39.

9. Campos-Outcalt D, England R, Porter B. Reporting of communicable diseases by university physicians. *Public Health Rep* 1991;106:579–583.

10. Alter MJ, Mares A, Hadler SC, et al. The effect of under reporting on the apparent incidence and epidemiology of acute viral hepatitis. *Am J Epidemiol* 1987:125:133–139.

11. Brackbill RM, Sternberg MR, Fishbein M. Where do people go for treatment of sexually transmitted diseases? *Fam Plann Perspect* 1999;31:10–15.

12. Kimball AM, Thacker SB, Levy ME. *Shigella* surveillance in a large metropolitan area: Assessment of a passive reporting system. *Am J Public Health* 1980;70:164–166.

13. Rosenberg ML, Marr JS, Gangarosa EJ, Pollard RA, Wallace M, Brolnitsky O. *Shigella* surveillance in the United States, 1975. *J Infect Dis* 1977:136:458–460.

14. Birkhead G, Chorba TL, Root S, Klaucke DN, Gibbs NJ. Timeliness of national reporting of communicable diseases: the experience of the National Electronic Telecommunications System for Surveillance. *Am J Public Health* 1991;81:1313–1315.

15. Koobatian TJ, Birkhead BS, Schramm MM, Vogt RL. The use of hospital discharge data for public health surveillance of Guillain-Barre Syndrome. *Ann Neurol* 1991;30:618–621.

16. Huff L, Bogdan G, Burke K et al. Using hospital discharge data for disease surveillance. *Public Health Rep* 1996:1111:78–81.

17. Annest JL, Mercy JA. Use of national data systems for firearm-related injury surveillance. *Am J Prev Med.* 1998;15:17–30.

18. Rotz LD, Koo D, O'Carroll PW, Kellogg RB, Lillibridge SR. Bioterrorism preparedness: Planning for the future. *J Public Health Manag Pract* 2000;6:45–49.

19. Barrows RC, Clayton PD. Privacy, confidentiality, and electronic medical records. *J Am Med Inform Assoc* 1996;3:139–148.

20. National Research Council, Computer Science and Telecommunications Board, Commission of Physical Sciences, Mathematics and Applications. *For The Record: Protecting Electronic Health Information.* Washington, DC: National Academy Press; 1997.

21. Halamka JD, Szolovits P, Rind D, Safran C. A WWW implementation of national recommendations for protecting electronic health information. *J Am Med Inform Assoc* 1997:4:458–464.

22. Harman J. Topics for our times: new health-care data—new horizons for public health. *Am J Public Health.* 1998;88:1019–1021.

23. Chute CG, Cohn SP, Campbell JR, et al. A framework for comprehensive health terminology systems in the United States: development guidelines, criteria for selection, and public policy implications. *J Am Med Inform Assoc* 1998;5:503–510.

24. Dolin RH. Advances in data exchange for the clinical laboratory. *Clin Lab Med* 1999;19:385–419.

25. Dolin RH, Rishel W, Biron PV, Spinosa J, Mattison JE. SGML and XML as interchange formats for HL7 messages. *Proc AMIA Symp* 1998;720–724.

26. Lasker RD, Humphreys BL, Braithwaite WR. *Making a Powerful Connection: The Health of the Public and the National Information Infrastructure.* Washington, DC: Public Health Data Policy Coordinating Committee, US Public Health Service; 1995.

27. Dick RS, Steen EB, eds. *The Computer-Based Patient Record: An Essential Technology for Health Care.* Washington, DC: National Academy Press; 1991.

28. Gostin LO, Hodge JG. Balancing individual privacy and communal uses of health information. White paper prepared for the workshop on The Implications of HIPAA's Administrative Simplification Provisions for Public Health and Health Services Research; November 2-3, 1998; Washington, DC. Available at http://www.cdc.gov/nchs/otheract/phdsc/presenters/gostin.htm. Accessed April 2, 2002.

29. Gostin LO. Health information privacy. *Cornell Law Rev* 1995;80:451–528.

30. Gostin LO, Lazzarini Z, Neslund VS, Osterholm MT. The public health information infrastructure. A national review of the law on health information privacy. *JAMA* 1996;275:1921–1927.

31. US Department of Health and Human Services. 45 CFR Parts 160 and 164. Standards in privacy of individually identifiable health information; final rule. Federal Register 2000;65:82462–82829.

32. The Consolidated Appropriations Act, 2000. Pub. L. No. 106-113. § 514 (1999).

33. Braude RM. People and organizational issues in health informatics. *J Am Med Inform Assoc* 1997;4:150–151.

34. Lorenzi NM, Riley RT, Blyth AJ, Southon G, Dixon BJ. Antecedents of the people and organizational aspects of medical informatics: review of the literature. *J Am Med Inform Assoc* 1997;4:79–93.

35. Southon FCG, Sauer C, Dampney CN. Information technology in complex health services: organization impediments to successful technology transfer and diffusion. *J Am Med Inform Assoc* 1997;4:112–124.

36. Yasnoff WA, O'Carroll PW, Koo D, Linkins RW, Kilbourne EM. Public health informatics: Improving and transforming public health in the information age. *J Public Health Management Practice.* 2000;6:67–75.

37. O'Carroll PW, Yasnoff WA, Wilhoite W. Public health informatics: A CDC course for public health program managers. In: Christopher G. Chute, MD, DrPh, ed. *A Paradigm Shift in Health Care Information Systems: Clinical Infrastuctures for the 21st Century. Proceedings of the 1998 AMIA Annual Symposium.* Bethesda, MD:American Medical Informatics Association; 1998:472–476.

38. Effler P, Ching-Lee M, Bogard A, Ieong M, Nekomoto T, Jernigan D. Statewide system of electronic notifiable disease reporting from clinical laboratories. Comparing automated reporting with conventional methods. *JAMA.* 1999:282:1845–1850.

39. Centers for Disease Control and Prevention. Electronic reporting of laboratory information for public health. Summary of meeting proceedings; January 7-8, 1999; Atlanta, GA. Available at: http://www.cdc.gov/od/hissb/act_elr.htm. Accessed April 2, 2002.

40. White MD, Kolar LM, Steindel SJ. Evaluation of vocabularies for electronic laboratory reporting to public health agencies. *J Am Med Inform Assoc* 1999;6:185–194.

41. National Immunization Program. *Implementation Guide for Immunization Data Transactions Using Version 2.3 of the Health Level Seven (HL7) Standard Protocol: Implementation Guide Version 2.0.* Atlanta, GA: Centers for Disease Control and Prevention; 1999. Available at: http://www.cdc.gov/nip/registry/lnip/registry/hl7guide.pdf.

42. Centers for Disease Control and Prevention. Working toward implementation of HL7 in NAACCR information technology standards. Meeting summary report; October

1998. Available at: http://www.cdc.gov/nccdphp/dcpc/npcr/npcrpdfs/hl7mtg8.pdf. Accessed April 2, 2002.

43. National Center for Injury Prevention and Control. Data Elements for Emergency Department Systems, Release 1.0. Atlanta, GA: Centers for Disease Control and Prevention; 1997.

44. DEEDS Writing Committee. Data Elements for Emergency Department Systems, Release 1.0 (DEEDS): A summary report. *Ann Emerg Med* 1998;31:264–273.

45. Kohn MA, Zechnich AD, Jui J, et al. Using electronically transmitted clinical data from emergency rooms for emerging infections surveillance. Presented at the International Conference on Emerging Infectious Diseases: ICEID 2000; July 16–19, 2000; Atlanta, GA.

46. Yokoe DS, Subramanyan GS, Nardell E, Sharnprapai S, McCray E, Platt R. Supplementing tuberculosis surveillance with automated data from health maintenance organizations. *Emerg Inf Dis* 1999;5:779–787.

47. Jernigan DB, Koski E, Shoemake HA, Mallon RP, Pinner RW. Evaluation of laboratory test orders and results in a national laboratory data repository: Implications for infectious diseases surveillance. Presented at the International Conference on Emerging Infectious Diseases: ICEID 2000; July 16–19, 2000; Atlanta, GA

48. Nolte KB, Yoon SS, Pertowski C. Medical examiners, coroners, and bioterrorism. *Emerg Infect Dis* 2000;6:559–660.

49. National Committee on Vital and Health Statistics. *Toward a National Health Information Infrastructure. Interim Report*; June 2000. Available at: http://ncvhs.hhs.gov/NHII2kReport.htm. Accessed April 2, 2002.

50. Ministry of Health/Australia. Agreement Between the Health Authorities of the Commonwealth of Australia, the States and Territories of Australia, the Australian Institute of Health and Welfare, and the Australian Bureau of Statistics. National Health Information Agreement, established 1993. Available at: http://www.aihw.gov.au/html/nhiaagre.htm. Accessed April 2, 2002.

51. National Health Service Information Authority, United Kingdom. The Background to the Health-care Modeling Programme. June 24, 1999. Available at: http://www.standards.nhsia.nhs.uk/hcm/htmldocs/fs-background.html. Access April 2, 2002.

52. Health Canada. National Conference of Health Infostructure, February 8–10, 1998. Available at: http://www.hc-sc.gc.ca/ohih-bsi/cnics/nchi_cnis_e.html.

20

New Means for Increasing Data Accessibility

ROBB CHAPMAN

Learning Objectives

After studying this chapter, you should be able to:

- List and define the characteristics of the three basic forms of data access.
- Explain why data are an expensive and a valuable resource, and list the reasons that an organization that owns data might want to share them and might not want to share them.
- Explain the characteristics of data access trends in the 1970s, 1980s, and 1990s.
- List and discuss at least five present-day considerations that an organization must make in building public health data access systems.
- Explain the characteristics, advantages, and disadvantages of using a data warehouse approach to sharing data.
- Explain why Web-based deployment of databases is a popular choice, and list at least six drawbacks or limitations inherent in Web-based deployment as it generally exists today.
- Define the concept of the data web, listing and explaining at least seven characteristics that render a data web approach to data access desirable.

Overview

Increasingly, organizations are finding that data are an expensive and valuable resource that needs to be husbanded carefully. Today, access to data takes several forms; the form varies according to the type of data analysis to be performed. Although there are many reasons that an organization might not want to share data, there are also benefits that an organization can derive from data sharing. The history of data-sharing technology over the past three decades has led to today's Web-based approach to database deployment. Although the current Web-based approach to data sharing has undeniable advantages, it also features certain disadvantages that render the approach less than ideal. The concept of a data web as a means of providing data access holds promise of providing an architecture that overcomes the limitations of today's Web-based approaches. It also accommodates the increasing need to examine data from socioeconomic, criminal justice, and environmental domains in conjunction with public and private health provider and payer data.

Introduction

The practice of public health can be considered, somewhat simplistically, as a three-stage process. First, data pertaining to some aspect of a health issue is gathered. Second, the data are studied and analyzed, and in the process they are transformed from data into information. Third, this information is used to guide a course of action aimed at changing, hopefully for the better, some social health condition.

The first of these steps comprises the varied data-gathering activities of public health: disease surveillance, surveying the populace, compiling of vital statistics, etc. The second step, data analysis, is predicated upon data access, the focus of this chapter. For our purposes, *data access* is access to data already gathered and compiled, for purposes of analysis and reporting, outside the context of any particular program, health area, or application. Here, we will regard data access not only as a technical problem, but also as an administrative, an organizational, and a political problem.

In this chapter, we will first differentiate among the common forms of data access. We will then discuss data as a business resource, including why organizations do and do not want to share data. After a brief treatment of the history of data access over the past three decades, we will discuss present-day considerations for building data access systems in public health. After a discussion of considerations in choosing an architecture to facilitate data sharing, we will point out some of the shortcomings inherent in a Web-based approach to providing data for use by healthcare and public health workers. We will conclude the chapter with a discussion of a data-sharing development mentioned in the previous chapter, the data web, including its characteristics and advantages.

Forms of Data Access

Data access can take several forms, and the types of data analysis that data support can vary correspondingly.

- *Access to fundamental data.* This level of access to data in all its detail and complexity supports exploratory data analysis. Researchers looking for new relationships or trying to illuminate poorly understood relationships between cause and effect in public health issues would be candidates for this level of access. The need of such researchers is for very flexible access to very detailed data and for precise data documentation. This type of analysis requires considerable sophistication in understanding and manipulating data—data used for such issues as survey methodology, choosing the correct weight to apply, calculation of confidence intervals, and measuring statistical significance.

- *Access to pre-interpreted data.* Pre-interpreted data might include aggregated data, data otherwise processed to enhance integrity and accuracy, or data processed to provide confidentiality. This kind of data is appropriate for what might be termed *guided data analysis*. Health program planners, policy makers, or health issue advocates who are looking for metrics on the size or severity of a well-defined, well-understood problem would be a typical audience for this level of access. Pre-interpreted data provide decision support. The need here is for somewhat flexible access to fairly detailed data. This type of analysis requires less sophistication in understanding and manipulating data.
- *Access to presentations based on data, such as reports, graphs, and maps.* This level of access is appropriate for the public, who are targeted with educational information, easily digested summaries and reports, and public health messages.

As is true in other areas of informatics and information technology, data access over the last several decades has become easier, more powerful, and available to a wider and less technically sophisticated audience.

The Business of Data

Data are an expensive and valuable resource. Data have market value; they represent a revenue stream for many academic and governmental agencies. Whether in the form of actual data sets on disk or of hardcopy reports bound in volumes, data are sold by many data-gathering organizations, even publicly funded ones. This should not be surprising, considering the effort and expense that go into gathering, compiling, cleaning, integrating, and storing some of these data sets. Businesses, political groups, and other organizations need and are quite happy to pay for information that supports their activities. Researchers at some organizations have significant personal and professional investment in their data; in fact, some have built their careers upon expertise in one or a few data sets, and many of these data sets are large and complex enough to require years of study and experience to interpret and utilize. Such resources are not something one gives away.

Why Organizations Do Not Want to Share Data

Even where data has been compiled through use of public funding, as in most government and academic settings, provision for general access to data is not often a priority. Although taxpayers, with legislatures behind them, increasingly see it as their right to see and use data that they have already paid for with tax dollars, it is a simple fact that most government and academic organizations, already pressed for funding, cannot afford to give away what they have struggled to obtain. Table 20.1 provides an overview of the typical reasons that organizations may not want to share data with the general public or with groups or individuals.

Possession of the data and authority over the interpretation of it may constitute the basis of an organization's authority; the idea of general public access to data can be perceived as an actual threat to an organization's continued existence. On a more fundamental level, it costs real money to publish and mail disks, to publish books, to create and maintain Web sites, and to pay staff to perform these tasks. Disseminating data to the wider world may or may not be one of the primary mandates, and more to the point, one of the funded mandates of the organization. Some organizations address this problem by charging for data simply to cover their costs of distributing it.

Another reason that organizations hesitate to provide general access to their data is that it may be dangerous to provide general access to uninterpreted data. After all, data can be misused and misinterpreted, either intentionally or because of simple ignorance. An organization may see the public and all organizational outsiders, justifiably or not, as unfit to interpret data properly, even if the outsiders have access to computers to assist in interpreting the data. After all, it is notoriously difficult to capture heuristics and such "right-

TABLE 20.1. Typical reasons that organizations do not want to share data

Reasons for Not Sharing Data	Comment
Organizational authority	Release of the data may pose an actual threat to the organization's continued existence.
Cost	Expenses of sharing include staff costs, mailing costs, publishing costs, Web site maintenance costs.
Funding	The organization may not be receiving a funding mandate to share data, and thus such data sharing is not a priority.
Ethical considerations	The organization may not perceive the general public as fit to interpret data properly, and thus there is a risk of misinterpretation.
Data security	The risk that providing general access to data may expose the data to hackers or malicious intruders, or else users may mistakenly modify or delete data fields or leave data pathways unguarded. Alternatively, providing general access to the data may run afoul of laws protecting the confidentiality of information about private citizens.

brained" abilities as "interpretation" in a computer system. The effort and expense required to capture and present institutional knowledge about data may be too daunting to contemplate.

In fact, it is dangerous to provide general access to data, period. Data security obviously is or ought to be a major concern to organizations that make their livelihood from data. It is an inescapable fact that the security of a data set is indirectly proportional to the number of persons who have access to it. Aside from the obvious concern over hackers and malicious intruders, as discussed in Chapter 10, bona fide users can mistakenly modify or delete fields, records, or files; overwhelm systems with too much work; introduce viruses; and leave privileged access pathways unprotected. Data access should never be attempted without tightly coupled attention to data security.

Finally, it may be unethical or illegal to provide general access to data. This can be particularly the case in the public health arena, where health information about private citizens is the subject and where personal privacy and confidentiality issues are common.

Why Organizations Want to Share Data

Nonetheless, despite the reasons for not wanting to share data, there is at the same time a genuine interest among health organizations in providing access to their data. These organizations view data as a product, a positive contribution that the organization makes to society, and a marketing tool. Possession of data and standing as an authoritative source of data bestows worth and value on an organization. Thus, organizations trade or give away data as a strategy to build up constituencies and clienteles, to attract business, to impress legislatures and funding sources, and to prove their value as organizations: Witness the stacks of CD-ROMs being handed out at health conventions and the eager proliferation of Web sites featuring data access.

Progress in Data Access over the Last Three Decades

The trends in data access over the last 30 years show that data access capability has migrated (1) from a technically adept few to the technically unsophisticated masses; (2) from organizational insiders to significant partners to the general public; and (3) from application-specific formats to "open architecture" formats (e.g., HyperText Markup Language [HTML], eXtensible Markup Language [XML]), and (4) from proprietary networks to the Web.

The 1970s

During the 1970s, businesses, governments, and other organizations moved from paper-based systems to mainframe computer systems. This transition was a direct result of the maturation and increased cost-effectiveness of magnetic tape and disk storage technology, the greater availability and decreasing cost of large database management systems, the replacement of punched cards with terminals as primary input devices, and the development of a computer-literate workforce. The first large-scale computerized government and private health-related information systems appeared in this decade.

During the 1970s, the Internet was unknown outside the defense and academic communities, and dial-up modem access was too slow for applications involving any appreciable volume of data. Access to computerized information, therefore, more or less depended on access to a terminal directly connected to a central computer via a proprietary network. Terminals usually existed exclusively in offices of the organization that owned a system. Access to data, therefore, depended on organizational affiliation and physical proximity to the machine. In practical terms, only employees of the organization or of direct partners had real-time access to an organization's data.

The formatting and structuring of databases were unique to each system. Proprietary databases and the proprietary computer programs that fed and cared for them evolved together in an inbred, incestuous manner. The databases were virtually inaccessible without special computer code unique to a database structure, and the computer code was usually incapable of accessing other databases. Writing, compiling, and executing this code required considerable programming skill and experience. Computer programmers—a very small minority of the organizational workforce—were the only available intermediaries to data access. For most users, data access was more or less limited to reports printed on hardcopy or displayed on 80 x 25 terminals and containing tables of aggregated data or detailed listings of fields from individual records. A given report could generally be executed with a small number of parameters that could be set at run time, the only control that could be exerted by the nonprogrammer. Nonprogrammers—users—could request new reports in support of some new business requirement, but in large organizations the waits of weeks to months or even years for these new reports to materialize became the stuff of sardonic cartoons and office legend.

The 1980s

During the 1980s, relational database technology and the structured query language (SQL) gained acceptance. This was a significant step toward establishment of what would eventually become universal database interfaces that encapsulate (hide) the particulars of a database implementation.

The personal computer revolution swept businesses and government, along with graphical user interfaces, user-friendly software, and the heretical notion that ordinary users could store, process, and present their own data without the services of a staff programmer. Spreadsheet software, in particular, with its highly flexible applicability and its built-in graphics, proved extraordinarily popular among business users and data users. However, PCs of the time lacked the sheer storage capacity and computing power required for large-scale database applications; therefore, significant efforts began to front-end the massive storage and computing power of the mainframe, along with the existing sophisticated mainframe application code base, with the user-friendliness and the compelling graphical capabilities of the PC.

Local-area networks (LANs) and the LAN-based file servers appeared. Dial-up modem access speeds reached 2400 bits per second. It became practical to provide remote dial-in access to an organization's internal systems from across a campus or from across the country.

Another major innovation of this decade was the advancement of report writers and statistical analysis software targeted at nonprogrammers—not ordinary users, perhaps, but knowledge-domain experts such as statisticians and epidemiologists. Such products as SAS, SPSS, and other packages required significantly less than full-fledged computer programming ability and shielded the user from much of the arcana of the computing environment. At the same time, these products enabled users to employ the superior storage and processing capabilities of the mainframe. Using a scaled-down set of commands that often mimicked the words and syntax of normal language, users were now able to write their own sorts, merges, data extraction procedures, and analysis routines and to produce analyses and reports. Users could build up their own libraries of reports and processing routines, modify them at will, and share them for use by others. Although much simpler than traditional computer programming, in any but the most trivial applications these products unavoidably drew their users into considerations such as conditional execution, loops, variable names, and other esoterica previously considered the domain of computer programming, and therefore required a considerable amount of educational investment to use. But the bang was worth the buck, and a huge number of scientists, epidemiologists, and statisticians made the investment in learning to use an analysis or reporting system. Using these systems, users obtained results much faster, and the domain expert was in control of the programming and had the liberty of trying different approaches—of playing with the data. Exploratory data analysis on the computer was now possible.

The 1990s

During the 1990s, the World Wide Web made the Internet a household word and became a dominant force in all aspects of commerce and government. In addition, important principles of open system design were advanced, giving rise to the object-oriented design paradigm and open architecture standards and technologies such as Java, ODBC, JDBC, XML, and CORBA/RMI. These technologies actually represent a profound shift in the business model of many information technology companies, away from attempted solo domination of the market and toward market share advancement through the building of symbiotic, mutually beneficial relationships.

Present-Day Considerations for Building
Public Health Data Access Systems

Today, there are many issues to consider in building public health data access systems. Before a builder of a system designs it, and well before a system architecture and a set of development tools and methods are selected, the nature of the system—its overall intent, the nature of its content, and the nature of its users—should be considered in a methodical way. The first and most pivotal issues to resolve are these: What data are to be presented, why are the data being presented, and who is the target audience? The answers to these questions inform virtually all aspects of the system design, from the layout and behavior of the user interface to the network architecture and database design.

On one extreme, the intent may be to provide the public at large with health statistics of general interest, such as birth and death counts, disease incidence, and hospital utilization data. Here, the emphasis needs to be on making the query interface clear and understandable and the presentation of the data such that results cannot be misinterpreted, even if this means sacrificing flexibility, functionality, and detail available in the data. For example, a system developer should give thought to selecting the most appropriate population denominators and precalculating rates, or perhaps use age-adjusted rates, so that naive users do not draw mistaken conclusions by comparing incidences of health events between unlike populations. Fast response times are also imperative; the public is easily bored and will quickly abandon a system perceived to be unresponsive. Gearing presentation toward the interests of specific communities and populations helps to generate interest. Thus, business graphics and maps will be highly desirable. An overall useful approach to such a system is to ascertain which views of the data are likely to be most sought after, and then, for performance reasons, to generate presummarized data sets containing no more detail than is required to deliver these views.

On the other extreme, the intent may be to serve the needs of the scientific community by providing researchers with access to original, detailed data. For example, the owner of an extensive health survey data set may be charged with providing access to researchers in the academic community. Here, it can be assumed that the system's users will be comfortable with the intricacies of complex data sets and will want to perform their own calculations and data manipulations. The system, therefore, should make as few assumptions as possible about how the data are going to be used and should process the data as little as possible, or perhaps only under direct command of the user. For example, the system can provide rate calculations, weighted averages, etc., as processing options at the discretion of the user. The system should also deliver as much data detail as possible at the expense of response time; researchers who have serious need of the data will tend to be computer savvy. will appreciate the demands they are placing on a system, and should be willing to wait for minutes or even hours to obtain what they need. Detailed documentation—metadata—about how and by whom the data were collected, sampling methods used, data element definitions, and explications of all data element values are a hard requirement. Graphics and maps, however, are not a high priority in such a system; in fact, little attention need be paid to beautiful presentation of the data at all. On the contrary, it should probably be assumed that users will import the data into a favorite sophisticated analysis program, which will vary from user to user; therefore, the data access system should emphasize file export capability more than data presentation capability. Table 20.2 summarizes the contrasts in the types of data access suitable for use by the general public, on the one hand, and by the research-oriented scientific community on the other.

What data are to be presented? Generally, organizations choose to put up their own data. But in some instances, they put up complimentary data originating in other organizations as well. For instance, community health indicator data can be complimented with economic and demographic data. Moreover, community health indicators can tell a more interesting story if they are compared against comparable indicators at the state level and national level. An organization today may find itself in a position to acquire and use data from another organization and also decide to present these data jointly with its own in one system. Such an idea is compelling, but before an organization embarks on such a venture, it is critical to establish some form of long-term agreement with the outside organization to help insure that updates for the imported data will be available in the future, in a form that is consistent with the present form of the data, so that data do not become quickly outdated or else change to such an extent that the system requires rewriting. Failure to establish such an agreement could result in an expensive failure—a system that becomes rapidly outdated or that must be revamped frequently.

Once an organization knows what data are to be presented, it must consider the scope of the data over the dimensions of geography and time. What geographic areas are to be included? How many years of data should be presented? The jurisdictional authority of the organization usually answers the question of geography. Determining how many years of data to offer requires weighing the relative value of performing trend analysis over time against the increasing cost, in both hardware and system performance, of housing more data. Many health applications are really interested only in the most current available data or data covering the last five years or so. On the other hand, public health programs have been known to need systems holding 20 or 30 years' data. One significant difficulty that arises with a requirement for many years of data is that the structure or content of data sets tends to change

TABLE 20.2. Contrasting data access needs of the general public and the scientific community

System Characteristic	General Public Need	Scientific Need
Data type	• Health statistics of general interest, presented by use of presummarization and in a way in which results cannot be misinterpreted	• Original, detailed data without presummarization and without processing, with options available to the user to perform rate calculations, weighted averages, etc.
Data interface	• Clear and understandable, with no assumption made about user familiarity with the interface	• Assumption that user will be computer savvy and will understand interface
Response time	• Speed at the expense of detail is a necessity	• Detail, even at the expense of speed
Data presentation	• Use of graphics and maps to help users interpret data • Emphasis on gearing data toward interests of the community	• Graphics and maps not a priority; priority is providing complete data and detailed documentation, including information about data collection, sampling methods, data element definitions, and explications of all data element values • Comprehensive presentation of data and data sets

over time. New variables are introduced, old ones are retired, or the categorical values or variables can take on change.

One simple example of this problem occurs in the Census population estimates over spans of decades. The race and ethnicity categories employed in these population estimates vary significantly over time, from "white/nonwhite" in the early 1960s, to "white/black/other" in the 1970s, to the 2000 Census in which respondents were allowed to classify themselves as any combination of dozens of newly recognized race and ethnicity categories. A researcher relying on Census estimates spanning these decades would have to make difficult choices before these population counts could be presented in a consolidated fashion by race. For example, either the number of race/ethnicity classifications would need to be collapsed into a set that is common across all years, or else the scope of years would need to be constrained. It is not possible to ferret out more granularity than existed in the original older data, and it would be presumptuous to impute what the race/ethnicity ratios might have been decades ago. This same type of comparability problem crops up when the "same" data from multiple regions are compiled; the various regions are likely to display local variations in the precise data elements collected, in the data element definitions, and in the data element values encoded. It is a phenomenon that is certain to occur whenever the scope of data is extended along any dimension: As the scope of the data increases, the probability of a breakdown in the comparability of data increases.

An additional design consideration emerges around the issue of data content. If the intent is to put up more than one data set in the system, then code reuse and consistency of functionality and system behavior from the user's point of view is important. Nothing is more frustrating to users than having to learn a new interface and a new set of behaviors for each content area. The system needs to be designed to reuse code and enforce consistency across content areas.

Are the data sensitive in any way? Are all the data sets appropriate for public access, or are there data that must be restricted to access only by the public health research community or trusted associates? If access control is necessary, the complexity of both developing and operating the system increases significantly. The best and surest solution, if it is possible, is to constrain the system to an enclosed network, such as the organization's LAN, and to use the existing network and server security facilities to restrict access. However, if the system must be made available to users on a public network, then the system developers have no choice but to become immersed in the security business. This is a topic that exceeds the scope of the present chapter. Suffice it to say that it is imperative that system security proceed from a security model that delineates roles and authorities—what system functions must be restricted and what roles will be defined with authority to perform them—and that an organization must give significant thought to how the system's security will be managed and operated over the long haul. And if the organization is going to use the Internet to provide access to a public network, it is necessary to recognize that the traditional method of authenticating users with user ID accounts and passwords is woefully inadequate in an age of sophisticated hackers. The system's security should instead be based on the best practical Internet security technology available and integrated with the organization's network security plan (see Chapter 10).

What desktop systems do the intended users typically operate? Are they all Windows users running on Intel-based computers, or is there a mix of operating systems and platforms? Do they tend to have up-to-date, powerful machines or are there older, slower machines in the mix? Is it practical to ignore the constraints of the slowest machines, or is it important to be as inclusive of slower machines as possible?

Are the intended users generally computer literate and comfortable in installing, configuring, and troubleshooting software, or will they need support to install or gain access to and use the intended system? Does the organization have the ability to provide this support if it is needed? A system that is inadequately supported is a system that users by definition will not be able to use. Support does not necessarily mean staffing a help desk and supplying toll-free phone support. Depending on the system, it can be as simple as adequate documentation and a "frequently asked questions" document.

By no means least important of the issues to consider before embarking on a system design is the question of overall organizational support for a data access system. It is important to realize that providing data access successfully requires some degree of institutional investment and commitment. The host organization needs to make a clear decision as to what it intends to deliver, assess whether it has the resources to deliver it, and determine whether the organization is able to bear the cost. Is the intent to provide access "24 x 7 x 365," or simply during normal business hours?

Does the organization have sufficient technical staff available to develop, maintain, and operate the system? The almost-universal experience is that systems are much more difficult and expensive to develop than expected. And chances are that as soon as the system is released, requests for changes will start to arrive. Systems tend to require a lot of modification during the first two to four years of life. It is not generally wise to bank on outsourced development's leading seamlessly to maintenance-free operation. If the system is considered an important organizational asset, somebody on staff will have to be tasked with its care and feeding.

Are there sufficient server capacity and network capacity to handle the projected workload and perform adequately? System response times tend to vary exponentially with utilization. Systems can become victims of their own success and thus become overwhelmed with demand volume, effectively rendering systems unavailable as response times increase to unacceptable levels. It is important to develop best-guess estimates of audience size and workload volume well ahead of time, to plan for acquisition of sufficient hardware, and to take into account the hard realities of the budget and procurement process. This process, known as capacity planning, is fraught with uncertainty and guesswork and is perhaps as much art as science, but is critical nonetheless to the prevention of embarrassing failures. Creative contingency planning is often the best approach, especially in government organizations that are not known for their ability to react quickly to the unexpected.

Choosing an Architecture

It is really only at this point that the typical activities of system design should begin. Having addressed the much larger questions of the precise intent and purpose of the system, the nature of the data itself, the characteristics of the user community, and the level of organizational capacity and commitment, an organization can make an informed decision about whether and how to proceed.

For a variety of reasons, most new systems being developed today are targeted for deployment over the Web. This is a simple economic decision. HTML and the Web browser provide a simple means of presenting applications on virtually any kind of computing platform anywhere in the world. The widest possible audience is reachable. Software distribution and version management problems disappear. Attractive user interfaces can be designed and deployed with a fraction of the effort required for using thick client approaches.

Even where a thick client is employed, if there is any telecommunication involved in the system, the universal choice today is to employ TCP/IP (Transmission Control Protocol/Internet Protocol) or one of the communication protocols built on top of it, usually HTTP. The public Internet is so ubiquitous that any other choice becomes extremely difficult to justify. HTTP is often the best choice of protocol because it has the least problem in communicating through other organizations' firewalls.

Web-based deployment is an increasingly popular choice for applications intended only for the organization's Intranet. Web-based deployment simply takes advantage of (1) what is often already-existing infrastructure, (2) the fact that most workstations come with a Web browser installed, and (3) the fact that users are already comfortable and familiar with the Web paradigm.

The main drawback to Web deployment on the public Internet is performance. Whenever significant amounts of data must flow, and especially where the connection is via dial-up modem, response times on Web applications very quickly reach unacceptable levels. Even lean applications running in a high-speed connection environment are subject to the unpredictable and uncontrollable performance of the public Internet. If predictable, consistent, high performance is a high priority, an organization clearly needs to avoid the Internet. In fact, a high-speed data access system today is probably best deployed as an Intranet or a LAN-based application, because the performance of an organizational Intranet is generally better and presumably controllable. Otherwise, the system needs to be a stand-alone application running only on the client's workstation. The trade-off is that this approach creates data synchronization problems. Infrequent updates—say, annual or less frequent—are probably best handled by sending an entire new copy of the database to the client site, either on compact disk through the mail or by means of a single, large download. Frequent updates might best be handled by downloading only the changes made to the master database to each slave copy, but in doing so it will be critical to insure that all updates are received and applied in the correct sequence; otherwise, data integrity can be lost.

The limitations of the browser-based interface is the second most serious drawback to Web deployment, whether Internet or Intranet. Consider the problem of performing edits on input fields. The browser-based HTML form has no ability to execute instructions; therefore, all edits have to be performed on the server side. This limitation means that the form has to be transmitted to the server. Any error messages must be returned on a copy of the form. While all this is going on, the user experiences an awkward delay. Various technologies have been introduced to circumvent such limitations by essentially embedding executable instructions within the HTML pages and providing the means to execute them on the client side. Notable among these are Java applets and JavaScript, supported on all platforms and browsers, and ActiveX and DCOM, supported only on the Microsoft platform and browser. These technologies can work within limited circumstances—that is, if employed for simple problems and/or if only certain platforms and browsers are to be supported. But the difficulty is that none of these technologies are universally supported or behave consistently on various platform and browser combinations.

In spite of the limitations, the most popular approach to data access in public health today, as in many other fields, is to develop simple browser-based Web applications that provide real-time access to health databases. The number, variety, and sophistication of development tools available to construct such systems have skyrocketed in recent years. The amount of developer effort and level of developer expertise required to use these tools has correspondingly diminished and can be expected to continue to do so.

The Shortcomings of Today's Rush to the Web

The current rush to put up health databases on the Web is clearly a step forward, both for the public and for the practice of public health. It is hard to argue with the value of more data being made available to more users of data. There is a sense of excitement over the possibilities of the new Web technology, and even a spirit of competitiveness as sites attempt to outdo each other in functionality, usability, and clever interface design. This competitiveness can lead only to better systems. Through these systems, in turn, members of the public are able to apprehend directly the purpose and function of public health and of the local health department, to see the fruits of tax dollars more clearly, and to enjoy direct access and use of information about public health issues affecting their families and their communities.

At the same time, the fact remains that there are serious limitations inherent in the Web-enablement approach being pursued today. These limitations are summarized in Table 20.3.

It is a disjointed, unorganized effort, devoid of overarching plan or purpose. There is a great need for a more coherent approach. Below, we will address some of the limitations that public health and other domains need to recognize in adopting a Web-based approach to sharing data.

For example, there is no systematic directory service for data. To find health data on the Web today, one has to know that it exists and know where to go to access it. One has to have the data's URL (Uniform Resource Loca-

TABLE **20.3.** Limitations of current Web-based approaches to making data available

Web-Based Characteristics	Limitation(s)
Data location	Lack of systematic directory service for data. Normal Web search engines are useless for locating data because content is not present as text in Web pages
Data mounting	Data not mounted according to scientific need or importance and usefulness, but rather according to whether an organization has the resources to develop Web-based database systems
Functional capability	Lack of continuity; many systems serve up data only in a very limited manner, with no support for exploratory analysis, and others present data featuring a confusing and inconsistent array of offerings
Data coverage and comprehensiveness	Many systems focus on data compiled for one or another single political region, with many different sites presenting the data; lack of data comparability
Data standards and documentation	Differ from one system to another, rendering comparability difficult

tor). The situation is particularly glaring at a large institutional Web site like the CDC's: One has to know the organizational structure of the agency in order to locate the database systems put up by various program areas. Normal Web search engines are useless for mapping the location of these sites, because, for the most part, the content of interest is not present as text in Web pages, but rather is encoded inside the database in such a way that search engines cannot parse it. A Web-enabled hospital discharge database may contain records containing *International Classification of Diseases (ICD)* codes that represent myocardial infarction, but the phrase "heart attack" probably does not appear as text in any Web page where a search engine could pick it up. A typical Web search would therefore not locate this resource.

Another limitation of the Web approach is that there is no plan for mounting data on the Web according to scientific need. Rather, availability of data on the Web today is a function of the distribution of wealth among health agencies, not of the relative importance and usefulness of the data. Those organizations blessed with technical resources can afford to develop Web-enabled database systems. Poorer organizations cannot. Yet, it is hardly the funding level of an agency that determines the usefulness of its data to the larger public health community.

A third major limitation of the Web-based approach is that there is no continuity of functional capability across these systems. Some of the systems being developed simply offer preprepared tables of statistics derived from one or a few underlying database systems. These are essentially book pages published on the Web, not true data access systems. Although often useful, and certainly better than no Web presence at all, such systems by their nature can serve up data only in a very limited manner; they cannot support exploratory analysis at all. Some systems present data in simple HTML tables. Some offer graphs and maps. Some offer the ability to reformat data into a variety of popular file formats and download it to the desktop for import into any number of analytic packages—a useful feature for exploratory analysis, more serious research, or the incorporation of data into presentations and reports. But because there is no continuity of functionality across systems, users of public health data are presented with a confusing and inconsistent array of offerings, an array that hampers their ability to use the data.

A fourth limitation is that most public health data are compiled for one or another single political region—a state, a city, a county, a planning region—by whatever health organization is authorized or positioned to perform the collection. As a result, the data are presented by separate systems at separate sites that reflect these political divisions. But diseases and social problems do not respect political boundaries; in public health, data for adjoining or comparable regions often need to be compiled or compared. Unfortunately in many cases, the data are not directly comparable across systems. As we have previously pointed out, this lack of comparability is often a function of the lack of comparability in the underlying data as a result of differences in the data elements being collected, the method of collection, the categorical values into which data are encoded, etc., stemming directly from a lack of data standards. Or it may be an artifact of differences in the systems themselves, whether in the manner and degree of data summarization and aggregation being performed, in the method of rate calculation, or in something as trivial as the form of the output. Without comparability of data, the task of characterizing public health issues across jurisdictional boundaries remains very difficult.

Finally, there is an overall lack of data standards and data documentation accompanying many of these Web database systems, and as a result there is, again, a lack of comparability of data documentation. Public health has been slow to adopt data standards and metadata standards. An effective metadata standard adhered to across the public health enterprise is key to addressing the data comparability issues.

The Data Web

In response to these current challenges and shortcomings, some individuals have proposed approaches to public health data access that take a more overarching, enterprise-wide perspective, as discussed in the previous chapter. It is significant to note that similar pressures are being experienced in other social science domains as well, and parallel solutions are being advanced there. Because these social science domains, such as economics, demographics, and environmental science, share so much in common with public health (collaboration of government, academic and private entities, huge holdings of statistics housed primarily in publicly funded institutions, similar budgetary and resource constraints), it is exciting to contemplate joint solutions that can serve many needs as well as promote multiple reuse of data across disciplines.

One approach that has been advanced in many quarters is to build data warehouses. It is an attractive idea that derives from the success of data warehouses in many commercial enterprises.

Data warehouses integrate formerly disparate data for purposes of discovering otherwise invisible relationships and increasing the potential of data to communicate information about the underlying reality it is intended to represent. Certainly there are huge dividends to be reaped from data warehouses targeted at public health issues. Particularly of interest would be warehouses that explore the intersection of public health and clinical medical practice— such an exploration would provide public health disease surveillance capability, allow for much timelier assessment of therapies and interventions, and lead to better informed prevention programs. But it remains to be seen whether such a data warehouse approach will begin in earnest or bear fruit. After all, data warehouses are very large, expensive and relatively risky projects that tend to require very significant ongoing support for long periods before they become productive. It is not clear at the present time that the public health enterprise possesses the means and the perseverance to succeed with one.

Another approach is to build a common, integrated set of services to provide access to data sources distributed across the Internet. The intent here is to build a data web analogous to the existing World Wide Web, with services aimed at locating and serving up statistical content instead of text and image content. This web can be thought of as a remote data access infrastructure, on top of which specific application systems designed to serve the needs of public health programs, environmental scientists, economists, demographers, urban planners, or private businesses could be built. A major advantage of this approach over a data warehouse is that it is a much less daunting and complex project: It is built up from a series of relatively simple components and standards, it distributes the burden of management and maintenance across collaborating partners, and it requires no attempt to enforce a semantic model—that is, it requires no presumption about how data will be used. *Data Web*, as discussed in the previous chapter, is in fact the name of a research project under joint development by the Centers for Disease Control and Prevention and the US Census Bureau. Whether this particular effort succeeds or whether it proves simply to be an initial attempt that informs later successful attempts, it is an idea that is so logical as to be inevitable. The Web is clearly the new public forum and global communication platform, superior to the telephone and to mass media in its versatility and its provision for two-way and collective communication. Government and public services are clearly destined to move to the Web. Public health and the other social sciences are publicly funded activities built upon publicly funded data-gathering activities. In turn, publicly funded data are a public resource; it therefore needs to be on the very public Web. Government, despite its nay-sayers (who forget that the present Internet would not exist had it not been built by government), is uniquely capable of establishing cohesive, standard protocols and mechanisms that can be implemented at no cost or even free to the user.

What Are the Characteristics of a Data Web?

A data web has numerous characteristics, and in those characteristics reside its advantages as a data access device. These characteristics are listed below.

Data Can Be Accessed at Its Authoritative Source

The organization that "owns" a data set should be the organization responsible for its management. The data set should therefore reside at its home organization. Systems in other organizations that need read access to that data should go to the data's home site. The alternative—permitting external systems to import and store local copies of the data—is duplicative: It immediately engenders data synchronization problems. After all, data change over time. In fact, as a rule, data get more accurate over time. For example, the Census Bureau's population estimates for any given point in time are revised several times over the years; public health disease surveillance reports trickle in over a period of months; *ICD* codes and Federal Information Processing Standards (FIPS) codes are revised approximately yearly. The Census Bureau, where Census data reside, is in a position to update the data. However, if multiple copies of base data exist in various external systems, it is inevitable that these copies will become outdated and unreliable. In short, the most accurate, timely, and authoritative source for data is at the home organization. In a data web architecture, replication of databases is avoided; instead, queries are dynamically directed to the most authoritative source.

Such an architecture does not, however, rule out the possibility of caching local copies of data for performance reasons, so long as the caching mechanism can determine when the cached copy is out of date and needs to be refreshed from the master. Such a local caching mechanism is simply a network-level analogy to the in-memory caching of disk storage systems to improve input-output response time within a single machine.

This approach has the added benefit of minimizing and distributing the work of managing data. After all, data management is not an insignificant task when the number of databases being managed begins to number in the dozens. Operators of large systems should be grateful for the opportunity to offload this task as much as possible. Moreover, no one is more appropriate or more qualified to perform the data management work than the organization responsible for creating the data set to begin with.

Data Can Reside on Any Platform

Currently, there is no reason that the user, or the application system, needs to be concerned about the type of computer, the operating system, or the data base management system on which the data of interest reside. Relational tables are the de facto standard for public health and social science data, and there are a number of tools—American National Standards Institute (ANSI), structured query language (SQL), Java Database Connectivity (JDBC), Java—that encapsulate the data repository and provide platform independence.

Data Can Be Readily Located

Every network requires a directory to assist in locating the contents of the network. At its most basic level, a data web directory would have to consist of data source names linked to network addresses. Thus, a user or an application system could access a data source without knowing anything more about it than its name.

But this basic level is of limited usefulness. It is analogous to requiring users to know a Web site's URL in order to access the site. For example, users need to be able to search the World Wide Web by topic of interest in order to discover unknown sites. Similarly, users will want to search the data web by topic to discover data sources of interest to them. At its next level, then, the data web directory needs the ability to associate "topical terms" with data sources. One simple approach to providing this capability is to collect all parseable text associated with a data source—the data set documentation, a list of words one might want to associate with the data set, and descriptions of all variables—to form an index.

But this next level is also of limited usefulness. After all, it is one thing to know that a hospital discharge database contains a field for diagnosis expressed as an *ICD* code. But it is more interesting to know that there are records in the database wherein the diagnosis field contains the *ICD* code for "myocardial infarction." In other words, it is more interesting to know that this data set contains information about cases of heart attack. To provide a user with ready access to this kind of information would require collecting all the text associated with the definitions of all data element values into the index.

But there is one final level of usefulness that has an analogy familiar to anyone who has ever failed to get results with a Web search engine. That level of usefulness requires building a thesaurus into the index. Such a thesaurus would accommodate multiple definitions of data element values. For example, users will tend to search the data by using the phrase *heart attack* more often than they will use the phrase *myocardial infarction*, even though the latter phrase is the precise definition of the *ICD* code value. A thesaurus would accommodate both.

Clearly, what this discussion points to is the necessity of highly structured, highly complete, and accurate metadata for each data set, metadata that can be used not only to document the content of data sets but also to provide a semantic directory. Admittedly, generating such metadata is no small task.

Data Are Accessed in Real Time

The purpose of the data web is to provide direct access to "live" databases. Preprocessed summaries and reports are not components of the data web, any more than they would be considered part of a database management system.

Data Support a Wide Variety of Applications

The data web is intended to function as a data access infrastructure, on top of which a wide variety of data applications may be built. The data access infrastructure should make no presumptions about how the data will be used or presented in the application layer.

Data Can Be Recoded

Different databases employ different coding schemes to express meaning. Categorical data attributes—such as race, gender, state, smoker/nonsmoker—are encoded in any number of ways. Specific application systems built on top of the data web may require translation of codes from one scheme to another in order to present data from a distant source in a familiar form. A facility to support requests for recoding at query time therefore belongs in the data access infrastructure.

Data Are Appropriate for All Audiences

In a well-conceived data web, data access is not constrained to a certain level of aggregation, to a maximum-sized result set, or to a maximum response time. Data queries can, in principle, be as large and as effort-intensive as necessary to serve the needs of the user or application. Data queries can also involve more than one data source. The data web therefore supports the exploratory data analysis needs of researchers. But less intensive queries are, of course, also possible.

Data Can Be Presented in Multiple Interchange Formats

This data access layer is capable of presenting data in a number of formats suitable for data interchange with other systems, including systems using XML, popular file formats such as Excel and delimited ASCII, and via JDBC and Open Database Connectivity (ODBC) interfaces. The intention is to permit the data access process to integrate seamlessly with the data analysis/data visualization/reporting process, regardless of what the latter might be.

Data from Multiple Sources Can Be Conjoined

An important consequence of the ability to resolve differences in database location and in platform and data-coding scheme is the ability to co-tabulate data from separate systems into a single result table with exponentially less effort than is required today. It is true that there are significant restraints on the number of variables by which and the circumstances under which such co-tabulations can validly be performed. However, even the ability to link on a few of the most common and obvious geographic and population variables (date, state, county, age, race, sex) opens potentially significant new frontiers for exploring data relationships and vastly reduces the cost and effort of doing so.

Appropriate Data Manipulations Can Be Associated with Data

Certain data manipulations—such as the application of weights in the tabulation of survey data or the calculation of age adjusted rates in the presentation of incidence of health events—are so fundamental to the data that they may be considered to be "behaviors" of the data. These manipulations ought to be consistent from one application to the next. Therefore, they are not a feature of the application, but rather of the data layer. In an object-oriented sense, they are methods of the data sets. The metadata might well tag data sets with these manipulations and the circumstances under which they may be performed and build into the data web the ability to invoke these manipulations when they are needed or requested.

Access to Data Can Be Controlled

Digital certificates and other public key infrastructure technology may be employed in the data web to authenticate users strongly and to encrypt their data transmissions across the public net. Pending development of a workable security model that allows data set owners to control access to their data, it may become practical to mount non-public user data on the data web and provide restricted access to authorized users.

Expanding Data Needs of Today and the Future

The information needs of public health and of other social sciences are changing in significant ways. The needs are growing in scope and complexity, and they increasingly involve partners outside the traditional domains. For example, public health programs increasingly need to examine data from the socioeconomic, criminal justice, and environmental domains, just as they need to examine public and private health provider and payer data. Programs in these other domains, in turn, also increasingly express need for public health data, such as data related to disease incidence and data regarding natality and mortality. There may be no limit to the number and variety of computer applications that can derive benefit from cross-system data exchange. Indeed, it can be argued that the primary value of the enormous existing volume of information, gathered originally to study various separate aspects of populations and communities, will be tapped only when this information is merged, linked, and compared.

Advances in information technology have made it possible to imagine developing an integrated suite of services that would serve to bridge the gap between data in all its disparate forms and applications that might make use of it. Public health and the other social sciences may be positioned to make great strides forward in capacity, capability, and efficiency as a result of these advances. In this chapter, we have presented some concepts for increasing the accessibility and usefulness of data to accommodate those disparate needs.

Questions for Review

Questions 1 through 10 are based upon the following information:

The Department of Public Health of State X maintains a database that contains fundamental raw data relating to physician diagnoses of AIDS cases of state residents. The department maintains a Web site at which it provides simplified graphs and charts related to the incidence and prevalence of the disease in the state, along with AIDS-prevention guidelines. These graphs and charts compare the incidence and prevalence to national levels. The department also provides restricted Web-based access to data that have been manipulated to enhance the data's security and integrity; this data, for example, exclude geographic region and age at diagnosis. The data are updated every three months.

1. Which of the Web features would be appropriate for general public access? For access of health program planners, policy makers, or health issue advocates looking for metrics on the size or severity of AIDS incidence and prevalence? For researchers needing detailed data?
2. Explain why the Department of Public Health of State X might be reluctant to provide general access to all the data.
3. In what sense might it be beneficial to the department to share the data with the general public?
4. In what sense could it be illegal or unethical to provide public access to all the data?
5. Explain why full organizational support is essential if the department is to provide AIDS diagnoses data that are both current and accurate? What technical support will the department need to provide to users?
6. What are the drawbacks and limitations to the department's Web-deployment approach to providing access to the data, assuming the department maintains a typical Web-based database system and assuming the current state of technology? What are the advantages and limitations?
7. Explain why a data warehouse approach to integrating the AIDS data with data related to all diagnoses of disease in the state might be beneficial. What are the drawbacks to such an approach?

8. Why might it not be a good idea for the department to permit researchers and other state departments to download and maintain their own AIDS diagnoses databases from the department's Web site?

9. Explain how use of a data web to house the AIDS data might provide the department with advantages (provide at least six advantages of this approach over traditional Web-based approaches).

10. In what ways would the characteristics of the data access systems of the department need to be different if the primary purpose of the department's Web site was to (a) provide overall information about AIDS prevalence and causes to the general public and (b) serve the needs of the scientific community interested in conducting research?

21
Geographic Information Systems

Carol L. Hanchette

Learning Objectives

Upon completing this chapter, you should be able to:

- Describe the uses and value of the application of geographic information systems (GIS) to public health.
- Discuss the history and the theoretical foundations of GIS.
- Understand the functional development of GIS and how it works.
- Analyze the organizational models and the respective hardware/software/ personnel requirements for GIS along the continuum from a single individual user to community use.
- List and discuss the social/institutional issues that individual and organizational users of GIS must address.
- Describe the limitations of GIS software and spatial data.
- Discuss the emerging technologies that have implications for GIS use in public health.

Overview

Geographic information systems are powerful tools that can enable public health practitioners to analyze and visualize data. A system of computer hardware and software that allows users to input, analyze, and display geographic data, GIS permits the manipulation and display of both spatial and attribute data. GIS now exists at various levels, ranging from small-scale systems for individual users to enterprise-wide systems. The advent of Internet map servers and client-server applications has made GIS more widely available and accessible. However, users of GIS need to have the proper training in order to use such systems properly. They also need to be aware of the social/institutional issues that can influence GIS use. Finally, users need to be aware of the limitations in GIS software and in data sets, limitations that can, if ignored, result in reliance on incomplete and inaccurate data.

Introduction

During the past few years, the contribution of information technology to the practice of public health has become increasingly apparent and has led to the emergence of the discipline of *public health informatics*. Public health informatics has been defined as "the application of information science and technology to public health practice and research."[1(p1)] (also see Chapter 1). Until very recently, there has been a general perception that the use of information technology in the health sciences is 10 to 15 years behind its use in other fields. Historically, the use of information systems in public health has focused on the storage and retrieval of data. This focus is changing as the healthcare industry increases its use of electronic medical records, upgrades hospital information systems, and uses the Internet for distributing health-related information and providing remote diagnostics.[2,3] In addition, with the shift of the U.S. healthcare system toward a managed care model, the role of public health agencies is becoming strongly oriented toward the provision and use of information and efficient access to it.

At a time when computer hardware and software are becoming more affordable, powerful, and user-friendly, public health agencies and service providers are scrambling to develop the technological infrastructure that will allow them to make use of information technology. Recognizing the importance of a strong information infrastructure in providing public health professionals with access to technical information, the Centers for Disease Control and Prevention (CDC) in 1992 initiated the Information Network for Public Health Officials (INPHO) program, which has provided funding to public health agencies to acquire and upgrade information resources. This program is administered by the Public Health Practice Program Office (PHPPO), which is dedicated to improving systems that manage public health information and knowledge.

One of the emerging technologies being adopted by public health professionals is that of geographic information systems. A GIS is a computer mapping and analysis technology consisting of hardware, software, and data allowing large quantities of information to be viewed and analyzed in a geographic context. It has nearly all of the features of a database management system, with a major enhancement: Every item of information in a GIS is tied to a geographic location. Lasker et al. have identified three basic types of information needs essential to public health services: (1) data collection and analysis, (2) communication, and (3) support in decision making.[4] GIS has enormous potential to contribute to the analysis of population-based public health with its ability to support all three types of information needs.

Although medical geographers have been mapping disease and conducting spatial analysis for decades, the use of GIS among public health professionals is a relatively recent development. The fact that two 1999 editions of the *Journal for Public Health Management and Practice* were devoted entirely to GIS applications attests to its emerging importance in health sciences. With GIS, public health professionals can manage large quantities of information; map the distribution of diseases and health care resources; analyze the relationships among environmental factors and socioeconomic environments and disease outcomes; determine where to locate a new hospital or clinic; and even make decisions about the development or implementation of health policy.

In this chapter, we will define the nature of a GIS. We will trace its theoretical foundations and its development and discuss the importance of GIS, particularly with regard to its contribution to public health. We will then discuss how GIS concepts work—their treatment and representation of data, GIS organizational models, and issues related to implementation and uses of GIS. We will conclude the chapter with a discussion of the implications of emerging technologies such as Web-based applications and data warehousing for GIS as a public health tool.

What Is GIS?

What is a GIS? Dozens of definitions exist. Essentially, it is a system of computer hardware and software that allows users to input, analyze, and display geographic data. More specifically, it is ". . . a computer system that stores and links non-graphic attributes or geographically referenced data with graphic map features to allow a wide range of information processing and display operations, as well as map production, analysis and modeling."[5(p281)]

Clarke refers to GIS as (1) a toolbox, (2) an information system, and (3) an approach to science.[6] As a toolbox, GIS is a software package that contains a variety of tools for processing and analyzing spatial data. Public health professionals might use these tools to map infant mortality rates across a state, identify areas with underserved populations, maintain an infectious disease surveillance system, or model environmental exposures to toxic substances.

As an information system, a GIS consists of a series of databases that contain observations about features or events that can be located in space and, hence, mapped and analyzed. GIS also functions as a means of spatial data storage.[7] Information that for centuries was stored on paper maps can now be stored in digital format in a geographic information system.

In some circles, the meaning of GIS is gradually shifting from "geographic information system" to "geographic information science," sometimes referred to as GIScience.[8] GIScience refers to the science behind the technology and the study and understanding of the disciplines and technologies that have contributed to the development of today's GIS software. These disciplines include geography, cartography, geodesy, photogrammetry, computer science, spatial statistics, and a wide range of physical and social sciences. Goodchild has categorized these disciplines and provided a more extensive list of them.[8]

Theoretical Foundations and the Development of GIS

GIS owes its current level of functionality to developments in a wide range of disciplines and technologies. As a "science," its theoretical roots lie in geography, cartography, and spatial analysis. Ties to cartography are obvious, and some of the basic cartographic principles critical to GIS use are discussed later in the chapter. Certain paradigms in the discipline of geography have had a strong impact on the development of GIS technology. In the mid-1950s, geography experienced a shift from integrated, regional science approaches to a paradigm that embraced logical positivism (with its deductive vs. inductive reasoning), laws of probability, and the quantitative revolution. Emerging computer technology contributed to this shift by providing faster computations and a means of storing and retrieving vast quantities of information.[9] During this time, methods of spatial analysis that had been developed earlier in the century were automated, and many new spatial/statistical methods were developed. Other schools of thought in geography, such as the landscape and human ecology schools, had an impact on the development of automated mapping techniques to store and map environmental information.

In 1959, Waldo Tobler published a paper about the use of computer programming to automate cartography.[10] Over the next decade, Tobler's ideas led to the development of several computer programs and mapping packages, many written in FORTRAN, for map production and spatial analysis. Faculty and students at the Laboratory for Computer Graphics and Spatial Analysis at Harvard University Graduate School of Design developed the most widely used of these programs and packages. The Laboratory was directed by architect and city planner Howard Fisher, who developed SYMAP, a computer-mapping program for analyzing data and producing maps on a line printer. Other early mapping programs include GRID, IMGRID, CALFORM, and SUR-FACE II (the latter developed by the Kansas Geological Survey). These software packages all ran on mainframe computers and were still in widespread use on university campuses until the mid- to late-1980s.

In 1969, landscape architect Ian McHarg published his book *Design with Nature*, which described the process of using transparent overlays for making siting decisions and for analysis of spatial relationships among features. McHarg was not the first to use and overlay map transparencies, but his book had a widespread audience. In fact, the ability to superimpose and overlay maps is one of the strengths of GIS. One of the first programs to perform polygon (area) overlay analysis was the ODYSSEY program, developed at Harvard in early 1980s.[11]

Some of the earliest geographic and database management systems also evolved during the 1960s. Roger Tomlinson's Canada Geographic Information System was capable of providing nationwide geographic analysis with map data layers on agriculture, forestry, wildlife, recreation, census/demographics, and land use. In 1967, the Land Management Information Center was established at the University of Minnesota and began development of a statewide GIS database. Parallel traditions in automated mapping and facility management (AM/FM) systems by gas and electric utilities and other important contributions, such as the development of computer-aided drafting (CAD) systems, are described in detail in Antenucci et al.[5]

Although many of the early computer mapping and GIS programs were quite powerful, they appear primitive by today's standards. The maps they produced were nowhere near as aesthetic as hand-produced maps; the software had a much longer learning curve (which included learning mainframe Job Control Language and commands specific to the software), and digital data were difficult to come by.

Many U.S. federal government agencies were important to the evolution of GIS technology and the development of digital cartographic data, perhaps most notably the U.S. Bureau of the Census. In 1967, the agency piloted the use of digital geographic files (streets and census blocks) for a study in New Haven, Connecticut. These files, the Geographic Base File Dual Independent Map Encoding files (otherwise known as GBF/ DIME files), were used in urban areas for the 1970 and 1980 censes. Military use of geographic data technology in the 1960s led to development of digital databases such as the World Databank, which could be used in some of the early mapping programs.

In the late 1980s, the move away from mainframe computers and toward workstation and PC technologies resulted in dramatic changes to GIS software and functionality. Most notably, software became increasingly easy to use with the development of graphical user interfaces and menu-driven systems, and large collections of digital datasets were developed for use with the software. Today, computer users with a day's training or less can easily begin using GIS. Such a facility of use has obvious advantages, but there are drawbacks as well. After all, geographic data are complex. Without a sound knowledge of basic geographic principles, data issues, and map design, it is easy for an uninformed user to make errors, to mislead, and to be misled.

The Importance of GIS and Its Contribution to Public Health

Many introductory texts on medical geography and the use of GIS in public health begin with a reference to John Snow, the London physician who mapped cholera cases in the Soho District of London during the cholera epidemic of 1854 (see also Chapter 2.) Snow was able to show that these cases clustered around the Broad Street pump. The closure of the pump, through the removal of the pump handle, and subsequent reduction in cases supported Snow's contention that cholera was a water-borne disease.

Perhaps more interesting than Snow's map, however, was his "medical detective" work preceding the 1854 epidemic and following the epidemic of 1849, which helped him to recognize the association between contaminated water and cholera. The cholera epidemic of 1849 killed over 52,000 people in Great Britain and over 13,000 in London alone.[12] While Snow published a brief account of this epidemic in 1849, he continued to carry out research over the next few years, leading to a second edition, published in 1854, that was a more substantial work.

In his second account, Snow noted the association between cholera, poverty, elevation, and the water supply of the various London districts. A fascinating reconstruction, mapping, and geographic analysis of these associations is provided by Cliff and Haggett.[12] As the authors have noted, "these associations result in some striking geographical distributions" such as the higher mortality rates in areas adjacent to the River Thames and the relationship between cholera and the water supply of London districts. At that time, a number of metropolitan water companies were supplying water to the city from a myriad of sources—some directly from the Thames, others from reservoirs. Cholera mortality was linked to contaminated water supplies provided by companies drawing their water directly from the Thames.

Snow also investigated the relationship between elevation and cholera incidence and observed that cholera was more likely to occur in low-lying areas than in higher ones. There was some dispute over whether this was the result of water contamination or of soil type, but it was actually a product of a combination of the two factors: Lower lying areas had poorer drainage (soil type), resulting in water stagnation and contamination. The alkalinity of water also played a role in the transmission of cholera, as the microbe *Vibrio cholerae* likes water with a high pH.

Although many of us would prefer to be in the field, rather than at a desk, today's technology makes it possible to carry out an analysis such as Snow's in a very small amount of time, at the desktop. Imagine Dr. John Snow at his desk with a powerful computer mapping and information system. On his computer screen, he has maps of London districts, their water supplies, and the locations of cholera cases. In addition, his water supply map database contains information about characteristics of the water, such as pH factor and water source. He also has a map of soils, with information about their characteristics and an elevation model to work with. With the tools available in a geographic information system (provided that he has spatial data in digital format), Dr. Snow could do point mapping of cholera cases, calculate distances to water sources, and examine the relationship of cholera incidence to water source, water type, soils, and elevation.

Snow's work provides an indication of how a GIS can benefit public health practice. Medical geographers, epidemiologists, and other health practitioners have been carrying out mapping and spatial analysis for centuries, but have been doing it "longhand," so to speak. Some of the classic geographic research on probability mapping,[13] disease diffusion and modeling,[14] the spatial organization of cancer mortality,[15] cardiovascular disease,[16] and the allocation of health services[17] would have benefited from the use of GIS, or, more specifically, from the combination of GIS and statistical analysis software—all used some combination of mapping, spatial analysis, and statistical analysis.

Obviously, GIS is needed for more efficient processing and analysis of geographic data. It is also needed to integrate public health data from a wide range of sources, to perform population-based public health analyses, and to provide sound information on which to base decisions. Geography is a great integrator: Nearly every entity of public health information is located somewhere in space, whether it be a county, a ZIP code, a dot on a map, a hospital room, or even a point within the human body. GIS provides a means of integrating all this information through a spatial referencing system.

GIS technology, then, has much to offer public health practitioners. Perhaps most importantly, the analysis and display of geographic data is an efficient and effective means of providing data for decision-making. As an example, Hanchette has demonstrated the use of GIS by North Carolina state health agencies to implement the 1997 CDC lead screening guidelines and perform eligibility testing for reimbursements under federal welfare reform legislation.[18]

Richards et al. have provided an excellent discussion of the advantages of GIS technology, examples of its potential use by public health practitioners, and constraints on its use.[19] In addition to the advantages noted in the preceding paragraphs, GIS permits the development of new types of data, the establishment of data partnerships and data sharing, and the development of new methods and tools for use by public health professionals.

An additional benefit or function of GIS is that it can be used to carry out quality control procedures for health datasets. Geographically based logical consistency checks can be carried out to verify the accuracy of geographic identifiers in health datasets. An example of this application is the use of city/zip/county lookup tables to determine correspondence of geographic data variables. Any records that do not have correspondence should be a red flag. Geocoded patient residences or clinics can be overlaid with county or zip code boundaries to ascertain whether their county or zip codes are correct. Although such quality control procedures may appear to be an insignificant role for GIS, an example cited later in this chapter confirms their importance.

How Does GIS Work?

GIS has in common concepts related to data association and display.

Spatial and Attribute Data

Although recent developments in hardware and database management software have led to the development of many new data structures, we can think of GIS data as having two components. The first component is *spatial data*, consisting of geographic coordinates that provide information about the location and dimensions of features on earth and the relationships among these features. These spatial data are stored in a *topologic* data structure—a data structure that maintains information about the spatial relationships among features, such as adjacency, connectivity, and containment.

The second component is *attribute* or *statistical data*, such as census variables or health outcomes, that describe the non-spatial aspects of the database. Attribute and geographic data are linked through a geocode, a geographic identifier that is contained in both data components. This geocode can be a county name or a state name, a zip code, a street address, or some other numeric code.

Figure 21.1 displays a map of Missouri that shows the number of persons age 65 and over, by county. The spatial data on the map are the Missouri county boundaries. Attribute data are contained in the table below the map and are represented on the map by a series of shading patterns. Each record contains information for a single county; in this case it includes county name, state name, 1997 population, and the population age 65 and older. The table also contains standard numeric codes (geocodes) for counties and the state of Missouri. These codes were developed by US government agencies as part of the Federal Information Processing Standard (FIPS).

The record for Saline County is highlighted, and the corresponding county is highlighted on the map. The FIPS code for Missouri is 29, and the FIPS code for Saline County is 195, providing a combined FIPS code (and a unique identifier for Saline County, Missouri) of 29195. This value is contained in the table's FIPS field. The Missouri county boundary file has a FIPS code associated with each county, and the attribute data are linked to the appropriate boundary through this geocode.

Most federal geographic data, such as census data, use a set of FIPS codes. However, the federal codes are not always used by state agencies or other organizations. Geographic files, such as the county boundary file in Figure 21.1, often contain more than one set of geocodes. If health agencies in the state of Missouri coded health data by county name, these data could be mapped using county name as a geocode, so long as that information was also contained in a field in the spatial database.

Attribute data originate from a variety of sources and come in a wide range of formats. One of the challenges of using health and demographic data in a GIS is working with different data formats and structures. Attribute data are typically stored in tables, where columns represent fields or variables and rows represent cases or observations. These tables or files are often stored in a database, defined as "a collection of related data items stored in an organized manner."[20] The original data may be stored in mainframe legacy systems; SAS, SPSS or Access databases; Excel spreadsheets; or a number of other formats. Linking these data to spatial data usually requires importing them

Population Age 65 and Over
Missouri Counties, 1990

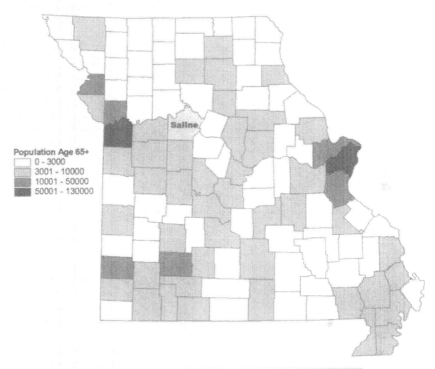

FIGURE 21.1. Spatial and attribute data for Missouri counties. (Data source: US Census, 1990. Map Source: ESRI Redlands, CA.)

into GIS. Most data tables can be converted to ASCII or dBase (.dbf) format, for easy incorporation into GIS. Spreadsheets and databases are not the same, and importing spreadsheets into GIS software can be problematic, although it is often done. Many GIS users view dBase as a preferred file transfer format because it is readable by many GIS software applications and requires little or no formatting. Recent developments in both GIS and database management software allow direct, live linkage among some GIS applications and database management systems.

For years, the main database management system utilized by GIS applications has been the relational model, where two or more tables can be linked easily via a common identifier, or key. This is how attribute data are linked to spatial data using a common geocode. The new trend in the larger GIS software applications is toward object-oriented databases, which are capable of modeling complex spatial objects. These spatial objects contain not only attributes, but the methods and procedures that operate on them. A more detailed discussion of database management systems is beyond the scope of this chapter, but readers are referred to Jones[7] for more information about database models in the context of geographic information systems.

Map Projections and Coordinate Systems

In a GIS, all geographic features, such as hospital location, county boundaries, and street networks, must be defined in terms of a common frame of reference, or coordinate system. Coordinates are defined by their distance from a fixed set of axes. In general, an *x-coordinate* refers to an east/west location; a *y-coordinate* defines a north/south location. Features on the earth can be located with the *geographic coordinate system*, which uses latitude for a north/south position and longitude for an east/west position. However, this system pinpoints location on a spherical earth. Maps, on the other hand, are flat. Therefore, the transformation of features from a three-dimensional sphere to a two-dimensional surface, known as a *map projection*, must take place in order for the system to produce accurate mapping and analysis. Because degrees of longitude vary in actual distance across the globe (i.e., they converge at the poles), projections are used to establish a grid system with uniform units of measurement and to reduce the distortion in unprojected map coordinates.

Map projection is a science in and of itself. Projections are mathematical transformations of endless variety and, although they reduce the distortion inherent in geographic coordinates, they all involve some sort of distortion of shape, area, direction or distance. Imagine drawing a map on the entire outside of an orange, then trying to remove and flatten the peel and maintain the integrity of the map features. While it takes time and experience to learn which projections are best suited for a particular application, it is important for the new GIS user to understand that all map layers to be used in an application must use the same projection and coordinate system. Indeed, this is one of the strengths of GIS: Multiple map layers can be overlaid and relation-

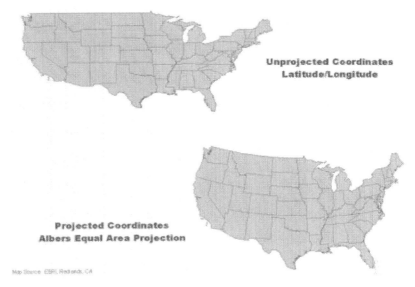

FIGURE 21.2. Unprojected and projected coordinates. (Map source: ESRI Redlands, CA.)

ships among them can be analyzed and displayed when they are tied to a common coordinate system.

Many geographic databases are stored as unprojected data—that is, as latitude/longitude coordinates. Indeed, latitude/longitude coordinates are a sort of *lingua franca*, a standard data exchange format, and must be projected by use of the projection capabilities available in most GIS software products. Projections and/or coordinate systems that are commonly used in the United States include (1) state plane coordinate systems, (2) Albers Equal Area projection, (3) Lambert Conformal Conic projection, and (4) Universal Transverse Mercator (UTM) projection. Good descriptions of map projections and coordinate systems can be found in Clarke[6] and Robinson et al.[21] Figure 21.2 displays a map of the continental United States in latitude/longitude coordinates (unprojected) and in Albers Equal Area coordinates (projected).

Representations of Spatial Data

Most spatial data in a GIS are either feature-based or image-based, often referred to as *vector* or *raster*, respectively. Vector data are represented by feature types that resemble the way we visualize and draw maps by hand—by use of (1) *point*, a single *x,y* location (example: a residence); (2) *line*, a string of

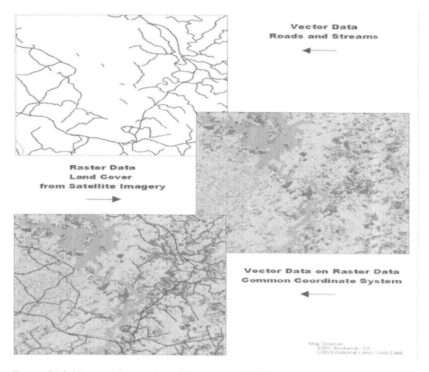

Figure 21.3. Vector and raster data. (Map source: ESRI Redlands, CA: USGS National Land Cover Data.)

coordinates (example: a road): and (3) *polygon*, a chain of coordinates that define an area (example: a county boundary).

Satellite images, digital aerial photography, and other forms of remotely sensed data are the most commonly used raster data. These data are stored, not as features, but as a series of pixels or grid cells. Both types of data can (and should) be registered to a real-world coordinate system for display and analysis. Figure 21.3 displays examples of feature (vector) and image (raster) data and the ability of the GIS software to overlay these by use of a common coordinate system.

Scale

Scale refers to the ratio of a distance on a map to the corresponding distance on the ground. A scale of 1/100,000 (usually represented as 1:100,000) means that 1 inch on the map is equal to 100,000 inches on the real earth. The ratio is true for any unit of measurement (1 centimeter on the map is equal to 100,000 centimeters on the ground). Large-scale maps show more detail than small-scale maps. The concept of scale can be confusing because the larger

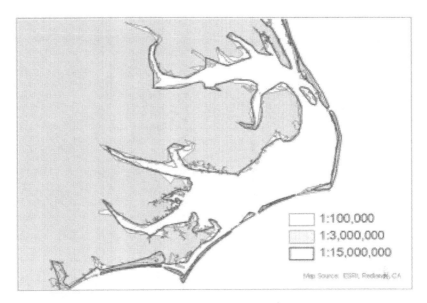

FIGURE 21.4. An area of coastal Carolina, shown at several map scales. (Map source: ESRI, Redlands, CA.)

the denominator in the fraction is, the smaller the scale is. In other words, a map at a scale of 1:12,000 is a larger-scale map than one at 1:2,000,000. Smaller-scale maps are generally used to show a larger area (such as the world or the United States), whereas larger-scale maps can be used to "zoom in" to a smaller area (such as a city or a neighborhood). Because many map details are lost in smaller-scale maps, scale has an important effect on the precision of location. Figure 21.4 shows an area of coastal North Carolina represented at different scales. It is important to remember that, although GIS software allows users to zoom in and out to different scales, the amount of detail in a map depends entirely on the scale of the original map!

Functionality: Mapping and Spatial Analysis for Health Applications

A discussion of GIS functions used for public health applications can be found in Vine et al.[22] Some of the more generic functions are described below. For the beginning GIS user, the most heavily utilized application of GIS probably will be the display of map layers and the production of thematic maps, most likely shaded (choropleth) maps.

Choropleth mapping assigns different shades or colors to geographic areas, according to their values; it was, in fact, the technique used to produce the map in

Figure 21.1. In health applications, it may be used with counties, zip codes, health service areas, census tracts, or other geographic units to show the distribution of health outcomes, socio-demographic characteristics, health services, or other relevant variables. Because correct interpretation of the message or pattern displayed on a choropleth map is so critical to analysis and decision-making, a more detailed discussion of choropleth map production is provided in a later section in this chapter concerning visual display of spatial data.

Automated address matching can be used to map clinics, patient residences, and other locations that contain street addresses. *Address matching* is a term that is often used synonymously with *geocoding*, but it is actually only one of many methods of geocoding. Essentially, an address, such as 525 Fuller Street, is a geocode—it refers to a specific location along Fuller Street. Address matching works by comparing a specific street address in a database to a map layer of streets. If the map layer contains relevant information about the street name and the range of addresses along that street, the software can interpolate the location of the address and place it along the street. An example is shown in Figure 21.5. In this case, the street network data contain fields with information about the beginning and ending address for the 500 block of Fuller Street. Even addresses are on one side; odd addresses on the other. The address, 525 Fuller Street, falls about 25% of the distance from the beginning of the block. Issues of privacy and confidentiality that arise from address matching are discussed later in the chapter.

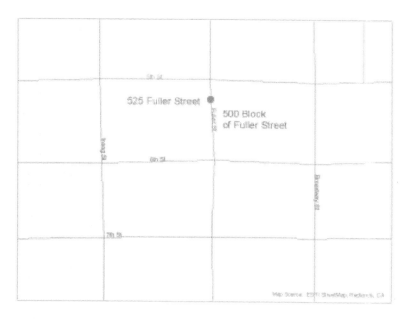

FIGURE 21.5. Address matching. (Source: ESRI Street Map, Redlands, CA.)

Most GIS software allows the user either to enter addresses interactively, one at a time, or to process an entire database of addresses in batch mode. Although the concept of address matching is very straightforward, there are many limitations and problems that can be encountered. These are described in a later section.

Distances among geographic features can be determined with nearly all GIS/mapping software. In health applications, distances are often needed to analyze access to health care or to model exposure to an environmental contaminant, among other things. Most GIS software allows users to determine distances either interactively or in batch mode through the use of a distance function. In the case of the latter, the distance calculation is stored in a variable that may be used for later analysis, such as regression or some sort of exposure modeling.

Spatial query allows a GIS user to query the attribute database and display the results geographically. For instance, a user could make a query to display the location of all rabies cases that have occurred in a county during the past year, or to show all census tracts in which more than 50% of households have a household income below the poverty rate. Queries can also be based on distance: A GIS can be used to display all zip codes within a 25-mile radius of a particular health clinic or to show all patients within 15 miles of a field phlebotomist.

Buffer functions can define and display a region or "ring" of specified radius around a point, a line, or an area. GIS software allows the user to define the width of the buffer—that is, the distance of the outside edge of the buffer from the feature boundary. A 150-meter buffer might be created to determine the number of residences close to a toxic release event. A 25-meter buffer zone around major roads could identify areas with potential lead hazards in soil from past use of leaded gasoline. Figure 21.6 shows buffers of 25, 50 and 75 miles from Saint Charles Medical Center in Bend, Oregon. Another hospital is located within 25 miles of Saint Charles Medical Center and there are three hospitals within 50 miles of the center.

Overlay analysis allows GIS users to integrate feature types and data from different sources. It is not to be confused with visual overlay, which occurs when several map layers are registered to a common coordinate system and displayed together, as in Figure 21.3. Overlay analysis involves some spatial data processing and results in the creation of new data or modification of existing data. Two commonly used types of overlay analysis are *point-in-polygon overlay* and *polygon overlay.*

Point-in-polygon overlay is used to determine which area, or polygon, a point or set of points lies in or whether a point lies inside or outside a particular geographic area. For example, a point map of patient residences might be overlaid on a map layer of census tracts to determine the census tract of the residence of each patient. This application is important when a user is examining the association of census variables, particularly socioeconomic ones, with health outcomes.

Polygon overlay can be used to create a new map layer from two existing polygon map layers, when their boundaries are not coincident. For example,

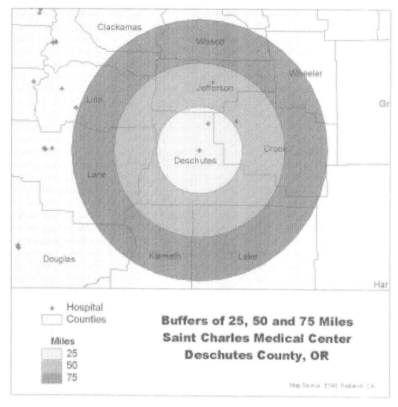

FIGURE 21.6. Buffer function. (Source ESRI, Redlands, CA.)

a zip code map layer can be overlaid on a layer of primary sampling units to obtain a map layer showing all ZIP codes and partial ZIP codes within a sampling area. This application can be used to create a lookup table that can be linked to addresses. Polygon overlay is sometimes used to estimate populations within a geographic area whose boundaries differ from census boundaries; it operates in a "cookie cutter" fashion to create new polygons. Population is then prorated by comparison of the area of the new polygon to that of the original.

While these are only a few examples of GIS functions, they are all commonly used in health applications and are easy to learn. Many other functions exist, ranging from relatively simple techniques such as suitability analysis and creation of Thiessen polygons to complex methods of spatial modeling. A good source of information on GIS modeling is Bonham-Carter.[23] Kulldorff has described some statistical issues and methods pertinent to public health data,[24] and Buescher has warned about computing and using rates based on small numbers.[25]

There are many time-honored spatial analysis techniques used by geographers for decades that are not yet incorporated into the more widely used GIS software products. Furthermore, GIS software has always been lacking in statistical analysis functions. Using statistical or more advanced spatial analysis techniques usually requires additional programming, often incorporating a GIS software macro language, or reformatting GIS data for use with statistical software, such as SAS or SPSS. One statistical software package, S-PLUS, can be used with ArcView software developed by Environmental Systems Research Institute (ESRI). Other statistical software has been developed for very specific applications, such as SaTScan (which can be obtained from the National Cancer Institute at no charge) for analysis of disease clusters.[24] Those unfamiliar with spatial analysis and spatial statistics may want to refer to Unwin[26] or Cressie.[27] Anyone with a strong interest in exploring spatial analysis methods for use in health applications is urged to read *Atlas of Disease Distributions: Analytic Approaches to Epidemiologic Data*.[14]

Visual Display of Spatial Data

The proper display of spatial data requires an understanding of cartographic design, of levels of measurement, and of the wide range of symbols and color schemes that can be used to represent feature, and image data. A thorough treatment of this subject is beyond the scope of this chapter, but it can be found in cartography references such as Robinson et al.[21] and Monmonier.[28] Unfortunately, the proliferation of GIS and the development of user-friendly interfaces to GIS software has made it easy for the "cartographically illiterate" to produce bad maps. Bad maps can result from the improper use of map projections, unfamiliarity with basic principles of map design, lack of understanding of data type and distribution, and poor symbol choice.

Because choropleth maps are so frequently produced and they convey such a powerful image of the distribution and quantity of phenomena, two critical aspects of their production are discussed briefly in this chapter: (1) grouping data into classes for mapping and (2) appropriate use of symbols for choropleth mapping.

Grouping Data into Classes for Mapping

The way in which data are grouped or classified has a strong effect on the appearance of the map and can result in maps that look very dissimilar but use the same set of data. The mapmaker must determine how many categories or classes to use and the intervals, or cut-off points, for each class. Most shaded maps use from three to six classes that are represented in the legend. Most GIS/mapping software

Equal Interval

The range of the data is determined by subtracting the lowest value from the highest value. The range is then divided by the desired number of classes, usually four or five, to determine the beginning and end values for each class.

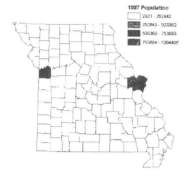

Quantiles

The data are arranged in sequence from low to high values. The observations are then separated into the desired number of classes so that each class contains the same number of observations, or geographic units.

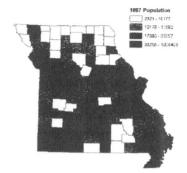

Natural Breaks

Natural breaks are points where there are gaps in the distribution of the data, i.e. fewer or no observations. These break points are often used as dividing points for the classes

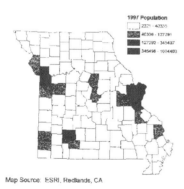

Mean and Standard Deviation

The mean is computed and established as the center of the data distribution. Class intervals are determined by the standard deviation, a measure that determines the spread of the data around the mean.

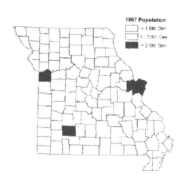

Map Source: ESRI, Redlands, CA

FIGURE 21.7. Data grouping methods for choropleth mapping. (Map source: ESRI, Redlands, CA.)

provides users with a number of options for classifying numeric data. Four commonly used methods are (1) equal interval, (2) quantile, (3) natural breaks, and (4) mean and standard deviation. Figure 21.7 provides examples of these methods, using the data from Figure 21.1 for illustrative purposes.

Generally, there is no consistent "right" or "wrong" classification method to use for classifying data, but some methods are more appropriate for certain data distributions. The mean and standard deviation method is probably used least, because the general public may not understand the concept of standard deviation. A disadvantage of using the equal interval method is that, because classes are determined by dividing the range of data, and not by data distribution, it is possible to have data classes with no observations. In this case, a class (and associated shade) would be represented in the legend, but not on the map. Probably the best rule of thumb for those who are uncertain is to use the natural breaks or the quantile methods.

Appropriate Use of Symbols for Choropleth Mapping

With the availability of color in computer hardware and software, it is tempting to use a wide range of colors in map production. However, a user working with numeric data should choose colors and shading patterns that communicate the map's message as clearly as possible and reflect the value of the data so that the patterns on the map are intuitive to the viewer.

In color terminology, *hue* refers to the name of the color (e.g., red, blue, green) and *value* is the lightness or darkness of a hue.[21] In general, it is best to use light colors for low data values and intense or dark colors for high data values. A gradation of values for one hue works well with numeric data, as does a range of hues from light to dark. These configurations of colors are often available in GIS/mapping software as *color ramps*, a range of hues or colors set up in the software that the user can quickly apply to numeric data. In the past, cartographers used white to indicate missing data. However, it is sometimes difficult to develop a full range of colors that are distinguishable from one another and that print out well, so white is often used out of necessity to represent the class of lowest data values. When a user is producing a series of maps, it is important to standardize color and shading patterns so that their interpretation is consistent across the series. Examples can be found in two recently published health atlases: The *Atlas of Cancer Mortality in the United States, 1950–94* [29] and *Women and Heart Disease: An Atlas of Racial and Ethnic Disparities in Mortality*.[30] Figure 21.8 provides examples of both appropriate and inappropriate use of symbols.

Maps are often produced for publications or reports. When color maps are too expensive to produce, the map's message often can be conveyed as effectively in black and white. Gray shades, ranging from low to high value, can be used in place of a range of colors. However, gray shades do not always print or copy well, and solid black can obscure boundaries, text, and other features. Dot and hatch patterns can be a more effective way to present the information. Lower density patterns, such as sparse dots or hatch patterns with wider line spacing, should be used for classes with lower data values.

Visual displays of spatial data often incorporate tables, charts, and graphs to show data distributions and other important statistical information. A wonderful example of this is the *Atlas of United States Mortality*,[31] which uses a two-page layout for each cause of death. A series of maps, charts, and box plots displays information about the significance of rates (known as probability mapping), distribution of data, smoothed death rates for specific ages, and predicted regional rates with confidence limits.

Use of Map Symbols for Choropleth Mapping of Numeric Data

Different values of the same hue, a progression of hues, or black and white shading can be used to show patterns that are intuitive to the viewer. Dot and hatch patterns also can be used effectively. The map in the lower right corner shows a pattern resulting from a poor choice of shades.

Black, White and Gray Shading

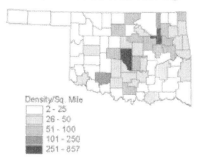

Density/Sq. Mile
- 2 - 25
- 26 - 50
- 51 - 100
- 101 - 250
- 251 - 857

Dot and Hatch Patterns

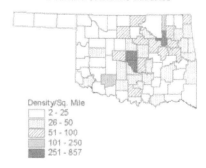

Density/Sq. Mile
- 2 - 25
- 26 - 50
- 51 - 100
- 101 - 250
- 251 - 857

Inappropriate Use of Symbols

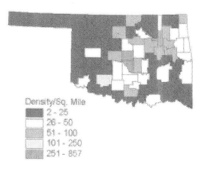

Density/Sq. Mile
- 2 - 25
- 26 - 50
- 51 - 100
- 101 - 250
- 251 - 857

Map Source: ESRI, Redlands, CA

FIGURE 21.8. Use of map symbols for choropleth mapping of numeric data, (Map source: ESRI. Redlands, CA.)

GIS Implementation and Use

Getting Started: GIS Organizational Models

In the late 1980s and the early 1990s. GIS implementation strategies focused on the acquisition of hardware and software, the collection of data, and aspects of managing the system, including organization and staffing.[5] Although all of the considerations addressed by formal implementation strategies remain important today, the technology has evolved to the point at which many GIS software development companies offer a wide range of products that accommodate a variety of approaches or models.[32] This flexibility provides the technological basis for a continuum of organizational models and implementation strategies. At one end of the continuum, a single individual uses GIS (small-scale GIS); at the other extreme, the entire organization uses GIS and, in some cases, with the advent of the Internet, even the community uses GIS (large-scale GIS). For purposes of the discussion that follows, we will describe several "discrete" models along this continuum, but the reader should keep in mind that the boundaries between the "discrete" models are quite fuzzy. In addition, these models can overlap, and more than one model may exist in any organization.

Smaller-Scale GIS

Since the early 1990s, there has been a trend toward the use of desktop GIS, a concept that involves making GIS and mapping accessible to people who use computers in their everyday work environment. The advent of desktop GIS has been concomitant with the development of powerful personal computers and user-friendly, Windows-based software environments. A variety of desktop GIS software packages have menu-driven graphical user interfaces and are easily integrated with office computer hardware.

Departmental GIS

A second organizational model is the departmental GIS. An example is a GIS in a state health department, where project and mapping support are provided on an as-needed basis to state and local public health agencies and where multiple GIS analysts work under the supervision of a GIS manager. Larger GIS operations such as these often use a wider range of GIS software products and store large amounts of data on Unix or Windows-based servers.

Enterprise GIS

Larger-scale GIS operations use an enterprise GIS model that provides GIS capabilities to an entire organization or a corporation and involves the use or development of multiple data types and applications and coordination among many departments. With an enterprise GIS, an organization's data are spatially enabled (i.e., geocoded and available for GIS and mapping applications) and accessible to the entire organization as a resource for analysis and decision-making. Data are usually stored on powerful servers within the organization and served to users across a network. For example, the city of Wilson, North Carolina houses an enterprise GIS that is used by employees in many departments, including fire, police, public utilities, public works, and planning and community development.[33] Environmental Systems Research Institute (ESRI), Inc. has developed a white paper on the development of enterprise GIS in health and social service agencies.[34]

Internet Map Servers

In recent years, a revolution has occurred in GIS technology with the advent of the Internet map server (IMS). This technology provides access to mapping capabilities through the use of a Web browser such as Netscape or Internet Explorer. It requires some behind-the-scenes set up and/or programming (depending on the product being used) by the organization providing the service, but it is accessible to anyone with a Web browser. This technology differs from the desktop GIS products discussed earlier, in that Internet map servers have no software or data storage requirements and can be accessed from any computer platform.

Three-Tier Client Server

Many agencies are using a three-tier client-server architecture to provide geographic information and services to clients. Tier 1 refers to a data server or data warehouse. Tier 2 is an application server that accesses data from Tier 1 and uses the data in an application, such as an Internet map server, to provide the data to Tier 3, the client. As an example, the Research Triangle Institute's GIS program uses this architecture to provide project management support for an epidemiology project. This project uses phlebotomists located throughout the United States to draw blood samples from survey respondents. Project management staff members need dynamic data and maps showing the location of field staff (phlebotomists) and their geographic relationship to survey respondents so that phlebotomists can be allocated to respondents efficiently. Additional information, such as percentage of respondent surveys completed by primary sampling unit or identification of all respondents within a 60-mile buffer of phlebotomist location, have been incorporated into the application. These types of applications use a Unix or Windows-based data server for data storage and retrieval (Tier 1), a PC running ESRI's ArcIMS Internet map server software to serve the data via a Web-based application (Tier 2), and a client—the epidemiologist/project manager, who accesses the application through a Web browser (Tier 3).

Hardware and Software Requirements

GIS has been developed for a variety of computer platforms. The trend has moved from minicomputers (mid-1980s) and powerful Unix workstations (late 1980s/early 1990s) to personal computers. While Unix workstations are used to run more complex GIS applications and still function as GIS data servers, most GIS/mapping software applications used today are available for the PC environment.

In recent years, GIS software has moved away from command line interfaces to a Windows environment with easy-to-use graphical user interfaces consisting of menus and tool bars. Many inexpensive, user-friendly GIS/mapping software products are now available, and product reviews are frequently published in *GeoWorld* and *Geospatial Solutions* (formerly *Geo Info Systems*). A recent comparison of selected GIS software products can be found in Thrall,[35] and Richards et al.[19] have provided information about costs.

In order to evaluate hardware and software needs, GIS users in public health must determine which GIS organizational model meets their needs, the availability and format of digital geographic data, and how their GIS activities will be integrated with other research or operational units. In many cases, a powerful PC with desktop software will be sufficient. With more sophisticated systems, such as those used in a departmental or an enterprise GIS, larger investments in data servers and software will be necessary. No matter which GIS system is purchased, spatial data is always space-intensive. Geographic data files are large. A user should purchase more hard drive space than anticipated need indicates.

Spatial Data Collection, Development, and Distribution

In the 1980s and early 1990s, the primary bottleneck in GIS implementation was the need to develop and/or acquire high-quality geographic data, a factor that was, and still is, often underestimated. Fortunately, during the past several years, there has been a proliferation of available spatial data in digital form as a result of improvements in technology, the ever-increasing use of GIS, and coordination efforts by federal, state, and local government agencies, such as the Federal Geographic Data Committee (FGDC). Many of these spatial data layers are free or can be purchased at a minimal cost from federal or state agencies. Others are sold by private vendors who have either created spatial data themselves or else added value to spatial data from government and other sources. Due to the recent acts of terrorism in the United States, public access to some spatial data has become more restricted.

Probably the most commonly used spatial data in the country are the U.S. Bureau of the Census TIGER/Line These files, usually referred to as simply TIGER/Line (Topologically Integrated Geographic Encoding and Referencing system) files. These files were first produced for the 1990 census and contain map layers for census geography, physical landmarks, rivers and streams, transportation networks, and other features. These geographic files can be linked with the census data files for mapping and analysis of census variables. In urban areas, the street network data can be used for address matching. Most states have several repositories for census data. The US Bureau of the Census Web site available at http://www.census.gov provides information about accessing these data sets.

Tiger/Line files are updated on a regular basis. The Census 2000 TIGER/Line files are now available. These files contain all of the geographic census entities, including a new statistical unit, the Zip Code Tabulation Area (ZCTA), that consists of an aggregation of census blocks but closely approximates a post office ZIP code area. Such a combination is a dream come true for many health professionals because it will allow them to link the ZIP code information in many health datasets with census socio-demographic data with greater accuracy than has been possible in the past. Of course, ZIP codes are relatively small geographic units, so users will need to take even greater caution when dealing with rates and small numbers or issues of confidentiality. One of the projects of the Federal Geographic Data Committee has been to implement a national Geospatial Data Clearinghouse, which functions as a data catalog and is accessible via the Internet at http://www.fgdc.gov/clearinghouse/clearinghouse.html. The University of Arkansas' Center for Advanced Spatial Technologies maintains a guide to online spatial and attribute data on its Web site available at http://www.cast.uark.edu/local/hunt/index.html. Environmental Systems Research Institute (Redland, CA) maintains a Geography Network site that is a global network of GIS users and data and service providers. Users can search for spatial data via this link: http://www.geographynetwork.com/.

GIS data for public health applications are often created by linking health attribute data from state and local government agencies to geographic boundary files by geocode. For instance, county-level mortality data can be linked to a state's county boundary file by county code. Health datasets that contain zip code fields can be linked to a zip code boundary file by the zip code field in both databases. Many public health datasets are created through the address matching process, described in a previous section. A thorough review of GIS data sources for community health planning can be found in Lee and Irving.[36]

Often, local public health community planning efforts require relatively detailed data in order to permit development of maps at the sub-county or neighborhood level of geography.[37] Given the requirement to protect the confidentiality and privacy of individual medical record information, many existing state or federal spatial databases typically do not provide a sub-county level of detail—the smallest geographic unit of analysis is often at the county level. Thus, in addition to whatever data may be available at the state and federal level, local health agencies need capabilities to geocode and import their own data. Depending on the nature of a specific health problem being addressed, the local public health agency also may need to develop local spatial data partnerships with other local government agencies and community organizations (e.g., the department of transportation for motor vehicle accidents, the police department for teenage crime data.)

Spatial data are critical for GIS operations, but so is information about those data. The Federal Geographic Data Committee (FGDC) has spent several years developing a standard for *metadata* that describes the content and quality of a spatial database, or, in FGDC's words, "data about data." Metadata provide important information about who developed the database, the scale of the original data, the time period of the content, and attribute and positional accuracy. While metadata does not guarantee the quality of the data, they do provide important information with which a user can determine appropriateness of the data's use. Metadata are usually in the form of text stored in a separate file. They are available for many of the datasets developed by federal agencies and are gradually being developed by other agencies as well.

Today, it is of critical importance to have knowledge of existing GIS coordination efforts at the federal, state, and local levels. Most organizations need more data than they can afford to develop. Even though one organization may not collect a certain type of spatial data, another organization may have those data. And, for certain types of data (e.g. aerial photography), the total cost for an entire state base-map may be sufficiently expensive that multiple organizations need to contribute to the funding.

Personnel and Training Issues

All organizational models of GIS require personnel with high levels of technical competence to develop the databases and applications that provide analysis and results for decision support. Somers has made a distinction between (1) full-time GIS users, (2) part-time GIS users, and (3) support staff.[38] On the whole, one would expect full-time GIS users to be technicians, analysts, or managers who have educational backgrounds in geography or GIS; part-time users might have backgrounds in a field of expertise, with training in the use of GIS.

GIS practitioners come from all walks of life, however, and personnel classification schemes for GIS positions are not always clear-cut. In some cases, the classification schemes do not exist at all. For full-time GIS staff, an organization may access a number of position and salary surveys available from private vendors and associations. These surveys provide job classification guidance with respect to salary, educational and experience requirements, and responsibilities. For example, Geosearch, Inc. conducts an ongoing wage and salary survey for GIS and related professions and makes information available on its Web site at http://www.geosearch.com. The Urban and Regional Information Systems Association (URISA) also conducts salary surveys, available at http://www.urisa.org. Rather than hiring and attempting to retain full-time GIS practitioners, some organizations find it more cost-effective to contract out their GIS work to other organizations or to hire contract employees to conduct GIS work.

Many public health professionals—in epidemiology and disease surveillance, environmental health, and community assessment—are using GIS as a tool for analysis and decision-making. Although the educational background of such professionals often does not include GIS, it is important for these GIS users to understand basic geographic/GIS concepts and to be able to interpret and critically analyze GIS maps created by others.

Eventually, as such part-time GIS users become more familiar with the technology and its wide range of applications, they will go beyond mapping and begin to use GIS for more sophisticated forms of spatial analysis. The collection of maps recently published in the *Journal of Public Health Man-*

agement and Practice[39] indicates that the use of GIS in health applications is headed in this direction. This evolution in GIS use will necessitate a higher level of training and education for the part-time GIS user.

For the most part, learning how to use GIS/desktop mapping software is not difficult or time-consuming, a fact that can be deceptive because it obscures the complexity of GIS. GIS software vendors often offer their own training courses, some of which are even available as distance learning options. As GIS users become more advanced in their analyses, it is imperative that they have an understanding of coordinate systems, map projections, geocoding, data development and conversion, metadata, and spatial analysis. The National Center for Geographic Information and Analysis (NCGIA) has been developing a core curriculum for GIS education. Topics in the core curriculum are listed on the Web at http://www.ncgia.ucsb.edu/pubs/core.html.

GIS users in the public health fields have additional concepts that they must master. Many of these concepts can be gleaned from a course in epidemiology or biostatistics. These concepts include the use of rates, statistical variation involving the use of small numbers in either the numerator or denominator, the concept of rate adjustment (e.g., age, race, sex) and the impact of different standard populations (e.g., 1940 vs. 2000) on rates. In addition, state and local public health GIS users need to have a sound understanding of the ecological fallacy in the analysis of cause-and-effect relationships and of issues involved in modeling exposure to environmental factors or using proximity as a surrogate.[22]

Fortunately, universities and community colleges are rising to the challenge of providing GIS education to a range of users. Many of them now offer GIS-related courses in the evening or over the World Wide Web, making them accessible to "mid-career professionals" who wish to enhance their GIS knowledge. Many are also offering certificate or degree programs in GIS.

Social Institutional Issues

Individual and organizational users of GIS typically need to address a number of social and institutional issues. These issues include confidentiality, security and data access, coordination with other agencies, and organizational politics.

Confidentiality

Many health datasets contain sensitive information. Consequently, public law mandates that many agencies maintain the confidentiality of patient records and health statistics. Databases often contain addresses that serve as individual identifiers—the location of a point on a map could be used to identify a person. GIS users should be cautious about which maps are produced for internal use vs. those that are distributed to the public or shown in presentations. Some methods used to protect privacy in GIS applications are to (1) aggregate patient data to zip code or county level (in some cases, small population numbers in these units may pose confidentiality concerns); (2) use smaller-scale maps that show less detail; (3) avoid including the street network on the map, as this provides the most familiar means of locating an address; or (4) displace point features through the use of a random displacement algorithm, thus offsetting x,y coordinates but maintaining geographic integrity.[40]

Security and Data Access

Many of the security and data access concerns are closely related to data privacy and confidentiality issues discussed in Chapter 10. All of the major computer operating systems have security features that can restrict access to files and data through the use of log-ins and passwords. In addition, firewalls are often set up to limit access from outside an organization. The epidemiology project management IMS application, discussed in an earlier section, uses a map database of respondents that contains identifying information needed by the epidemiologists. For this reason, the application runs behind the Institute's firewall and is accessible only to epidemiology/project management staff. Data access and security are serious issues. It is critical to have competent system administration and information technology staff to handle them. All organizations that handle confidential or sensitive data should have a set of procedures in place to cover digital and non-digital data. In fact, public law mandates that agencies protect vital statistics and health data. As discussed in Chapter 10, some agencies require employees to sign confidentiality agreements and conform to an established set of procedures.

Coordination with Other Agencies

In an earlier section, we have noted the importance of coordination activities in the development and sharing of digital spatial data. In addition to federal coordination agencies, such as the FGDC, many states and regions are involved in data sharing and coordination activities. Coordination activities provide GIS users with opportunities for sharing data and applications; for keeping abreast of developments in the technology; for training; and for access to important information for decision-making, such as the proper software product to purchase. As an example, North Carolina has a well-developed GIS coordination infrastructure that embraces state and local government agencies, universities, and the private sector. The state's Geographic Information Coordinating Council, first established in 1991 by an executive order, oversees the coordination efforts. Many of the state's coordination activities are carried out by a state agency, the North Carolina Center for Geographic Information and Analysis. The agency provides geographic data and Internet mapping capabilities via its Website (http://www.ncmapnet.com).

Organizational Politics

The impact of organizational politics on GIS operations should not be overlooked. For example, upper-level managers might veto GIS applications that address politically sensitive or controversial issues. In addition, reorganization in government agencies, common and usually political, can have either a positive or an adverse impact on GIS operations. Moreover, GIS is a technology that nearly everyone wants. Consequently, the location of a GIS unit in the organizational structure in an agency can affect which projects receive priority and/or funding.

Limitations and Lessons Learned

Although GIS is a powerful tool that is increasingly easy to use, GIS users must recognize the limitations of the software and of the spatial data and make attempts to work around those limitations. In this section, we will describe some of the common limitations that GIS users face.

Accuracy and Completeness of Spatial Data

Mapping and spatial analysis can be severely impacted by the quality of the geographic data. Entire books have been written on this topic.[41] In addition, errors can be propagated during data processing or modeling activities.[42] Coordinate precision, that is, the number of significant digits that are stored for each coordinate, plays a role in some of these errors, as does the use of different map projections. Three good rules to follow are (1) never to assume that a geographic database is free of error; (2) to acquire the metadata and read it to obtain information about the creation of the data, and (3) whenever possible, to develop methods of assessing data quality.

Accuracy and Completeness of Attribute Data

Inaccuracies also exist in non-spatial databases. Character fields may have misspellings, and numeric fields may have data entry errors. As with spatial databases, quality control procedures should be developed to the extent possible. In 1998, the author conducted extensive mapping and geographic analysis using one of the public health screening databases maintained by the state of North Carolina. During this process, it became apparent that many of the county geocodes in the database were incorrect. For the most part, staff members of the laboratories doing blood sample analysis keyed in the geocodes. The author compared data from 1994 to 1996, consisting of 265,492 records, to a master lookup table containing CITY, COUNTY and ZIP CODE fields to check for city/county/zip correspondence in the screening database. The shocking discovery was that only 158,552 records (59.72%) contained accurate and/or complete information. Many counties had incorrect geocodes. Some resulted from data entry errors (i.e., typos), which are easy to make, because most geocodes are numeric; others resulted from confusion over city and county names: many North Carolina towns and counties have the same names but very different locations. For example, the town of Henderson, located in Vance County, often gets coded to Henderson County, which is over 200 miles to the southwest. These types of errors are by no means limited to this particular dataset in North Carolina. They went unnoticed until these data were used in a GIS. With the use of GIS, North Carolina health agencies have gained an increased awareness of the geocoding data issues affecting their databases and have taken steps to address them.

Currency/Time Period of Data Content

One data characteristic that is often neglected is that of time. When were the data collected? When were they last updated? It is easier to obtain funds to create GIS databases than to maintain and update them. Currency is a serious issue when a user is working with census data, which are commonly used in health analyses. Because a census is conducted only every ten years, census data can become seriously out of date. Moreover, while population projections and intercensal estimates are routinely computed for states, counties and large municipalities, many analyses require data for small geographic units or information about socioeconomic factors. Fortunately, projections for smaller units can sometimes be purchased from private vendors. In 2003, the full implementation of the American Community Survey by the U.S. Census will result in more up-to-date data products, but it will be several years before these data are available for small units such as census tracts.

Address Matching Issues

Address matching is commonly used with health datasets to create a map layer of points showing facility locations or patient residences. Whereas address matching works well in urban areas, in which complete map layers of named streets with address ranges exist, its success rate in rural areas is usually lower. Address matching does not work for addresses that consist of P. O. boxes or rural routes. Many counties across the nation are implementing enhanced 911 (E911) systems for the routing of emergency vehicles. This process involves the assignment of numbered street addresses to every building in the county—including buildings in rural areas—and the development of GIS databases to maintain this information.

Finally, a clinic or patient address does not always reflect the building or residence location. Many health surveys obtain information about mailing address, which sometimes differs from address of residence. For epidemiologic studies, it is important to remember that address of residence does not always infer location of exposure. Also, an address provides no indication of residential mobility. Information about previous addresses or length of residence at current address is rarely contained in health datasets.

Use of Zip Codes

Many health datasets do not contain an address field, and attempts to conduct sub-county analyses may therefore be limited to the use of ZIP codes. When a user is mapping or analyzing ZIP code data, it is extremely important to remember that ZIP codes were developed by the U.S. Postal Service for the delivery of mail, *not for geographic analysis and mapping*. Unlike census units (e.g., tracts, block groups) ZIP codes were not intended to be homogeneous with respect to socio-demographic variables. Although census data are provided for ZIP codes, the heterogeneity of populations within a specific ZIP code can lead to averaging of values. In other words, demographic characteristics may vary widely within a ZIP code, but this variation will not be detected with ZIP code data. The use of the Census 2000 Zip Code Tabulation Area (ZCTA) should alleviate some of these problems.

One additional problem with ZIP code boundaries is that they change over time. Therefore, health data from 1999, for example, should not be mapped by use of a 1994 ZIP code file. Because the post office does not develop digital ZIP code boundary files, in the past, they have been acquired from private vendors, and purchasing them for a time period of several years could be expensive. This situation will be improved with the release of Census 2000 TIGER/Line files with ZCTAs. Sometimes, because of economic constraints, there is no choice but to use available data. In such a case, a user should always document the source of the data and its time period.

Scale and Precision of Location

We have already noted the importance of metadata for assessing the quality of a database. The FGDC metadata standard also includes information about the processes used to create the database. For example, the scale of the source map has a great impact on the coordinate precision of a feature's location. The location of features digitized from a large-scale map will be more precise than those obtained from a small-scale map. The precision of point data is dependent on the method used to locate the points. Points that have been address matched to a street network will generally be more precise than points matched to a ZIP code centroid.

Proximity Versus Exposure

In epidemiologic studies, it is important to remember that proximity to a feature, such as a hazardous waste site, does not always imply exposure. Beware of associations gleaned from map overlay or geographic analysis. GIS is a wonderful tool for understanding relationships among features and for generating hypotheses about etiology, but GIS must be supplemented with standard epidemiological methods when analyzing spatial correlates of health outcomes.

Emerging Technologies and Their Implications for GIS

Innovations in technology are making GIS less costly, easier to use, and more widely available. These innovations include the Internet and Web-based applications, along with data warehousing.

The Internet and Web-based Applications

Internet map server technology was discussed briefly in an earlier section. A more technical discussion can be found in Foresman.[43] Internet applications are highly varied; they range from viewing geographic data catalogues to sophisticated geoprocessing activities. Harder has developed a categorization scheme for geographic resources over the Internet,[44] including:

- Maps that show only location—static images that are imbedded in an HTML document. These maps are usually produced by use of GIS software and saved as GIF or JPEG files.
- Maps that show change, such as weather or traffic maps. These maps are frequently updated. A program running in the background replaces the map image when a new one becomes available.
- Interactive maps, or maps that the user creates. These maps are technologically more complex than the first two categories, as they require the use of an Internet map server. The user sends a request to the map server and a map is produced "on the fly."
- Maps that perform spatial analysis—examples are maps that compute the shortest distance and route between two points, or that locate all facilities within a specified area.
- Maps that perform geoprocessing. These maps are less common than all other categories. These are sites that process raw geographic data.
- Public data sites and commercial data sites that point to or provide access to geographic data. In some cases, on-line data can be downloaded directly, or, it can be provided on CD-ROM. In general, data available through public data sites tend to be free or else available at low cost. Many commercial data sites accept credit card orders.

Although Internet map server technology is promising, there are technological limitations to be overcome during the next several years. First and foremost, map data are space-intensive, and serving them over the Web takes time. Many IMS applications are slow, and they include only basic functions, such as turning map layers on or off and zooming in or out. As the technology evolves, more sophisticated geoprocessing functions will become increasingly available.

Data Warehousing

GIS software products are incorporating developments in database management technology. One of these developments is data warehousing, a term that implies more than a large central database. The term is used to describe a central repository of all types of data used by an organization or enterprise. These data warehouses provide high-speed access to databases by many users, and they allow transactions, such as editing, to occur without interrupting the normal flow of work. In the future, warehouses for spatial data will become more common. Currently, few exist, but examples include CubeWerx of Canada, MrSID image data warehousing, and ESRI's Spatial Data Engine.[45]

Conclusion

GIS is an information system, an approach to science, and a powerful set of analysis and visualization tools that can be used by public health professionals to enhance their analysis and understanding of public health issues and to provide a basis for sound decision making. GIS is deceptively easy to use; however, geographic data, spatial/epidemiologic analysis, and GIS information systems are more complex than they appear to the casual user. The effective use of GIS requires a combination of good training and experience. In the years ahead, that training and experience will become even more important as GIS becomes an increasingly powerful and common tool in the practice of public health.

Questions for Review

1. List at least five disciplines underlying the practice of "geographic information science."
2. Explain why GIS is needed in the practice of public health and how it can assist epidemiologists and other practitioners in performing their duties.
3. Differentiate between *spatial* and *attribute* data as components in a GIS.
4. Explain why map projections and coordinate systems are important to the use of GIS in displaying geographic features and why data obtained from a *geographic information system* must be transformed before it can be used for accurate mapping and analysis.

5. Differentiate between *unprojected* and *projected* coordinates in the use of a GIS, and differentiate between *vector* and *raster* data, providing an example of each data type.
6. Define (1) *choropleth mapping* and (2) *automated address matching* in the use of a GIS, and describe at least three potential limitations and pitfalls in the use of automated address matching.
7. Explain the principles underlying (1) the use of colors in maps that display data and (2) the principles for appropriate use of black and white.
8. Describe the capabilities and the nature of (1) Internet map servers and (2) three-tier client servers in GIS applications.
9. Describe the limitations inherent in using census data produced before the year 2000 in GIS applications, particularly with respect to the need to display data covering sub-county areas, and explain how a GIS user can overcome these limitations.
10. Explain why *metadata* is important to the proper application of GIS systems.
11. Explain why the apparent ease of use of modern GIS systems can be deceiving to the uninformed user.

Questions 12–13 are based on the following short case.
A public health researcher wants to use a GIS to analyze an apparent increase in lead levels in well water in two small communities in a county during the year 2001. The researcher is relying, in part, on use of a local dataset produced in 1994 to display historic lead level measurements. County health employees directly input the data in the dataset. This dataset covers the years 1988–1994. It does not contain address fields, but it does contain postal zip codes.

12. Explain why reliance on the postal zip codes contained in this dataset may result in maps that display inaccurate or inconsistent data.
13. Explain why the data in the dataset may be inaccurate.

Acknowledgments

The author wishes to acknowledge the Research Triangle Institute for its support, in the form of a Personal Development Award, during the development of materials for this chapter.

References

1. O'Carroll P. Informatics Training for CDC Public Health Advisors: Introduction and Background. http://faculty.washington.edu/~ocarroll/infrmatc/home.htm, posted July 1997.
2. Cesnik B. The Future of Health Informatics. *International Journal of Medical Informatics.* 1999: 55:83-85.

3. Raghupathi W, Tan J. 1999. Strategic Uses of Information Technology in Health Care: a State-of-the-art Survey. *Topics in Health Information Management.* 1999;20:1-15.
4. Lasker RD. Humphreys BL. Braithwaite WR. Making a Powerful Connection: The Health of the Public and the National Information Infrastructure. Report of the U.S. Public Health Service Public Health Data Policy Coordinating Committee; 1995. Also available at: www.nnlm.gov/fed/phs.powerful.html.
5. Antenucci JC, Brown K. Croswell P, Kevany MJ, Archer H. *Geographic Information Systems: A Guide to the Technology.* New York:Van Nostrand Reinhold; 1991.
6. Clarke KC. *Getting Started with Geographic Information Systems.* Upper Saddle River, NJ: Prentice-Hall; 1999.
7. Jones C. *Geographical Information Systems and Computer Cartography.* Essex, England: Longman; 1997.
8. Goodchild MF. What is Geographic Information Science? *NCGIA Core Curriculum in GIScience*; http://www.ncgia.ucsb.edu/giscc/units/u002/u002.html, posted October 7, 1997.
9. Haggett P. *Geography: A Modern Synthesis.* New York: Harper & Row Publishers; 1983.
10. Tobler WR. Automation and Cartography. *Geographical Review.* 1959;49:526-534.
11. Burrough PA. *Principles of Geographical Information Systems for Land Resources Assessment.* Oxford: Oxford University Press; 1986.
12. Cliff AD, Haggett P, Ord JK. 1983. Forecasting Epidemic Pathways for Measles in Iceland: the Use of Simultaneous Equation and Logic Models. *Ecology of Disease.* 1983;2:377-396.
13. Choynowski M. Maps Based on Probabilities. *Journal of the American Statistical Association.* 1959;54:385-388.
14. Cliff AD. Haggett P. *Atlas of Disease Distributions: Analytic Approaches to Epidemiological Data.* Oxford: Blackwell Publishers; 1988.
15. Glick BJ. The Spatial Organization of Cancer Mortality. *Annals of the Association of American Geographers.* 1982:72:471-481.
16. Meade MS. Cardiovascular Disease in Savannah, Georgia. In: McGlashan ND, Blunden JR, eds. *Geographical Aspects of Health: Essays in Honor of Andrew Learmonth.* London: Academic Press; 1983:175-196.
17. Gould PR, Leinbach TR. An Approach to the Geographical Assignment of Hospital Services. *Tijdschrift voor Economische en Sociale Geographie.* 1966:57:203-206.
18. Hanchette CL. GIS and Decision Making for Public Health Agencies: Childhood Lead Poisoning and Welfare Reform. *Journal of Public Health Management and Practice.* 1999;5:41-47.
19. Richards TB, Croner CM. Rushton G, Brown CK, Fowler L. Geographic Information Systems and Public Health: Mapping the Future. *Public Health Reports.* 1999;114:359-373.
20. Jennings R. *Special Edition: Using Microsoft Access 2000.* Indianapolis, Indiana: Que Corporation; 1999.
21. Robinson AH, Morrison JL. Muehrcke PC, Kimerling AJ. Guptill SC. *Elements of Cartography (6th Edition).* New York: John Wiley and Sons; 1995.
22. Vine MF, Degnan D, Hanchette C. Geographic Information Systems: Their Use in Environmental Epidemiologic Research. *Environmental Health Perspectives.* 1997;105:598-605.

23. Bonham-Carter GF. *Geographic Information Systems for Geoscientists: Modelling with GIS.* Tarrytown, NY: Pergamon Press (Elsevier Science); 1994.
24. Kulldorff M. Geographic Information Systems (GIS) and Community Health: Some Statistical Issues. *Journal of Public Health Management and Practice.* 1999;5:100-106.
25. Buescher PA. *Problems with Rates Based on Small Numbers. Statistical Primer No. 12.* Raleigh, NC: State Center for Health Statistics; 1997. (available at http://www.schs.state.nc.us/SCHS/pdf/primer12.pdf)
26. Unwin DJ. *Introductory Spatial Analysis.* INSERT PUBLISHER LOCATION: PUBLISHER; 1981.
27. Cressie NA. *Statistics for Spatial Data.* New York: John Wiley and Sons; 1993.
28. Monmonier M. *How to Lie with Maps.* Chicago: The University of Chicago Press; 1991.
29. National Institutes of Health (NIH), National Cancer Institute (NCI). *Atlas of Cancer Mortality in the United States, 1950-94.* NIH Publication No. 99-4564. Bethesda, Maryland: NIH; 1999.
30. Casper ML, Barnett E, Halverson JA, Elmes GA, Braham VE, Majeed ZA, Bloom AS, Stanley S. *Women and Heart Disease: An Atlas of Racial and Ethnic Disparities in Mortality.* Morgantown, West Virginia: Office for Social Environment and Health Research, West Virginia University; Atlanta, Georgia: National Center for Chronic Disease Prevention and Health Promotion, Center for Disease Control and Prevention; 2000.
31. Pickle LW, Mungiole M, Jones GK, White AA. *Atlas of United States Mortality.* Hyattsville, Maryland: National Center for Health Statistics; 1996.
32. Environmental Systems Research Institute (ESRI). Arc GIS Scales to Fit Your Organization (http:www.esri.com/software/scalable_arcgis.html).
33. Hinton C. North Carolina City Saves Time, Lives and Money with Award-Winning GIS. *Geo Info Systems.* 1997;7:35-37.
34. Environmental Systems Research Institute (ESRI). Enterprise GIS in Health and Social Service Agencies. White paper available at http://www.esri.com/library/whitepapers/addl_lit.html; July 1999.
35. Thrall SE. Geographic Information System (GIS) Hardware and Software. *Journal of Public Health Management and Practice.* 1999;5:82-90.
36. Lee CV, Irving JL. Sources of Spatial Data for Community Health Planning. *Journal of Public Health Management and Practice.* 1999;5:7-22.
37. Melnick A, Seigal N, Hildner J, Troxel T. Clackamas County Department of Human Services Community Health Mapping Engine (ChiME) Geographic Information Systems Project. *Journal of Public Health Management and Practice.* 1999;5:64-69.
38. Somers R. Organizing and Staffing a Successful GIS: Organization Strategies. *URISA Journal.* 1995;7:49-52.
39. Richards T, Croner C, Novick L. Atlas of State and Local Geographic Information Systems (GIS) Maps to Improve Community Health. *Journal of Public Health Management and Practice.* 1999;4:2-72.
40. Armstrong MP, Rushton G, Zimmerman DL. Geographically Masking Health Data to Preserve Confidentiality. *Statistics in Medicine.* 1999;18:497-525.
41. Goodchild MF, Gopal S eds. *Accuracy of Spatial Databases.* London: Taylor and Francis; 1989.

42. Heuvelink GBM. *Error Propagation in Environmental Modelling with GIS.* London: Taylor and Francis; 1998.
43. Foresman TW. Spatial Analysis and Mapping on the Internet. *Journal of Public Health Management and Practice.* 1999;5:57-63.
44. Harder C. *Serving Maps on the Internet: Geographic Information on the World Wide Web.* Redlands, CA: Environmental Systems Research Institute, Inc.; 1998.
45. Lowe JW. Data Warehouses and Spatial Web Sites. *Geospatial Solutions.* September 2000.

22
Immunization Registries: Critical Tools for Sustaining Success

ROBERT W. LINKINS

Learning Objectives

After studying this chapter, you should be able to

- Understand the challenges to sustaining current high immunization coverage and to reaching the unimmunized and under-immunized populations in the United States.
- Define the concept of an immunization registry and describe the benefits of a registry to (1) parents, (2) immunization providers, and (3) the public.
- Describe the history of the development of immunization registries and the issues raised during the development of immunization registries in the United States.
- Describe the current status of the development of population-based immunization registries in the United States and identify the challenges that must be met if public health officials are to succeed in widespread implementation of such registries.
- Discuss the future role of immunization registries in the improvement of public health in the United States.

Overview

Widespread, population-based immunization registries hold the promise of increasing immunization rates in the United States and of effecting a reduction in the rates of morbidity and mortality attributable to vaccine-preventable disease. Such registries also provide both direct and indirect benefits for parents, school officials, providers of vaccination services, and public health organizations. In recent years, public health officials have made considerable progress in assisting states and communities to build such registries. Funding and sponsorship, development of standards, and production of guidelines are only a few of the steps that public health organizations have taken to assist state and local health departments to develop and implement immunization registries. Still, the widespread implementation of population-based immunization registries faces many hurdles in the years ahead. Progress in increasing the participation of immunization providers, ensuring the confidentiality of registry information, integrating immunization reporting with provider systems, and securing funding must continue if immunization registries are to deliver the full range of their potential benefits. As support from healthcare organizations and members of the public continues to grow, meeting the registry objective set forth in the publication *Healthy People 2010* is clearly realizable.

Introduction

Immunizations have been described as one of the greatest public health triumphs of the 20th century, and the U.S. immunization delivery system "a national treasure that is too often taken for granted."[1,2] Disease morbidity rates have declined dramatically for nine vaccine preventable diseases—smallpox, polio, diphtheria, pertussis, tetanus, measles, mumps, rubella, and *Haemophilus influenzae* Type b,[2] and the United States now has record-high immunization coverage levels[3,4] as a result of the enormous effort and dedication of our immunization providers and public health workforce.

Despite this success, approximately 300 U.S. children die each year from diseases that can be prevented by immunizations, and an estimated one million two-year-old children still need one or more vaccine doses to be fully immunized.[2] Disparities in immunization coverage exist for the most critical childhood vaccines, with the lowest coverage among urban and low-income populations.[5-7] Despite unprecedented success in protecting the population from vaccine-preventable diseases, these "pockets of need" have not been completely reached by current immunization delivery strategies.

Sustaining this coverage in the 11,000 babies born on average each day, as well as reaching those population groups that continue to be at risk for vaccine-preventable diseases, is a continuing challenge threatened by several factors:

- *An increasingly complex childhood immunization schedule.* Currently, 15–20 vaccine doses are recommended for a child by 18 months of age.[8] By the year 2020, this number is expected to triple.[2] Already, parents[9-14] and providers[15] find it difficult to assess whether a child needs an immunization, potentially missing an opportunity to vaccinate or else vaccinating when a child is already up-to-date. More recommended vaccines would likely compound this problem.
- *Provider overestimation of immunization coverage in their practices.* Several studies have shown that providers tend to think that the

immunization coverage in their practice is better than it truly is.[16] In California, for example, providers thought coverage was approximately 90% for their patient population when the actual rate was below 70%.[17,18] In Massachusetts, providers estimated 85%–100% coverage among two-year-old children in their practices, whereas actual coverage rates were as low as 19%.

- *Incomplete immunization records scattered across health care providers.* By two years of age, more than 20% of children have seen more than one provider.[19,20] Accurately assessing immunization needs can be difficult if records are scattered among different providers and the available immunization history is incomplete.[21-24] In addition to missed opportunities for immunization, children who receive care from multiple providers may receive too many immunizations.[25] It has been estimated that 21% of children 19–35 months of age receive at least one unnecessary dose of vaccine.[26]

- *Inconsistent use of effective immunization strategies.* Recently, the Task Force on Community Preventive Services conducted an extensive literature review to identify effective public health strategies.[27,28] Among the immunization interventions identified were (1) reminder and recall systems operated to notify parents about needed immunizations; (2) the "AFIX" evaluation system implemented by public health departments to Assess providers' immunization coverage, provide Feedback on results, supply Incentives, and eXchange information to boost coverage and avert missed immunization opportunities; and (3) linkages between immunization programs and WIC (the Special Supplemental Nutrition Program for Women, Infants, and Children) services to insure that a child's immunization status is assessed at every WIC visit. Although 75% of WIC agencies were reported in a 1994–1995 survey to be assessing the immunization status of WIC children,[29] a 1995 survey showed that only 35% of pediatricians and 23% of family physicians routinely operated reminder and recall systems,[2] and a 2000 study showed that only 48% of public and 6% of private clinics nationwide conducted AFIX evaluations.[30] Some studies have shown that providers have difficulty implementing patient reminders and AFIX evaluations, suggesting that the administrative burden associated with these activities may be a barrier to their use.[27] Lack of accurate information about vaccination status, as well as an adequate information infrastructure, may also inhibit their use.[2]

- *Fluctuating federal resources to support demonstrably effective, but resource-intensive immunization strategies.* During the early 1990s, federal dollars to support state immunization program infrastructure grew substantially. Funding levels were at an all-time high of approximately $261 million in fiscal year 1995. However, federal funding decreased during the late 1990s to a low of $139 million in fiscal year 2000. As a result, states reported that they reduced efforts to implement effective immunization interventions.[2,30] More recently, federal support for state immunization programs is on the rise. Congress appropriated $181.9 million in fiscal year 2001 for state operations/infrastructure grants (K. Lane, personal communication).

- *Growing public complacency about the need for childhood immunizations as a result of the record low levels of vaccine-preventable disease.* With record-high coverage levels achieving significant disease reduction, there is little to remind parents and providers of the seriousness of vaccine-preventable diseases.[31] In the near-absence of disease, concerns about the risks of vaccines versus the risks of disease have grown.

Together, these factors are making it more and more difficult to insure that all children get the immunizations that they need. Community- and state-based immunization registries may provide a sustainable tool to overcome these ongoing challenges by providing an automated immunization delivery infrastructure.

This chapter will provide a definition of an immunization registry, emphasizing the benefits of immunization registries. It will next discuss the developmental history of immunization registries in the United States, including an overview of the involvement of various public health organizations in the development and implementation of population-based registries. This chapter will then discuss some of the challenges associated with developing and implementing immunization registries, including the need to create immunization provider demand, the need to ensure the confidentiality of registry information, the need to identify necessary resources, and the need to promulgate registry standards. After a discussion of the current status of immunization registries in the United States, the chapter will conclude with a look at the future role of such registries.

A Definition of Immunization Registries

Immunization registries are confidential, population-based, computerized information systems that contain data about children's vaccinations.[31] Ideally, after consent is obtained from a parent or guardian, a child is enrolled in an immunization registry at birth, often through registry linkage with the electronic birth record or at first contact with the health care system. Identifying data and immunization information is recorded at enrollment and transferred electronically from the provider's office to the registry database, typically located at a county or state health department. At each immunization encounter, the child's immunization record is electronically retrieved by the provider's office from the registry. If more than one provider has been seen since the last visit, or if the child is a new patient, all records of immunization are aggregated by the registry to generate a complete and accurate immunization history for the provider. An automated algorithm is used by the registry to assist the provider in assessing the child's current immunization needs, identify children who are due or late for an immunization, produce reminder and recall notices, and calculate immunization coverage levels in the provider's practice or geographic area. When the child begins school or day care, official immunization records can be automatically generated by the registry, hence saving office time and resources.

Some of the potential benefits of immunization registries for parents, providers, and public health officials are described in Table 22.1. Registries have been used to increase immunization rates by as much as 45% in children.[32-41] More limited evaluations of registries that target adults demonstrate similar effectiveness at increasing immunization coverage.[15]

Registries also can play an important role in increasing vaccine safety and monitoring vaccine-associated adverse events, and consequently they can increase the public demand for immunization. Tracking valid vaccine contraindications can help ensure that children get only indicated vaccines. Registries can also facilitate timely and accurate reporting of adverse events and provide public health officials with population denominators necessary to calculate and track adverse event rates. Registry data have been used to help identify a cluster of vaccine-associated adverse events,[42] to identify and recall children who received immunizations from sub-potent vaccine lots or inadequate dosages of vaccine,[43,44] and to monitor the implementation of new vaccine recommendations.[44-48]

Immunization registries that are integrated with a broader public health information system have even greater benefits. Such registries have assisted in increasing immunization rates in underserved WIC populations, in delivering non-immunization-related public health care, including screenings for lead, tuberculosis, and anemia, and in identifying high-risk families for home visits and nutrition counseling.[49-56]

Developmental History of Immunization Registries

In the 1960s, many US immunization programs began developing infant immunization tracking systems that used birth certificates to monitor all children in their catchment areas. However, these systems were abandoned by most states because they were primarily manual, expensive to maintain, and not integrated within the broader public health delivery system. With the assistance of the National Immunization Program (NIP) at the Centers for Disease Control and Prevention (CDC) in 1974, Delaware became the first state to develop an immunization registry that recorded immunization data from all pediatric and family practice providers in the state.[2]

In 1980, NIP developed an Automated Immunization Management System (AIMS) that ran on a microcomputer. From 1980 through 1985, this system was installed and operated in 10 states or cities. Included among the features

TABLE 22.1. Potential benefits of immunization registries

Beneficiary	Potential Immunization Registry Benefits
Parents	• Assemble in one site all immunizations a child has received to create an accurate and complete immunization history.
	• Help ensure that a child's immunizations are up-to-date through computerized decision support.
	• Provide reminder and recall notices when an immunization is due or late.
	• Prevent unnecessary (duplicative) doses of vaccine.
	• Produce an accurate, official copy of a child's immunization history for personal, day care, school, or camp entry requirements.
Providers	• Consolidate immunizations from all providers into one record to serve as a source of complete and accurate immunization histories for any child, whether a new or continuing patient.
	• Help interpret the complex immunization schedule by providing computerized immunization decision support.
	• Identify immunizations due or overdue, and produce reminder and recall notices.
	• Produce official immunization records for schools, camps, and day cares.
	• Reduce a practice's paperwork.
	• Facilitate introduction of new vaccines or changes in the vaccine schedule.
	• Help manage vaccine inventories.
	• Generate quality assurance reports (e.g., Health Plan Employer Data Information Set [HEDIS] for managed-care organizations).
	• Reinforce the concept of the medical home by facilitating vaccination and referral back to the medical home.
Public health officials	• Help control vaccine-preventable diseases.
	• Provide information to identify unimmunized and under-immunized populations, target interventions and resources, and evaluate programs.
	• Promote reminder and recall of children who need immunizations.
	• Reduce missed immunization opportunities by ensuring providers follow the most up-to-date recommendations.
	• Integrate immunization services with other public health functions.

Source: Adapted from Report of the National Vaccine Advisory Committee. Development of Community- and State-Based Immunization Registries. January 12, 1999. Available at http:www.cdc.gov/nip/registry/nvac.htm.

of AIMS were immunization tracking and recall, immunization status assessment, and vaccine inventory and accountability. Among the lessons learned from this experience was the vital role that end-users and management staff played in the development process. Ease-of-use and integration with office routines were critical to system acceptance.

Several managed care organizations began to develop immunization registries following the AIMS effort. Group Health, Puget Sound's registry, included its 350,000 enrollees in the late 1980s, and in the early 1990s several managed care organizations began developing registries and tracking systems for vaccine-adverse events in collaboration with NIP.[2]

Today's concerted registry activity was motivated by a nationwide resurgence of measles in 1989. From 1989 through 1991, 55,622 measles cases and 123 deaths were reported in the United States.[57] Because of the difficulty in estimating measles vaccine coverage in the population, CDC convened a group of experts in 1991 to provide advice on measuring immunization coverage. These experts recommended that a national registry system be created to provide immunization coverage at the state and local level.[58] The desired outputs of this network of these state-based tracking systems were threefold: (1) assessment of the immunization status of individual children; (2) estimation of immunization coverage of provider practices for self-evaluation; and (3) provision of local and state-based immunization coverage estimates to enable effective targeting of immunization delivery efforts.[59]

At about the same time, The Robert Wood Johnson Foundation established the All Kids Count Program to work with other national efforts to develop computerized monitoring and follow-up systems. With assistance from five other private foundations, 24 states and communities were funded in 1992 to assist in the development of immunization registries in states and local communities.[60]

In 1993, NIP began awarding planning grants to develop state-based immunization registries in every state. These state-based systems were to be populated from birth registry databases and used to collect immunization histories on all children resident in the state. As proposed by CDC's panel of experts in 1991, it was conceived that all the systems would be linked together for the exchange of definitive immunization histories for children who moved from one state to another. Considerable flexibility was allowed in the development of these systems. In particular, NIP supported the concept of integrating state-based registries within more comprehensive information systems at the state level.

In 1993, the Director of NIP stated, "The immunization registry system, therefore, is the means to institutionalize vaccination of each succeeding birth cohort and will be vital to maintaining high levels of immunization coverage."[59] Shortly thereafter, in 1994, a National Vaccine Advisory Committee (NVAC) Subcommittee on Vaccination Registries recommended expanded funding and new federal policies for a system of immunization registries to support national immunization goals. The members determined that "Immunization registries are essential to reaching and sustaining coverage levels at the national goal."[61] In 2000, the Institute of Medicine echoed NVAC's members when noting, "with the increasing importance of population-based approaches to health system planning and evaluation, immunization registries offer one of the most useful instruments for assessing population-specific effectiveness of health and medical care programs."

Since 1994, NIP has allocated $181.9 million for the development and implementation of a nationwide network of community- and state-based immunization registries to its 64 immunization grantees (50 states, the District of Columbia, Chicago, Houston, New York City, Philadelphia, San Antonio, American Samoa, Guam, Marshall Islands, Micronesia, Northern Mariana Islands, Palau, Puerto Rico, and the U.S. Virgin Islands) that receive federal immunization funds under the Public Health Service Act. The Robert Wood Johnson Foundation, with a second phase of funding for 16 projects through the All Kids Count Program, has provided an estimated $20 million for registry development.[31] Federal funds account for approximately 56% of dollars spent on immunization registries. Other sources of funding include state (19%), in-kind (12%), other (8%), private (5%), and local (<1%) sources (G. Urquhart, personal communication).

Initiative on Immunization Registries

In 1997, the President of the United States directed the Secretary of the Department of Health and Human Services (DHHS) to work with the states on developing immunization registries.[62] In response to this charge, the Initiative on Immunization Registries was launched, led by NVAC, with support from NIP and the National Vaccine Program Office. Members of the Initiative's Workgroup on Immunization Registries (WIR) included representatives of provider organizations, managed care plans, state and local health departments, parent and consumer groups, and the health information system community. The WIR considered four key issues critical to registry development:

1. *Protecting the privacy of individuals and the confidentiality of information*—Public health practice often requires access to health information on individuals. Balancing the need for this information with the need to protect the privacy of individuals is one of the greatest challenges in registry development.
2. *Overcoming technical and operational challenges*—Since 1993, NIP has encouraged the development of immunization registries to meet the local needs of states and communities. This approach has resulted in a diversity of registry systems that operate in different electronic environments using a variety of front-, middle-, and back-end technologies and differing in functionality. For example, population-based registries may be seeded

through hospital birth data, vital records data, or newborn screening records, or include only records that have received parental approval for registry inclusion. System architectures include Web-based, client/server, or distributed database designs, with central databases typically located in smaller geographic areas. Larger areas tend to have hubs that connect several smaller population-based registries together. Data entry occurs through a variety of approaches (e.g., direct data entry, replication, batch transfer, or bar codes), and data may be transported electronically via Internet/intranet, dial-up connections, fax, interactive voice response, or mail. Enabling these systems to exchange information with other registries in secure environments to generate complete and accurate immunization information on children is a continuing challenge.

3. *Insuring recipient and provider participation*—To be useful immunization tools, registries must include immunization histories on a large percentage of the target population. Consequently, they must have active participation from all or nearly all public and private immunization providers. Currently, only 24% of children in the United States have their immunization histories included in a population-based registry,[63] despite anecdotal reports that less than 1% of parents choose not to participate when given the option.[64] Focus group research indicates that although most parents are very positive about immunization registries, they tend to follow their doctor's advice regarding participation.[65] Data on the 32 population-based immunization registries operated by federal immunization grantees in 2000 indicated that 56% of public provider sites compared with 41% of private provider sites are enrolled, a disparity due in part to the initial targeting of registries to the public sector.[66] Focus groups have indicated that barriers to registry use in private practices include staff concerns about dual record systems, slowing of patient flow, and the high costs for small practices with a high staff turnover.[67,68] One study estimated annual provider costs associated with registry participation from $0.65 to $7.74 per child vaccinated.[69] Other studies have shown that private providers are willing to participate if (1) registry data are accurate; (2) participation costs are offset by cost savings[5,70]; (3) registry data are kept confidential[71,72]; (4) the time required for personnel to enter and retrieve immunization data is not significant[73]; (5) there is no liability for data entry errors[2,63]; (6) the data are useful in improving clinical practice[73]; and (7) providers understand the purposes and benefits of the registry.[73]

4. *Determining the resources needed to develop and maintain immunization registries*—The identification of stable funding sources, as well as better information on the costs and cost-effectiveness of developing and implementing registries, is critical to insure continued registry development.[74,75] Federal funds for registries have declined from a high of approximately $50 million in 1995 to approximately $15 million in 2000 (K. Lane, personal communication).

CDC Activities in Response to NVAC Recommendations

Results from the hearings, from 21 focus groups with African American, Non-Hispanic White, Hispanic, Native American, and Asian parents, and from WIR deliberations resulted in the development of the recommendations that were approved by NVAC in 1999 (see Appendix A). Since then, substantial progress by CDC has been made in each of the four key issues in response to the recommendations.

Protecting the Privacy of Individuals and the Confidentiality of Information

In response to the WIR's recommendations, NIP and partner organizations developed minimum specifications to protect the privacy and confidentiality of immunization registry information.[76] These were approved by NVAC in 2000 and are consistent with recommendations made by the Secretary of DHHS to Congress for privacy legislation and with privacy regulations now required by the Health Insurance Portability and Accountability Act of 1996.[77] The minimum specifications cover the following critical areas:

- *Confidentiality policies:* All registries must have a written confidentiality policy that applies to everyone who has access to the registry. This policy must be consistent with applicable federal, state, and local laws.
- *Agreements to protect confidentiality:* Authorized registry users must agree in writing to comply with the written confidentiality policy.
- *Notification:* Patients and/or their parents must be informed of the registry, and be told what data the registry will store, what the data will be used for, with whom the data will be shared, and the procedures for data review and correction.
- *Choice:* Patients and/or their parents must be allowed to choose whether or not to participate in the registry, and be allowed to change this decision at any time. Parents and children must not be penalized for choosing not to participate.
- *Use of registry information:* All authorized registry users and parents must be told why registry information is collected. Registry information must be used only for its intended purpose.
- *Access to and disclosure of registry information:* Policies must define who has access to registry information, and to what information they have access. Law enforcement access to registry information must be limited to extraordinary circumstances.
- *Penalties for unauthorized disclosures:* Policies must define what constitutes a breach of confidentiality. Penalties for inappropriate information use or disclosure must be defined and enforced.

- *Data retention and disposal:* Policies must identify the length of time that registry information will be retained, and what will happen to the data at the end of that period.

Survey data collected from each state and the District of Columbia as of October 2000 indicated that 24 (47%) of the 51 jurisdictions had legislation specifically authorizing the establishment of an immunization registry.[64] Twelve (24%) jurisdictions mandated provider reporting to the registry, but only 4 (8%) had penalties for failing to report to the registry. Eleven (22%) jurisdictions provided some type of immunity for providers who report in good faith, and 8 (16%) had penalties for improper disclosure of information. Of the 51 jurisdictions, 14 (27%) required explicit consent to be in a registry, 35 (69%) had implied consent, and the remaining 2 (4%) jurisdictions had not yet addressed this issue. Thirty-five jurisdictions (69%) provided or were planning to provide notice of the registry; however, 13 (25%) did not provide notice. The remaining 3 (6%) jurisdictions had not addressed the issue of notice.

Future NIP activities related to privacy and confidentiality protection include ongoing monitoring of state legislation. Confidentiality policies are being modified by several states to comply with the specifications. It will be critical to insure conformity of the minimum specifications with future federal privacy regulations. NIP also intends to monitor the impact of these protections on immunization registry development. One barrier already identified is related to the interstate exchange of immunization information. Because federal legislation will not preempt stricter state laws,[78] interstate exchange of registry information between two states with different levels of legislative stringency may be problematic. Solutions must be identified to insure that providers have access to accurate and complete immunization histories, even when this requires sharing immunization information across state lines.

Overcoming Technical and Operational Challenges

One of the WIR's technical/operational recommendations was the development of functional standards considered essential for immunization registry operation. Work on identifying these standards began in 1997 through a survey of immunization program managers and registry developers. Approximately 35 potential functions were listed in the survey, and the managers and developers were asked to identify which of these functions was required for an electronic tracking system to be considered an "immunization registry." The functions that were identified as "core" by 75% or more of the respondents were considered minimum immunization registry functions. Focus group research was then conducted with immunization program managers and registry developers to insure consensus on these functional standards. Key elements associated with each standard were then proposed to create more sensitive progress measures of registry development and implementation.

At the recommendation of the WIR, a Technical Working Group (TWG) was created by NIP in 1999 to (1) serve as a consultant body to NIP to insure the appropriate technical functioning of registries; (2) reach agreement on registry data transfer standards; (3) assist in identifying a registry certification process and provide ongoing registry data quality monitoring; and (4) recommend ways to facilitate integrating registry functions into existing information systems. The first achievement of the TWG was its review of and agreement with the functional standards, as indicated in Table 22.2.

One of the approved functional standards is the storage of the required core data elements: patient name, patient birth date, patient sex, patient birth state/country, mother's name, vaccine type, vaccine manufacturer, vaccination date, and vaccine lot number. These core elements were identified in 1995 by NIP and subsequently approved by NVAC. They represent the data necessary for identifying individuals and describing immunization events and are thus considered essential for the record exchange process. Each registry must have a method to receive and store all of these elements, even if the registry does not routinely collect the information. In this way, if a registry receives a record from one system and subsequently transfers it to another, no required core data elements will be lost in the process. Data from 2000 indicate that only 15 population-based registries reported storing data on each of the required core data elements.[66]

Also included in the functional standards is the ability of a registry to automatically determine the vaccine(s) needed, based on recommendations made by the Advisory Committee on Immunization Practices (ACIP), when a person seeks immunization. Despite the release of NIP's "Programmer's Guide to the Automated Immunization Evaluation Process" in 1995,[79] creation of computerized, immunization decision support algorithms by registry developers has been problematic. Current ACIP recommendations are not computer-friendly. For example, there is a lack of clarity and consistency about the meaning of terms such as *minimum age at vaccination* and *minimum interval between doses*, and there is a lack of guidance on the need for re-vaccination when minimum ages/intervals are violated. These factors have resulted in confusion among providers, public health program officials, and information system developers. In recognition of the need for uniformity, an ACIP workgroup was created and staffed by an NIP team for standardization of vaccination decision rules; draft rules are currently under review. In the meantime, NIP has developed and released a public domain algorithm and installation program as an ActiveX component, as well as a corresponding set of test cases, to validate recommendations made by algorithms created by registry developers.[80]

Progress has also been made in enabling registry data exchange through the use of standard codes and transmission rules identified by the Health Level 7 (HL7) organization (see Chapter 11). In 1995, NIP developed standard HL7 messages and an implementation guide for immunization record transactions. These were approved by the HL7 organization in 1997. The guide's first version was intended to familiarize registry developers with HL7 message definitions and

TABLE 22.2. Functional standards of immunization registries

The approved functional standards for immunization registries include:

1. Electronic data storage of all NVAC-approved core data elements.

2. Establish a registry record within 6 weeks of birth for each newborn child born in the catchment area.

3. Enable access to and retrieval of immunization information in the registry at the time of encounter.

4. Receive and process immunization information within 1 month of vaccine administration.

5. Protect the confidentiality of medical information.

6. Ensure the security of medical information.

7. Exchange immunization records using Health Level 7 (HL7) standards.

8. Automatic determination of the routine childhood immunization(s) needed, in compliance with current recommendations of the Advisory Committee on Immunization Practices, when an individual presents for a scheduled immunization.

9. Automatic identification of individuals who are due/late for immunization(s) to enable the production of reminder/recall notifications.

10. Automatic reporting of immunization coverage by providers, age groups, and geographic areas.

11. Produce official immunization records.

12. Promote accuracy and completeness of registry data.

Source: S. Abernathy, Chair, Technical Working Group, personal communication, 2001.

encoding rules and to explain how standard HL7 messages could be used for immunization. However, as developers created HL7 implementations, they discovered that built-in flexibility resulted in data transactions that were not "plug and play." Before data exchange could successfully occur, site-specific negotiations were necessary to harmonize different implementations. Commercial vendors of clinical, computer-based information systems encouraged developers to create one nationally consistent implementation.

In 1999, collaboration between NIP and representatives from six registries resulted in a new implementation guide for data exchange entitled "Immunization Data Transactions Using the Health Level Seven (Version 2.3.1) Standard Protocol."[81] This guide defines four HL7 immunization messages in detail. It used existing HL7 defined code sets, when such use was appropriate, and requested the addition of new codes to the HL7 standard when needed. New

LOINC (Logical Observation Identifiers, Names, and Codes) codes were also obtained to allow for more specialized reporting of clinical data related to the immunization event. Additionally, NIP developed and maintains code sets for vaccines administered (CVX codes) and vaccine manufacturers (MVX codes) that are now part of the HL7 standard.[82]

The Committee on Immunization Registry Standards and Electronic Transactions (CIRSET) evolved out of this effort. CIRSET is an association of immunization registry developers who are actively developing data exchange capability with other registries and providers and have agreed to follow the HL7 implementation guide. Currently, only two population-based registries in the United States are able to exchange records using HL7 standards.[66] However, CIRSET may increase this capacity though the establishment of common implementation policies and provision of technical assistance to other developers. In addition, CIRSET intends to approach vendors about building the HL7 specification into their information systems. To assist with CIRSET's efforts, NVPO has provided funds for NIP to develop a public domain HL7 parser for intended distribution to registry developers. Pilot testing of this tool is planned for 2002.

Currently, much of NIP's technical focus is on identifying methods to monitor progress in reaching the *Healthy People 2010* objective of increasing to 95% the proportion of children aged <6 years who are enrolled in a fully operational population-based immunization registry.[83] Currently, the key elements associated with each of the functional standards are being reviewed. Measurable criteria will be identified for milestone years prior to 2010. Annual NIP site visits are planned to collect data on these criteria for review. Projects will be evaluated based on their progress in reaching these criteria, and recommendations and feedback will be made to insure success.

Insuring Recipient and Provider Participation

In an effort to increase registry participation, several research projects were funded by NIP in 1997 to (1) identify strategies to encourage private provider participation; (2) improve registry data quality by developing generalizable de-duplication methods to insure no more than one record per child in a registry's database; and (3) assess the feasibility of avoiding dual record systems in provider offices by enabling pre-existing provider systems to electronically report vaccines administered directly to an immunization registry.

One of the greatest challenges identified from these projects is insuring the quality of registry data. Record de-duplication is required to enable an accurate assessment of a child's need for immunization. Duplicate registry records have consistently been noted to pose a serious challenge to the integrity of registry databases; one developer estimated that up to 50% of records in her registry's database were duplicates. While 100% of population-based state registries report methods in place for resolving duplicates,[84] no national criteria currently exist for evaluating the effectiveness of these methods. NIP is currently developing a set of test cases for evaluation of these de-duplication methods.

De-duplication is critical to the feasibility of using billing systems to report immunizations to registries, thus minimizing the administrative burden on providers. Although NIP-funded research projects demonstrated the potential for billing systems to function as registry reporting tools, the utility of these systems was found to be dependent on their data quality.[85–87] In one project, research had to be halted until the registry's database could be de-duplicated. An additional barrier to the use of billing data was the lack of specificity of immunization billing codes used for immunization reporting. Without increased billing code specificity, algorithms could not be developed that provided valid immunization decision support. To overcome this problem, NIP worked with the American Medical Association (AMA) to increase the specificity of the AMA's Current Procedural Terminology (CPT) billing codes. In 1997, the AMA agreed to NIP's request and published the modified CPT codes in 1999.

Much of NIP's future efforts to increase registry participation will focus on improving registry data quality and creating parental and provider demand. NIP is now evaluating one promising method of monitoring data quality.[88,89] Immunization coverage estimates generated from registry databases are being compared with estimates generated from the National Immunization Survey (NIS), a nationwide, random digit-dial survey of children's immunization coverage in states and selected large metropolitan areas. High concordance rates between registry estimates and these "gold standard" estimates should identify registries with complete and accurate data.

Related to this effort is the identification by NIP of eight registries that include a large proportion of their target populations or sub-groups of this population and that are thought to have high quality registry data. Immunization coverage estimates from these "sentinel sites" are regularly reported to NIP and compared with NIS estimates. If these sites can consistently demonstrate that registries with high data quality are useful in providing valid and reliable estimates of vaccine coverage, the NIS survey in its present form may eventually become obsolete. Sentinel sites will also be used to monitor the impact of vaccine recalls and the implementation of new vaccine recommendations.

Improved data quality and demonstrated usefulness should generate increased demand by parents and providers that registries become part of normal immunization practice. Registry participation offers multiple incentives to parents and providers (Table 22–1). A key challenge will be to insure that these incentives are appropriately marketed to all registry stakeholders.

Determining Resources Needed to Develop and Maintain Immunization Registries

Several efforts have been made to estimate the costs to develop and maintain an immunization registry. After pilot testing a survey instrument in three registries, NIP categorized registries developed by its 64 immunization grantees by level of registry development (low, medium, and high) and the proportion of the target population enrolled (low, medium, and high.) Four registries were randomly selected from each of the six strata containing at least one registry. After reviewing the 24 sampled registries, NIP estimated that the mean cost per child (0–<6 years of age) per year was $4.13.[89] The All Kids Count Program estimated registry costs of $3.91 per child per year, based on data from each of the Program's 16 projects. NIP-funded research projects of registries in Boston and Atlanta estimated annual costs of $10.00 and $5.26 per child, respectively (V. McKenna, written com-munication 2000).[90] Based on NIP's $4.13 estimate, reaching the *Healthy People 2010* registry objective will require an estimated $76.1 million annually (2002 dollars).

States and communities have used different approaches to generate sufficient registry funds. One state created a private, non-profit corporation of large health plans to help underwrite registry costs,[91] and another state used tobacco tax revenues to supplement registry funds.[72] Several states have charged providers and/or managed care organization for registry-related services such as generation of immunization coverage reports, HEDIS measures, and lists of children who need immunizations.[72,92,93]

In 2000, the Centers for Medicare and Medicaid Services (CMS), formerly the Health Care Financing Administration, agreed to fund up to 90% of registry development and implementation costs, and up to 75% of ongoing registry support costs for its Medicaid population. Several states have already received CMS funding for their registries, including Maine, Michigan, Minnesota, Missouri, New Hampshire, New Mexico, Oregon, and Wisconsin (A. Salazar-Martini, personal communication). Other options for registry funding are also being evaluated, including using Vaccines for Children funds to ensure that registries enroll children eligible for this entitlement program.

Estimated annual fiscal savings of $273.5 million associated with registries include avoiding manual record pulls for school/day care entry ($58 million); changes in immunization providers ($16.2 million); managed care reporting requirements ($4.8 million); preventing duplicative immunizations ($26.5 million); and negating the necessity to review vaccination records for school entry requirements compliance ($168.0 million).[60,94]

Other unaccounted cost savings include decreased no-show appointment rates through the use of reminder/recall notices, and decreased rates and complications associated with vaccine-preventable diseases. NIP-funded research showed that registries in three sites in California increased worker productivity up to 50% and saved $8 for each $1 spent on registries.[43] Cost savings may be even greater for immunization registries that are integrated within broader public health information systems.

Current Registry Status

To assess the current status of immunization registry development, data from the calendar year 2000 Immunization Registry Annual Report (IRAR) were analyzed for the 50 states and the District of Columbia. The IRAR is a self-administered questionnaire that measures the degree of enrollment of children 0-<6 years of age living in a registry's catchment area, and the achievement of the functional standards. Because IRAR information is self-reported, NIP has validated progress reported through annual site visits since 2001.

Calendar year 2000 data from the 32 areas that reported operating population-based registries indicated that nearly 50% of the children aged <6 years in these areas were enrolled in a registry.[66] Extrapolating to the US population suggests that 24% of the children in the United States are currently participating in a population-based immunization registry. Four (13%) of the 32 areas with population-based registries reported implementing at least one key element in each of the functional standards. No area reported implementing all key elements of all of the functional standards.

The Future Role of Registries

Findings from the 2000 IRAR indicate that substantial progress has been made in developing and implementing community- and state-based immunization registries since the 1960s. However, with less than a decade remaining, approximately 16 million children need to be enrolled in fully functional immunization registries before the *Healthy People 2010* registry objective is met. Recruitment efforts targeted at private providers, in addition to the provision of technical support to enable full registry functionality, will be critical in reaching this goal. Additional work must also focus on insuring the confidentiality of registry information as well as on identifying broad-based, sustainable financial support for a nationwide immunization registry network.

Much of the success of these efforts will depend upon the creation of a noticeable demand for immunization registries. Parents must continue to recognize the benefits of vaccines, even in the absence of disease, and become convinced that registries are critical tools both for insuring that their children return for immunization and for insuring that their children miss no immunization opportunities when they do return. Providers and professional organizations must recognize the value of automated medical information systems and incorporate these tools in their office settings. Registry developers must understand the importance of seamless integration of their products into pre-existing office software and work toward developing systems that maintain the highest quality of data and reduce the burden of providing immunization services in the medical home. Public health officials must understand that registries provide vital information for identifying under-immunized children and targeting scare resources. Finally, political leaders must understand that immunization registries are critical tools for maintaining our current record-breaking levels of immunization coverage in the United States and that funding levels must reflect that these information tools are costly to develop and maintain.

Demand for registries is already being created. Key parent and professional organizations have formally endorsed immunization registries, and immunization programs are increasingly incorporating national registry standards of functionality and confidentiality in their registry development efforts. Some registries are beginning to reach a mature level of development at which a large percentage of their target populations are enrolled and the data quality is high. In addition to insuring that children are getting the immunizations they need on time, these public health tools have enabled the estimation of provider- and geography-based coverage, the targeting of public health prevention efforts, and the tracking of the implementation of new vaccine recommendations and recalls. Perhaps most importantly, sources that may provide sustainable funding streams for registries well into the future are being identified.

Nonetheless, the sustainability of immunization registries may be dependent upon their ability to integrate with other health information systems. Vertical systems supported by categorical program funds have proven to be only one more challenge to the overburdened health care provider. Because these "silo" systems have only a limited public health scope, they have been difficult to market and sustain. Children often have multiple health needs that would benefit from coordinated, electronic health information systems.

Immunization registries have been described as the first step in creating such systems. Population-based health registries could be used to insure that children get the immunizations they need on time and that children are targeted for a variety of non-immunization related public health interventions, including screening for lead exposure, hearing defects, and metabolic disorders. These electronic tools could also make it easier for public health practitioners to fulfill their mission to assess the health of the public, insure their access to health care, and develop effective policies to insure a healthy population.

Recent developments indicate that the United States is well under way in developing such a comprehensive electronic system. As discussed in Chapters 11 and 20, the 1996 Health Insurance Portability and Accountability Act mandates the standardization of health data and the development of unique identifiers for insurers, providers, and individuals. Such standardization has been critical to the successful development of immunization registries by enabling maximum flexibility at the local and state level without jeopardizing data sharing between registries.

Since 1993, NIP has funded health departments to develop integrated public health information systems through Integrated Network for Public Health Officials (INPHO) grants. The second phase of these INPHO grants focused on the integration of immunization registries with broader public health information systems. Other efforts are under way at the CDC to develop a public health data model with standard data elements and methods of uniquely identifying individuals (see Chapter 19.) These efforts, along with federal dollars to support the development of integrated disease surveillance systems, are a giant step toward the creation of a comprehensive public health information infrastructure. Non-profit organizations are also involved in the creation of this infrastructure. A third phase of the All Kids Count Program has recently been funded to promote the development of integrated public health information systems.

Lessons learned through efforts to build immunization registries should enable more efficient development of a public health information infrastructure that serves the total public health needs of our population.

Appendix A: National Vaccine Advisory Committee Recommendations[31]

Protecting the Privacy of Individuals and the Confidentiality of Information

1. Protection of privacy and maintenance of confidentiality are essential to the successful development of immunization registries. Registry developers must give careful consideration to privacy and confidentiality issues to reflect the values and special needs of the communities they serve.

2. Registry developers must give special consideration to the privacy and confidentiality needs of immigrant communities.

3. Federal legislation to establish a minimum set of privacy/confidentiality standards would be very helpful. To assist in the development of registries that can exchange data while also ensuring privacy and confidentiality, the federal government should work with key stakeholders to develop and disseminate model privacy and confidentiality policies and legislation for registries.

4. At a minimum, immunization registries should:
   - Ensure that patients/parents are notified of the existence of the registry and of the information contained in the registry;
   - Inform patients/parents of the purpose and potential uses of the registry;
   - Permit patients/parents to review and amend information in the registry;
   - Accept responsibility for reliability and protection of registry information.

5. Parents must be given the option to decide whether or not their children will participate in a registry. In some communities, parents are informed of the registry and its purposes and potential uses during routine educational sessions offered at the birth hospital. At this time, or at any later time, parents should be allowed to opt out of a registry. In communities where the "opt in"/informed consent approach is most consistent with community values, this is the option that should be offered. Parents should not be penalized for choosing not to participate in a registry for religious, philosophical, privacy, or other reasons.

6. Registry developers should limit access to registry information and maintain audit trails to monitor access to records. Individuals should have access to their own records and to these audit trails.
7. Strong penalties for the unauthorized use of registry data should be in place and consistently enforced.
8. Use of registry data in a manner that is punitive to parents/patients (e.g., denial of health insurance/coverage, Immigration and Naturalization Service tracking of immigrants, other law enforcement purposes) must be prohibited.
9. If registries are to be integrated with larger health information systems, protection of privacy and confidentiality must be ensured.
10. The federal government should support an ongoing independent assessment of the benefits, risks, and costs of registry development and implementation with regard to issues including privacy and confidentiality.

Overcoming Technical and Operational Challenges

1. CDC, in cooperation with state and local health agencies, provider groups, software/hardware vendors, and national standard-setting organizations, should take the lead in developing, implementing, and maintaining standards pertaining to immunization registries, including:
   - Defining essential registry system functions and attributes;
   - Defining core data elements;
   - Certifying clinical decision-support functions;
   - Certifying the registry's ability to consolidate multiple records on the same individual;
   - Enabling intra- and inter-registry record exchange with standard (e.g., HL7) messages;
   - Adopting system security standards to address both technical and administrative issues and to ensure that access is limited to authorized persons;
   - Certifying registry functions.
2. The initial target group for inclusion in immunization registries should be children from birth through five years, although many registries will want to continue the registry beyond school entry and/or include other age groups (e.g., adolescents, older adults).

Ensuring Recipient and Provider Participation

1. Providers and interested community groups should be involved throughout registry development and implementation, beginning at the initial planning stages.
2. Registries should be simple to use and should be designed to minimize the administrative burden on providers. When possible, registries should

capitalize on data already being collected and used in providers' practices for billing or other purposes thereby avoiding duplicate data entry. This could be done using billing or encounter information systems, although some modifications might be necessary to ensure data completeness and quality. Initial and subsequent training should be provided; technical and non-technical support should be readily available.

3. Registries should include reminder/recall functions to improve adherence to recommended immunization schedules. Whether both reminders and recalls will be used will depend on local circumstances.

4. Data in immunization registries should be used to improve immunization services and immunization coverage; they should not be used to "punish" providers whose immunization coverage is low.

Determining Resources Needed to Develop and Maintain Immunization Registries

1. CDC should immediately pursue further study to characterize start-up and maintenance costs of registries and compare these to costs of alternative systems. Information about the prospects for state and local health agencies to secure funding to partially or fully support their immunization registries should also be gathered and evaluated.

2. NVPO should coordinate discussions leading to a recommendation about appropriate mechanisms for long-term funding of registries.

3. A short-term (3–5 year) federal appropriation should be sought to support the further development and initial implementation of registries, with evaluation of costs and benefits an integral part of these efforts. This funding would provide time to establish a mechanism for long-term funding.

Questions for Review

1. List at least four factors that account for the fact that, even in the 21st century, many children in the United States remain unimmunized or else under-immunized.

2. Explain how widespread implementation of population-based immunization registries would reduce or eliminate the incidence of morbidity and mortality attributable to infectious diseases.

Questions 3–11 are based on the following short case:

State X has no immunization registries in place, although the state's Department of Public Health hopes to implement a statewide registry within the next three years. State law currently requires that all children presenting themselves at either public or private schools provide certificates of vaccinations against smallpox, polio, diphtheria, tetanus, measles, mumps, and rubella.

Health care providers in the state handle vaccination certification, and school nurses are responsible for verification. Although the Department of Public Health has announced its long-term plans to implement a statewide registry, many providers and parents have objected to the scheme. The providers have pointed out that such a registry would impose additional labor and costs on their offices. Parents have registered objections to the burden placed on them and to the threat to privacy and confidentiality that a registry might entail. School nurses and other school officials have been generally supportive of the concept, but they have expressed concern about the additional workload and resources that a statewide registry might entail.

3. What sources of assistance are potentially available to State X in planning and implementing a statewide registry?
4. Explain why the present method of certifying and verifying vaccinations against the diseases may result in overlooking individuals who have not been immunized or else result in duplicate vaccination of children?
5. How would implementation of a statewide registry benefit the parents of children in the state's schools? Health care providers? School nurses and other school officials responsible for adhering to state law regarding vaccinations? Public health, in general, in the state?
6. How could the Department of Public Health address the objections of health care providers to the plan to implement a statewide immunization registry? How could the department address the concerns of parents and school nurses/officials?
7. Explain why it is important that a statewide immunization registry be compatible with (a) other health information systems and (b) immunization registries in other states and localities.
8. What provisions will State X need to incorporate in the immunization registry in order to conform to the recommendations of the National Vaccine Advisory Committee regarding the privacy and confidentiality of individual health information that the registry includes?
9. Explain how State X can address any technical and operational challenges to making its registry compatible with other registries and with other health information systems.
10. How can State X help insure the participation of health care recipients and health care providers in the immunization registry, other than by making participation legally mandatory?
11. Assuming that the registry will be phased in over time and will eventually include all school-age children, what target group should be included first? Why?

References

1. Ten Great Public Health Achievements—United States, 1990–1999. *MMWR Morb Mortal Wkly Rep* 1999;48:241–243.

2. Institute of Medicine. *Calling the Shots—Immunization Finance Policies and Practices*. National Academy Press, Washington, D.C., 2000.

3. Herrera G, Smith P, Daniels D, et al. National, state, and urban area vaccination coverage levels among children aged 19–35 months—United States, 1998. *MMWR Morb Mortal Wkly Rep CDC Surveill Summ*. 2000;49(9):1–26.

4. Impact of vaccines universally recommended for children—United States, 1990–1998. *MMWR Morb Mortal Wkly Rep* 1999;48(12):243–248.

5. National, state, and urban area vaccination coverage levels among children aged 19–35 months—United States, July 1996–June 1997. *MMWR Morb Mortal Wkly Rep* 1998;47(6):108–116.

6. Williams I, Dwyer D, Hirshorn E, et al. Immunization coverage in a population-based sample of Maryland children. *Arch Pediatr Adolesc Med* 1994;148:350–356.

7. Vaccination coverage by race/ethnicity and poverty level among children aged 19–35 months—United States, 1996. *MMWR Morb Mortal Wkly Rep* 1997;46(41):963–969.

8. Notice to Readers: Recommended Childhood Immunization Schedule—United States, 2002. *MMWR Morb Mortal Wkly Rep* 2002;51(2):31–33.

9. Goldstein K, Daum R. Counting immunisations. *Lancet* 1994;344:144–145.

10. Wood D, Halfon N, Sherbourne C, et al. Assessing the accuracy of parental recall of child immunization in an inner city population. *Ambul Child Health* 1997;4:319–328.

11. Goldstein K, Kviz F, Daum R. Accuracy of immunization histories provided by adults accompanying preschool children to a pediatric emergency department. *JAMA* 1993;270:2190–2194.

12. Bates A, Fitzgerald J, Dittus R, Wolinsky F. Risk factors for underimmunization in poor urban infants. *JAMA* 1994;272:1105–1110.

13. Joffe M, Luberti A. Effect of emergency department immunization on compliance with primary care. *Pediatr Emerg Care* 1994;10:317–319.

14. Basco W, Recknor J, Darden P. Who needs an immunization in a pediatric subspecialty clinic? *Arch Pediatr Adolesc Med* 1996;150:508–511.

15. Nordin J. Impact of implementation of a fully functioning immunization registry on immunization rates. Presented at the All Kids Count Annual Immunization Registry Conference; April 1999; St. Paul, MN.

16. Buschnell C. The ABC's of practice-based immunization assessments. Presented at the 28th National Immunization Conference; 1994;Washington, DC.

17. Bordley W, Margolis P, Lannon C. The delivery of immunizations and other preventive services in private practices. *Pediatrics* 1996;97:467–473.

18. Szilagyi P, Roghmann K, Campbell J, et al. Immunization practices of primary care practitioners and their relation to immunization levels. *Arch Pediatr Adolesc Med* 1994;148:158–166.

19. Rodewald L, Peak R, Ezzati-Rice T, Zell E, Thompson K. Who are the immunization providers for U.S. children: Findings from the 1994 National Health Interview Survey (NHIS) Provider Record Check (PRC). *Ambul Child Health* 1997;3:168.

20. Fowler M, Simpson G, Schoendorf K. Families on the move and children's healthcare. *Pediatrics* 1993;91:934–940.

21. Hamlin J, Wood D, Pereyra M, Grabowsky M. Inappropriately timed immunizations: Types, causes, and their relationship to record keeping. *Am J Public Health* 1996;86:1812–1814.

22. Ortega A, Andrews S, Katz S, et al. Comparing a computer-based childhood vaccina-

tion registry with parental vaccination cards: A population-based study of Delaware children. *Clin Pediatr* 1997;36:217–221.

23. Szilagyi P, Rodewald L, Humiston S. et al. Missed Opportunities for Childhood Vaccinations in Office Practices and the Effect on Vaccination Status. *Pediatrics* 1993;91:1–7.

24. Watson M, Feldman K. Sugar N. et al. Inadequate History as a Barrier to Immunization. *Arch Pediatr Adolesc Med* 1996;150:135–139.

25. Murphy T, Pastor P, Medley F. Factors associated with unnecessary immunization given to children. *Pediatr Infec Dis J* 1997;16:47–52.

26. Feikema S, Klevens R, Washington M, Barker, L. Extraimmunization among U.S. children. *JAMA* 2000;283:1311–1317.

27. Briss P. Rodewald L, Hinman A. et al. Reviews of evidence regarding interventions to improve vaccination coverage in children, adolescents, and adults. *Am J Prev Med* 2000;18(1S):97–140.

28. Shefer A. Briss P, Rodewald L. et al. Improving immunization coverage rates: An evidence-based review of the literature. *Epidemiol Rev* 1999;21:96–142.

29. Shefer A. Maes E, Brink E. Mize J, Passino J. Assessment and related immunization issues in the Special Supplemental Nutrition Program for Women, Infants and Children: A status report. *J Public Health Manage Pract* 1996;2:34–44.

30. LeBaron C, Massoudi M, Stevenson J. Dang H, Lyons B. The status of immunization measurement and feedback in the United States. *Arch Pediatr Adoles Med* 2000;154:832–836.

31. National Vaccine Advisory Committee. Development of community- and state-based immunization registries. January 12. 1999. Available at: http://www.cdc.gov/nip/registry/nvac.htm. Accessed April 2, 2002.

32. Mack S, Carlson R, Ryan A, Hughes G. Prendergast T. Crude trend analysis of the average age children receive selected immunization in San Bernardino County. Presented at the 2000 Immunization Registry Conference; March 2000; Newport, RI.

33. Kempe A. Steiner J, Beaty B. et al. How much does a regional immunization registry increase documented immunization rates in a rural private practice? Presented at the 34th National Immunization Conference; July 2000; Washington, D.C.

34. McChesney M. Use of Arizona's Health Links Registry. Presented at the Western Governors Association meeting; June 1999; Jackson Hole, WY.

35. LaVenture M, Olson M, Brand B. et al. Creating a statewide immunization registry: A tool for physicians and public health. *Minn Med* 1997;80:50–52.

36. Tormey P. McConnell P, Coppola D, et al. Changes in immunization rates and practices over time: Data from a collaborative citywide immunization registry. Presented at the 31st National Immunization Conference; May 1997; Detroit, MI.

37. Yawn B, Edmonson L, Huber L, et al. The impact of a simulated immunization registry on perceived childhood immunization status. *Am J Managed Care* 1998;4:185–192.

38. Brooks D. Johnson K. Livingston L. Can computer-based immunization tracking aid in improving age-appropriate immunization rates for low income urban children in a managed-care setting? Presented at the 31st National Immunization Conference; May 1977; Detroit, MI.

39. Lieu T, Black S. Sorel M, Ray P, Shinefield H. Would better adherence to guidelines improve childhood immunization rates? *Pediatrics* 1996;98:1062–1068.

40. Payne T, Kanvik S. Seward R, et al. Development and validation of an immunization tracking system in a large health maintenance organization. *Am J Prev Med* 1993;9:96–100.

41. Van Acker B, McIntosh G, Gudes M. Continuous quality improvement techniques enhance HMO members' immunization rates. *J Healthcare Qual* 1994;20:36–41.

42. Murphy T, Gargiullo P, Massoudi M, Nelson D, et al. Intussusception among infants given an oral rotavirus vaccine. *New Engl J Med* 2001;344:564–572.

43. Fowler K. An immunization registry provider feedback module—the missing link in registries: An Arkansas case example. Presented at the 2000 Immunization Registry Conference; March 2000; Newport, RI.

44. Fontanesi J. A cost-benefit analysis of electronic immunization registries. Presented at the 33rd National Immunization Conference; June 1999; Dallas, Texas.

45. Blose D. Using registries to monitor the implementation of new vaccine recommendations. Presented at the 2000 Immunization Registry Conference; March 2000; Newport, RI.

46. Boyd R. Using immunization registries to speed public acceptance of changes in vaccine usage. Presented at the 2000 Immunization Registry Conference; March 2000; Newport, RI.

47. Canavan B. Using registry data to assess the impact of changes in the vaccine schedule. Presented at the 2001 Immunization Registry Conference. July 2001; Little Rock, AR.

48. Poydence K, Balter S, Stevenson J, et al. Utilization of a metropolitan immunization registry to examine implementation of Heptavalent Pneumococcal Conjugate Vaccine (PCV7). Presented at the 2001 Immunization Registry Conference; July 2001; Little Rock, AR.

49. Bean L, Kontuly T, Schulthies S, Xu W. Linking Utah WIC and immunization information systems. Presented at the 2000 Immunization Registry Conference; March 2000; Newport, RI.

50. Metroka A, Walker D, Arzt N, Salkowitz S. Integration of the New York Citywide Immunization Registry and LeadQuest. Presented at the 2000 Immunization Registry Conference; March 2000; Newport, RI.

51. Brackbill R, Walker D, Metroka A. The role of an immunization registry in community health assessment. Presented at the 34th National Immunization Conference; July 2000; Washington, D.C.

52. Gubernick R, Boclair L, DeAngelo-Cashman S. Community partnerships: A key factor in the deployment of an immunization registry. *Am J Prev Med* 1997;13(suppl): 86–89).

53. Hoekstra E, LeBaron C, Megaloeconomou Y, et al. Impact of a large-scale immunization initiative in the Special Supplemental Nutrition Program for Women, Infants, and Children (WIC), Chicago 1996–1997. *JAMA* 1998;280:1143–1147.

54. Wood D, Halfon N. Reconfiguring child health services in the inner city. *JAMA* 1998;280:1182–1183.

55. Hall K, Zimmerman A, Samos J, et al. Coordinating care for children's health: A public health integrated information systems approach. *Am J Prev Med* 1997;13(suppl): 32–36.

56. Pease J. Maine's experience partnering with Medicaid. Presented at the All Kids Count Conference; April 1998; New Orleans, LA.

57. Atkinson W, Orenstein W, Krugman S. The resurgence of measles in the United States, 1989–1990. *Annu Rev Med* 1992;43:451–463.

58. National Vaccine Advisory Committee. Strategies to sustain success in childhood immunizations. *JAMA* 1999;282:363–370.

59. Orenstein W. Immunization registries. Presented at the American Academy of Pediatrics Meeting; October 1993; Washington, D.C.

60. Watson W, Saarlas K. Hearn R. Russell R. The All Kids Count National Program: A Robert Wood Johnson Foundation initiative to develop immunization registries. *Am J Prev Med* 1997;13(suppl):3–6.

61. National Vaccine Advisory Committee Subcommittee on Vaccination Registries. *Developing a national childhood immunization information system: registries, reminders, and recall.* Washington, DC: US Department of Health and Human Services; 1994.

62. The White House. Office of the Press Secretary. Remarks by the President in Immunization-Child Care Announcement; July 23, 1997. Available at: http://clinton4.nara.gov/WH/New/html/19970723-2969.html. Accessed April 2, 2002.

63. Linkins R. Current status of registries. Presented at the 2001 Immunization Registry Conference; July 2001: Little Rock, AR.

64. Horlick G, Beeler S, Linkins R. A review of state legislation related to immunization registries. *Am J Prev Med* 2001;3:208–213.

65. Immunization Registry Clearinghouse. Focus group research on immunization registries—Fall 1998. Available at: http://www.cdc.gov/nip/registry/fg/fg.htm. Accessed April 2, 2002.

66. Immunization registry use and progress. United States, 2001. *MMWR Morb Mortal Wkly Rep* 2002;51(3):53–56.

67. Bordley W, Dempsey-Tanner T, Freed G. Lister M. Challenges to private provider participation in immunization registries. *Am J Prev Med* 1997;13(suppl 1):66–70.

68. Pappas M, Baker B, Appelbaum D, et al. Immunization registries: Provider recruitment and participation. *Am J Prev Med* 1997;13(suppl 1):71–76.

69. Rask K, Wells K, Kohler S, et al. The cost to providers of participating in an immunization registry. *Am J Prev Med* 2000;19:99–103.

70. Sinn J, Kroneburg M, Morrow A. The purpose and functions of immunization information systems within health care organizations. *Arch Pediatr Adolesc Med* 1997;151:615–620.

71. Stoltman G, Swanson B, McLaury D. Privacy, confidentiality and other concerns of parents and providers. Presented at the All Kids Count Conference; April 1999; St. Paul, MN.

72. Wood D. Saarlas K, Inkelas M, Matyas B. Immunization registries in the United States: Implications for the practice of public health in a changing health care system. *Annu Rev Public Health* 1999;20:231–255.

73. LaVenture M, Gatewood L, Roody M. Olson M. Key factors supporting provider participation in immunization registries. Presented at the 2000 Immunization Registry Conference; March 2000; Newport, RI.

74. Slifkin R, Freeman V, Biddle A. Costs of developing childhood immunization registries: Case studies from four All Kids Count projects. *J Public Health Manage Pract* 1999;5:67–81.

75. Pratt H. Goun B. Alexander L, et al. A cost-effectiveness analysis model for immunization registries: The New Jersey experience. *Am J Prev Med* 1997;13(suppl 1):115–119.

76. Centers for Disease Control and Prevention. National Immunization Program. Community Immunization Registry Manual. Chapter II: Confidentiality. Available at: http://www.cdc.gov/nip/registry. Accessed April 2, 2002.

77. US Department of Health and Human Services. Standards for privacy of individually identifiable health information: Final rule, December 28, 2000 [45 CFR parts 160 through 164]. Federal Register 2000;65:82462–82829.

78. US Department of Health and Human Services. *Confidentiality of individually identifi-*

able health information. Washington, DC: US Department of Health and Human Services; 1997.

79. Centers for Disease Control and Prevention. National Immunization Program. Programmer's Guide to the Automated Immunization Algorithm. Available at: http://www.cdc.gov/nip/registry. Accessed April 2, 2002.

80. Centers for Disease Control and Prevention. National Immunization Program. Immunization decision support algorithm and test cases. Available at: http://www.cdc.gov/nip/registry. Accessed April 2, 2002.

81. Centers for Disease Control and Prevention. National Immunization Program. Implementation Guide for Immunization Data Transactions using Version 2.3.1 of the Health Level Seven Standard Protocol. Available at: http://www.cdc.gov/nip/registry. Accessed April 2, 2002.

82. Centers for Disease Control and Prevention. National Immunization Program. CVX and MVX codes. Available at: http://www.cdc.gov/nip/registry. Accessed April 2, 2002.

83. US Department of Health and Human Services. *Healthy People 2010* (Conference ed., vol 1). Washington, D.C.: US Department of Health and Human Services; January 2000. Available at http://www.health.gov/healthypeople. Accessed April 2, 2002.

84. Progress in development of immunization registries. United States, 2000. *MMWR Morb Mortal Wkly Rep* 2001;50(1):3–7.

85. Walker D, Papadouka V, Huie S, et al. Effect of time and feedback on the quality of data reported via billing systems. Presented at the 2000 Immunization Registry Conference; March 2000; Newport, RI.

86. Blosberg J. Immunization billing audit—quality data in registry + improved clinic practice. Presented at the 2000 Immunization Registry Conference; March 2000; Newport, RI.

87. Fairbrother G, Papadouka V, Walker D. New York Citywide Immunization Registry: Accuracy and completeness of data extracted from billing systems. Presented at the 34th National Immunization Conference; July 2000; Washington, D.C.

88. Bartlett D, Urquhart G, Linkins R. The relationship between immunization registry operational status and accurate vaccination coverage estimates among children aged 19-35 months. Presented at the 2000 Immunization Registry Conference; March 2000; Newport, RI.

89. Horne P, Saarlas K, Hinman A. Costs of immunization registries. Experience from the all kids count II projects. *Am J Prev Med.* 2000;19:94–98.

90. Stevenson J, Wright B, Huggins V. The National Immunization Survey registry validation study. Presented at the 2000 Immunization Registry Conference; March 2000; Newport, RI.

91. Rask K, Wells K, Kohler S, et al. Measuring immunization registry costs—promises and pitfalls. *Am J Prev Med* 2000;18:262–267.

92. Canavan B. Sustaining immunization registries through innovative funding strategies. Presented at the 2000 Immunization Registry Conference; March 27, 2000; Newport, RI.

93. Berg T. Marketing HEDIS data to supplement registry revenue. Presented at the 2000 Immunization Registry Conference; March 2000; Newport, RI.

94. Xu W, Williams S, Harston D, Hasbrouk D, Lewis T. Methodology of developing a cost-sharing funding formula for a statewide immunization registry. Presented at the 2000 Immunization Registry Conference; March 27, 2000; Newport, RI.

95. Horne P, Saarlas K, Hinman A. Update on immunization registries [letter]. *Am J Prev Med* 2001;20:174.

23
Decision Support and Expert Systems in Public Health

WILLIAM A. YASNOFF AND PERRY L. MILLER

Learning Objectives

After studying this chapter, you should be able to:

- Define and describe the purpose of decision support and expert systems.
- List and explain the three reasons that decision support and expert systems are needed in public health.
- Differentiate among (1) tabular knowledge, (2) rule-based knowledge, and (3) procedural knowledge in decision support and expert systems, as illustrated by the IMM/Serve system.
- Describe decision support and expert system testing through (1) automated tools for knowledge testing, (2) testing with hand-crafted sets of test cases, and (3) testing with pilot use, as illustrated by the IMM/Serve system.
- Describe the goals for choosing knowledge representation in encoding health knowledge in a computer to be used for decision support, and indicate the uses and limitations, if any, of (1) tables, (2) rules, (3) flowcharts, (4) semantic networks, (5) model-based knowledge, and (6) procedural knowledge.
- Describe the characteristics of an environment in which development and implementation of a decision support or an expert system is likely to be successful, and list the steps that a development team must take in building such a system.

Overview

The expanding quantity of health data and the complexity of its applications are pointing to the need for greater application of computer resources to provide support for decision-making in public health and clinical practice. Decision support and expert systems, as illustrated by the immunization-forecasting program IMM/Serve, offer such support, both now and in the future. Would-be developers of such systems, however, must recognize that the systems are both inherently complex and work-intensive in development. Successful decision support and expert systems require incorporation of comprehensive knowledge and sound logic, extensive testing by use of a variety of methods, and consideration of the nature of the decision making to be supported and the appropriateness of the environment in which such systems will be placed, including the willingness of users to participate in the development process. Clearly, decision-support systems can be appropriate for a number of potential applications in public health practice, including analysis of surveillance data, resource management, and the dissemination of practice guidelines.

Introduction

Information systems that assist in the analysis of data to assist decision making are known as decision support and expert systems. While it may be difficult to distinguish clearly between these two types of systems, *decision support systems* generally incorporate simpler and more straightforward knowledge. *Expert systems*, on the other hand, usually include substantial and complex representations of policies, rules, and facts that are important in evaluating alternative courses of action or recommendations. In any case, the goal of such systems is to bring external knowledge to the process of data analysis in an effort to improve the speed, accuracy, and consistency of human decision making.

Why are decision support and expert systems needed in public health? There are three basic reasons:

- increasing quantities of data;
- the need for more rapid decision making; and
- the need for better dissemination of best practices.

As we move into the 21st century, the sheer quantity of public health data is expanding rapidly. We are working on improving our surveillance systems so that a larger proportion of reportable diseases are actually reported. In addition, the development and dissemination of electronic laboratory reporting systems and electronic medical record systems will greatly increase the volume of case reports to the public health system. Increasingly, state and local governments are collecting and disseminating community health status information at greater and greater levels of detail. In addition, performance data about the health system and from health plans is becoming more abundant. There is certainly no shortage of data, although accurate, complete, and timely data are still difficult to obtain. It can be argued that the application of computer-based information systems to public health is, to some extent, responsible for this explosion of data. Nevertheless, we must increase our capacity to handle such data and analyze and act on them. Existing methods, mostly manual, are not sufficient to permit the public health system to cope. Decision support systems can provide preliminary analysis that allows scarce human resources to focus on the key problems while ignoring a vast sea of irrelevancy.

Public health is also facing major new challenges that require more rapid decision-making. Foremost among these challenges is the threat of bioterrorism. It is clear that the earlier a bioterrorism event is detected, the more effective the response can be in limiting both the associated morbidity and mortality. Another key threat involves emerging infections. Tracking these new and sometimes confusing diseases requires very quick responses. We are also facing increasing demands from policy makers for information and for justifications for both existing and proposed public health initiatives.

Public health also is challenged to be more effective in dissemination of best practices. Such a challenge requires public health to possess the ability to both discover and disseminate successful programs and interventions. By sharing knowledge and experience effectively, we can avoid the unnecessary rediscovery of successful practice strategies and help insure more uniform performance of the public health system.

We also need to improve compliance with preventive medicine guidelines. Although most physicians are very supportive of preventive measures for their patients, it is not a primary focus of their practice. The increasing use of electronic medical records (EMR) systems provides an opportunity to deliver reminders at the point of care in order to improve compliance. In addition, guidelines that require specific patient data can obtain this input directly from EMR systems, thereby relieving providers of an administrative obstacle to their use.

In addition to the clear need for decision support and expert systems in public health, we are fortunate that the delivery mechanisms for these systems are improving rapidly. The increasing use of EMR systems has already been mentioned with respect to dissemination of clinical preventive guidelines. We are also seeing a substantial investment in electronic infrastructure for public health in the form of both computers and networks. The Health Alert Network program at the Centers for Disease Control and Prevention (CDC), for example, has already funded tens of millions of dollars of such badly needed infrastructure and is expected to continue to do so for some time.

Finally, the Internet provides a common network and user interface for public health information systems of all types. Decision support and expert systems can both access data and deliver recommendations by use of the Internet. Furthermore, the availability of this common network can both reduce the cost of system development and ease widespread deployment. In such an environment, the cost of an expensive system may be more easily justified through its nationwide dissemination and use. Finally, the continuing improvement of the price-performance characteristics of computer systems allows the cost-effective use of extremely sophisticated and complex algorithms. Whereas, in the past, application of certain expert systems was limited by the speed and cost of computation, such limitations are increasingly disappearing.

An Example of the Use of Decision Support Systems: Childhood Immunization Forecasting

There is a wide range of potential applications for computer-based decision support within public health. This section uses the IMM/Serve immunization forecasting program[1] to illustrate many of the issues involved. IMM/Serve is a computer program built to provide patient-specific recommendations for childhood immunization, based primarily on the guidelines of the CDC's Advisory Committee on Immunization Practices (ACIP). IMM/Serve currently handles seven vaccine series: diphtheria tetanus pertussis (DTP), hepatitis A (HepA), hepatitis B (HepB), *Haemophilus influenzae* Type b (Hib), measles mumps rubella (MMR), polio, and varicella (Var).

Childhood immunization is a particularly good domain in which to implement decision support because (1) many different organizations nationwide are building immunization registries[2] (see Chapter 22), (2) national panels maintain detailed guidelines that are quite complex, and (3) many clinicians will benefit if these recommendations can be produced automatically based on data contained in a registry database. IMM/Serve is currently being used in several settings. For example, the US Indian Health Service (IHS) is currently using IMM/Serve in a rapidly growing number of its 300+ clinics nationwide.

IMM/Serve takes as its input a child's vaccination history, together with a small amount of additional information. Table 23.1 shows a case that might be submitted to IMM/Serve. This input specifies the vaccine doses the child has received as well as the date of each vaccination. For the Hib series, the vaccine brand is also specified (PRP-OMP). The input also specifies the child's date of birth, the "forecast" date for which recommendations are desired, any vaccines that are contraindicated, and other facts, such as whether the child's mother is "HBsAg positive," that could affect the schedule for Hepatitis B vaccination. IMM/Serve processes this input and produces the output seen in Table 23.2.

IMM/Serve's output indicates (1) which vaccinations are due "now" (i.e., as of the requested forecast date), (2) when the next dose for each vaccine series will be due, and (3) which series are complete. It also indicates which doses are covered by the national Vaccine for Children (VFC) Program for economically eligible children.

TABLE 23.1. An example case to be analyzed by IMM/Serve

Date of birth: 7/10/1999

Date used for forecast: 10/1/2000

Contraindicated vaccines: none

Other facts: none

HepB: 7/10/1999, 9/12/1999, 1/20/2000

DTaP: 9/12/1999, 11/15/1999, 1/20/2000

Hib: PRP-OMP 9/12/1999, PRP-OMP 11/15/1999

IPV: 9/12/1999, 11/15/1999

MMR: 7/14/2000

Sources of Complexity in the Immunization Domain

IMM/Serve's goal is to take the recommendations produced by the ACIP expert panel and encode those recommendations into computer-based form so that they can be automatically delivered to a clinician in the context of a

TABLE 23.2. The output produced by IMM/Serve for the case shown in Table 23.1

The following immunization(s) are due on 10/1/2000:
    DTaP 4
    Hib 3 (PRP-OMP)
    IPV 3
    MMR 2 or Me 2
    Var 1

The following immunization(s) will be due:
    D/T series dose 5, on or after 7/10/2003 but before 7/10/2004
      (if DTaP 4 is given on 10/1/2000)
    IPV 4, on or after 7/10/2003 but before 7/10/2004
      (if IPV 3 is given on 10/1/2000)
    HepA 1, on or after 7/10/2001 but before 1/10/2002

The following vaccine series are either complete or no longer relevant for this case:
    HepB

Note: For the doses due today, the Vaccine for Children (VFC) Program will pay for the following doses:
    DTaP
    Hib
    IPV
    MMR
    Var

patient's care. There are a number of sources of complexity that make this process much more complicated than it might first appear.

A major source of complexity is the guideline logic itself. When the guideline logic is published in paper form, there is typically a time chart for each vaccine series indicating when each vaccination should be given, augmented by a detailed set of footnotes dealing with various special circumstances in which this basic logic must be modified. When a child is brought to the clinic on a regular basis and when no special circumstances apply, the relevant logic is quite straightforward. However, when the child has been receiving irregular care, the relevant logic can be quite complex. Examples of complexity in the guideline logic include the following:

1. *Minimum ages and wait-intervals for immunization forecasting.* For each dose in each vaccine series, there is a set of associated ages and wait-intervals to be used for forecasting that dose. For example, there are minimum ages at which the dose can be given. The minimum recommended age is the age at which the child should be scheduled for the dose. The minimum acceptable age is usually a younger age: If the child is already at the clinic, the dose may be given as of that age. There is also an age at which the dose becomes "past-due." In addition, for most doses there are minimum "wait-intervals." One type of wait-interval indicates how long one should wait from the previous dose in that series. Even if the child is over the minimum age for a dose, the dose should not be given until this wait-interval is past. For live vaccine doses, there may also be wait-intervals from previous live vaccine doses in other series. Other wait-intervals are also used, including a minimum wait-interval between dose 1 and dose 3 for Hepatitis B, and wait-intervals before a dose becomes past due.

2. *Logic variation for different clinical conditions.* For most vaccine series, the logic of the recommendations varies in different clinical conditions. For example, if the child's mother is HBsAg positive, there may be an accelerated HepB vaccination schedule. In other series, there is special logic for "late starts." For example, in the Hib vaccine series, there is different logic for later doses if the age at dose 1 is under 7 months, or if it occurs at 7–11 months, 12–14 months, or 15 months or more. In each of these four circumstances, there may be different minimum ages and wait-intervals for subsequent doses and/or a different number of doses needed to complete the series. In addition, in the Hib vaccine series, the schedule and number of doses required varies with the brand of vaccine used. These are just a few examples of the many different variations in the guideline logic. As a result of these variations, each dose of a vaccine series may have several distinct sets of minimum ages and wait-intervals. The clinical logic determines which set of parameters applies to a particular child at a particular time.

3. *Invalid doses based on immunization screening.* In addition to the forecasting parameters described above, there is a similar set of screening parameters (minimum ages and wait-intervals) for each vaccine dose. Any

dose that is given too early based on these screening parameters is not counted as part of the series for purposes of forecasting. If an invalid dose involves a live vaccine, however, it may still impose a wait-interval for other live vaccine doses.

4. *What is a month?* Another interesting complexity concerns the definition of a month. Sometimes it makes most sense to consider a month to be a calendar month, but at other times it makes more sense to consider a month to have a fixed length, such as 28 days.

These are just a few examples of the complexity inherent in the immunization guidelines logic. A further source of complexity arises because the recommendations produced by the panel of clinical experts typically contain "logical gaps." Clinical experts are accustomed to treating patients one at a time, but they are usually not adept at specifying logic that responds appropriately to all possible combinations of conditions that could conceivably arise. Examples of such gaps include the following.

- The ACIP guidelines do not currently make a distinction between minimum ages and wait-intervals to be used for screening vs. forecasting, even though it is clear that these frequently are not the same.
- At one point, the ACIP guidelines recommended a "sequential" approach to giving polio vaccine, an approach that involved giving two doses of inactivated polio vaccine (IPV) followed by two doses of oral polio vaccine (OPV). The guideline did not specify, however, whether IPV or OPV should be used for dose 2 with a child who had already received OPV as dose 1.

Frequently, these logical gaps become apparent only in the process of converting the logic into computer-based form, a process that forces one to think through all the implications in a systematic fashion. Some gaps become evident only when one is running the program with real patient data.

The only way to fill in these gaps in the logic is to work with clinician users (e.g., a group of immunization registry staff) to discuss all such gaps and decide how the guideline should deal with each. This work involves a great deal of iterative discussion and is very time-consuming.

Another source of complexity arises because of the need for local customization. Different users of the system may want their own customized versions of the recommendations. This problem is discussed in more detail later in this section.

These complexities are further compounded by the fact that the national panel produces a new version of its recommendations roughly once a year. The new version typically contains important revisions or additions. As a result, approximately once a year, a significant portion of the logic must be changed, new gaps may need to be resolved, and any local customization may need to be adapted. Then, the entire program must be thoroughly retested. If this process is not performed in a rapid, timely fashion, the program will never be up to date.

Encoding IMM/Serve's Immunization Knowledge

IMM/Serve uses three different approaches to represent its immunization domain knowledge: (1) tabular knowledge (tables), (2) rule-based knowledge ("if–then" rules), and (3) procedural knowledge (conventional computer programming.)

Tabular Knowledge

IMM/Serve uses tables to represent all of the forecasting parameters for each dose—for example, the minimum acceptable age, the minimum recommended age, and the minimum wait-intervals from previous doses, etc. For each dose of each vaccine series, IMM/Serve may store several sets of such parameters, corresponding to the different clinical conditions in which different sets of parameters apply to that dose. Table 23.3 illustrates how this tabular forecasting knowledge is stored. For purposes of this illustration, the information seen in Table 23.3 has been somewhat simplified. In fact, even more parameters are stored for each dose. Each line of this table contains one set of related parameters. Each line shows three minimum ages (acceptable, recommended, and past-due), and also the minimum wait-interval for each dose after the previous dose. Two doses (Hib 1 and Hib 4) have only a single parameter set. Doses Hib 2 and Hib3, however, each have two different parameter sets. The child's age at Hib dose 1 and the Hib brand received can determine which of these parameter sets will apply.

IMM/Serve also uses tables (a) to store the screening parameters that allow it to recognize when a dose has been given too early and should be considered invalid, and (b) to define which live-vaccine interactions should be enforced and what wait-intervals to use for each.

TABLE 23.3. A simplified table of immunization forecasting parameters

Immunization	Acceptable Age	Recommended Age	Past-Due Age	Wait-Interval
Hib1	6 weeks	2 months	3 months	—
Hib2	10 weeks	4 months	5 months	Hib1 1 month
Hib2_final	12 months	15 months	16 months	Hib1 2 months
Hib3	18 weeks	6 months	7 months	Hib2 1 month
Hib3_final	12 months	15 months	16 months	Hib2 2 month
Hib4	12 months	15 months	16 months	Hib3 2 months

TABLE 23.4. Example of if–then rules used by IMM/Serve to represent the clinical logic that determines which set of tabular parameters applies to a particular case

if:	Hib.prior = 1 and not Hib_inactive and Hib1_age_in_months ≥ 12 and Hib2_final_parameters_met
then:	due.Hib2_final
if:	Hib.prior = 1 and not Hib_inactive and Hib1_age_in_months < 12 and Hib2_parameters_met
then:	due.Hib2
if:	Hib.prior = 1 and not Hib_inactive and Hib1_age_in_months ≥ 12 and not Hib2_final_parameters_met
then:	next.Hib2_final
if:	Hib.prior = 1 and not Hib_inactive and Hib1_age_in_months < 12 and not Hib2_parameters_met
then:	next.Hib2

Rule-Based Knowledge

IMM/Serve uses if–then rules to store the clinical logic that determines when a dose should be given and which set of tabular parameters applies to a particular child at a particular time. The rules also determine other factors, such as which vaccine brand or preparation should be recommended, if alternatives exist. (For example, there are four different vaccine preparations in the DTP vaccine series: DT, DTP, DTaP, and Td.)

Table 23.4 shows example rules that partially specify the clinical logic for Hib dose 2. The first rule says "if there has been one previous Hib dose (Hib_prior = 1) and the Hib series is active and the Hib dose 1 was given at over 12 months of age and the Hib2_final parameter set is met (e.g., the minimum ages and wait-interval criteria are satisfied), then dose Hib 2 is due, and the parameters in the Hib2_final parameter set apply." The other three rules test different combinations of (1) whether the child is over 12 months of age, and (2) whether the Hib2 or Hib2_final parameter sets are met. IMM/Serve's knowledge base contains roughly 300 rules.

Procedural Knowledge

Procedural logic (conventional computer programs) is used to represent aspects of the immunization knowledge that is complex but not expected to change very much over time. For example, the temporal logic that combines dates, minimum ages, and several wait-intervals (which may be expressed in a combination of days, weeks, months, and years) to determine when a dose is due (accommodating the different lengths of different months, including the effect of leap years) is written procedurally. As long as we continue to use our current calendar, this logic is not likely to require major change.

The goal in combining these different forms of knowledge representation is to make it easy to modify and test the knowledge as that knowledge evolves over time. The biggest advantage of IMM/Serve's tabular knowledge is that it is very easy to modify parameter tables. Similarly, the complex clinical logic is written by use of if–then rules to better separate it from the rest of the IMM/ Serve program (which consists of several hundred pages of C programs), so that the rule-based logic can be more easily inspected, tested, modified, and refined.

The Development Process

IMM/Serve was developed by a collaborative interdisciplinary team. This team included (1) a computer programmer who implemented the major programming components of IMM/Serve, (2) a "knowledge engineer" who had experience building a wide range of different clinical consultation programs, (3) several clinical domain experts who had extensive clinical experience with childhood immunization and immunization registries, and (4) a project manager responsible for coordinating the project as a whole. The project manager worked closely with the clinical domain experts to discuss the various issues (e.g., how the guidelines should be interpreted, how any gaps in the guidelines should be resolved), to translate the results of these discussions into table entries and rules, to explain any nuances to the knowledge engineer and programmer, and to conduct iterative testing of the knowledge. This process of development, refinement, testing, and maintenance has extended over a period of years, involving many extensive conference phone calls, electronic mail exchanges, and testing of IMM/Serve at different sites.

Testing

IMM/Serve has been tested in several ways. A high-priority goal is to develop a set of computer-based tools to assist in this knowledge testing process.

Automated Tools for Knowledge Testing

Two automated tools that have been quite extensively used for knowledge testing are IMM/Def and IMM/Test.[3,4] IMM/Def is designed to help the knowledge engineers double-check IMM/Serve's rule "kernel," the most complex part of the knowledge in which the logic must react appropriately to a range of different combinations of conditions. IMM/Test is designed to generate automatically a set of test cases that are intended to exercise all meaningful combinations of clinical conditions contained within the rule kernel.

Testing with Hand-Crafted Sets of Test Cases

Although IMM/Def and IMM/Test are designed to help test the most complex portion of IMM/Serve's logic, there are many other parts of the logic that these tools do not handle. To help test these portions of the logic, sets of test cases have been constructed by hand.

Testing with Pilot Use

Once a new version of IMM/Serve has been thoroughly tested as described above, the next step is further testing in the context of pilot use. Here, IMM/Serve is linked to a real immunization database and run on real patient records, either in test mode or in monitored operational use by a member of the development team. Real patient data may well expose additional unanticipated issues and problems.

Implementation

When IMM/Serve is run operationally, it currently runs on the local computer of an immunization registry as a callable module. The patient data are extracted from the registry database and passed to IMM/Serve for its analysis. The actual input to and output from IMM/Serve is a coded form of the information shown in Tables 23.1 and 23.2. The coded output produced by IMM/Serve can be used in different ways. To generate recommendations for a single case, the output is passed to a report generator. Table 23.2 shows the output produced by one such report generator. Specific users may wish to use a different report generator that presents this information in different ways. Alternatively, if IMM/Serve is being used to generate a list of patients for a forthcoming clinic, IMM/Serve might be run on a set of patients and its output used to construct a list showing patients who will have vaccinations due, which vaccinations will be due for those patients, and which vaccinations will become due in the near future. Staff can then use this list to determine which patients should be called in for that clinic and which might best be delayed to allow more vaccinations to be given at one time.

Another potentially valuable strategy for using IMM/Serve operationally is to run it on a powerful central server on the Internet and to allow many registry computers to link to that single version of IMM/Serve remotely. The advantage of this approach is that as IMM/Serve needs to be modified, the modification need only be performed on a single machine.

Local Customization

Clinics that use IMM/Serve frequently want to use customized versions of the logic.[5] The US Indian Health Service (IHS) provides an interesting case study of this phenomenon. Seven versions of IMM/Serve's tabular knowledge are

currently defined for use by different IHS clinics. (A single version of IMM/
Serve may contain several different versions of each table, as well as several
variations of the rules. When IMM/Serve is run, a version name is passed in
on a case-by-case basis, indicating which version of the knowledge should be
used.) These seven versions of the tables define alternative sets of forecasting
parameters for six vaccine series. The number of such sets of tabular knowledge for each series is as follows: DTP (2), HepA (1), HepB (2), Hib (4), MMR
(2), Polio (3), and Var (2).

In addition, the IHS requested a specific variant of the Hib rule-based
knowledge for use at two clinics and two changes in the DTP rule-based logic
that differ from the national ACIP guidelines for use at all IHS clinics. Another
capability that the IHS requested was the ability to accommodate incomplete
vaccination histories. The IHS registries store a dose number with each vaccine dose. (Many other registries do not store dose numbers.) The registries
frequently show missing doses—for example, because a child has moved
from one location to another. As a result, IMM/Serve's underlying engine was
modified to allow the system to operate in the presence of certain types of
incomplete IHS vaccination histories.[6]

Maintenance

It has been an exciting challenge to build IMM/Serve and to refine it as an
operational tool. It will be at least an equal challenge to maintain IMM/
Serve's knowledge as the field evolves over time and as increasing numbers
of users request local customizations. As described previously, the national
ACIP panel typically makes major changes in its recommendations every
year. These changes will need to be rapidly incorporated into IMM/Serve and
thoroughly tested. As a result, maintaining the knowledge requires a continuing collaboration between IMM/Serve's developers and its domain experts.
Computer-based tools will be particularly important to assist in this knowledge maintenance process.

Design Considerations

Designing a decision support system requires consideration of how knowledge is
to be represented and of how the system will interface with data sources.

Knowledge Representation

Once one has decided to encode health knowledge in the computer to be used
for decision support, a major decision concerns what form of knowledge representation to use. The desirable goals in choosing a knowledge representation are:

1. To make it easy for computer-unsophisticated health experts to understand the encoded knowledge;
2. To make the knowledge easy to modify as the health domain evolves;
3. To facilitate building computer-based tools to help test and validate the knowledge; and
4. To separate as cleanly as possible the complex health-related logic from the rest of the computer program required for implementation of the application as a whole.

The choice of the best knowledge representation to use will vary with the nature of the domain. In general, one would like to use a technique that is as simple as possible, yet powerful enough to solve the problem. For example, tables, which are very simple and easy to modify, can be a very straightforward approach. On the other hand, it may become clear that different parts of the problem will most naturally fit different knowledge representation approaches. If so, as was the case with IMM/Serve, one may choose to combine several approaches. We will discuss examples of different knowledge representations.

Tables

As we have indicated, tables are probably the simplest form for knowledge representation. Tabular knowledge can be used in many ways. In IMM/Serve, tables were used to store parameter values. Tables can also include decision logic as well. These are called *decision tables*. A decision table might contain a set of rows, each containing a condition and a set of actions. For a given case, each row whose condition is satisfied by the input describing the case specifies a set of actions that should be performed.

Rules

If–then rules have been widely used in health-related decision support programs. Rules provide a simple way to encode small atomistic "chunks" of logic. A potential advantage is that the action of each rule can be readily understood and modified. New rules can easily be added. A potential drawback in a large, complex, interrelated domain is that it can be difficult to anticipate the interactions of a large number of rules operating together.

Flowcharts

Flowcharts have been extensively used to represent computer logic, and they may provide a convenient way to structure certain domains to help make the logic easy to understand and visualize.

Semantic Networks

When complex interrelated knowledge needs to be stored in the computer, semantic networks can be used to explicitly represent the various relationships between data items in a flexible fashion.

Model-Based Knowledge

Certain decision support systems contain within them one or more models that operate on the data. These might be statistical models, simulation models, or models of scientific processes. When one or more models of this type can be combined with other knowledge representations, the result is a potentially powerful system.

Procedural Knowledge

Conventional computer programming is widely used to build many computing applications. Certain decision support systems may be most easily built by use of a conventional programming language. In systems such as IMM/Serve, a part of the domain knowledge may most easily be built by use of conventional programming.

Interface with Data Sources

As increasing amounts of health data are placed into computer-based form and as increasing numbers of software tools are developed for analyzing those data in different ways, it will be essential to develop standards for describing that data. Without standards, data will not readily be passed from one health database to another and to the growing set of software tools. There are a variety of levels at which health data standards are being developed. Chapter 11 contains additional information about these topics.

System Development Strategies

Development of decision support and expert systems requires some special considerations in addition to the usual issues related to creating any information system. First and perhaps most important of these is consideration of the sources of knowledge to be incorporated in the system. Ideally, existing written guidelines are already in place, along with a system to revise and maintain them. This was the case, for example, with the childhood immunization forecasting expert system just described. Unfortunately, however, the existence of such written guidelines is the exception, rather than the rule.

More commonly, there are no written guidelines to explicitly guide decision making. In such cases, extensive efforts will be required to capture the relevant knowledge prior to system development. If the guidelines exist but are not written, it may be possible to convene and work with a group of experts to formally express consensus rules and procedures. Such work itself can be a long and tedious process.

If decision rules do not really exist, development of a decision support system is probably premature. A useful alternative is to develop mechanisms for integrating and presenting information to decision makers in an improved fashion—either faster or more easily interpretable, or some combination. Once such information is available, it may lead to the development of informal decision rules that can later be incorporated in a more advanced system.

The development of a decision support or an expert system is most likely to succeed in an environment where written guidelines are already in place. On the other hand, if the knowledge is well known but not codified, development efforts can be successful but are much more difficult. However, in cases in which decision rules are largely unknown or else there is substantial controversy as to the best approach, attempts to develop decision support systems should be avoided, as they are likely to be futile.

As with all public health information systems, the development of decision support and expert systems should be led by an interdisciplinary team. This team should include experts in public health practice, in the subject matter of the system, and in *knowledge engineering*, the subspecialty of computer science that deals with the formal encoding of knowledge. Naturally, there should be a steering committee composed primarily of users to guide the development process.

The first step in the development process is to define the overall architecture of the system, requiring primarily making a determination of how the knowledge will be delivered. The key consideration in this first step is the limitations in the user environment. Developers must address such issues as time, space, needed level of detail, and requirements for explanations and references. Of course, the infrastructure to deliver the recommendations, such as computer systems connected to a network, must be in place. Furthermore, the user must have access to the relevant systems at the time and in the place where decisions are made. Another key architectural consideration that should be considered from the outset is maintenance. Knowledge is not static over time. Without a mechanism in place for maintaining and updating the knowledge, development of a system is merely an academic exercise.

During system development itself, the use of existing tools will greatly increase productivity. There are many tools available for encoding and processing knowledge. We have already described several examples of such tools in the discussion of childhood immunization forecasting. Sometimes, it is necessary to create new tools where none are available. In the childhood immunization forecasting system, for example, new tools were necessary—tools such as the tool for automatic generation of test cases to revalidate the system when changes are made.

As with other information systems, dividing the problem domain into segments and then implementing and testing those segments independently is one of the best approaches to development. For each segment, an iterative approach involving the creation of multiple rapid prototypes is typically very effective. When the various independent segments of the system are combined, interactions between them can be identified and addressed appropriately.

It is also important to anticipate specific problems that are likely to occur in the process of creating a decision support or an expert system. The first of these problems relates to the significant demands on the time of the subject matter experts. For example, even when written guidelines are already in place, development of an expert system is likely to reveal many gaps in the knowledge base, gaps that have not been previously considered. These gaps can occur, for instance, because of unanticipated or unusual combinations of inputs. These gaps—and other ambiguous situations—require subject matter experts to make many decisions about the desired system output.

In addition, it is extremely important for system developers to conduct rigorous testing. One reason is that it is easy for developers to become overly confident in the initial output of a decision support or an expert system. The output tends to have the aura of accuracy and authority because it is formatted nicely and produced quickly. However, more detailed testing involving the creation of test cases that exercise every portion of the system's knowledge base may reveal flaws in the output. For this reason, developers should undertake both manual and automatic testing at every stage in the development process. The creation and verification of an extensive library of test cases for such testing is itself a substantial effort. Nevertheless, it is highly inadvisable to shortchange or circumvent this aspect of system development work.

As always, user feedback throughout the system development process is crucial to success. After all, the goal is not to produce the "perfect" system. Rather, the goal is to provide meaningful assistance in decision making for the users. Therefore, the users must be involved in the creation and refinement of the system at every stage. In particular, they must be comfortable with the mechanism and with the formatting for delivery of both the information and the recommendations derived from that information. Typically, users must have the ability to override the system when other factors supervene. In addition, adequate explanations of the recommendations must usually be accessible to reassure the users and provide justification for the output of the system.

Criteria for Determining the Desirability of Decision Support and Expert Systems

In light of these considerations, it is possible to suggest criteria that may be used to determine whether a decision support or an expert system would be desirable in a given environment. There are two major factors in making such a determination: the decision characteristics and the nature of the user environment.

With regard to the decision characteristics, the decisions to be made should be complex or least not trivial in order for a decision support system to be useful. In the decision-making, there should be well-defined rules or algorithms that are subject to relatively rapid and continuous change. Naturally, the existence of a high degree of consensus with respect to the appropriate criteria for decision-making will greatly ease the system development process.

The second of the criteria requires that the user environment include a convenient delivery mechanism for recommendations generated by a decision support or an expert system. Ideally, this delivery mechanism should (1) already be in place and (2) provide easy and inexpensive access for users. In addition, the environment should include multiple applications sites for the system, allowing the costs, which can be substantial, to be widely distributed. (However, even when multiple application sites exist, system developers need to keep in mind that while customization of decision support and expert systems for specific sites is certainly possible, it adds to the cost of the system, both initially and in the maintenance phase.) In addition, it is very positive for the user community to recognize that the decisions to be supported by a proposed system could be improved through the use of technology. After all, it is much easier to enlist the cooperation of users in the development of a decision support or an expert system when they are the ones demanding the help that such a system can provide.

Illustration of the Criteria

To illustrate these criteria, here are some examples of potential applications of decision support in public health practice.

The analysis of surveillance data to detect aberrations that may represent outbreaks is an obvious application of decision support. Here, the justification is the expected increase in surveillance data received by public health without a concomitant increase in personnel available for its analysis. Another area related to outbreaks that might benefit from decision support is the preparation of outbreak-specific surveys that can be used in interviews that accompany disease investigations.

Resource management is another area in which decision support might be helpful. System estimation of cost/benefit ratios for specific public health programmatic interventions could be used to generate recommended priorities for expenditures. Of course, using such a system would require much better baseline information about both the expenditures and the results of various public health programs.

Finally, decision support is clearly applicable to the dissemination of practice guidelines, as described in the example of childhood immunization forecasting. By encoding such guidelines in computable form and delivering them to public health clinics and other relevant healthcare settings, we should be able to increase greatly the delivery of effective preventive services. While development of decision support and expert systems based on clinical prevention guidelines is clearly a substantial undertaking, the results of many previous studies indicating the benefits of clinician reminders in improving compliance provide a substantial body of evidence for the expectation that the benefits of this work would be well worth the effort.[7-9]

Questions for Review

Questions 1–11 are based on the following short case.

The head of a state public health department wants to build a decision support system for use by public environmental specialists who are responsible for monitoring contaminants in well water, streams, and lakes in the state. The decision support system would provide the environmental specialists with access via laptop computers to toxicological profiles of the Agency for Toxic Substances and Disease Registry (ATSDR) and to the Environmental Protection Agency's Reference Dose Media Evaluation Guide (RMEGs) comparison values. It would provide recommended action levels through incorporation of the EPA's Maximum Contaminant Levels (MCLs). As conceived by the head of the department, the system would permit public environmental specialists to enter data related to contaminant measurements, then send that data via remote hookup to the state's contaminant databases. This data would be site-specific. The system would then compare this data to the RMEG comparison values and to the MCLs and generate an action to be taken by an environmental specialist at the site. These specialists have used laptop computers in their work for many years, and they have complained frequently about the slowness of the current assessment processes, which require manual collection of data and then a considerable wait before agency officials analyze the data and provide recommended courses of action. However, many of the specialists are not schooled in the use of databases. In addition, some have expressed concerns that the proposed decision support system might not meet all their needs or else would by-pass their judgment. Finally, the guidelines to be incorporated in the system change over time.

1. What data in the proposed decision support system would lend themselves to being represented by tables?
2. What knowledge would best be represented by if–then rules?
3. In what ways might the guideline logic of this system, as conceived by the department head, fail to recognize all the applicable conditions to be encountered by an environmental specialist in addressing contaminant levels found in water?
4. How would testing via automated tools, hand-crafted sets of test cases, and pilot use help to address any gaps in the guideline logic?
5. Suppose the environmental specialists charged with measuring contaminant levels in community wells want a customized version of the proposed system. What challenges would such customization present?
6. What difficulties are likely to be inherent in maintaining the decision support system, assuming it is developed?
7. What knowledge representation goals should a development team establish in building the proposed decision support system?
8. What criteria should already be in place within the department's functions in order to maximize the likelihood that the decision support system will be successful if it is built?
9. What is the first step in the development process for the decision support system?
10. What should be the composition of the system development team? Explain why the team should have this composition.

11. To what extent has the department met the criteria for determining the desirability of the decision support system?

References

1. Miller PL, Frawley SJ, Sayward FG, Yasnoff WA, Duncan L, Fleming D. Combining tabular, rule-based and procedural knowledge in computer-based guidelines for childhood immunization. *Comput Biomed Res* 1997;30:211–231.
2. Cordero JF, Guerra FA, Saarlas KN, eds. Developing immunization registries: Experience from the All Kids Count Program. *Am J Prev Med.* 1997;13(Suppl).
3. Miller PL. Tools for immunization guideline knowledge maintenance I: Automated generation of the logic "kernel" for immunization forecasting. *Comput Biomed Res* 1998;31:172–189.
4. Miller PL, Frawley SJ, Brandt C, Sayward FG. Tools for immunization guideline knowledge maintenance II: Automated Web-based generation of user-customized test cases. *Comput Biomed Res,* 1998;31:190–208.
5. Miller PL, Frawley SJ, Sayward FG. Informatics issues in the national dissemination of a computer-based clinical guideline: A case study in childhood immunization. In: *Proceedings of the 2000 AMIA Annual Fall Symposium, Los Angeles, CA.* 2000:580–584.
6. Miller PL, Frawley SJ, Sayward FG. Exploring three approaches for handling incomplete patient histories in a computer-based guideline for childhood immunization. In: *Proceedings of the 1999 AMIA Annual Fall Symposium, Washington, DC*; 1999:878–882.
7. McDonald CJ. Protocol-based computer reminders, the quality of care and the nonperfectability of man. *New Engl J Med.* 1976:295:1351–1355.
8. Litezelman DK, Dittus RS, Miller ME, and Tierney WM. Requiring physicians to respond to computerized reminders improves their compliance with preventive care protocols. *J Gen Intern Med* 1993:8:311–317.
9. Shea S, DuMouchel W, Bahamonde L. A meta-analysis of 16 randomized controlled trials to evaluate computer-based clinical reminder systems for preventive care in the ambulatory setting. *J Am Med Inform Assoc* 1996;3:399–409.

24
Promoting the Delivery of Preventive Medicine in Primary Care

LARRY L. DICKEY AND JOHN D. PIETTE

Learning Objectives

After studying this chapter, you should be able to:

- Describe the components that constitute clinical preventive services.
- Explain why preventive medicine has received less emphasis, to date, than curative medical service.
- Explain the value of information technology for improving preventive care.
- Discuss the uses and potential value of the electronic medical record, the comprehensive computerized risk assessment, and interactive voice response systems in preventive care assessment.
- Discuss the uses and potential value of telephone counseling services and interactive Internet-based tools such as the Comprehensive Health Enhancement Support System (CHESS) in improving the delivery of preventive services.
- Explain the value of electronic systems for providing preventive care reminders to both providers and patients and for providing auditing of preventive care services.
- Discuss the future challenges for increasing the use of information technology in the practice of preventive care.

Overview

For a number of reasons, medical services have tended to put more emphasis on curative than on preventive functions. Yet, a number of forces, including costs, are refocusing medical services toward prevention—at primary, secondary, and tertiary levels. The application of technology to preventive medicine demonstrated the ability of informatics to improve the timeliness and quality of preventive care in a cost-effective manner. For preventive care assessment, effective tools include the computerized health risk assessment, the electronic medical record, and interactive voice response systems. For preventive service delivery, tools ranging from the relatively low-tech telephone counseling services to the sophisticated Comprehensive Health Enhancement Support System (CHESS) are helping to improve the quality of life of patients. Technology has also become important to the improvement of preventive care reminders and auditing. Although the application of technology to preventive medicine faces many challenges and barriers, there seems to be little question that, with creativity and care, clinicians and patients can learn to use technology-based tools to promote health and prevent disease much more effectively and efficiently than ever before.

Introduction

To many people, *preventive medicine* may seem to be a contradiction in terms. After all, medicines are used primarily to cure illness, not to prevent it. If people are not ill, then why would they need medicines or medical attention? Such an assumption is an example of the power and influence of the curative model of health care, which grew exponentially during the 20th century with the rapid development of the pharmaceutical industry and advances in critical care technology. This enterprise has, however, been very costly—with 27% of Medicare payments and 10–12% of our country's total healthcare dollars devoted to care at the end of life.[1] In fact, advances in curative technology are outpacing the ability of our healthcare system to pay for them.

This chapter explores an alternative use for technology, to help prevent rather than cure disease, and to help control the large amount of dollars going into curative medicine. Advances in human genetics may hold the greatest potential for the advancement of disease prevention in the 21st century.[2-4] However, many currently available interventions have the ability to prevent much disease and promote health, if they are fully implemented. By one estimate, roughly half of all deaths in 1990 in the United States were premature and preventable to some degree.[5] Counseling interventions have the ability to improve lifestyle choices related to smoking, nutrition, and unsafe behaviors that lead to the greatest amount of unnecessary morbidity and mortality.[6] In addition, immunizations prevent a growing list of infectious diseases and can save up to $5 in treatment costs for every $1 expended.[7] Screening tests, such as mammography, help prevent the progression of many illnesses and death from cancer—and often at much less cost and suffering than medical treatment.[8]

Clinical Preventive Services

Counseling, screening, and immunizations constitute the core armamentarium available to healthcare providers to prevent disease and promote health. Collectively, these are called *clinical preventive services*. They address the three levels of intervention: primary, secondary, and tertiary prevention. *Primary prevention* (vaccinations, counseling) intercedes even before precursor signs of disease are detectable. *Secondary prevention* (screening tests and examinations) detects diseases before symptoms develop, thus enabling interventions for early eradication or control. *Tertiary prevention* involves treatment and counseling for symptomatic diseases (such as diabetes) to prevent progression and the development of complications.

Full implementation of clinical preventive services has proven to be an elusive goal for the US healthcare system. A 1994 survey of patients in California health plans found that for most behavioral health risks, less than 20% of patients with a risk factor had spoken with a health professional about it in the preceding three years.[9] A 1997 study of US citizens over 50 years of age found that less than 20% reported using a fecal occult blood test in the last year, and less than 30% reported having a sigmoidoscopy in the preceding five years.[10] Nationally, only about 75% of children are up to date with all immunizations on their second birthday,[11] and only about 50% of persons over 65 years of age have received a pneumococcal vaccination.[12]

There are multiple reasons for failures in the delivery of preventive services. Lack of medical insurance is undoubtedly a major factor for many patients.[13,14] However, even in populations where financial factors are not present, preventive service delivery is usually suboptimal. A 1990 study of breast cancer screening found that women reported that lack of knowledge and not having been told by their physician that they needed a mammogram were the most important barriers.[15] When asked to estimate their preventive service delivery, physicians tend to report rates much higher than can be verified by review of their patients' charts.[16,17] Good intentions and wishful thinking seem to be common characteristics of physicians when it comes to delivering preventive care.

Some studies have identified the competing demands of medical practice as constituting the most important barrier to the delivery of preventive care.[18,19] In a busy office or clinic, it is understandable that sick patients will demand and receive immediate attention, while the provision of preventive services to well or not acutely ill patients is often overlooked or delayed. In contrast, preventive services are delivered at increased rates during health maintenance or wellness clinic visits, where the competing pressures and distractions of acute care medicine can be avoided.[20–22] Unfortunately, the infrastructure to support dedicated wellness clinics does not exist in most locations, and check-up or wellness visits are not utilized or available to many patients. This situation has led many authorities, including the US Preventive Services Task Force, to recommend that clinicians use every opportunity to deliver preventive services, including delivering these services at the time that patients come in for treatment of illnesses.[23]

Incorporating preventive care delivery into the cramped time frame of a 10- or 15-minute acute care visit is very difficult. Information technology can help address the problem by efficiently automating many of the steps of preventive care in the busy clinical setting. These steps are (1) assessment, (2) preventive service delivery, (3) reminding, and (4) auditing.

Using Information Technology for Preventive Care Assessment

The first challenge clinicians face is simply determining what preventive care a patient has already received and what they additionally need. Patients' needs vary according to age, gender, and risk factors (such as family history). Most practices determine their own protocols for preventive service delivery and post the protocols in a printed form in patient charts. Unfortunately, such printed protocols are often misplaced and not consistently utilized in a busy practice settings.[24,25] Several types of electronic assessment tools have been developed to meet the need for current and consistent preventive service delivery protocols. These tools include the electronic medical record, the comprehensive health risk assessment, and interactive voice response systems.

The Electronic Medical Record

Some electronic medical record (EMR) applications are able to assess a patient's need for screening and immunization services based on age and gender information that is input by clinicians or support staff. Many such programs have the flexibility to allow providers to customize the protocol of preventive services according to the needs of the individual practice. This is a highly desirable feature because, despite guidelines issued by national authorities such as the US Preventive Services Task Force and the American Cancer Society, most practices choose to utilize a protocol tailored to the needs and preferences of their patients and providers.[26] Some assessment programs utilize direct patient data entry through keyboards, touch screens, or other devices. The optimal methods for data entry have not be established, although systems that are not components of EMRs may not be well maintained because of the need to also enter data into a paper record.

The Comprehensive Health Risk Assessment

Assessment of behavioral risk factors (such as tobacco use, drug and alcohol use, and sexual behavior) is a complex task that involves gathering information from patients regarding a wide variety of specific and often personally sensitive behaviors. Over the last 30 years, much work has been devoted to developing and testing electronic tools for this purpose. Most study has been carried out with the comprehensive health risk assessment (HRA), first developed by the Centers for Disease Control and Prevention in 1977 and subsequently released in an updated form as *Healthier People, Version 3.0* by the Carter Center of Emory University in 1988.[27,28]

In addition to gathering important patient data for use by clinicians, HRAs are able to use data from epidemiologic studies to estimate the risks of adverse events (e.g., reductions in life expectancy or the probability of a heart attack) based on patients' behavioral risk factors, medical histories, and sociodemographic characteristics. This feedback may be helpful in conveying the importance of behavioral changes to patients.[29]

Computerized HRAs have several advantages over printed or verbal assessments. They can improve data quality by insuring that all appropriate questions are included and answered. They can be administered by allied health workers or self-administered by patients, thereby minimizing their impact on staffing costs or clinicians' time. Moreover, repeated administrations can be easily stored in patients' EMRs, thus allowing clinicians to track patients' progress toward health behavior goals. HRAs may be more readily accessible at the point-of-care than paper forms, and they can provide data supporting population-level analyses useful in identifying priority areas for health counseling and evaluating the effectiveness of preventive services.

Investigators have examined the impact of HRAs on physicians' preventive service delivery, as well as on patients' health behaviors and health status. In a study conducted by Geiger and colleagues,[22] intervention patients received an HRA followed by face-to-face discussions of the results. Outcomes were measured through subsequent medical record reviews. These outcomes indicated that individuals receiving the HRA were more likely to be counseled about risks (e.g., those related to diet, exercise, substance abuse, and injury prevention) than patients in a comparison sample. However, improvements in these areas were difficult to attribute exclusively to the HRAs, because the HRAs were administered in conjunction with other important services, such as outpatient visits specifically focusing on health promotion.

Computerized HRAs make it possible to provide feedback tailored to the personal characteristics and needs of patients. Kreuter and Strecher found that patients who received such personalized feedback were more likely to change risk behaviors than patients who received generic feedback or no feedback at all.[30] These results are consistent with the broader literature, demonstrating that tailored counseling is more likely to result in positive behavior changes than a generic, didactic approach.

In addition to promoting primary preventive counseling for healthy populations, HRAs can be used to improve self-care education for patients with chronic health problems. Glasgow and colleagues studied the effects of a brief HRA administered via a touch-screen computer located in physicians' waiting rooms.[31,32] The assessments focused on patients' diet, barriers to behavior changes, and attainment of goals for incremental dietary improvements. The HRA then generated reports summarizing the session for both the patient and the provider. These reports were then used to structure dietary counseling sessions and promote behavioral adherence between office visits. Compared with patients receiving usual care, those receiving this intervention improved on several outcome measures at the three-month follow-up, and they maintained these improvements for one year after entry into the study. Compared with controls, follow-up cholesterol levels were lower among intervention patients, and these patients reported consuming fewer calories. The proportion of calories from fat was lower among intervention than among control patients, especially calories from saturated fat.

These investigators estimated the cost-effectiveness of this HRA-based intervention and found that, on average, the annual cost was $115–$139 per patient, or $8.40 per unit reduction in serum cholesterol. By way of context, cholesterol-lowering medications can cost from $350 to $1400 per patient per year and can be less cost-effective and cause more adverse reactions. In a follow-up study,[33] Glasgow and Toobert examined whether additional services such as follow-up telephone calls and community resource information increased the impact of the intervention just described. They found that neither of these services, either alone or in combination, improved patients' outcomes.

In summary, studies suggest that HRAs may be useful tools for improving primary prevention counseling. Studies conducted to date suggest that the amount of impact associated with HRAs seems to depend on the characteristics of follow-up counseling. Although studies suggest that counseling following an HRA should be tailored rather than generic, more intensive face-to-face counseling or long-term follow-up appears to yield minimal incremental benefits.

Interactive Voice Response Systems

The prevention of chronic disease progression (tertiary prevention) requires the timely reporting and assessment of patient signs, symptoms, and tests. Innovative information technology approaches hold promise for facilitating this assessment process. Interactive voice response (IVR) systems can bring health technology into the homes of people who have difficulty coming to clinic visits in person and who lack the ability to access or utilize computers.[34] IVR enables patients to interact with computers by using a standard telephone to respond to queries for information through the touch-tone keypad or through voice recognition technology. IVR systems have been evaluated for the assessment of patients with depression,[35] cancer,[36,37] heart failure,[38] and diabetes.[39] A comprehensive review of IVR systems has been published by one of the current chapter authors.[40]

IVR systems can increase a provider's ability to monitor patients between clinic visits and identify individuals with health and behavioral problems requiring early intervention. This use may be important because in-person treatment encounters provide relatively infrequent opportunities to assess patients' health status. As a result, many opportunities to prevent short-term acute illness episodes and health crises are missed.

Studies consistently indicate that patients provide clinically useful information during IVR health assessments. In a study of 229 managed care patients with low-back pain,[41] investigators found that scores on the SF-12 Health Status Survey[42] were similar among patients using IVR reporting and those reporting information during a "live" telephone interview. IVR assessments often identify more health problems than standard modalities for gathering patient information, perhaps because patients report less embarrassment when reporting sensitive information to a computer than to a clinician.[43,44]

Compared to "live" interviews, patients are more likely to report alcohol abuse[45,46] as well as psychiatric symptoms[47] during IVR assessments. Millard and Carver[39] found that patients with low-back pain reported more psychiatric symptoms during an IVR administration of the SF-12 than patients who completed the SF-12 during a "live" telephone call. IVR assessments of patients' mental health status have been used to determine psychiatric diagnoses that are comparable to those obtained by clinicians using a structured clinical interview.[48,49] Baer et al.[35] used IVR assessments to administer a standard, multi-item survey to screen for depression. Of the 1,812 callers, 88% completed the entire 20-item questionnaire. More than one third of callers met criteria for "moderate," "marked," "severe," or "extreme" depression; and most of those identified as depressed had received no prior treatment.

IVR assessments of patients' preferences for cancer treatment can identity important disparities in understanding between patients and their clinicians.[50] IVR assessments of frail elders can be a useful screening tool for detecting functional decline, although they identify fewer problems than in-home assessments by a case manager.[51] IVR assessment data can also be used to identify patients with diabetes who are at a heightened risk of developing health problems.[52]

Outcome studies indicate that interventions based on IVR assessments can have moderate effects on patients' health and health behavior. Alemi and colleagues randomized 179 pregnant cocaine-using women to usual care or usual care supported by IVR health assessment, mutual support, and health education.[53] The intervention increased patients' use of drug treatment services, although it had no measurable impact on their health status or drug use. Other investigators have randomized hypertensive patients to usual care or weekly IVR monitoring with feedback of their assessment data to physicians.[54] After six months, antihypertensive medication adherence improved among intervention patients compared with usual care controls, and diastolic blood pressure levels decreased more in the IVR group than in the control group. Among patients with the poorest baseline medication adherence, diastolic blood pressure decreased among IVR users but increased slightly among patients receiving usual care.

Studies also indicate that IVR assessments influence the health of diabetes patients. In a pretest/post-test study,[55] patients with diabetes used an IVR system to obtain health information, report changes in their glycemic control, and access a decision-support system for making insulin dose adjustments. At follow-up, investigators observed a threefold decrease in diabetic crises and a significant improvement in measures of long-term glycemic control. In a randomized trial of IVR-supported diabetes care,[56,57] intervention patients at follow-up reported greater improvements in self-care and fewer symptoms of poor glycemic control than patients receiving usual care. Compared with usual care patients, patients receiving the intervention also reported fewer symptoms of depression and days in bed due to illness, greater self-efficacy to perform self-care activities, and higher levels of satisfaction with their health care. End point glucose control was better among intervention than control patients, and more than twice as many intervention patients had end point glucose levels within the normal range.

Similar findings were observed in a follow-up study among patients with diabetes treated in Department of Veterans Affairs clinics.[58] At 12 months, intervention patients reported more frequent glucose self-monitoring and foot inspections than patients receiving usual care. In addition, these intervention patients were more likely to receive recommended clinic services such as foot exams. Intervention patients were also more likely than control patients to have had a cholesterol test. Among patients with especially poor baseline glycemic control, end point values among intervention patients were lower than values for control patients. At follow-up, intervention patients reported fewer symptoms than control patients and greater satisfaction with their health care.

The utility of IVR is probably dependent on the nature of the chronic illness, a patient's sociodemographic characteristics (particularly those impacting access to care), and the healthcare system in which the IVR system is implemented. Some studies have used a centralized nurse to evaluate IVR assessment reports, make initial follow-up calls, and serve as the interface between the IVR monitoring system and patients' overall care,[59] whereas others have simply reported IVR data back to patients' physicians.[34] Finer points about the process of IVR assessment, such as the relative effectiveness of patient-initiated versus clinician-initiated assessment systems, the optimal length of IVR calls, and the use of random assessments to characterize health behavior patterns,[60] are also important and should be evaluated in controlled studies.

Using Information Technology for Preventive Service Delivery

Once patients have been assessed as needing preventive care, the actual in-office delivery of needed services, particularly counseling, can be very time-consuming. As previously discussed, time is a scarce commodity in primary care, and the pressures of managed care may make the time pressure even worse. Information technology has shown much promise for making the actual delivery of preventive services more efficient, particularly for counseling. It should be acknowledged that separating behavioral risk *assessment* from *counseling* is somewhat artificial and, as describe above, HRA and IVR tools usually have some counseling utility in addition to their more developed assessment capabilities.

Although relatively "low-tech" by today's standards, telephone counseling services are a good example of how information technology can be used to augment or replace clinician services. The California Smoker's Helpline has been operational since 1992 and has assisted over 100,000 smokers in six different languages in their attempts to quit.[61] Counselors using well-tested protocols in up to seven sessions over a period of two months provide counseling proactively. Tobacco abstinence rates at one year for users of the helpline are almost double that for smokers receiving only self-help materials (26.7% vs. 14.7%).[62] By participating in this program, patients in the state's Medicaid program are considered to have fulfilled behavior modification program requirements needed to qualify for obtaining prescription smoking cessation medications.

Interactive Internet-based tools are now being tested to assist patients with the tertiary prevention efforts for chronic diseases. The Comprehensive Health Enhancement Support System (CHESS) project represents one of the major efforts in this area. CHESS developers constructed Web sites that allowed patients to access medical information, use decision-support tools, and communicate with other chronically ill patients via e-mail and "chat" rooms. CHESS applications have been developed for a number of populations, including patients with breast cancer and HIV infection. Additional modules addressing substance abuse, Alzheimer disease, and heart disease are under development.

Patients with HIV disease used CHESS daily, with little difference in usage across demographic groups. CHESS users reported quality-of-life improvements, improved cognitive functioning, fewer ambulatory care visits, and both fewer and shorter hospitalizations.[63] Comparison of intervention patients who did and did not improve on quality of life scores suggested that the total amount of CHESS use was less important than whether patients accessed medical information and decision-support tools.[64] In a separate study, investigators found that women with breast cancer used CHESS regularly, even when they had incomes below the poverty level.[65,66]

Investigators at the Oregon Research Institute are evaluating the use of a Web-based diabetes self-management support system focused on personalized goal setting, feedback regarding progress toward behavioral goals, and social support.[67] Feasibility data indicate that a broad range of users frequently access the site. Data indicate that 111 patients logged on to the system more than 21,000 times over a 10-week period, including some individuals up to 77 years of age. The most popular area of the site was the social support section, which allowed patients to exchange information, share coping strategies, and provide emotional support. The health information pages, which allowed patients to access articles on topics such as healthy eating, were also popular. Effects of this Web-based diabetes support system on health and behavior outcomes are currently being analyzed in a randomized, controlled trial.

Using Information Technology for Preventive Care Reminders

Because of the complexity of preventive service guidelines and the unavoidable distractions of busy professional and personal lives, providers and patients frequently need to receive reminders about preventive care. Various paper-based tools for this purpose, such as printed flow-sheets and "shoe box" tickler files, have been developed and tested. Unfortunately, such tools can be difficult to maintain and generally result in only modest improvements in preventive care delivery rates.[68]

Numerous studies have demonstrated the utility and effectiveness of electronic reminding and prompting systems for preventive care.[69–73] A 1996 meta-analytic study of randomized controlled trials of such systems found that their use almost doubled the odds that preventive services in general would be delivered appropriately (odds ratio = 1.77).[74] For certain types of preventive services, the improvement was even higher (vaccinations: odds ratio = 3.09; colorectal cancer screening: odds ratio = 2.25). When electronic reminder systems have been added to practices with existing paper-based systems, significant additional improvements resulted. A similar effect was not found for the addition of paper-based reminder systems to electronic systems—leading the researchers to conclude that electronic systems are more robust.

Electronic systems have the ability to generate reminders automatically for both providers and patients. Provider reminders in the form of paper printouts or computer-posted alerts cue the busy clinician about preventive care that is not up to date for patients. These cues are most useful when issued at the time of patient visits, when the needed tests, immunizations, and counseling can be immediately provided. Computer-screen alerts can be used when electronic medical records are the primary or only mode of patient data storage. Many electronic medical record programs have preventive care tracking systems capable of generating physician preventive care alerts.

Unfortunately, even when using electronic tools, providers still often have trouble finding the time and motivation for preventive care. Some studies have found that providers may ignore the preventive care tracking functions of electronic medical records.[75,76] This tendency has prompted some electronic medical record designers to require users to actively turn off or respond to preventive medicine reminders before using other aspects of the record. The success of this strategy is unknown, although computer users may quickly develop the ability to bypass such road blocks. Also, there is evidence that the effectiveness of reminders decreases with time—perhaps because clinicians learn to tune them out.[77]

Patient reminders are most useful as outreach tools between visits—to help bring patients in for needed preventive care. Perhaps the greatest advantage of electronic reminder/recall systems over paper-based reminder/recall systems is the ability to generate and send patients reminder messages automatically. Usually such messages are in the form of mailed letters. Some research indicates that the use of patient-specific information (individual risk factors, habits, etc.) to generate personalized letters may increase potential effectiveness.

Recently, automated telephone systems (autodialers) have been successfully tested to deliver preventive care reminder messages to patients. Immunization reminder messages delivered by a computer-controlled autodialer were found in a recent study of urban private practices to be much more cost effective than mailed postcards in bringing pediatric patients in for needed immunizations ($4.06 vs. $12.82 for each additional immunization delivered).[78] Even at $4.06 per each additional immunization, patient reminding can mount up to be a considerable cost for a large practice or clinic, since provider reimbursement for immunization delivery and other preventive care is generally low ($9 for Medicaid patients in California). Unfortunately, the use of reminder systems to bring patients in for preventive care may be marginally profitable for practices because of the low rate of reimbursement for preventive care.

Using Information Technology for Preventive Care Auditing

Because of clinicians' tendency to consistently overestimate the amount of preventive services they deliver,[16,17] a number of authorities have recommended that providers periodically audit patient records in order to determine service delivery rates accurately and to identify the success or failure of quality improvement efforts.[79–81]

A number of studies have demonstrated improved rates of preventive care when auditing is employed to give feedback to providers and practices.[82,83] A recent review of randomized trials using auditing to provide feedback to providers about immunization delivery found significant improvements in 12 of 15 studies.[84]

Most electronic reminder systems, whether independent or incorporated into an electronic medical record, have the advantage of being able to generate ongoing practice-wide reports of preventive care delivery, obviating the need for time-consuming and costly patient chart audits. This function may become increasingly attractive to clinicians as they receive more and more pressure from quality improvement efforts, such as the Health Employer Data and Information Set (HEDIS) audit process.

In addition to reminder systems and electronic medical records, other types of electronic tools have been developed to aid providers in this process. One such tool is the Clinical Assessment Software Application (CASA) program developed and distributed free of charge by the Centers for Disease Control and Prevention.[85] Providers can enter childhood immunization data derived from patient chart review or other sources into the CASA program, which will analyze the data and produce detailed reports on the percentages of their patients who are up to date for each of several childhood immunizations based on various criteria, including the Advisory Committee on Immunization Practices and HEDIS. The CASA program, although primarily an audit tool, can also be used as a reminder system.

Although most providers use electronic billing and accounting systems, these lack standardization—a problem that has hindered the development of software for reminding and auditing preventive service delivery by use of administrative and billing data. This situation may improve over the coming years with implementation of the Health Insurance Portability and Accountability Act (HIPAA) standards for electronic patient data exchange. With this standardization, auditing of preventive service delivery using preexisting billing data may become much easier and make the laborious task of performing patient chart reviews unnecessary.

Beyond auditing of individual practices and health plans, many public health authorities believe that population-wide auditing is necessary. Practices and health plans should not only use their audit data for internal quality improvement purposes, but share the data with public health authorities for surveillance and healthcare planning activities as well.[86] Currently, only large health maintenance systems with computerized medical records, such as Kaiser Permanente in California, have been able to begin undertaking such collaborative efforts. Kaiser Permanente data is frequently utilized by state and local public health officials to help monitor preventive service delivery and disease outbreaks. The development and widespread implementation of medical care tracking and auditing systems one day should make population-wide preventive care efforts easier to implement and monitor.

The Future

It is difficult to fully envision how clinical preventive care will change in the next century, because there are so many opportunities. One thing seems certain, however: It will become much more complex and targeted. Using genetic analysis, we may be able to determine precisely which patients need which types of screening, immunization, prophylactic use of medications, or even counseling. The age- and gender-based protocols now used to target these services may appear quite crude in retrospect. As a consequence, clinicians' need for assistance in assessing, reminding, delivering, and auditing preventive care activities will become even more acute. The use of printed checklists, "shoe box" tickler systems, and audits of paper charts will be obviously inadequate for the task at hand. Information technology solutions will become a necessity, rather than an option.

"Stand-alone" reminder and recall systems probably won't be widely adopted so long as paper-based patient charts remain the standard of practice. The burden of entering data both digitally and manually will remain too great. The future of electronic reminder and recall systems rests with the development and widespread deployment of an electronic medical record in community and private practices.

Many barriers remain to widespread use of EMRs in community clinical practice. Perhaps the most basic of these is the continuing cottage-industry nature of many medical practices. Most small practices do not yet use computers, except for billing purposes. A recent survey of family physicians in Iowa found that only 26% had computers in their offices.[87] In addition to "hardware" inadequacy, many attitudinal barriers of clinicians will have to be overcome.[88] These barriers may prove more challenging than software standardization issues such as those currently being addressed by the efforts of Health Level 7 (HL7) and other organizations.[89]

As electronic tracking and reminding systems expand in prevalence and scope (e.g., one can imagine registries not only for childhood immunizations but for all types of preventive care), issues of control and access will become much more important. Will patients give over all control to large centralized systems? Certain automobile manufacturers today advertise the ability to access a car's repair and maintenance history by satellite link at any of their dealers nationwide. The technology exists to create similar systems for human healthcare maintenance, but will there be the political will to employ or oppose them?

Options for decentralized systems do exist. Smart cards, which utilize computer chips embedded in a plastic card, are currently used for healthcare purposes in some European countries.[90,91] Such smart cards could potentially enable individual patients to retain their own electronic medical records or control access of others to those records.[92] Just as smart cards have been used in some projects to track medication use,[93] so might they be used to track and remind patients and providers about preventive care. The use of smart cards or more powerful patient-retained electronic data management devices may be tools to empower patients to compete with large centralized systems for the locus of control of their health care and privacy.

It is both inevitable and desirable that patient education and counseling services become more available electronically. Currently, many providers are beginning to use the Internet to communicate appointment and other simple information to patients. It is only a short step from there to Internet referrals to health promotion and education sites. For providers treating ethnic minorities for whom appropriate health education materials may not be available locally, the ability to refer to resources nationally and internationally may be of great help.

It is doubtful that computers or information technology will ever replace the health-promoting relationships of primary care clinicians with their patients. However, with creativity and care, the tools will be developed that will empower clinicians and patients to promote health and prevent disease much more effectively and efficiently than ever before.

Questions for Review

Questions 1–8 are based on the following short case:
The Valley Medical Clinic provides both curative and preventive medicine to patients who live within a 40-mile distance in the surrounding rural area, although it has placed more emphasis on curative rather than preventive services. Recently, the management of the clinic has decided to increase emphasis on the delivery of preventive services to patients, offering a dedicated wellness clinic. Although the current clinic uses computers for billing purposes, it does not use technology for preventive care assessment, delivery of preventive services, preventive care reminders, or preventive care auditing. Management has decided to invest several million dollars for the purpose of acquiring technology in order to improve preventive care services.

1. List some of the factors that may have led the Valley Medical Clinic to concentrate on the delivery of curative services, rather than preventive services, to patients in the past.
2. Explain how incorporating technology in its preventive care services can help the clinic to overcome the obstacles typically imposed by a 10- to 15-minute clinical visit by a patient.
3. Explain how the use of the following computerized applications could help the clinic to lower the costs of preventive care assessment while improving its efficiency and effectiveness:
   a. Electronic medical record applications
   b. Computerized health risk assessments
   c. Interactive voice response systems
4. Explain how the use of the following technologic applications could help the clinic to improve its delivery of preventive care:
   a. Telephone counseling services
   b. Interactive Internet-based tools to assist patients with chronic diseases
5. Explain why the use of electronic systems to generate reminders for both clinic providers and clinic patients is superior to the current system of "shoe box" tickler files used by the clinic. What benefits does an electronic reminder system offer that the shoe box system cannot?

6. How would the use of an automated telephone system (autodialer) help as a reminder system?
7. Explain why clinical assessment software might be more effective in measuring the quality of preventive care delivery than a manual system.
8. Explain why an electronic medical record system is a prerequisite to an effective reminder and recall system for the clinic.

References

1. Emanuel EJ. Cost savings at the end of life. What do the data show? *JAMA* 1996;275:1907–1914.
2. Coughlin SS. The intersection of genetics, public health, and preventive medicine. *Am J Prev Med* 1999;16:89–90.
3. Van Ommen GJ, Bakker E, den Dunnen JT. The human genome project and the future of diagnostics, treatment, and prevention. *Lancet* 1999;354(Suppl 1):SI5–SI10.
4. Collins FS. Shattuck lecture—medical and societal consequences of the Human Genome Project. *N Engl J Med* 1999;341:28–37.
5. McGinnis JM, Foege WH. Actual causes of death in the United States. *JAMA* 1993;270:2207–2212.
6. US Preventive Services Task Force. Recommendations for patient education and counseling. In: *Guide to Clinical Preventive Services*. Baltimore, MD: Williams & Wilkins Co.; 1989.
7. Hinman AR. Economic aspects of vaccines and immunizations. *C R Acad Sci III* 1999;322:989–994.
8. Stone PW, Teutsch S, Chapman RH, Bell C, Goldie SJ, Neumann PJ. Cost-utility analysis of clinical preventive services: published ratio, 1976–1997. *Am J Prev Med* 2000;19:15–23.
9. Schauffler HH, Rodriguez T, Milstein A. Health education and patient satisfaction. *J Fam Pract* 1996;42:62–68.
10. Bolen JC, Rhodes L, Powell-Griner EE, Bland SD, Holtzman D. State-specific prevalence of selected health behaviors, by race and ethnicity—Behavioral Risk Factor Surveillance System, 1997. *Mor Mortal Wkly Rep CDC Surveill Summ* 2000;49:1–60.
11. Teitelbaum, Edmunds M. Immunization and vaccine-preventable illness, UnitedStates, 1992 to 1997. *Stat Bull Metrop Insur Co* 1999;80:13–20.
12. Janes GR, Blackman DK, Bolen JC, Kamimoto LA, et al. Surveillance for use of preventive health-care services by older adults, 1995–1997. *Mor Mortal Wkly Rep CDC Surveill Summ* 1999;48:51–88.
13. Woolhandler S, Himmelstein DU. Reverse targeting of preventive care due to lack of health insurance. *JAMA* 1988;259:2872–2874.
14. Lurie L, Manning WG, Perterson C. Preventive care: do we practice what we preach. *Am J Public Health* 1987;77:801–804.
15. NCI Breast Cancer Screening Consortium. Screening mammography—a missed clinical opportunity? *JAMA* 1990;264:54–58.
16. McPhee SJ, Richard RJ, Solkowitz SN. Performance of cancer screening in a university general internal medicine practice: Comparison with the 1980 American Cancer Society Guidelines. *J Gen Intern Med* 1986;1:275–281.
17. Montano DE, Phillips WR. Cancer screening by primary care physicians: A compari-

son of rates obtained from physician self-report, patient survey, and chart audit. *Am J Public Health* 1995;85:795–800.

18. Jaen CR, Stange KC, Nutting PA. The competing demands of primary care: A model for the delivery of clinical preventive services. *J Fam Pract* 1994;38:166–171.

19. Stange KC, Fedirko T, Zyzanski SJ, Jaen CR. How do family physicians prioritize delivery of multiple preventive services? *J Fam Pract* 1994;38:231–237.

20. Belcher DW. Implementing preventive services: success and failure in an outpatient trial. *Arch Intern Med* 1990;159:2533–2541.

21. Sox CH, Dietrich AJ, Tosteson TD, Winchell CW, Labaree CE. Periodic health examinations and the provision of cancer prevention services. *Arch Fam Med* 1997;6:223–230.

22. Geiger WJ, Neuberger MJ, Bell GC. Implementing the US Preventive Services guidelines in a family practice residency. *Fam Med*. 1993;25:447–451.

23. US Preventive Services Task Force. *Guide to Clinical Preventive Services, Second Edition.* Washington DC: US Government Printing Office; 1996.

24. Prislin MGD, Vandenbark MS, Clarkson QD. The impact of a health screening flowsheet on the performance and documentation of health screening procedures. *Fam Med* 1986;18:290–292.

25. Battista RN, Williams I, Boucher J, et al. Testing various methods of introducing health charts into medical records in family medicine units. *Can Med Assoc J* 1991;141:1469–1474.

26. Frame PS. Computerized health maintenance tracking systems: A clinician's guide to necessary and optional features: A report from the American Cancer Society Advisory Group on Preventive Health Care Reminder Systems. *J Am Board Fam Pract* 1995;8:221–229.

27. Defriese GH, Fielding JE. Health risk appraisal in the 1990: Opportunities, challenges, and expectations. *Ann Rev Public Health* 1990;11:401–418.

28. Carter Center. *Healthier People, Version 3.0.* Atlanta, GA: Emory University; 1988.

29. Gemson DH, Sloan RP. Efficacy of computerized health risk appraisal as part of a periodic health examination at the worksite. *Am J Health Promot* 1995;9:462–464.

30. Kreuter MW, Strecher VJ. Do tailored behavior change messages enhance the effectiveness of health risk appraisal? Results of a randomized trial. *Health Educ Res* 1996;11:97–105.

31. Glasgow RE, Toobart DJ, Hampson. Effects of a brief office-based intervention to facilitate diabetes dietary self-management. *Diabetes Care* 1996;19:835–842.

32. Glasgow RE, La Chance PA, Toobert DJ, Brown J, Hampson SE, Riddle MC. Long-term effects and costs of brief behavioural dietary intervention for patients with diabetes delivered from the medical office. *Patient Educ Couns* 1997;32:175–184.

33. Glasgow RE, Toobert DJ, Hampson SE. Brief computer-assisted diabetes dietary self-management counseling: Effect on behavior, physiologic outcomes and quality of life. *Med Care*. 2000;38:1062–1073.

34. National Telecommunications and Information Administration. *Falling Through the Net: Defining the Digital Divide.* Washington, DC: Department of Commerce; 1999. Available at: http://www.ntia.doc.gov/ntiahome/digitaldivide/. Accessed April 3, 2002.

35. Baer L, Jacobs DG, Cukor P, O'Laughlen J, Coyle JT, et al. Automated telephone screening survey of depression. *JAMA* 1995;273:1943–1944.

36. Christ G, Siegel K. Monitoring quality-of-life needs of cancer patients. *Cancer* 1990;65:760–765.

37. Siegel K, Mesagno P, Karus DG, et al. Reducing the prevalence of unmet needs for concrete services of patients with cancer. *Cancer* 1992;69:1873–1883.
38. Patel UH, Babbs CF. A computer-based, automated, telephonic system to monitor patient progress in the home setting. *J Med Syst* 1992;16:101–112.
39. Piette JD, Mah CA. The feasibility of automated voice messaging as an adjunct to diabetes outpatient care. *Diabetes Care* 1997;20:15–21.
40. Piette JD. Interactive voice response systems in the diagnosis and management of chronic disease. *Am J Manag Care* 2000;6:817–827.
41. Millard RW, Carver JR. Cross-sectional comparison of live and interactive voice recognition administration of the SF-12 Health Status Survey. *Am J Manag Care* 1999;5:153–159.
42. Ware JE, Kosinski M, Keller SD. A 12-item short-form health survey: Construction of scales and preliminary tests of reliability and validity. *Med Care* 1996;34:220–233.
43. Kobak KA, Reynolds WM, Greist JH. Computerized and clinician assessment of depression and anxiety: Respondent evaluation and satisfaction. *J Pers Assess* 1994;63:173–180.
44. Kobak KA, Greist JH, Jefferson JW, Katzelnick DJ. Computer-administered clinical rating scales: A review. *Psychopharmacology* 1996;127:291–301.
45. Kobak KA, Taylor LV, Dottle SL, Greist JH, Jefferson JW, Burroughs D, et al. A computer administered telephone interview to identify mental disorders. *JAMA* 1997;278:905–910.
46. Searles JS, Perrine MW, Mundt JC, et al. Self-report of drinking using touch-tone telephone: Extending the limits of reliable daily contact. *J Stud Alcohol* 1995;56:375–382.
47. Kobak KA, Taylor LV, Dottle SL, Greist JH, Jefferson JW, Burroughs D, et al. Computerized screening for psychiatric disorders in an outpatient community mental health clinic. *Psychiatr Serv* 1997;48:1048–1057.
48. Kobak KA, Taylor LV, Dottle SL, Greist JH, Jefferson JW, Burroughs D, et al. A computer-administered telephone interview to identify mental disorders. *JAMA* 1997;278:905–910.
49. Kobak KA, Taylor LV, Dottle SL, Greist JH, Jefferson JW, Burroughs D, et al. Computerized screening for psychiatric disorders in an outpatient community mental health clinic. *Psychiatr Serv* 1997;48:1048–1057.
50. Temple W, Toews J, Fidler H, Lockyer JM, Taenzer P, Parboosingh J. Concordance in communication between surgeon and patient. *Can J Surg* 1998;41:439–445.
51. Mahoney D, Tennstedt S, Friedman R, Heeren T. An automated telephone system for monitoring the functional status of community-residing elders. *Gerontologist* 1999;39:229–234.
52. Piette JD, PcPhee SJ, Weinberger M, Mah CA, Kraemer FB. Use of automated telephone disease management calls in an ethnically diverse sample of low income patients with diabetes. *Diabetes Care* 1999;22:1302–1309.
53. Alemi F, Stephens RC, Javalghi RG, Dyches H, Butts J, Ghadiri A. A randomized trial of a telecommunications network for pregnant women who use cocaine. *Med Care* 1996;34(Suppl 10):OS10–20.
54. Friedman RH, Kazis LE, Jette A, Smith MB, Stollerman J, Torgerson J, Carey K. A telecommunications system for monitoring and counseling patients with hypertension. Impact on medication adherence and blood pressure control. *Am J Hypertens* 1996;9:285–292.

55. Meneghini LF, Albisser AM, Goldberg RB, Mintz DH. An electronic case manager for diabetes control. *Diabetes Care* 1998;21:591–596.
56. Piette JD, Weinberger M, McPhee SJ, Mah CA, Kraemer FB, Crapo LA. Do automated calls with nurse follow-up improve self-care and glycemic control among vulnerable patients with diabetes? A randomized controlled trial. *Am J Med* 2000;108:20–27.
57. Piette JD, Weinberger M, McPhee SJ. The effect of automated calls with telephone nurse follow-up on patient-centered outcomes of diabetes care (a randomized controlled trial). *Med Care* 2000;38:218–230.
58. Piette JD, Weinberger M, Kraemer FB, McPhee SJ. The impact of automated calls with nurse follow-up on diabetes treatment outcomes in a Department of Veterans Affairs health care system. *DM Care* 2001;24:202–208.
59. Piette JD. Moving diabetes management from clinic to community: Development of a prototype based on automated voice messaging. *Diabetes Educ* 1997;23:672–679.
60. Collins RL, Morsheimer ET, Shiffman S, Paty JA, Gnys M, Papandonatos GD. Ecological momentary assessment in a behavioral drinking moderation training program. *Exp Clin Psychopharmacol* 1998;6:306–315.
61. Zhu S, Anderson CM, Johnson CE, Tedeschi G, Roeseler A. A centralized telephone service for tobacco cessation: the California experience. *Tobacco Control* 2000;9(Suppl II):ii48–ii55.
62. Zhu S, Stretch V, Balabanis M, Rosbrook B, Sadler G, Pierce J. Telephone counseling for smoking cessation: effects of single-session and multiple-session interventions. *J Consult Clin Psych* 1996;64:202–211.
63. Gustafson DH, Hawkins R, Boberg E, Pingree S, Serlin RE, Graziano F, Chan CL. Impact of a patient-centered computer-based health information/support system. *Am J Prev Med* 1999;16:1–9.
64. Smaglik P, Hawkins RP, Pingree S, Gustafson DH, Boberg E, Bricker E. The quality of interactive computer use among HIV-infected individuals. *J Health Commun* 1998;3:53–68.
65. McTavish FM, Gustafson DH, Owens BH, Hawkins RP, Pingree S, Wise M, Taylor JO, Apantaku FM. CHESS (Comprehensive Health Enhancement Support System): An interactive computer system for women with breast cancer piloted with an underserved population. *J Ambul Care Manage* 1995;18:35–41.
66. Owens BH, Robbins KC. CHESS: Comprehensive health enhancement support for women with breast cancer. *Plas Surg Nurs* 1996;16:172–175.
67. McKay HG, Feil EG, Glasgow RE, Brown JE. Feasibility and use of an Internet support service for diabetes self-management. *Diabetes Educ* 1998;24:174–179.
68. McPhee SJ, Detmer WM. Office-based interventions to improve delivery of cancer prevention services by primary care physicians. *Cancer* 1993;72:1100–1112.
69. McPhee S, Bird JA, Fordham D, Rodnick J, Osborn E. Promoting cancer prevention activities by primary care physicians. *JAMA* 1991;266:538–544.
70. McDonald C, Hui S, Tierney W. Reminders to physicians from an introspective computer medical record. *Ann Intern Med* 1984;100:130–138.
71. Frame P, Zimmer J, Werth P, Hall J, Eberly S. Computer-based vs. manual health maintenance tracking. *Arch Fam Med* 1994;3:581–588.
72. McDowell I, Newell C, Rosser C. Use of reminders for preventive procedures in family medicine. *J Fam Pract* 1989;28:420–424.
73. Burack RC, Gimotty PA. Promoting screening mammography in inner-city settings: The sustained effectiveness of computerized reminders in a randomized controlled trial. *Med Care* 1997;35:921–931.

74. Shea S, DuMouchel W, Bahamonde L. A meta-analysis of 16 randomized controlled trials to evaluate computer-based clinical reminder systems for preventive care in the ambulatory setting. *J Am Med Inform Assoc* 1996;3:399–409.

75. Ornstein SM, Garr DR, Jenkins RG, Musham C Hamadeh G, Lancaster C. Implementation and evaluation of a computer-based preventive services system. *Fam Med* 1995;27:260–266.

76. Dickey LL. Computer system to improve delivery of preventive care. *Fam Med* 1995;27:630.

77. Demakis JG, Beauchamp C, Cull WL, Denwood R, Eisen SA, Lofgren R, Nichol K, Woolliscroft J, Henderson WG. Improving residents' compliance with standards of ambulatory care. *JAMA* 2000;284:1411–1416.

78. Franzini L, Rosenthal J, Spars W, Martin HS, Balderas L, Brown M, et al. Cost effectiveness of childhood immunization reminder/recall systems in urban private practices. *Pediatrics* 2000;106:177–183.

79. Dietrich AJ, Woodruff CB, Carney PA. Improving and maintaining preventive care: the preventive GAPS approach. *Arch Fam Med* 1994;3:176–183.

80. US Department of Health and Human Services. Implementing preventive care. In: *Clinician's Handbook of Preventive Services*. Washington, DC: US Department of Health and Human Services; 1998.

81. Leninger LS, Finn L, Dickey L, et al. An office system for organizing preventive services. *Arch Fam Med* 1996;5:108–115.

82. McPhee SJ, Bird J, Jenkins CNH, Fordham D. Promoting cancer screening: a randomized controlled trial of three interventions. *Arch Int Med* 1989;149:1866–1872.

83. Winickoff RN, Coltin KL, Morgan RC, Buxbaum RC, Barnett GO. Improving physician performance through peer comparison feedback. *Med Care* 1984;22:527–533.

84. Bordley WC, Chelminski A, Margolis PA, Kraus R, Szilagyi PG, Vann JJ. The effect of audit and feedback on immunization delivery: a systematic review. *Am J Prev Med* 2000;18:343–350.

85. National Immunization Program, Centers for Disease Control and Prevention. *Clinical Assessment Software Application.(CASA)*. Available at: www.cdc.gov/nip/casa/Default.htm. Accessed April 3, 2002.

86. Scutchfield FD, Harris JR, Koplan JP, Gordon RL, Violante T. Managed care and public health. *J Public Health Manag Pract* 1998;4:1–11.

87. Ely JW, Levy BT, Hartz A. What clinical information resources are available in family physicians offices? *J Fam Pract* 1999;48:135–139.

88. Dansky KH, Gamm LD, Vasey JJ, Barsukiewicz. Electronic medical records: are physicians ready? *J Healthc Manag* 1999;44:440–454.

89. Dolin, R. The HL7 patient record architecture. *MD Net Guide* 2000;2:24–27.

90. Mitchell P. The role of smart cards in France. *Health Data Manag* 1998;6:54,56.

91. Walsworth-Bell JP, Horsley SD. The use of smart cards in the NHS. *Health Trends* 1988;20:86–88.

92. Neame R. Smart cards—the key to trustworthy health information systems. *BMJ* 1997;314:573–577.

93. Ognibene PJ. Smart Pharmacy Cards to automate patient records for prospective drug utilization review. *Proc Annu Symp Comput Appl Med Care*. 1991:906–908.

Part V
Case Studies: Applications of
Information Systems Development

Introduction

The promise of information technology is widely appreciated. but the true value of information technology lies in bringing that promise to fulfillment. This section presents a variety of real-world case studies, each of which is designed either to exemplify a particular kind of value derived from the deployment of actual information systems (e.g., the value of using scientific data to drive policy). or to illustrate critical issues associated with the development of new information systems (e.g., dealing with the policy and privacy issues raised by electronic disease surveillance). This section is intended to illustrate the value of applying informatics principles and practices as well as cutting-edge information technologies to both new and traditional public health information applications.

Common threads among these case studies include (1) the importance of involving users in the design, construction. and implementation of systems and (2) the necessity of adequate planning in all phases of systems development.

The section begins with Chapter 25, "Policy Issues in Developing Information Systems for Public Health Surveillance of Communicable Diseases." In this chapter, the authors introduce the concepts and issues associated with public health surveillance systems, stressing the importance of an information architecture that provides for ease of use. centralized control of data resources. use of national data and coding standards. and provisions for security and confidentiality of surveillance information. The authors illustrate these concepts by reference to the New York State Department of Health's Health Information Network and Health Provider Network. They then present three cases involving the development and implementation of disease surveillance systems. The lessons learned from the experience with each case have the following in common: (a) the importance of involving prospective users and other stakeholders in system design; (b) the importance of developing an information infrastructure and an architecture that facilitates ease of use. control and confidentiality of data, and ready sharing of information; (c) involving executives, program managers, prospective users, and knowledgeable information technology professionals in system design, testing, implementation, and user training; and (d) most of all, focusing on the needs of users of the systems first, rather than permitting perceived cost constraints to drive activities.

In Chapter 26, Ron Seymour and Fran Muskopf relate the story of the development of a state information network for public health officials. The INPHO project, an initiative of the Centers for Disease Control and Prevention, was developed to assist state health organizations in the development of information networks. The project in the state of Washington faced numerous challenges in its attempt to link local health jurisdictions (LHJs) and counties to state networks. Through involvement of the LHJs and the counties in system design, through conferring ownership of the developed systems on the LHJs, through recognizing political realities and addressing them, and through the exercise of INPHO project team ingenuity, the INPHO project team succeeded beyond reasonable expectations in securing LHJ and county buy-in and enthusiastic support for the project—this despite a long history of LHJ mistrust of state agencies. The lessons learned by the INPHO project team during this venture included the need to (1) stay focused on a project's vision and avoid the distractions of other issues; (2) use proven, but not old, technology; (3) use national standards, but avoid entanglements about minor issues; (3) avoid preconceptions and stereotyping regarding the capabilities and needs of LBJs and counties; (4) recognize political realities; and (5) build systems to last. With regard to the practice of informatics, the INPHO project taught the lesson that fancy technology may be attractive to system developers, but the true value of an information system resides in the access to relevant information it provides to users.

In Chapter 27, Richard D. Rubin discusses the long, circuitous route that the community health information movement, itself an illustrative case study, has taken. Rubin points out that early efforts to develop community health information systems failed for a variety of reasons, and these reasons themselves constitute valuable lessons to would-be developers of community health-oriented information systems. Among the lessons taught by the history of the community health information movement is the need of system developers to concentrate on needs, rather than wants; on building community health information systems on a solid business foundation that offers benefits to partners in proportion to the funding required; on going beyond merely offering another network; on using a competitive, rather than a collaborative model, to build systems; on clearly defining the roles of the various players in a community health information system; on narrowing a project's scope and avoiding creeping incrementalism; and on addressing privacy matters. Offering examples of successful community health information initiatives, Rubin concludes the chapter by stating that only by using partnerships of enterprises, vendors, and community groups can community health information initiatives hope to succeed.

In Chapter 28, Garland Land, Nancy Hoffman, and Rex Peterson present an overview and an analysis of the Missouri Health Strategic Architectures and Information Cooperative (MOHSAIC), a massive project of the Missouri Department of Health to design and build a statewide integrated public health system that would meet the information needs of public health practitioners at both the state and the local level. Through solid planning and well-reasoned choices, the MOHSAIC team succeeded in the face of daunting challenges involving funding, politics, resistance to change, staffing, and the existence of numerous existing legacy systems. The authors point out that among the keys to success and the lessons learned during this project were the need to provide sufficient resources, the need to address politics as an inevitable force encountered in building an integrated system, and the need to secure top-level promotion and support for building an integrated system. Equally important are developing and following a strategic plan to guide the project, centralizing information systems, beginning construction in areas where support already exists, and involving users at all levels in system design.

Chapter 29 focuses on the National Turning Point Initiative, a major project dedicated to improving population health through an investment in strengthening and transforming the public health infrastructure at the state and the community level. The development of a Public Health Improvement Tool Box to provide support tools for those engaged in improving the public health infrastructure is a major focus of the chapter. The PHI Tool Box provides users with access to information, connectivity to other users, and distance education. The project is ongoing, and it is too early to state the lessons learned from this initiative.

Chapter 30 focuses on the development and the promise of the Comprehensive Assessment for Tracking Community Health (CATCH) data warehouse system by the University of South Florida. A state-of-the-art tool, CATCH serves as the gold standard for community health assessment. Although its current applications focus on Florida community health issues, CATCH as a concept has implications for community health decision making on a national scale. The authors illustrate the utility of CATCH by demonstrating its use in a sample case study of racial disparity in infant mortality. CATCH, too, is a work in progress.

In Chapter 31, Ann Marie Kimball and Tiffany Harris put an international focus on public health informatics by describing the Emerging Infections Network (EINet), a telecommunications network in the Asia Pacific geographic region. EINet provides a good example of the challenges inherent in developing and maintaining an international electronic network that connects nations with differing views and practices regarding data sharing. The authors point out, however, that international networks such as EINet offer untold benefits for epidemic investigation and control of infections that cross international boundaries.

Chapter 32 provides a first-person account of a successful effort to link private providers to an existing immunization registry in the state of Oregon.

Dr. William A. Yasnoff traces, from start to finish, the tasks and challenges associated with such a public health informatics project. Among the lessons learned during this project is the need to secure user input in the design of a system, the need for system designers to develop a thorough understanding of user requirements, and the importance of being willing to respond effectively to user concerns. Also important among the lessons learned during this project are (1) the importance of developing alternative solutions in the event that a preferred solution proves unacceptable to users, (2) the need to avoid a bias in favor of highly technical approaches to problems that may lend themselves to simpler solutions, and (3) the importance of comprehensive planning in all phases of system design, development, and implementation.

Chapter 33 provides a description of the development and the nature of the National Health and Nutrition Examination Survey (NHANES) as an example of the use of technology and systems to connect users in diverse locations and to collect and make available crucial data related to public health. The authors focus on the development of NHANES IV and its Integrated Survey Information System (IRIS). NHANES IV provides an innovative example of achieving apparent real-time data flow while also making data available to users with diverse interests. In discussing NHANES IV, the authors focus on several issues that have been addressed successfully, including quality assurance and control, data editing, security and confidentiality, and reporting results to survey participants. The state-of-the-art capabilities of NHANES IV and IRIS offer implications for future data collection efforts.

This part of the textbook concludes with Chapter 34, a look forward at the challenges facing the discipline and the practice of public health informatics. The challenges include developing coherent, integrated national public health information systems; developing closer integration between public health and clinical care; and addressing pervasive concerns about the impact of information technology on confidentiality and privacy. Moreover, if the contribution of informatics to public health is to be maximized, organizational leaders will need to communicate the need for public health informatics to all public health workers, to provide training in its nature and its use, and to provide the physical infrastructure/architecture to accommodate the practice of public health informatics. Through such efforts, public health has the opportunity not only to improve the efficiency and effectiveness of public health practice, but also to transform fundamentally some aspects of public health practice itself.

25

Policy Issues in Developing Information Systems for Public Health Surveillance of Communicable Diseases

Ivan J. Gotham, Perry F. Smith, Guthrie S. Birkhead, and Michael C. Davisson

Learning Objectives

After studying this chapter, you should be able to:

- Define public health surveillance and discuss the purposes of surveillance.
- Using the case examples, explain the opportunities and challenges that information technology provides to public health surveillance.
- List and describe the general policy issues that need to be considered in establishing a new surveillance system.
- Describe the information infrastructure requirements for a surveillance system.

Overview

In many respects, the New York State Department of Health's Health Provider Network (HPN) and its Health Information Network (HIN) stand as models of integrated public health networks. This chapter begins with a discussion of the nature and purposes of public health surveillance systems. It then provides an overview of the policy issues to be considered in establishing such systems and the characteristics of the underlying information infrastructure for surveillance systems. After treatment of the policy issues and architecture solutions applied in the development of the HPN and the HIN, along with the lessons learned in the development process, the chapter presents case studies involving HIV surveillance and partner notification, electronic clinical laboratory reporting, and West Nile virus disease surveillance. The lessons learned, as presented in these cases, emphasize the importance of involving users and stakeholders in system design, of keeping user needs at the forefront of considerations, of providing for user training, and of providing for the security and confidentiality of information. The cases also emphasize the need for careful planning and for providing adequate lead-time in the development of systems. Finally, the cases stress the importance of an information architecture that provides for interoperability, central control, and ease of use.

Introduction

Public health surveillance is the ongoing, systematic collection and analysis of public health data, including data on rates of disease, injuries, health-related risk factors, and environmental conditions that impact health, with dissemination of data to policy makers, public health program managers, and others who need to know.[1] Surveillance is a key part of public health assessment, one of the three core public health functions (assessment, assurance, and policy development) stated in the Institute of Medicine's landmark 1988 report *The Future of Public Health*.[2] Surveillance is information for action, the eyes and ears of public health, without which public health would be flying blind. Public health surveillance occurs in the United States at many levels: local county or city, state, and federal. This chapter views issues of informatics policy for surveillance primarily from the state and local level.

The purposes of public health surveillance include monitoring disease trends, guiding immediate public health action as well as public health prevention programs, suggesting hypotheses for disease occurrence and prevention, and detecting new and emerging public health problems.[3] The effectiveness of public health surveillance can be evaluated by examining factors such as the completeness of reporting, the sensitivity and specificity of reporting, the timeliness of reporting, and the usefulness of the data collected.[4]

A prominent method of infectious disease surveillance, and historically the first to be practiced, is the mandated reporting of cases of disease from physicians and hospitals to state or local health departments (also called notification). Increasingly, clinical laboratories also have been used as a source of infectious disease surveillance reports. Other surveillance methods that may not require notification include periodic surveys (e.g., the Behavioral Risk Factor Surveillance System) and use of data collected for other purposes, such as mortality, natality, and hospital discharge data.

Public health surveillance has been practiced in some form since the mid-1700s, beginning with requirements that health practitioners and others report cases of diseases of public health interest, such as plague, cholera, and smallpox, to local and state public health authorities in order to permit application of such measures as quarantine to protect the public health. The US Constitution leaves health matters to the states, and disease-reporting requirements are therefore the responsibility of state and in some cases local health departments. Today, most public health surveillance systems collect data under some kind of legal (legislative or regulatory) mandate, usually at the state level. Such mandates not only require the holders of data of interest to report the data to state health departments, but also specify the confidentiality protections that must be applied and the permissible uses of the data.[5]

Recently, the Centers for Disease Control and Prevention (CDC) revisited the criteria for evaluation of surveillance systems, taking into account, in part, the revolution in electronic information systems that took place in the 1990s.[6] The resulting new evaluation criteria include examining the security of data in electronic systems, reviewing the authority to collect data with electronic systems, and reviewing data access policies and requirements for storing data in archives or data warehouse. Of course, the ability to collect identifying information about persons with disease, to eliminate duplicate surveillance reports, and to enable linkage with other data systems are important considerations in surveillance system design.

As previous chapters have pointed out, ensuring the confidentiality and security of surveillance data is critical to effective public health efforts. One major reason is that physicians and other mandated reporters must be assured that the data they report will be held under the strictest security, that confidentiality will not be breached, and that the data will be used only for authorized public health purposes. After all, the cooperation of physicians and other health professionals in achieving complete and timely disease reports and in working with the patient to carry out public health measures such as identification, screening, and treatment of contacts who may be at risk of disease is critical. A breach or other unauthorized use of surveillance data can jeopardize the cooperation of physicians and other mandated reporters and ultimately impede public health efforts.

Information technology provides both an opportunity and a challenge to public health surveillance efforts. On the one hand, electronic data systems may permit public health workers to collect, distribute, share, manage, and analyze large amounts of data easily, accurately, and promptly. It offers the expectations of integration, "real-time" data acquisition, timely and easy access to information, simplification of business processes, increased productivity, and cost savings. On the other hand, the application of this tool to surveillance systems creates many new policy issues that not only feed back into design and technology, but also have significant organizational implications. Policy needs surrounding surveillance activities and related data systems dictate stringent quality control, compartmentalization, and strong protection and control over information access, perhaps even requiring built-in time lags for dissemination of information. These requirements result in business rules and information architecture designs that may lessen the expected benefits of information technology by increasing system cost and complexity as well as by impacting project completion time, usability, extensibility, training, and support. They also place increased burdens on public health workers to understand the uses and limitations of applying information technology to surveillance systems and in validating the data systems they support.

The successful electronic surveillance infrastructure is a blend of peer-based partnerships, organizational support, training, and information technology. A clear understanding of the policy issues and their implications, and of the required interactions with information technology, is a prerequisite to tuning an organization's expectations and commitment to establishing an infrastructure that is robust enough to support its policies.

Overview of Policy Issues to Be Considered in Establishing New Surveillance Systems

There are a number of policy issues that must be considered in establishing new public health surveillance systems. Several of these issues relate to the use of electronic data systems in surveillance system design.

The most important policy decision, often made by state legislatures or commissioners of health, is determining when and for which diseases to undertake required surveillance. Some of the considerations associated with this decision include determining whether the disease is of public health importance in terms of morbidity, mortality, incidence, and prevalence, and/ or whether surveillance is associated with a new or an emerging disease. Also important to consider is whether there is a clear public health purpose for conducting surveillance: For example, is there a public health intervention that can be applied or is there a need to monitor a newly emerging disease whose full public health impact is not known?

If a disease is deemed to be of public health importance and there is a public health purpose for conducting surveillance, the next policy issue is determining what overall surveillance methods should be employed. How should surveillance be conducted? The more general considerations in examining this issue include deciding whether medical provider reporting of individual cases of disease is necessary to meet the public health purposes of surveillance, or whether other, less invasive surveillance methods, such as employing periodic surveys or utilizing existing data being collected for other purposes—for example, administrative and billing data—may be sufficient. Are there legal mandates to be considered in determining who may have access to surveillance data or for what purposes it can be used? Such policy decisions are also usually made at the legislative or regulatory level.

Once the broader surveillance issues are addressed and the system's parameters are established, more specific issues in determining what surveillance methods to employ to match the purposes of the system must be addressed. These issues include:

- What information is required and from whom is it going to be collected?
- Do the holders and sources of the data have the information in a readily reportable form—for example, in either electronic or paper records?
- What degree of sensitivity, specificity, duplication, and timeliness are required to achieve the purposes of reporting?
- What protections must be built into surveillance system design to insure the security of the data and the confidentiality of persons reported to the

surveillance system. For what purposes may the data be used, and how is access to the data to be controlled? Reporting of individual cases of disease necessitates consideration of the confidentiality and data security requirements for collecting, analyzing, releasing, and storing such data.

Policy decisions of this nature are often made at the public health program level. The answers to these questions will determine the details of the surveillance system design.

Given the nature of the overall surveillance policy decisions we have discussed, system designers must address a series of logistical, organizational, and programmatic issues in order to move forward with the final design and implementation of the system. Ideally, an implementation team that includes representatives of different core public health disciplines—including epidemiologists, program managers, information system specialists, health department administrators, and legal counsels—addresses these issues and makes decisions. Each of these disciplines brings critical skills to the table, skills that are necessary for the successful implementation of a new surveillance system. Decisions that need to be made in system design and implementation include defining data standards for each class of reporting provider (physician, hospital, laboratory). Such standards should acknowledge existing healthcare industry and CDC data standards as well as HIPAA requirements. Standards should also reflect the need to integrate data from a number of different data sources and existing data systems.

A critical step in surveillance system design is defining the data system security requirements and information access and usage rules required to protect confidentiality. For example, for each public health worker, what is the level of detail and timing of access to information/data essential to the performance of that person's job, based on a legitimate need and right to know? How are these access rules to be accommodated in the system design? How are information security, confidentiality, and integrity protected during any transmission of data and during storage on host servers? Will the system use open architecture and open development environments or proprietary systems? Will databases be distributed or centralized?

In designing the hardware and software components of the system, it is also important to consider the anticipated useful life of the proposed system technology. Will the system be used for only a limited period of time? Will it be superceded by newer technology, or is the system expected to be installed and operated indefinitely—i.e., more than five years? Are there anticipated changes in the information infrastructure in the near future and, if so, how will those changes affect system planning and implementation?

Infrastructure support policies are also a key consideration in the design and implementation of new information systems to support public health surveillance. The organizational structure for the management, development, and operation of the system needs to be designed carefully. In larger health departments with offices for both information systems management and disease surveillance and control programs, the degree of shared responsibility for system development and management needs to be clarified early in the process. In addition, funding for system development and subsequent routine system management is a key issue to be addressed by the health department administrative team members. Further, technical support and training need to be considered from the beginning of program development. In particular, systems intended for use by public health field staff need to have particularly strong training and ongoing technical help-desk components.

Underlying Information Infrastructure for Surveillance Systems

Background

The New York State Department of Health (NYSDOH) has evolved an enterprise-wide architecture for secure electronic health (e-health) commerce. It was designed as the strategic infrastructure to support all the agency's information interchange with external agencies, including disease surveillance. Given this scope, it was critical that the architecture be sufficiently robust to address the core policy issues of all the data systems that would use the infrastructure.

The infrastructure has two functional segments and meets many of the key functional characteristics of the architectural components of the National Electronic Disease Surveillance System (NEDSS) of the CDC. Each segment is targeted at the specific needs of the information and data transactions between the NYSDOH and external partners. One of the two segments, the Health Provider Network (HPN), is targeted at providing information interchange with tens of thousands of health providers and professionals at regulated facilities, including hospitals and clinical laboratories. The HPN supports a wide range of applications, including disease surveillance and clinical lab reporting. Table 25.1 provides an overview of the HPN.

The second segment, the Health Information Network (HIN), is targeted specifically at data and information interchange between state staff and thousands of public health staff at local health departments. All 57 county health departments and the New York City Department of Health are connected to the HIN. The HIN also supports a wide variety of applications for local health, including electronic disease reporting and West Nile virus surveillance. Table 25.2 provides examples of state and local health information systems on the HIN.

Policy Issues and Architecture Solutions

Communications Access

Communications access had to be ubiquitous, easily accessible, noninvasive, and inexpensive. The cost of deployment and maintenance of a closed, stand-

TABLE 25.1. Examples of organizations and information exchanged with NYSDOH on the Health Provider Network

Electronic Data System	Participating Organization(s) or Function	Description
Inpatient hospital stays	NY State Hospitals (250 facilities)	Abstracts of medical records and bills
Patient incident reporting	NY State Hospitals (250 facilities)	Tracking system for reportable patient incidents
Cancer registry reporting	NY State Hospitals (250 facilities)	Cancer case reports
Hospital occupancy and quarterly report	NY State Hospitals (250 facilities)	Facility utilization data for planning and management
Birth records	NY State Hospitals (210 facilities)	Electronic birth certificates
Health Systems Management	NY state hospitals (250 facilities), nursing homes (800 facilities), home health care (300 facilities)	Cost reports, budget surveys, rate reports, patient reviews
Blood lead surveillance	Clinical labs (60)	Electronic reporting for blood serum lead levels
Electronic lab reporting	Clinical labs (200)	Positive test results for cancer, HIV, STD, TB, communicable diseases
Electronic laboratory approval program	Environmental labs (900 facilities)	Electronic certification
Electronic reporting of triplicate prescriptions	Pharmacies (100)	All prescriptions issued for class 3 substances
Managed care	Managed care organizations (100)	Provider network and ancillary care reporting
West Nile virus surveillance	External organizations involved in surveillance: NYS Wild Life Pathology Unit, NYS Dept of Agriculture and Markets, commercial contractors	Access to bird, mammal, mosquito surveillance reporting systems

alone network presence at and within each facility at this scale was prohibitive. It was also known from past experience that local health departments or local health facilities would not support such stand-alone networks. The in-

TABLE 25.2. Examples of state and local health information systems on the Health Information Network

---

Dynamic data queries
    Statistical reports: cross-tabulations, charts, graphs rates for
        Communicable diseases, sexually transmitted diseases (STDs), tuberculosis (TB)
        Inpatient hospital stays and diagnoses
        Death records
        Birth records
        Injuries
    Patient level registry data line listings, cross-tabulations for
        Communicable diseases, STDs, TB

Automated posting and distribution of electronic health alerts for
    Epidemiological outbreak/problem alert
    Public health alerts

Electronic disease case reporting
    County-based electronic reporting for communicable diseases, TB, and STDs
    Electronic distribution of physician reports of HIV/AIDS cases

Clinical laboratory data
    Blood lead surveillance—electronic distribution of blood lead laboratory reports to
        local county health departments
    Disease reports—electronic distribution of lab records for positive test results to
        local health departments for communicable diseases, HIV, STDs, and TB

Vital records
    Birth data—electronic distribution of birth record data to local health departments

West Nile surveillance system
    Human case surveillance
    Dead bird surveillance
    Sentinel bird surveillance
    Mosquito surveillance
    Electronic access to lab results for all surveillance systems

General utilities
    Secure file transfer—ad hoc person-to-person file exchange over encrypted Secure
        Socket Layer
    Secure discussion—secure, access controlled, discussion groups operating over en-
        crypted Secure Socket Layer

Examples of health program–related information
    Directory information systems
    Community health profiles
    Chronic disease
    Immunization registry
    AIDS
    Environmental health
    Family and local health

---

frastructure would therefore have to use public networks and interoperate with the existing local network infrastructure at county health departments and health facilities; it would logically function as an outbound connection from the local network. Given the success of the Internet, Transmission Control Protocol/Internet Protocol (TCP/IP) was chosen as the communications protocol, and the Internet would serve as the communications path to the e-health commerce system. For local health departments without Internet access, NYSDOH established an intranet connections network to provide these departments with outbound access to the Internet and access to the e-commerce Web system.

Vehicle for Application and Information Delivery

The vehicle chosen for delivery of applications, information, and data had to be easy to use, had to provide a common look and feel, and had to be platform-independent and readily available as a commercially supported product. Local health departments and health facilities vary widely in technical capacity, sophistication, and support. The workstation client software had to operate across these diverse environments and to be based on technology that the user is likely to be familiar with already or else can easily obtain training from local commercial providers. Given the rapid growth and success of the Internet and the World Wide Web, the thin client (i.e., an application designed to be small so that the bulk of data processing occurs on the server), Web browser model was chosen as the vehicle for delivery of HIN/HPN applications.

The model for application development and deployment also had to facilitate rapid development and large-scale deployment, maintenance, and support. Distribution and maintenance of customized software and local databases are prohibitive at this scale of endeavor. Customized software is also typically single-purpose, placing large support and training burdens on both central and local users. The Web browser/server model provided centralized development, deployment, and support for applications and static documents viewed through thin clients. The common look and feel of the browser model minimizes training efforts. It also facilitates rapid deployment of prototypes, new applications, changes and updates, and training materials from a central location.

Responsibility for Data and Quality Control

Statutory responsibility of the state for data requires centralized control over data, data quality, and application distribution. In the three-tier Web model employed in New York's e-commerce system, Web browser/client users interact via Web and application servers to exchange data from a central database. The central database insures state control over responsibility for confidentiality and security of the data as well as for backup and archiving. It also insures a standard, integrated data source and representation across all users.

Centrally managed business rules in the middle tier and client edits in the Web server/client insure centralized control over data quality and assurance. Central management of application development also guarantees uniform change control processes for application deployment as they are moved from development, to evaluation, to production systems.

Responsibilities for Security and Confidentiality of Information

NYSDOH is responsible for supporting the e-health commerce infrastructure. NYSDOH House Counsel and Security Units determined that through its statutory authority under public health law, NYSDOH was responsible for security and confidentiality of data, information, and resources on the e-commerce infrastructure. Thus, in order for an organization to use the infrastructure, the organization had to agree to the Agency's security and use policies. Two types of memoranda of understanding (MOU) were developed; county health department officials must complete both memoranda types to gain HIN access. The first of the memoranda of understanding is the Organizational Security MOU, which must be completed and signed by the commissioner or public health director of each county health department desiring its staff to have access to the HIN/HPN network. A second MOU, known as the Security and Usage Agreement, must be completed and signed by every prospective HIN user among county NYSDOH staff before the user is granted access to HIN resources. These MOUs define responsibilities for appropriate use of resources and confidentiality of information. The language in the MOUs was developed in collaboration with NYSDOH House Counsel, Security Unit and county health departments through the New York State Association of County Health Officials (NYSACHO). The MOUs were officially endorsed by NYSACHO, and the NYSDOH Commissioner of Health subsequently promulgated them as public health policy. Similar MOUs are required of health facilities and providers using the HPN.

The NYSDOH policies regarding responsibility for protection of confidentiality required protection of information in transit. Given the diversity and openness of networks and organizations connecting to the e-commerce system, it was critical to encrypt the information in transit by use of a strong encryption mechanism; at the same time, there was a need for ease of use and minimization of the cost and support issues associated with licensing and distributing encryption software. Once again, standardization on the Web browser/server model provided the solution.

US versions of Web browsers support strong encryption, using a technology known as Secure Socket Layer. To insure that the privacy of the information exchanged between Web client and server is protected, the Web server is configured to accept only HTTPS connections (the Secure Socket Layer encrypted protocol). This configuration functions to establish an encrypted pathway from the Web client browser software through to the server as the first step of establishing the connection to it. The encryption session is established transparently to the user, protecting data as the data traverse the network and obviating the need for the user to deal with separate encryption software and the need for the State to deploy, support, and train county users in using encryption software and the associated encryption keys.

To protect the information on the central servers from being compromised, the servers are isolated from the Internet by means of both router filters and a firewall (see Chapter 10 for a discussion of firewalls as security devices). Both the filters and the firewall are configured to assure that the HTTPS connection is the only permitted pathway and that users have only indirect access to the Web server. The HIN/HPN Web servers are separated from the database server by additional filters and firewalls to further guarantee that there are no direct connections to the database from the Web servers. Thus, HIN/HPN users do not have direct access to the central database. Rather, applications have access, and users have roles and access that the application may use on their behalf to provide them with the necessary functionality, such as reading, writing, or updating data through a Web form.

Control of Authentication and Access to Data and Applications

The scale of New York's e-health commerce system and the need to maintain central control over access to it requires a centrally administered system for authentication of users. This system enables users to authenticate themselves to the e-health commerce server with a single sign-on, using a strong ID/password system. The execution of organizational and individual security MOUs is a prerequisite for receiving an ID and a password from the central HIN/HPN accounts unit. All user validation and transfer of ID/password pairs occur via out-of-band mechanisms. For HIN access, the accounting unit calls the user and establishes the user's identity (known as authentication), using New York State Department of Motor Vehicles driver license information. The accounting unit then assigns an ID and a password to each user. The accounting unit calls the user and orally exchanges a series of pass phrases and pin numbers as a means of establishing HPN user identities. On the first log-in, users are immediately challenged for this ID and Password upon connection to the proxy. Whereas the user's ID is permanent (so long as the user is affiliated with the state or a county health department), the original password assigned to a user is valid for only the initial log-in, at which time it immediately expires and the user is forced to select a new password that only he/she would know. The system requires frequent changing of passwords, and password rules insure that users do not select passwords that are too "weak" (i.e., that are similar to a previous password or easy to guess). The proxy queries a central authentication server to check the validity of the ID and password pair; the system also provides for automatic account "locking" if an excessive number of failed attempts occurs. Thus, the authentication system provides for a means of preventing a user's ID and password from being determined by use of exhaustive attacks. Once authenticated, the user may access the HIN or the HPN Web server. However, the responsible NYSDOH program area still must separately grant specific access to information and data associated with functions such as electronic disease surveillance.

As the HIN/HPN infrastructure is an enterprise-wide initiative, the policies regarding control of access to data and information vary greatly according to health program areas and the nature of information exchanged between local health and state health program areas. The policies range from very narrowly defined access for highly confidential information, such as case reports for notifiable diseases, to broadly defined access for county information bulletins or statistical data queries. Implementing such a high level of access specificity required that the security system be designed to be user-specific; thus, a single ID and password pair authenticates access to precisely defined access roles and permissions with regard to data and information for all an individual county (or external HPN) user's information needs. Given the diversity of data access policies and roles, it is not feasible for a central authority within the NYSDOH to administer access. Thus, specific user roles and access permissions with regard to highly confidential areas of information are determined and administered separately by the specific NYSDOH program area governing those data. After all, the program areas are best able to know who should access their data and what the correct roles and access rights to be assigned to the user should be. Users may request access to secure applications and information via electronic forms supplied with each information system on the HIN. The requests are sent directly to the appropriate program area, which will follow its program-specific protocol for granting roles and access to its data. The permissions and roles for each user are stored in a central communications directory, along with contact information for the user. The users may update their own individual contact information, such as phone, e-mail, and fax numbers. Additionally, the HIN/HPN accounts control unit periodically generates automated letters to and from the central communications directory, asking the signatory on each organizational MOU to verify the organization's list of HIN/HPN users and to attest to those users' continued rights to access the system.

Involving Stakeholders, Training, and Help

The e-health commerce system and its related surveillance systems are dependent for completeness of reporting and for data quality on the active and enthusiastic participation of the local users who are the primary source of data entered into the system. It is key, therefore, that these users receive value from use of the systems and that they have the skill and capacity level to use it. As part of an effort to insure local input into the e-health commerce architecture and its applications, system designers established a joint state and local health automation committee under the auspices of NYSACHO. This committee was charged with approving proposals for applications, such as electronic disease surveillance. Through this approval process, the system meets local needs regarding data entry screens, reports, data access, data sharing, and compatibility with existing local systems.

The HIN also has a dedicated field-training unit, with training staff traveling to local health departments and to NYSDOH district, area, and regional offices (and to external agencies using the HPN). The function of this training staff is to build local capacity in the use of the HIN/HPN Web and the Internet. The training staff also assesses local technical and information needs and installs several PC workstations at each local health department. These staff members are available by phone, by secure discussion forum, and by e-mail to provide immediate user support. The HIN Web server system also provides an electronic version of the training course.

Lessons Learned

The responsiveness and utility of the architecture was demonstrated during a recent outbreak of West Nile virus (WNV) in the state in August 1999. During this outbreak, the architecture provided a reliable and timely source of information for both state and local health department staff.[7] The reliability of the architecture is also illustrated by the fact that New York was able to use it as the core of its response plan for dealing with the reemergence of WNV in 2000.[8] Moreover, the skill level in the use of the HIN/HPN (among an audience largely lacking computer skills) and the familiarity of users with HIN/HPN resources have increased dramatically in the last two years. Among users, anxiety about the use of such new systems has given way to a demand for replacement or integration of older, less functional information systems currently in use. Through their participation in design and implementation, local health agencies have developed a sense of co-ownership of the HIN/HPN. In turn, this sense of co-ownership has fully solidified support and recognition of the HIN/HPN as *the* health information infrastructure in New York State.

The evolutionary development process required significant initial investment in time and effort. However, the enterprise-wide approach to the Web-based authentication/access control system and the secure three-tiered, Web-based development model allows the agency to leverage existing infrastructure and to respond quickly to policy or surveillance needs. For example, during the WNV outbreak, public health authorities found that there was a great need for the ability for ad hoc file exchange and for professional dialogue relating to individual patient cases of suspected WNV. Plain text e-mail, however, is not private and was therefore not suitable for this purpose. NYSDOH was able to develop and deploy Web-based utilities for person-to-person secure file transfer and for holding secure group discussion forums within a matter of months, using its existing authentication and access control system.

The Web model facilitates responsiveness to user input. Test versions can be put out on the e-commerce Web, comments can be solicited, and agreed-upon changes can be implemented instantaneously over the entire user community.

The NYSDOH e-health commerce infrastructure has evolved over the past six years. This evolution attempts to insure an architecture that is robust enough to reflect agency data and information policy. This is a process of continual change that refines the architecture both to fit existing policy and to adapt to changes in policy. Although information policies and statutory authority/responsibility drive a significant portion of the design of the technical architecture, the success of the NYSDOH e-health commerce initiative to date has been based on organizational commitment—commitment to supporting this evolutionary process, to consensus building, to involving stakeholders as partners, and to insuring that programmatic needs regarding data access are met.

Case Studies of Surveillance Systems and Their Key Policy Issues

HIV Surveillance and Partner Notification Case Study: Data Security and Confidentiality

Information systems to conduct HIV surveillance, with or without linkage to partner notification activities, should represent the paradigm of data security and confidentiality because of the very sensitive nature of HIV information.

From 1998 through 2000, the NYSDOH developed an HIV surveillance and partner notification system in response to a legislative mandate that required the department to combine the highest degree of data security and confidentiality with a new program that involved partner notification staff in 13 county health departments and NYSDOH staff covering the rest of the state. These staff members had not been involved in such activities before. The lessons learned during the development and implement of the HIV surveillance and partner notification system relate to development of highly secure, yet functional, systems.

Background

Acquired immunodeficiency syndrome (AIDS) was recognized as a new disease in the early 1980s. AIDS is a clinical syndrome or a combination of signs and symptoms, the hallmark of which is opportunistic infections and certain cancers that result from immune system dysfunction. Human immunodeficiency virus (HIV) was identified as the cause of AIDS in the mid-1980s; at that time, blood tests to detect antibodies to HIV and HIV antigens were developed. HIV is spread by sexual contact, by blood-to-blood contact as in sharing of contaminated injection equipment among injection drug users, and by perinatal contact from mother to child. AIDS represents the end-stage of HIV infection. AIDS was first recognized in populations of gay men; however, it also heavily impacts injection drug users and minority populations in many areas of the country. All of these affected populations have suffered stigma and discrimination even before HIV came on the scene. Increasingly, too, heterosexual contact is a major route of HIV transmission.

AIDS has run a devastating course in the United States, with over 728,694 cases reported cumulatively and 426,619 deaths as of June 2000.[9] Approximately one million persons are estimated by CDC to be living with HIV, although only two thirds of these HIV-infected individuals are aware of their status. Since 1996, combination antiretroviral therapy (ARV) has been available to reduce the level of HIV virus to undetectable levels in many infected persons. However, ARV is not a cure for HIV, and many patients either cannot tolerate it or else the virus becomes resistant to therapy.

New York State, and particularly New York City, is one of the epicenters of the HIV/AIDS epidemic in the United States. In the initial years of the HIV/AIDS epidemic, New York State, along with all other US states and territories, conducted public health surveillance for AIDS by requiring physicians to report persons diagnosed with AIDS to the state health department. Because of the very sensitive nature of the disease reports and the stigma associated with AIDS and with the practices (gay lifestyle, injection drug use) that place persons at risk for HIV transmission, the decision was made in the mid-1980s in New York to have surveillance reports come only to the state health department and the New York City health department. The purposes of the original AIDS surveillance system were (1) to monitor the course and spread of the epidemic, (2) to identify the routes of transmission, and (3) to provide data to direct prevention and healthcare programs. For example, the Ryan White Care Act, the large federal program that offers funding for states and localities to provide health and supportive services for persons with HIV and AIDS, bases its funding formula on the number of living AIDS cases in each jurisdiction. Local county health departments, which have a primary role in the surveillance of other communicable diseases, including STDs, because of the need to notify and treat sexual partners of cases, were not involved in this original AIDS surveillance system.

Until the mid-1990s, AIDS surveillance was conducted primarily through a paper-based system of physician and hospital-based reporting, because AIDS frequently resulted in hospitalization. As a means of protecting the confidentiality of AIDS-related information, health department surveillance staff actively visited major hospitals to collect surveillance data directly.

In 1993, in recognition of the broadening clinical spectrum of AIDS and HIV, the national surveillance case definition for AIDS was expanded by CDC and the Council of State and Territorial Epidemiologists (CSTE) to include all persons with HIV infection who had levels of key immune system cells (CD4 cells) less than 200 per mm^3. This expanded definition provided a distinct laboratory marker for AIDS. In New York, clinical laboratories became an important source of AIDS surveillance data because (1) the laboratory test results of CD4 <200 provided definitive evidence of AIDS (in persons with HIV); (2) there are relatively few laboratories to monitor compared to the numbers of physicians and hospitals;

and (3) most clinical laboratories already had computerized health information systems, thus easing the transfer and management of large quantities of data. New York had the additional advantage of having strict regulatory oversight of clinical laboratories, even those outside its borders, thus enabling enforcement of reporting requirements.

Beginning in May 1994, New York established an electronic reporting system for two dozen laboratories that accounted for the majority of CD4 testing on New York residents. The state health department provided a personal computer software package with prescribed, standardized data elements, and a mechanism for encrypted, dial-up electronic transfer of data to the state health department. Because laboratory reporting could be both complete and timely within a short period of time, more than 90% of new AIDS cases reported in New York were reported through the laboratory-based system. The patient information provided by laboratories was highly accurate and complete, in large part because of the health department's requirements that laboratories directly bill patients for laboratory tests performed on them. New York is one of the few states with this requirement.

The advent of combination antiretroviral therapy in late 1995 profoundly changed the landscape of AIDS prevention and treatment in the United States and led to the recognition of new purposes and needs for public health surveillance for HIV infection itself. First, because ARV halted progression of immunosuppression (i.e., a decline in CD4 counts) in many persons with HIV, fewer persons with HIV progressed to AIDS. This development meant that AIDS surveillance began to be more incomplete, to present a more and more distant picture of trends in HIV transmission and risk factors, and therefore to provide a more and more incomplete picture of the HIV epidemic. Second, because the availability of effective therapy provided a strong rationale for persons to learn their HIV status in order to be treated, public health measures to encourage voluntary HIV testing became more important, including the practice, long used in the area of control of sexually transmitted diseases, of informing sexual and needle-sharing partners of persons with HIV of their possible exposure to HIV (partner notification). Surveillance data for HIV, as opposed to AIDS, could help to target these prevention efforts and to better measure the effectiveness of these prevention programs by providing a means of viewing the immediate impact on the number of reports of new HIV cases.

In 1998, the New York State legislature passed legislation requiring physicians and laboratories to report persons with HIV infection and HIV-related illness, in addition to AIDS, and to report the names of known partners or those the infected person wished to have notified through county health departments. In 1999, CDC formally recommended that all states begin to conduct HIV reporting.

Policy Issues and Architecture Solutions

A number of important program parameters were established in the HIV legislation. First, identifying information about persons with HIV was to be reported. Second, physicians and laboratories were both required to report. Third, county health departments had a role in conducting partner notification. Finally, stringent confidentiality requirements were placed on the data and the uses of the data. Penalties of up to $5,000 per violation plus a one-year prison sentence applied to breaches of confidentiality of the reported data. The State Health Commissioner, through regulation, placed additional requirements on the system as a way to improve the confidentiality of the data, including deleting the names of partners from the system when partner notification was completed. An additional concern of NYSDOH staff was that persons at risk for HIV might be reluctant to seek HIV testing and care if they felt that their data might not be secure. Similarly, physicians might be reluctant to cooperate with reporting if they felt the data might not be secure.

Therefore, the key surveillance policy issue in implementing the new program was the need to design a highly secure data system to insure confidentiality of the data while creating a functional system involving statewide public health staff who had not previously had access to HIV/AIDS surveillance information. Given the policy directives in the public health law and regulations, planners for program implementation immediately turned to electronic information system solutions for a number of reasons. First, the state had had a successful experience with reporting of low CD4 laboratory test results for AIDS surveillance. Second, a very large number of reports were expected; it was estimated that 140,000–180,000 persons were living with HIV in New York, with 10,000–12,000 new cases of HIV infection each year, though not all these persons would be diagnosed or receiving care. Third, those who were receiving regular health care might generate multiple reportable HIV test results each year. Any surveillance system would have to manage potentially tens or hundreds of thousands of reports easily each year. A final reason to consider electronic systems was the availability of highly secure hardware and software solutions.

The Department of Health designed the most secure electronic system possible by using the best technology available for each of the three major components of the program: laboratory reporting, physician reporting, and surveillance and partner notification follow-up by field staff.

The Electronic Laboratory Reporting System

The laboratory reporting system was built on the model used for AIDS surveillance. The first release of this system was a single purpose, telephone dial-up, electronic system that laboratories implemented solely for the purpose of reporting low CD4 reports. This system did not fit the current model of a multiple-use system built on existing infrastructure supported by the department. The system was therefore replaced with a more robust, multiple-purpose system, built on the Department's Health Information Network (HIN), that could handle the expanded laboratory reporting requirements in terms of number of different tests, number of reporting laboratories, and volume of test results. Members of the Electronic Clinical Laboratory Reporting System (see WNV case study, below) design team were involved in developing the new laboratory reporting system.

To insure the highest level of data security and confidentiality, system developers employed the following design parameters:

- Access controls were built so that authorized individuals have access only to information they need to perform their jobs.
- Information is encrypted, using a high-level encryption algorithm, during transmission from the laboratory to NYSDOH.
- At NYSDOH, the data management system conformed to the department's standards for safeguarding HIV/AIDS information.
- Laboratories could not access their data once those data were submitted to NYSDOH.
- Laboratories are required to have written confidentiality, security, and staff training policies for handling of HIV/AIDS information.

Physician Reporting

A paper-based reporting form was used to begin the physician reporting process, in as much as it was believed that most physicians who would be reporting HIV cases did not have office access to the equipment needed to report electronically. This form was produced in bulk and made available to physicians, hospitals, and clinics around the state. The form was designed so that the information written on the first page of the form wrote through to the second page. The second page contained only a basic layout of the first, without text or any other indication that the form contained HIV-related information. Risk information and other sensitive data were collected by use of check boxes, which again had no explanatory information on the second page. Physicians complete the form for cases that are to be reported and mail only the second page, devoid of any mention of HIV, to a post office box at NYSDOH. The address to be used provides no indication that the envelope might contain HIV information.

Training curricula and training videotapes for physicians were produced. This material discusses the use of the reporting form and stresses the need to keep information confidential at all stages, including in the medical record of the patient. Brochures and pamphlets explaining the confidentiality restrictions that applied to the data were also produced for physicians, test counselors, and patients.

Surveillance and Partner Notification Follow-up by Field Staff

Designing the secure data management system to enable state and county field staff to access the data to carry out their surveillance and partner notification follow-up activities was the most challenging part of program development. The system was built on the foundation of the state's already highly secure HIN system, but with additional security measures employed. Additional system requirements to maximize security included

- The ability to control access to information by only specified personnel with a need to know to carry out their jobs.
- The ability for supervisors to distribute case assignments to field staff and to monitor the status of assigned cases.
- The ability of field staff to access data and to input data on the outcome of surveillance and partner notification activities.
- A secure local computing environment with dedicated-use computers and printers in secure areas within local offices.
- Use of a simple user interface that does not require the users to install/ maintain applications software on remote computers.
- A prohibition on downloading of data at the local sites, accompanied by a restriction of access to such data only over the network.
- Use of a security token in addition to HIN password access controls.
- Recording of all transactions at the level of individual keystrokes to permit security audits.

In addition to these technical specifications, the program incorporated a rigorous series of training courses for staff in the use of the system and in the importance of the protection of the data. All staff members take a yearly confidentiality course and sign personal security and confidentiality statements attesting to their knowledge of the legal and programmatic requirements and the penalties for non-compliance. The staff-training component is as important as any other system design features in insuring the highest level of security and confidentiality for the system.

Lessons Learned

A number of lessons were learned in this process:

- *First, systems with high security requirements and complex business rules require a long lead-time for system planning and development, and this lead-time should be anticipated.* The information system described here took over two years to design and fully implement. A fully thought-through design is critical to the success of this type of system. This fact became obvious once the initial system was developed and design changes were being proposed. There was a significant challenge for the design team, as the legal protocols for implementation were being developed at the same time the system design was ongoing. Changes in the legal protocol required design changes in the system. If protocol changes occurred once the programming had begun, the resulting design changes ended up in additional project delays. As most public health professionals are very busy, finding the time to spend on the design can, in and of itself, be a challenge. Input from management was critical to setting priorities for the design team.
- *The time required to write down on paper how the workflow process was to operate was formidable, not just at the high level of design, but at the level at which all of the exceptions to the rules must be completely documented or else they could not be included in the system design.* The

system design was a major task, as representatives of two previously independent health programs were required to sit down at the table and design a single system that would meet the needs of both programs. Moreover, this system was to replace what were essentially manual processes for which the rules and exceptions were known but not well documented. The ripple effect of this process on the design had a significant impact on time required to work through the two process methods and how they were to be merged. Many of the modifications required redesign and modification of the forms currently being used. Additional security features were required to meet the mandates of the new system. These were designed, developed for this application, and built on top of the stringent security already incorporated in the HIN. The security enhancements had to be designed from the ground up, including evaluation of possible design problems and recognizing conflicts with existing security and working through them. It was not always possible to anticipate the problems that occurred or the time required to debug and fix problems.

- *The design team found that the longer a development project's duration, the greater the risk of the loss of key participants to projects with competing priorities or to the private sector.* The epidemiologists, information system designers, field staff, and legal staff all played critical roles in the system development process. Anticipating the loss of key participants was difficult to include in the planning, and loss of key staff had a significant impact on the project timeframe.

- *Finally, perseverance is important.* It can produce a system that successfully achieves the dual goals of security and functionality.

Electronic Clinical Laboratory Reporting System Case Study: Policy Issues in Organizational Roles, the Development Process, and Industry Standards

Background

One of the most effective tools available to public health staff for responding to communicable disease (CD) outbreaks is rapid access to information. To help insure effective control and intervention, information needs to be moved rapidly and accurately between providers, clinical laboratories, and local, state, and in some cases, federal public health officials. In New York State, there are some 60 reportable CDs, with 16 requiring immediate (within hours) notification of local public health staff when a diagnosis is made. There are currently two general processes by which CDs are reported to public health staff. One process involves clinical laboratories' (both commercial and hospital) reporting positive tests that are indicative of CD. The other involves providers or physicians who report suspect or confirmed cases. Currently, there are numerous modes of communication by which reports from providers and laboratories are transmitted to public health staff. The modes can take the form of telephone calls, fax transmissions, US mail, and, in limited cases, some form of electronic reporting. NYSDOH has elected to employ electronic technology as a strategic direction in reducing the delivery time of CD test results from clinical laboratories to public health staff.

Local public health staff members rely on provider and laboratory reports to identify possible outbreaks, determine what interventions are necessary, and follow the reports to assist in determining when the outbreak is contained. Providers and public health staff utilize laboratory reports to confirm a suspect case or actual cases of a CD. In both scenarios, rapid delivery of reports is critical to developing accurate/effective prevention intervention strategies, to minimizing costs, and to allocating resources through accurate, effective, and efficient utilization of staff.

The existing paper- and phone-based CD reporting system has been associated with recurring problems. For example, delays and late diagnosis have slowed and hampered the public health response to CD outbreaks. As a result, there have been continuing discussions in the NYSDOH and with the local public health department staff about the need for automating the CD reporting. Although it makes sense that public health should be able to utilize information technology to assist in the high-speed communications between all of the partners in public health prevention-intervention activities, understanding the details that need to be considered in a project of this scope is critical to its success.

There are a number of key issues involving the existing system of reporting for clinical laboratories. The first issue is the process of reporting between laboratories and local health departments (LHDs). In New York State (NYS), the laboratories currently report directly to the county public health staff. This reporting system places a burden on the 500-plus laboratories doing testing for NYS physicians to keep updated contact lists for each of the 57 counties plus New York City (NYC). The second issue is the method of reporting. Laboratories currently report by a variety of modes, with each laboratory having its own format. This variety of reporting modes places an additional burden on LHD staff; in many cases, there is a need to decipher the reports and the different coding formats used by laboratories. For some laboratories, reporting includes the use of laboratory-specific codes for the test performed, a coded identifier for the doctor submitting the request, and codes for very limited patient information. The third issue is the destination to which the report is to be sent. The laboratory is required to report by residence of the patient. This requirement is problematic if the laboratory staff members reporting the test result do not have ready access to the patient demographics at the time the reports are being submitted. Generally, the demographics are held in a separate billing system and not forwarded to the lab personnel performing the test. The laboratory may, and some do, elect to report to the county in which the laboratory resides, rather than locating the patient address and submitting the report to the county of the patient's residence. Such reports can make up as much as 20% of reports received by a county, placing added burden on local public health staff to determine where the report should go and then forward the report. Lastly, there is the issue of coordination. The coordinating agency must have the authority and capacity to coordinate with local health clinics and laboratories in the development and implementation of a large reporting system.

Policy Issues and Architecture Solutions

A number of key policy questions had to be addressed prior to embarking on the process of design and development of the electronic laboratory reporting system that will replace the existing system:

1. What are the role and responsibilities of the NYSDOH? Public health law states that reporting goes directly from the laboratory to the LHDs. Further, the NYSDOH has issued additional regulations for laboratory reporting of specified tests directly to the department in the instance of findings of cancer, lead, etc. How can the state provide the leadership and coordination between the counties and laboratories?
2. What is the role of the LHDs? Currently, there are 57 counties that receive reports from over 500 laboratories. How, and by whom, would communications be handled with the laboratories and counties?
3. What is the role of the commercial and hospital laboratories that perform testing for NYS physicians? Many of these laboratories are interested in a simplified system for communications; they do not want to build 57 different electronic systems for the counties.
4. What technology is available for connecting, and meeting the needs of, all partners involved? What is the expected lifetime of the technologies available? What are the costs associated with available technologies?
5. What are the security and confidentiality requirements of the system? Are the requirements of local/state/federal rules and regulations met through this technology? Will the system meet the HIPAA requirements?
6. Are the partners (local/state/laboratories) willing to work together to implement a new system?
7. How will the system be maintained? Currently, public health staff members utilize manual systems that they can maintain on their own; electronic systems, on the other hand, require a partnership with information technology staff.
8. Lastly, and the most important goal, what improvements in transmitting reports and in information contained in the reports are expected from a new system?

Discussions and debates about these issues occurred over a period of four to five years.

Ultimately, lengthy meetings within the NYSDOH, with the LHDs, and with laboratory staff were required for discussing and answering these questions. Many of the questions were resolved for the simple reason that each stakeholder stood to derive benefit from the solutions:

- The laboratories wanted a central repository to which they could submit reports, rather than the existing costly process of sending the reports directly to the counties.
- Both LHDs and the NYSDOH staff needed a system that will insure that laboratory reports are transmitted and received in a faster manner.
- Further, both state and local health staff wished to avoid multiple and different systems (some electronic) for laboratory reporting. In light of the fact that earlier versions of electronic reporting instituted by the NYSDOH required the laboratory to generate a special single purpose file for each reporting requirement, an early decision was made to focus on a system that would eventually meet all of the laboratory reporting requirements of state and local departments with a single protocol and a single reporting interface. Such a system is a tall order, requiring a secure communications protocol and a centralized reporting database with communications access to all users/partners of the system.

Prior to the HIN and HPN, one of the early underlying concerns for an effective and efficient laboratory reporting system was the need for a communications network that would easily allow all laboratories to obtain connectivity with the NYSDOH and with the counties. At a theoretical level, at least, everyone was able to agree on an electronic reporting system. However, a major early stumbling block was the lack of a robust communications infrastructure. During the early discussions, the Internet emerged as a communications platform that was universally accessible, stable, reliable, robust, and relatively inexpensive. The NYSDOH began building the HIN infrastructure to utilize the Internet as a platform for connecting all of the LHDs to NYSDOH. At the same time, the NYSDOH began building the infrastructure for the HPN, which permitted communication with hospitals, laboratories, and federal agencies. The HPN/HIN provided a solution to the basic system design questions regarding where a CD reporting system would be built and how the infrastructure would be maintained. The HPN/HIN met the goal of utilizing a common, robust, multipurpose, secure foundation for a communications/applications system.

The HIN/HPN provided for a common communications platform and execution of an application development philosophy that met state/county and commercial partner needs. The NYSDOH revisited the issue of automating laboratory reporting for CD and decided the time was right to move the project forward. A team of information technology specialists and epidemiologists was assembled within NYSDOH to oversee the project. The charge to the group was to develop a proposal to build an electronic CD reporting system that connected and met the needs of both the clinical laboratories and LHD staff. The system was labeled ECLRS, or Electronic Clinical Laboratory Reporting System.

The first step in developing the proposal was development of a clear statement of the overall objective of the project. That objective was:

Minimize the time it takes to transmit a reportable test result from the laboratory to the LHD staff.

It was important to keep the overall objective clearly in mind as the team proceeded through the design/development process. The ECLRS team held design sessions with its primary partners, the LHD staff. These design partners included large as well as small counties. In addition, commercial laboratories as well as staff members at the CDC were included in the design process. The overall focus of the design sessions was to build a "standardized" system. From these meetings came several high-level functional requirements for the system. The system must:

- Provide a standardized format for reporting that can be used for all laboratory-reporting requirements to the state and, if possible, to any other state—in short, it must offer a national standard;
- Utilize the existing NYSDOH HIN/HPN infrastructure;
- Provide standardized naming conventions for laboratory test methods and test results. This requirement is essential for comparing disease frequencies electronically. In the past, each laboratory used different test-naming conventions, making combined comparisons difficult without the use of significant and time-consuming recoding.
- Meet the request of laboratories for a single interface for distributing CD test results.
- Minimize the burdens placed on public health (at the county and state levels) and on laboratory staff in operating an electronic data system.
- Provide NYSDOH CD staff with access to incoming laboratory reports, thereby allowing staff to examine outbreaks in real-time as they occur in multi-county areas.
- Monitor laboratory-reporting patterns to insure that laboratories are reporting on a routine basis.
- Include security and confidentiality standards that insure that reports will be released only to authorized staff. The security would need to protect the confidentiality of individual data by limiting it to those county staff authorized to view it.

There would be other considerations in the use and deployment of the system as well:

- There would be adequate user training prior to implementation of the system.
- There would be dedicated, adequate, single-point-of-contact help desk support for the system.

The Design Process

The design team was then charged with developing specifications for the system. A critical design decision was made at this point: This project was not to be an interactive "design, code, review" project. The team would start by spending the time to design the system fully and completely *before any code was written*, including researching all possible methods of file formatting and lab test-naming conventions, both those currently in use and those to be incorporated in upcoming standards. Although the design team was charged with developing the technical specifications, the specifications had to be translated to an executive level proposal to NYSDOH senior management. Senior management would then decide either to go ahead with the project or to send it back with comments.

The design team spent six months identifying, designing, and developing the technical specifications for the system. This was an interactive process similar to the process used in joint application design sessions. The design team met with future users of the system on a routine basis. The team made assessments of existing workflow processes and of the strengths and weaknesses of the current system. Relying on the users' input, the team wrote the requirements for the system. Once drafted, the requirements document was distributed to the users for review and comment to insure that user intent was accurately reflected. Additional discussions were held on how the proposed system might require changes in workflow and processes of LHD, state, and laboratory staff. It was particularly important to hold discussions of the system design limitations with the LHD staff, because success of this system is ultimately dependent on the ability of LHD staff (as well as state and laboratory staff) to use this system efficiently and accurately. The team held discussions with the CDC to insure consistency of the system with plans being made at the national level. The laboratories also encouraged NYSDOH to confer with CDC in developing national standards that all states would adopt.

Most important in this process was continued, frequent communications with all future users and policy makers. These communications insured ongoing discussions, agreement on design plans, and awareness of upcoming events such as implementation and training. The communications also insured that the standards selected for communications and data would be consistent.

During these design activities, the issue of cost was kept in the background. The reason is that it is often too easy to base design decisions on expected costs, rather than on needs. Instead, the focus remained on designing the system according to the needs and requirements presented. If, in the final analysis, the cost of building and implementing the system proved too great, the team would reevaluate the design and determine what could be done within the fiscal constraints. This decision allowed the team the freedom to design the full system. Another benefit of this approach was that by staying focused on the system objectives, the team kept the design within its intended scope, with the ultimate result that the cost of the system remained within available funding.

The completed proposal was then submitted to senior staff at the department for review and approval. Additional approvals were also necessary from the NYS Office for Technology, which is responsible for approving technology projects and insuring that they are generally following state standards for development of new systems. Once approvals were obtained, the proposal was sent out to bid to private contractors. The design team was expanded to include local and state user communities when it came time to review the bid proposals.

Lessons Learned

The design team learned several valuable lessons during the process of developing the new system:

1. *Ongoing communications with all partners were essential to the success of a system.* As the design of the system proceeded, team members met daily. These meetings kept people involved and informed. Members were thereby able to approve or disapprove each of the design elements, thus insuring that the system met their needs and that these members would not return to request design changes later on. Such communications are important throughout the project, even when it does not seem there is much to communicate, but they are particularly important during the system construction phase. Routine meetings and written communications aid in keeping people involved until the system is ready for production.

2. *It was important to follow fairly strict guidelines for designing the system.* Formal joint application design sessions provided the forum for designing, reviewing, and accepting the design prior to development of any code. The common pitfall of writing programs, implementing and debugging while also trying to get everyone to use the system, is thereby avoided.

3. *There was a need for three teams to manage the project.* These were the design team, the guidance team, and the leadership team. The design team consisted of the project manager and members from the state department and the LHDs that oversaw the contract. These staff members were involved in the day-to-day work. The guidance team consisted of management staff from throughout the department; the guidance team therefore had a broader perspective on larger department needs. The guidance team reviewed the overall status of the project on a monthly basis and provided guidance as appropriate, as necessary, or upon request. The leadership team consisted of top NYSDOH executive staff. These executives were kept apprised of the project status on a semi-annual basis, thus insuring that all agency program areas in NYSDOH were familiar with the project.

4. *It was essential to select national data standards for the system.* Health Level 7 (HL-7 version 2.3) was selected as the standard file format that laboratories would use for reporting to the state. This format was selected because of its use nationally by larger medical institutions and laboratories for transferring information. In addition, CDC has recommended HL-7 as the format for use in communicating CD information. Selection of such a national data standard thus achieves the overall goal of selecting a format that could be widely used, and not merely one that was unique to NYS reporting requirements.

5. *National codes were necessary for the system.* LOINC/SNOMED codes (see Chapter 11) were selected as the test-naming and results-naming standard. Although at the time these standards were selected there was not widespread use of these coding schemes, the design team saw that they were most likely to become the standard for laboratory reporting.
6. *Providing adequate training and user support was a key element in providing necessary support to the LHD staff.*
7. *Involving IT professionals who can provide guidance concerning technology was very important.* Technology is constantly changing, and it is necessary to review the technology available for a system and to recognize likely adaptability to future developments. Such a review will insure that the solution is one that can be adapted to future changes in technology.

The West Nile Virus Surveillance System Case Study: Rapid Response for Data Integration and Sharing

Background

During the summer and fall of 1999, an unprecedented event occurred in New York State with the introduction of West Nile virus (WNV) into the Western Hemisphere for the first time. Not only did this event require the mobilization of hundreds of public health officials, but it involved the expenditure of millions of dollars on an emergency basis and the implementation of massive control measures, including wide-area spraying of mosquito adulticides.[10] It also urgently required the establishment of multiple new surveillance systems and the rapid exchange of accurate information throughout the involved region, the whole state, and the rest of the nation. This case study will focus on the issues of data integration and sharing when numerous staff in multiple agencies are involved in responding to a public health emergency and need to acquire surveillance information rapidly from multiple sources.

Prior to this outbreak, human cases of encephalitis and aseptic meningitis had already been reportable to local health departments by clinicians. However, reporting was markedly incomplete. Despite the fact that a statewide hospital discharge file suggested that there were approximately 700 to 800 cases of encephalitis hospitalized each year in New York State, physician-reported cases numbered far less than 100 per year. Even though this passive surveillance system resulted in incomplete reporting, it did lead one astute clinician in a hospital in Queens to report a cluster of four human cases of encephalitis to the New York City Department of Health in August 1999. An epidemiologic investigation by the city health department rapidly led to the recognition of four more cases that affected otherwise healthy, older adults living at home within a four square mile area of northern Queens. At the same time, there were increasing reports of dead birds in the same area. Subsequently, in September 1999, WNV was identified as the cause of this encephalitis outbreak and of the die-off in the bird population.

WNV was first identified in Uganda in 1937.[11] It had caused outbreaks in many parts of Africa, Asia, the Middle East, and parts of Europe.[12–18] The virus is carried by birds and transmitted to humans when they are bitten by mosquitoes that first become infected by feeding on infected birds. WNV causes a broad spectrum of illness in humans, from asymptomatic infection to meningitis (an inflammation of the lining of the brain and spinal cord) to severe life-threatening encephalitis (inflammation of the brain.) Symptoms can include abdominal pain, vomiting, rash, altered mental status, and weakness or paralysis in severe cases. The illness tends to be more severe in the elderly and probably in the very young and in persons with compromised immune systems. There is no specific treatment except for supportive medical care. Mortality rates in those with severe disease can be as high as 10–15%.

The most effective public health strategy to decrease morbidity and mortality from WNV is to prevent human infection through personal protective measures, through decreasing habitat conducive to the breeding of mosquitoes that spread the infection, through larviciding, and through spraying adulticides to decrease biting mosquitoes in specific areas where surveillance information suggests that WNV is likely to cause an outbreak of human illness.[19]

Personal protective measures include the avoidance of outside activities in locations and at times when mosquitoes are most actively feeding, wearing long sleeves and pants outdoors, and using insect repellent in situations when mosquito bites are likely. The primary vector for WNV is believed to be the common household mosquito, *Culex pipiens*, which breeds in stagnant water commonly found in populated areas. Thus, one of the most effective ways to reduce WNV transmission is through eliminating pools of stagnant water. As a last resort, ground or aerial spraying of adulticides that kill adult mosquitoes can be effective in decreasing the likelihood of infected mosquitoes biting humans. Precise surveillance information is necessary to detect the presence of WNV in specific geographic areas and to identify the number and species of mosquitoes prevalent in an area so that public health officials can decide which preventive measures to undertake and alert the public when and where the threat of WNV infection is occurring.

Before the WNV outbreak, there were few municipalities in New York State that conducted mosquito surveillance and control activities. Surveillance was directed mostly at the mosquito vector that transmitted another virus that caused a similar illness, eastern equine encephalitis. However, this mosquito surveillance system was very localized, targeted primarily at mosquito species other than *Culex pipiens*. Furthermore, not only was human encephalitis and mosquito surveillance incomplete, but also there had never been a surveillance system for monitoring bird die-offs prior to 1999. As the 1999 WNV outbreak evolved, it became apparent that large die-offs of birds, especially of American crows, were a sensitive indicator of WNV activity. WNV infection has a very high mortality rate among infected crows—probably well over 90%—and the testing of dead birds, especially crows, proved to be a very sensitive indicator of the presence of WNV in a region.[20]

In response to this outbreak, the New York State and City Health Departments and county health departments in the greater New York metropolitan area quickly developed active human surveillance for encephalitis, as well as surveillance systems for mosquitoes and dead birds. Through the use of this information, public health prevention efforts were directed at those areas most heavily affected during the outbreak, resulting in massive public health education campaigns throughout the greater metropolitan region, distribution of thousands of bottles of insect repellant, and aerial and ground spraying of adulticides throughout all of New York City and many of the surrounding counties. When the mosquito transmission season ended in October 1999, a total of 62 human cases had occurred in the greater New York City area, with seven deaths.[10] Without surveillance information that quickly guided public health prevention and response, it is likely that there could have been far more human illness and deaths.

Policy Issues and Architecture Solutions

The introduction of WNV into New York called for the rapid development of statewide systems for active surveillance for human encephalitis cases, reporting of bird die-offs, the submission of dead birds for testing at state and federal laboratories, mosquito trapping to determine the presence of *Culex pipiens* mosquitoes, testing of mosquitoes for WNV, and reporting of suspicious illness in domestic animals, especially horses, that might be another indicator of the presence of WNV. The NYSDOH response plan[8] to deal with the re-emergence of WNV in the spring of 2000 called for a single integrated surveillance system and database to be established on the HIN as the sole authoritative source of information and data for state and local health departments as well as for other agencies involved in the response to the outbreak. The plan, which was drafted in January 2000, called for the system to be designed and deployed and for local users to be trained in its use by April 2000, a period of only three months.

The need for rapid, accurate information on WNV created many challenges. First of all, there was a wide and diverse audience that needed this information on a daily basis. State, city, and county health departments issued almost daily press releases to an interested public to keep everyone informed of the most recent developments in this life-threatening outbreak and to alert neighborhoods where mosquito precautions were necessary and where adulticiding was scheduled to occur. At the same time, the security of this information was equally important to protecting the confidentiality of ill patients and their families and the owners of ill domestic animals. It was also necessary to control early access to critical information so that it could be assessed and interpreted first by the affected community officials who needed to be prepared to respond to the innumerable phone calls that would be generated from the concerned public once the information was announced. The data exchange system had to be designed in such a way that there could be differential transmission of information, so that those who needed to know first would receive the information before others who had a less urgent need to know.

Another challenge raised by this multifaceted surveillance system was the need to reach agreement regarding what agency or group of persons would maintain the databases, provide the appropriate matching of duplicate records, and establish the needed uniformity for data collection and surveillance instruments. Advancing technology has made rapid, almost instantaneous, widespread access to information possible. However, before establishing an information system, policy makers must decide what data will be gathered, who will have access to the data, when each user will have access to new information, who can edit the data, and who is responsible for maintaining it and training all users of the system once it is established. This process can be quite time consuming. From the start of the WNV outbreak in 1999 through 2000, as this surveillance system was developed and refined, NYSDOH employees devoted hundreds of hours on state and national conference calls and in meetings to resolve these issues.

Another challenge was the requirement to incorporate data from multiple surveillance systems and from different agencies at all levels of government. Unlike most other surveillance systems for communicable diseases, this system relies not only on reports of human cases, but also on reports of the number and species of dead bird sightings, test results on birds, reported numbers and species of trapped mosquitoes in different geographic areas, WNV test results on submitted mosquitoes, and WNV testing of numerous other animal species. Reports come from the public, from physicians and other healthcare providers, from local health departments, and from other agencies such as the New York State Department of Agriculture and Markets, which oversees the welfare of domestic commercial animals. In addition, testing for WNV was being conducted at numerous laboratories, including the New York State and City public health laboratories, the CDC, the National Wildlife Health Center, the National Veterinary Sciences Laboratory, and Cornell University. Some of these laboratories conducted testing at multiple locations. For example, within the New York State public health laboratory, the diagnostic immunology and viral isolation laboratories are at different locations several miles apart, each with its own laboratory database. Another important source of information is the necropsy reports on dead birds that were submitted for testing. This testing occurred at still another site, in the Wildlife Pathology Unit of the State Department of Environmental Conservation. An integrated and relational database was the only possible solution to manage such diverse sets of data while still providing rapid dissemination of information to the numerous partners that needed immediate access to critical information to guide public health action.

To provide the reader with an idea of the complexity of just one aspect of this surveillance system, we have included a diagram to illustrate the information flow in the dead bird surveillance system as Figure 25.1.

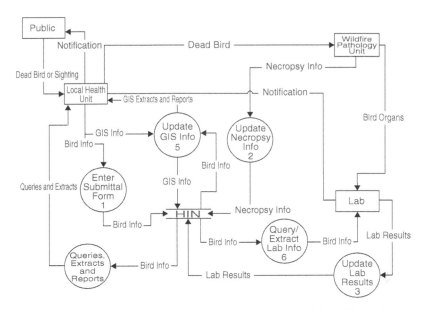

FIGURE 25.1. Information flow diagram for New York's Dead Bird Surveillance System.

This diagram shows how information comes into the system from such diverse locations as local health units, the Wildlife Pathology Unit, and laboratories, while at the same time the system provides selected information back to the laboratories, the local health units, and the public. Also, the bird information system must be integrated with the human surveillance, mosquito surveillance, and other animal surveillance systems already described. In 2000, the CDC developed a national surveillance system for WNV, with weekly uploads of New York State data into this system. With the integrated New York surveillance system, it was possible to accommodate this data interchange fairly easily.

Lastly, and of no trivial importance, is the need for adequate resources to develop and support a surveillance system of this magnitude. In addition to the resources needed for the field investigations and laboratory testing that generate much of the information, considerable staffing is essential for technical support to develop and maintain the communications system and databases. These kinds of resources can only be garnered when there is strong support from the highest levels of administration within every level of government.

New York's WNV surveillance system was built on the e-commerce infrastructure of the state health department's HIN/HPN. The system provides the capability of connecting all the local health units with the state health department, as well as with other important colleagues, such as commercial laboratories and other agencies. The HIN/HPN also provides user-specific privileges for accessing the central database according to each user's needs. Users may query the total database for aggregate data (i.e., summary tables), and they may manipulate their own county data. For example, in the case of the dead bird surveillance system, each local health unit has the capability of entering its own dead bird reports, utilizing common data entry screens. At the same time, the Wildlife Pathology Unit and different laboratories can submit results on birds that have been submitted for testing, with the linking of various results through a common bird identification number. When new laboratory results are added to the database by one of the laboratories, the system is programmed to allow each county to access its own results immediately, but not to view other counties' data until a predetermined lag period (usually several hours). This delay allows each responsible municipality to receive its own results first and prepare the appropriate public health response. In some cases, the information is entered on the HIN/HPN via data entry screens, whereas in other instances upload programs accommodate the rapid incorporation of data from other sources (e.g., results from the state laboratory information management systems).

The system also allows differential access to the central database at the individual staff person level. In applying for access to the WNV data system, each person must specify which privileges he/she is requesting and present a signed approval from his/her supervisor. Some individuals may need read-only privileges, whereas others will need both read and write privileges; still others may need to upload new data into the system or download portions of the database for local analysis. Table 25.3 illustrates the versatility that the HIN access control system needed to have in order to accommodate the various types of staff access to the system while protecting against unnecessary disclosure of confidential information or corruption of data files. The system allows the HIN access control officer to tailor specific privileges to the needs of each user.

Users who are granted access to the WNV system can see summary tables that include, in the case of bird surveillance, a listing of the number of positive, negative, and pending lab tests on birds, as well as the number of dead bird reports. There are also summary tables that include statewide totals, such as the tabulation of positive birds by different species. A county can also get a listing of all its own birds, with their identifying numbers, that have tested WNV positive, negative, or are pending.

On a weekly basis, summary tables are updated and posted on the HIN, as well as on the state health department's Web site for access by the public. In addition, specialized analyses are performed and uploaded as appropriate. For example, the human, bird, and mosquito data are entered into a geographic information system (GIS) in order to perform detailed mapping of the locations where positive WNV findings have occurred. This information is helpful for guiding public health action, for alerting the public to the introduction of WNV into new geographic areas, and for guiding prevention activities. Lastly, the HIN/HPN provides the capacity to conduct secure

TABLE 25.3. Examples of access levels to communicable disease information for HIN/HPN applications

Application	Read	White	Upload	Download	Delete
Problem alert	X	X			
Communicable disease summary data query (1993–1998, includes NYC data)	X				
Communicable disease confidential case query (1997–current) CD, TB, STD (includes West Nile)	D				
Communicable disease confidential case reports and supplemental data (1997–current, with names) CD, TB, STD (includes West Nile)	D	D	D	D	D
Rabies system	X	X			
West Nile integrated data reporting systems:					
Dead birds, sentinel birds, Wildlife Pathology Unit	X	X		X	
Lab results	X		X	X	
Geocoding			X	X	
Mammals	X	X	X	X	
Lab results	X		X	X	
Human: lab results	X		X	X	
Mosquito:	X	X	X	X	
Lab results			X		
Summary reports	X				

X, simple access permission; D, access limited by disease grouping (communicable disease [CD], tuberculosis [TB], sexually transmitted disease [STD]) and county with permission.

discussion forums, with controlled access for users. These discussion forums are important because many policy issues and questions arise that need to be confidentially discussed among only selected participants. In addition, when an issue arises in one county, its discussion is frequently relevant to other counties, and sharing of information through secure discussion forums provides an efficient opportunity for distributing information to those who need to know. Such a system can save staff time and reduce frustration.

The technical solution to the complex needs of the WNV surveillance system was based on a carefully orchestrated process that involved obtaining input from all affected parties and potential users of the system. Early and ongoing input from all users is important so that the appropriate system architecture can be determined from the start. This approach minimizes the likelihood of having to make costly and time-consuming changes to a system after it is built. Through a series of statewide meetings and conference calls, a preliminary design for the system was developed to meet the needs and challenges we have discussed. These user forums continued throughout the development of the system; in fact, they are continuing as the system is used, because they provide an important opportunity for continuing input on improving the system and identifying problems needing correction. In addition, six workgroups were formed early in the development process and charged with the task of addressing different aspects of the system; their discussions provided the more detailed architectural design for this system. These workgroups covered the following areas: human case surveillance, mosquito surveillance, bird and animal surveillance, WNV response and control activities, public relations, and information technology. These workgroups met in person, by telephone conferencing, and by the use of secure discussion forums on the HIN/HPN. They served the purpose of joint application discussion sessions and resolved detailed questions of system design. Participants in these workgroups included representatives of the state and local health departments, laboratories, information technology and programming staff, public relations staff, entomologists, disease control staff, epidemiologists, and representatives of the concerned public.

Lessons Learned

Advancing technology has increased everyone's expectations of immediate, easy access to accurate information. However, this same technology has raised numerous challenges as well. For example, the demand for rapid access to information has reduced the amount of time that epidemiologists have to confirm the accuracy of the data. The ability to connect many end users to the same surveillance system and central data bank carries with it the risk of jeopardizing data integrity, security and personal confidentiality. A related concern is the need to insure that selected officials are notified first of new information so that they have adequate time to prepare for the appropriate public health response. With increasing numbers of users of the same database, the importance of the uniformity of data structure and data elements is critical. Not the least of the implications of advancing technology is the tremendously increasing need for training of all users of a system. Lastly, there is the cost and time of establishing and maintaining the needed software, hardware, and connectivity for each user.

The WNV surveillance system illustrates several important lessons:

- *Any system is doomed if the stakeholders and users are not supportive of the system and are therefore not likely to use it. Early and continuing input from all stakeholders must be solicited, supported, and respected.*
- *Adequate resources in the form of staff and equipment need to be provided.* For a complicated information system to succeed, it needs to be everyone's top priority.

- *Technologic solutions to many of public health's needs are complicated by the large number of system users, who often work for different organizations and within different electronic information environments. Developing an information system takes time and can only be achieved incrementally.* The quick establishment of the WNV surveillance system was possible only because it was built on the structure of the previously existing HIN/HPN. It has been successful because its design was continuously driven by the needs of its different users and because it pulled together multiple sources of data to create "one-stop shopping" for reliable, timely, and essential information.

Conclusions

Effective modern surveillance systems require a carefully engineered information technology architecture that is based on open industry standards and that is robust enough to accommodate policy needs. The interplay between policy and technology can have synergistic and antagonistic effects on both architecture and the surveillance system. These interactions affect feasibility, complexity, cost, risk, time to deployment, usability, and information technology (IT) staffing requirements. Organizational commitment and expectations have to be attuned to these interactions, because the process of evolving a successful architecture and surveillance system is time-consuming and expensive. Understanding these interactions is therefore a key success factor in development, deployment, and continuity of both surveillance systems and their underlying IT architecture. This understanding comes from a process of exhaustive assessment of policy needs and from involvement of stakeholders and program area experts as partners with IT staff in the design process. The benefit of these investments will be a surveillance infrastructure that can respond to the needs of a health emergency such as West Nile virus, or that can accommodate a legislative mandate requiring a high degree of security/confidentiality, as in HIV reporting, or that can support an organizational initiative that changes the workflow process of paper-based laboratory reporting to a statewide electronic system.

Questions for Review

1. Explain why protecting the security and confidentiality of information gathered by public health surveillance systems is important. What methods are used in the cases presented in this chapter to insure the security and confidentiality of information?
2. What features do the surveillance systems described in this chapter have in common? Why are these features important?

3. What are the roles of (a) legislative and regulatory authorities and (b) program-level staff in developing surveillance systems? How do these roles differ?

4. What characteristics should a surveillance system that is used as a vehicle for information delivery among multiple levels of users possess? Why are these characteristics important?

5. Explain why it was important for a single entity, the NYSDOH, to control the security and confidential of information contained within the HIN and the HPN. Why was it important not to provide users with direct access to central databases? Why is the access system for the HIN designed in such a way that the ID and password of a user expire after the initial log-in? Why were decisions regarding access levels for employees delegated to local user organizations?

6. Why was involving prospective users of the HIN and the HPN important to the success of the system development efforts?

7. What reasons existed for emphasizing data security and confidentiality in the development of the HIV/AIDS surveillance system? Why were these reasons important to the success of the system?

8. Explain why data security and confidentiality were important factors in the design of the electronic clinical laboratory reporting system. Why was a determination of the role and responsibilities of the NYSDOH an important issue in the design and development of this system? What benefits did this system provide to users, compared to the old, largely paper-based system? To NYSDOH?

9. Why was the process of designing the entire clinical laboratory reporting system before writing any code a critical factor in the system's success? Why was keeping the focus on user needs, rather than on costs, an important success factor?

10. In what ways did frequent communications with future users and policy makers help insure the success of the electronic clinical laboratory reporting system? Why was there a need for three teams to manage the project? Why was the selection of national data standards and coding for the system important?

11. Explain how the presence of an existing information infrastructure enabled NYSDOH to respond so quickly to the West Nile virus emergency. Why was it important to provide for a delay in general access to county data? Why was securing input from all affected parties and potential users of the West Nile virus surveillance system important?

References

1. Langmuir, AD. The surveillance of communicable diseases of national importance. *New Engl J Med.* 1963;268:182–192.
2. Institute of Medicine. *The Future of Public Health.* Washington, DC: National Academy Press; 1988.

3. Birkhead G, Maylahn, CM. State and local public health surveillance. In: Teutsch SM and Churchill RE, eds. *Principals and Practice of Public Health Surveillance, Second Edition.* New York: Oxford University Press; 2001.

4. Klauke DN, Beuhler JW. Thacker SB. et al. Guidelines for evaluating surveillance systems. *MMWR Morb Mortal Wkly Rep* 1988;37:(S-5).

5. Privacy Law Advisory Committee. Model State Public Health Privacy Project. Model State Public Health Privacy Act. Washington, DC: Georgetown University Law Center, 1999. Available at: <http:www.critpath.org/msphpa/privacy.htm>. Accessed May 7, 2001. .

6. German RR. Horan JM. Lee LM. Milstein RL. Pertowski, CA. Waller MN, Birkhead GS. Updated guidelines for evaluating surveillance systems. *MMWR,* July 27, 2001:50(RR13);1–35.

7. Gotham IJ, Eidson M. White D, Wallace B, Chang H-G, Johnson G, Napoli J, Sottolano D. Birkhead G, Morse D. Smith P. West Nile virus: A case study in how NY State health information infrastructure facilitates preparation and response to disease outbreaks. *J Public Health Manage Pract* 2001;7(5):75–86.

8. New York State Department of Health. New York State West Nile virus Response Plan. May, 2000. Available at: http://www.health.state.ny.us/nysdoh/westnile/final.htm. Accessed April 3, 2002.

9. Centers for Disease Control and Prevention. *HIV/AIDS Surveillance Report.* 2000;12.

10. Novello, AC. West Nile virus in New York State: The 1999 outbreak and response plan for 2000. *Viral Immunol* 2000;13:463–467.

11. Smithburn KC. Hughes TP, Burke AW, Paul JH. A neurotropic virus isolated from the blood of a native of Uganda. *Am J Trop Med Hyg* 1940;20:471–492.

12. Ceausu E, Erscoiu S, Calistru P. et al. Clinical manifestations in the West Nile virus outbreak. *Rom J Virol* 1997;48:3–11.

13. Cernescu C. Nedelcu NI, Tardei G. Ruta S, Tsai TF. Continued transmission of West Nile virus to humans in southeastern Romania. 1997–1998. *J Infect Dis* 2000;181:710–712.

14. Cernescu C. Ruta SM, Tardei G. et al. A high number of severe neurologic clinical forms during an epidemic of West Nile virus infection. *Rom J Virol* 1997;48:13–25.

15. Lvov DK. Butenko AM, Gromashevsky VL, et al. Isolation of two strains of West Nile virus during an outbreak in southern Russia, 1999. *Emerg Infect Dis* 2000;6:373–376.

16. Platanov AE, Shipulin GA, Shipulina OY, et al. Outbreak of West Nile virus infection, Volgograd Region, Russia, 1999. *Emerg Infect Dis* 2001;7:128–132.

17. Tsai TF, Popovici F, Cernescu C. Campbell GL. Nedelcu NI. West Nile encephalitis epidemic in southeastern Romania. *Lancet* 1998;352:767–771.

18. Siegel-Itzkovich J. Twelve die of West Nile virus in Israel. *BMJ* 2000:321:724.

19. Guidelines for surveillance, prevention, and control of West Nile virus infection— United States. *MMWR.* 2000:49:25–28.

20. Eidsen M, Komar N. Sorhage F, Nelson R, Talbot T, Mostashari F, McLean R. Crow mortality as a sentinel surveillance system for West Nile virus in North America, 1999. *Emerg Infect Dis.* Jul-Aug 2001;7(4):615–620.

26

Networking/Connecting People in a Sustainable Way: Information Network for Public Health Officials

RON SEYMOUR AND FRAN MUSKOPF

Learning Objectives

After studying this chapter, you should be able to:

- Describe the challenges that any typical new public health information/communication system should expect to encounter and overcome.
- Understand the priority that collaboration among partners has in a successful implementation of a public health information system, using this Washington Information Network for Public Health Officials (INPHO) case as an example.
- Explain why a project team needs to take politics and the relationships between organizational users of a prospective public health information network into account.
- Analyze the lessons learned from the INPHO experience and describe the implications that these lessons have for other public health information systems.

Overview

The Information Network for Public Health Officials (INPHO), an initiative of the Centers for Disease Control and Prevention (CDC), formed its first project when representatives of the Washington State Department of Health (WSDOH) received a CDC grant to develop an information system for use by Washington counties and local health jurisdictions (LHJs) in connecting with the WSDOH. INPHO project team members were confronted with addressing challenges arising from unpleasant experiences of LHJs and counties with state agencies, with continuing funding issues, and with recognizing the importance of local politics in helping LHJs and counties to build an information network that would connect them with the state. The manner in which the INPHO project team organized the project and interacted with the LHJs and with local political entities is a model of how to proceed with an information network project. Solutions to the challenges encountered included involving LHJs and county officials in system planning and vesting ownership of the resulting systems in the LHJs. The solutions also included making provisions for training of users in system use and in network component maintenance. Finally, involving other state agencies in issues related to funding helped to resolve a funding crisis.

Introduction

In 1993, there was an *Escherichia coli 0157:h7* outbreak in the state of Washington. The Washington State Department of Health (WSDOH) went into action and collected information from Washington's Local Health Jurisdictions (LHJs) via faxes and telephone calls. In turn, WSDOH kept the LHJs informed of the rapidly evolving chain of events associated with the outbreak, using the telephone and employing fax messaging. This was an exhaustive effort by staff of the State Department of Health. The outbreak was identified and control measures were put in place in just slightly over a week. The outbreak was finally contained, but only after the death of one child and confirmation of 650 cases. The source of the outbreak was traced to undercooked hamburgers sold at Jack in the Box restaurants

In 1996, there was a similar *E. coli 0157:h7* outbreak in the state of Washington. This time, the source of the outbreak was Odwalla fruit juice. This outbreak was identified and control measures were put in place in 6 days and finally contained after 70 cases in Washington, Oregon, and Idaho. Although the time to identify and respond to this case was just slightly better than that of the 1993 outbreak, the methods of communications and control were significantly improved. When this outbreak occurred, the LHJs notified WSDOH by using e-mail and by exchanging important data relevant to these cases through use of secure electronic communications. The state used a public health listserve (e-mail distribution list) to send regular updates about the events to keep the state's public health officials informed of progress and findings. Also, by using a new DNA finger-printing technique, WSDOH was able to ship electronically the DNA results to the Centers for Disease Control and Prevention (CDC) in Atlanta; the CDC compared these samples to national samples and quickly determined that the fruit juice was the culprit.

What happened between 1993 and 1996 to permit such a rapid resolution of the 1996 outbreak? WSDOH, in partnership with CDC, created the nation's first of its kind high-speed data communications network connecting all of Washington's LHJs to each other, to the state, to the CDC, and to the Internet. The network-building process featured either installation of local-area networks (LANs) or augmentation of existing LANs; installation of e-mail capabilities; and the provision of T-1 speed Internet access for every LHJ. The project that made this quantum leap in technological capabilities possible was known as the Information Network for Public Health Officials (INPHO), an initiative of the CDC.

In 1992, CDC began INPHO as an initiative to strengthen the public health technology infrastructure in the United States. WSDOH had completed building its own agency network infrastructure in 1993 and was in the process of brainstorming how to expand that infrastructure to include the LHJs when CDC approached Washington with the concept of INPHO. In 1994, CDC awarded grants to 12 states to be part of the first INPHO project. Washington was one of those 12 states. So began the Washington INPHO project, which was fully completed in July 1997.

INPHO became much more than a network connecting public health organizations in Washington. It became the foundation for Washington's Inter-Governmental Network (IGN). In fact, the use and expansion of IGN was an explosive development made possible by the formation of partnerships with the state's Department of Information Services, with county information technology departments, and with other state agencies (such as The Administrator of the Courts, the Washington State Patrol, the Department of Social and Health Services, and others). The IGN today is a shared network being used by many state agencies, counties, cities, municipalities, Indian tribes, and other not-for-profit organizations. An estimated 80,000 users are now connected to IGN.

One obstacle encountered by WSDOH in implementing INPHO was county resistance—resistance resulting from the existing multiplicity of state-owned networks already installed at the county level. A 1994 study of existing state-owned networks located in the counties throughout the state had found that one small county with a population of 38,400 people had over 60 networks installed by various state agencies. Such a finding was typical throughout the state. The WSDOH itself had eight different LHJ-destined applications projects in the works, each with its own identified network components. The existence of these projects was, in fact, a major part of the motivation for WSDOH to begin the INPHO project. However, when INPHO project representatives came to discuss installing yet another network with county officials, the response from the county officials was a resounding no. Counties were tired of the state's proliferation of networks at the same time that the counties were in the process of planning and building their own networks.

Developing Partnerships

Throughout the INPHO project, many new partnerships were formed or else existing partnerships were used. Table 26.1 depicts the relationship between partners and what they brought to the table. The discussion that follows will delineate the roles played by the various partners.

TABLE 26.1. Partners in development of the INPHO system

Partner	Role in Project
Washington State Department of Health (WSDOH)	Provided overall responsibility for project management, design, construction, and coordination with partners for long-term support.
Centers for Disease Control and Prevention (CDC)	Provided the national public health vision, oversight, funding, and coordination with other state projects.
University of Washington, Northwest Center for Public Health Practice and Regional Library of Medicine (UW)	Provided Web development, e-mail and support, help desk functions, list server support, and training, both on-site and in classrooms.
Washington State Department of Information Services (DIS)	Provided installation coordination with vendors and network configurations and was instrumental in the coordination with other state and county agencies for using the network as a shared resource.
Washington State's Local Health Jurisdictions (LHJs)	Provided procurement of equipment and coordination of installation at the county level.
County information technology staffs	Facilitated equipment installations in the counties and WAN installation.
Association of City and County IS Managers (ACCIS)	Participated in the development of the guiding principles and was highly instrumental in pushing the state to use INPHO and a shared infrastructure.
Washington State legislature	Provided funding.
Washington's Customer Advisory Board (CAB)	Made up of state agency information technology directors. Accepted the IGN guiding principles and provided support for the state and local committee that dealt with the issues surrounding the use of a shared network infrastructure.
Northwest Portland Area Indian Health Board	Coordinated the effort to bring the Washington Tribes onto the IGN.

CDC and WSDOH

The CDC originally presented the concept and vision for a national network linking all public health officials and providing access to timely, authoritative, and accurate information to the WSDOH management. WSDOH management embraced this vision. With some seed money provided by CDC, WSDOH conducted an assessment of the information technology capacity of the state's

34 LHJs and developed a proposal for implementation of the CDC vision in the State of Washington. CDC then awarded one of 12 available grants to the state to begin construction of the network. CDC also assigned a public health advisor to Washington's INPHO project. This assignment proved to be extremely helpful in keeping the public health perspective within the project while network builders concentrated mainly on network construction.

University of Washington and WSDOH

The University of Washington's (UW) Regional National Library of Medicine and its Northwest Center for Public Health Practice provided Internet and e-mail training, Web publishing services and server support, listserve administration, and initial dial-in e-mail services for the LHJs. Staff of UW, WSDOH, and LHJs designed a Web page targeted at the needs of the LHJs. The UW staff set up dial-in e-mail accounts for the LHJs and provided on-site training for LHJs staff.

Department of Information Services and WSDOH

WSDOH contracted with Washington's Department of Information Services (DIS) to coordinate the actual construction of the wide-area network (WAN). DIS was supportive of the concept of the IGN and created a network that could be shared by multiple agencies. DIS management participated in the meetings with each county to discuss the implementation of INPHO and the eventual creation of the IGN.

County Information Technology Staff and WSDOH

In each county, the network was physically placed to maximize its ability to be shared by all county departments. This placement required coordination with the county's central information technology staff. In many cases, the placement task required a three-way partnership among the appropriate LHJ, the county, and WSDOH. Each county entered an agreement that WSDOH would provide free network access to the entire county for a period of two years in exchange for the county's housing and providing high-level support for the WAN equipment.

Customer Advisory Board and Association of City and County IS Managers

Washington's Customer Advisory Board (CAB) and the Association of City and County IS Managers (ACCIS) formed a subcommittee that developed the initial guiding principles for participation in the IGN and the templates for service level agreements for IGN services. This committee has also decided the rate structure for ongoing costs and is dealing with the security issues.

Northwest Portland Area Indian Health Board and WSDOH

The Northwest Portland Area Indian Health Board (NWPAIHB) had its own existing project to connect all the tribal clinics to a WAN. Through partnering with WSDOH, NWPAIHB installed a network/security design that allowed the tribes to be connected to the IGN, thus helping to bring the tribal health clinics to the same technical level as the state's LHJs.

Challenges

Throughout the project, the INPHO project had to address many challenges. In this section, we will discuss some of these challenges and how they were mitigated.

Challenge 1: Lack of Understanding of the Value of the Project

There was a lack of understanding of what another network, in this case the INPHO system, could do for an LHJ. This lack of understanding was itself understandable. After all, many of the LHJ staff had never used e-mail, and the Internet was something they had heard about only on the news. And that news was not always good.

Mitigation

To help educate the LHJ staff on the value of these tools, the INPHO project team took the approach of getting as much technology and as many services out to the LHJs as quickly as possible.

The INPHO team collaborated with the UW Regional National Library of Medicine and the NW Center for Public Health Practice staff to provide an interim solution: providing LHJs with access to e-mail, help desk services, World Wide Web services, and training in the uses of Internet tools at the LHJs. INPHO benefited from the university's extensive computer services and was able to create 130 e-mail accounts easily.

The UW provided dial-in connections very early in the process. The INPHO team wanted to give the LHJs "a taste" of what the INPHO project could do for them. A listserve was created for three or four public health practitioners in each LHJ. The listserve, called WSALPHO-L, is a forum for members of the Washington State Association of Local Public Health Officials. WSALPHO-L has become the primary mode of communication among local public health administrators. Many public health practitioners in remote counties have come to count on the listserve to keep them informed about what is happening elsewhere in the state; these practitioners use it as a tool to communicate with their peers. Previously, remote LHJs were "out of the loop" regarding legislative issues and other issues of immediate concern. Local health practitioners also use the listserve as an information-gathering tool. When confronted with a unique problem or a question, list members will frequently poll others for ideas about how best to approach a situation.

With just three months of collaboration, the INPHO team established a public health Web site for local public health practitioners. This site is the default home page for many LHJs, and local staff members use it daily. The site is well known in the Pacific Northwest, and many external agencies link to it as an excellent, comprehensive set of public health links. Another feature of the site is a calendar that contains updated information about public health happenings around the state and within the LHJ region.

Another early success for INPHO was the network connection to the state's birth certificate database. Before INPHO, LHJ staff needed to dial into the state's vital records database on a weekly basis via modem, then verify and print birth certificates. The modem process presented a security concern because it was not only inconsistent, but it also often disconnected the dialing computer. The result often was that the next person to dial into the same modem would receive the birth certificate file from the disconnected session. With the INPHO connection, in contrast, the entire process is not only secure but also requires less than 15 minutes for completion of a session. Customers are able to leave a session with a birth certificate in hand in one visit, rather than two. The reception of the new system was so positive that when the INPHO connection to the state's birth certificate database was installed on a test basis at an LHJ, the staff immediately began to lobby the program team not to take the new system away.

Challenge 2: Fear of the Internet

Many county officials and commissioners feared bringing the Internet into their county governments. They were afraid that staff would be wasting time by surfing the Internet for irrelevant topics and, even worse, by accessing pornography and other inappropriate material. Heightening these concerns even more, a news story broke about a county commissioner who had spent many hours of county time downloading hundreds of pornographic images from the Internet, using a county computer connected to the INPHO network. Though INPHO was not directly blamed for the incident, the issue certainly became a major topic of concern to county management. The county was unable to discipline the commissioner because it had no policies in place related to Internet usage.

Mitigation

To this point, the INPHO project staff had recommended that counties implement policies related to the use of the Internet, but the project staff had taken no further action. At the time, only about three counties actually had Internet use policies in place. Now, the INPHO team gathered policies from many different sources and made them available for counties to use as starting points for development of Internet use policies at the county level. Almost immediately, all the counties either implemented policies or began the process of developing them. This activity had an immediate positive effect on the INPHO project, because the activity began the process of addressing fears of what people could and could not do on the Internet. The newly developed and implemented policies provided a certain comfort level to the local officials.

Challenge 3: Fear of Network Attack by Hackers

There was also the fear among local officials that, once connected to the Internet, a county's networks would be vulnerable to Internet hackers.

Mitigation

This fear was addressed by bringing in security experts to sit down with the technical staff at the counties to design the network so that only outbound Internet traffic would be possible. E-mail would flow freely, both inbound and outbound, but all other inbound network traffic would be stopped at the county firewall. Once the county's technical staff members were convinced that the network would be secure from hacker attack, selling the security of the INPHO network to the county officials was no longer a problem.

Challenge 4: Lack of Trust Between County Agencies or Departments

In many counties, there was a history of poor communication between the county government and its LHJ. This poor communication resulted in a certain degree of mistrust and skepticism about collaboration. Some LHJs, in fact, had characterized their relationships with county information systems (IS) departments as lacking in responsiveness and cooperation. In some counties, the LHJ staff had never met the county IS staff. In other counties, in contrast, the two governmental entities had an excellent working relationship, and collaboration was a natural extension of their symbiotic relationship.

Mitigation

In cases in which there was a strained or else an absent relationship between an LHJ and county organizations, the INPHO project team worked very closely with LHJ staff members to assure them that ownership of the project rested with the LHJ and that the INPHO team was simply facilitating it. To reinforce this assurance, the INPHO team took a back seat during the negotiations between the LHJs and the counties. This stance allowed the LHJs to take ownership of the project; it also allowed them to be proactive with a county in presenting network proposals. Conferring project ownership on the LHJ worked out very well indeed. In many cases, according to communications of LHJ staff to the INHPO project team, an LHJ's presenting a network proposal to county officials became that very rare occasion when the LHJ could approach the county with something to offer, instead of habitually going to the county with a request for the county to offer something.

Challenge 5: Lack of County Trust in the State and Proliferation of State-Installed Networks

Another challenge was that counties had a long history of distrusting state-level agencies because of previous actions taken by the latter regarding network installation. In the past, many state agencies had shown little if any consideration for a county's infrastructure or standards in installing computers and networks in counties. Further, the state was perceived as having shown little respect for the technical capabilities of the counties. In addition, counties recounted instances in which state-level agencies had failed to honor commitments, in many cases costing the counties money.

Finally, state agencies had worked independently of each other, especially with regard to installing networks. The result was a proliferation of state-installed networks at the county level. For instance, one small county with a population of 38,400 people housed 60 networks that had been installed by state agencies. The WSDOH itself had eight different applications projects in the works, with each having a network component as part of its project and each identifying LHJs as customers. These planned applications, in fact, were a major component of the motivation for WSDOH to begin the INPHO project.

The history of mistrust of state agencies and the proliferation of state-installed networks at the county level had an initial negative effect on the INPHO project team. When INPHO team members approached county officials about installing what was perceived as yet another network, the quick response of county officials was "No!" This negative reaction was common among many of the counties. These counties were tired of the state's proliferation of networks at the same time that the counties were planning and building their own networks. Moreover, county officials feared that once the INPHO network was implemented, they would be stuck with the bill.

Mitigation

The INPHO team's approach of permitting county staff to install the associated networks eliminated the concern that INPHO was going to corrupt the county's network environment. Moreover, as a means of addressing the county concerns about costs, team members sent letters to each county stating that counties would not be held liable for long-term costs of network usage for state business. The letters pointed out that counties would eventually be charged for use of the network for county-specific business but that counties would also have the option of removing themselves from the network if they chose. In return for the cooperation and support of county staff in the installation of INPHO, this staff would be trained to support a county's LANs; moreover, county staff would receive two years of free access to the network—from July 1997 through June 1999. The costs of the network were broken into three categories: Initial network component costs and installation, monthly data circuits and maintenance, and an Internet access fee. Counties would have to pay for Internet access fees, but there would be no network fees during this period. In July 1999, all the counties decided to pay the minimal charge for using the network

Challenge 6: Lack of a Telecommunications Infrastructure in Rural Areas

In many remote areas of the state, the telephone companies lacked the infrastructure to support new high-speed networks.

Mitigation

The INPHO team worked very closely with the telecommunications firm US West to develop a detailed network design and project plan. US West committed to making its best effort to insure that the required telecommunications equipment would be in place to meet the project schedule. Even Mother Nature helped. In the early spring of 1996, record floods destroyed US West telecommunications equipment in a remote part of southeastern Washington. Because US West planned to meet future INPHO project requirements, it decided that rather than simply replace the existing destroyed equipment to get voice lines up and running, it would upgrade to fiber optic cable. Influenced by the prospect of working with INPHO, US West invested its own money at higher levels than might have been possible under different conditions.

In another situation during the design of the WAN, US West told the INPHO team that telecommunications capacity, including voice and data lines, in the small, remote town of Colville, Washington, had been "maxed out." Expanding existing capacity to the town would be prohibitively expensive. According to its prioritization plan, US West, the only telecommunications provider in the region, planned to address telecommunications capacity by laying new fiber optic cable or by adding to its microwave capacity in two years' time. The timeframe and expense level were incompatible with INPHO's goals.

Working with US West engineers, WSDOH learned what kind of equipment was currently in use and researched the equipment on the Internet, downloading the manufacturer's equipment manuals. Staff then consulted with the equipment manufacturer and US West, devising a way to split out and make available unused capacity in preexisting frame relay circuits, thereby expanding telecommunications capacity. WSDOH and US West engineers then wrote a proposal for procedural changes that met approval in three US West divisions before meeting final approval at the vice presidential level. This ingenuity and diligence saved the INPHO project large sums of money and also impacted how US West did business. WSDOH staff research thus allowed US West to increase its telecommunications capacity while also accommodating the needs of INPHO.

Challenge 7: Lack of Resources for Ongoing Support and Maintenance of the Networks

Maintenance of the network was always an issue. The monies provided for building the network were one-time funds, and there were no ongoing funds identified to keep the network running once installation was completed. The goal, therefore, became making the network as maintenance-free as possible.

Mitigation

To obviate the need for maintenance, fiber optic cable was used to connect facilities together wherever possible. Installed correctly, fiber optic cable requires very little if any maintenance. In a couple of counties, local utility districts agreed to run the fiber optic cable on their poles, and WSDOH connected the counties to the network without charge. This arrangement works out well: If the cable or the poles are damaged, the utility district has a vested interest in getting the cable repaired because the utilities use it, too.

LAN maintenance was a major concern, for LANs require maintenance almost daily. To mitigate the long-term costs of maintaining 40 LANs statewide, the INPHO team employed the approach of training local staff members to maintain their own networks from the beginning. The project offered to pay to train up to two people in each LHJ or county to become certified network engineers. The LHJ/county was permitted to designate who would be trained. The only stipulation was that the person trained would support the local LAN. In the smaller counties in which resources were scarce, INPHO trained the individual responsible for maintenance of the computers for the LHJ. In many cases, the person trained also occupied a position other than one normally associated with information technology support. In one county, for example, a deputy sheriff was trained. In another, a high school computer science teacher underwent training, since the LHJ is located in the elementary school adjacent to the high school in which the teacher worked. In all, 48 local health and county staff members took advantage of this training offer, becoming either Microsoft Certified Systems Engineers (MSCE) or Novell Certified Netware Engineers (CNE). Once the staff members were trained, they undertook the initial setup of the LAN for their LHJs, and the INPHO project provided a LAN expert who would visit to help an LHJ with any problems encountered. Through this method, the local staff not only received the necessary training but also gained hands-on experience with the LAN that they would be supporting.

The downside to this approach was the existence of turnover among staff members trained in LAN maintenance. When such turnover occurred, the LHJ had to decide whether to replace a departed incumbent with an information technology specialist or whether to fill the vacated position with a person possessing the same expertise as the person leaving may have been originally hired for. In most cases, LHJs chose to replace departing staff with other information technology specialists.

WANs also required provision for maintenance. There are two components of a WAN requiring maintenance. At the state level, there is the IGN for connecting the counties to the state, and at the county level, there is the network that supports the county offices. The county staff members are responsible for support of the network connecting the county offices. At the county level, the INPHO project team made sure that whatever was being built would fit in with the county's own network plans; in many cases, the INPHO network development became the beginning of a county's infrastructure plan. Another strategy to address the need for WAN maintenance was that the counties were encouraged to use the INPHO network to support other county functions as well. The underlying basis for this strategy was that the more people and organizations using the network, the better the chance of long-term support. The strategy was well accepted by the counties.

The Development Process

INPHO worked with each LHJ and county individually, avoiding stereotyping LHJ needs by population, size, geography, or economics. The INPHO team's negotiations with individual LHJs took place in five meetings over three days: (1) an LHJ technology assessment meeting, (2) a preplanning meeting, (3) an LHJ coordination meeting, (4) an LHJ and county meeting, and (5) a technical meeting. The collaboration that resulted from these meetings was the key to INPHO's local success. These meetings set the stage for the possible success or failure of INPHO. They determined LHJ buy-in and enthusiastic compliance with INPHO on all levels, qualities that were imperative for execution of such a large and complex information technology (IT) project.

Technology Assessment

The INPHO team began by performing a technology assessment at each of the 34 LHJs to determine what equipment was available on-site and what would need to be procured. At this time, the INPHO team began drafting a preliminary network design. This meeting was the initial exposure of the LHJ staff to the INPHO project. It presented an opportunity for the INPHO team to begin educating staff about the benefits of a statewide network and about network security issues.

The Preplanning Meeting

The preplanning meeting was a formal presentation of the INPHO project to the LHJ administration and staff. The focus of this meeting was on INPHO's preparing the LHJs for what was to come. These meetings focused on discussing the project schedule and on offering the LHJ the associated equipment, software, training, and support.

The LHJ Coordination Meeting and the LHJ and County Meeting

The LHJ coordination meeting and the LHJ and county meeting were typically held on the same day. The LHJ coordination meeting focused on determining how the LHJ would approach the county information technology management with the concept of the shared network.

In the meeting of the LHJ staff and county IT staff, the LHJ staff presented the project to the county, emphasizing the importance of the project as a public health initiative. INPHO encouraged the LHJ staff to take the lead in these discussions with the county about the proposed network. Topics addressed at this meeting included security concerns, funding issues, and support issues. The deliverables from the LHJ and county meetings were a high-level project plan, identification of staff to be involved and their project roles, a high level design, and a tentative project schedule.

The LHJ and county meeting included the management and information systems staff from the county and from the LHJ. This meeting focused on development of a cooperative approach to implementing INPHO within the county and the LHJ. If the county already had a network plan, INPHO insured that any work being done would build into or compliment the county's plan.

The Technical Meeting

The technical meeting included the INPHO team and LHJ and county technical staff. This meeting focused on development of an implementation plan for the WAN configuration in that county and for the interconnectedness of the physical computer networks. It created a detailed network design, including a list of hardware and software that needed to be purchased. The INPHO team approached these meetings with the intention of permitting the LHJ and the county to own the resulting county network. Accordingly, INPHO was not rigid about the LAN components or the configuration; INPHO gave the LHJ the freedom to choose hardware and software that the LHJ staff would be comfortable with. The only requirements from the INPHO team were that the LHJ adhere to the state standard TCP/IP (Transmission Control Protocol/Internet Protocol) protocol for its connection to the WAN for security reasons and that the e-mail system use Simple Mail Transport Protocol (SMTP). This flexibility allowed the LHJ to plan its network around its needs, with positive results. Some LHJs had sophisticated network plans already in place, whereas others were using stand-alone computers that were not on a network at all. The INPHO team tailored the amount of advice and help that it provided to the needs and situation of the individual LHJ.

After completion of this series of planning meetings, the INPHO project was considered to be under way in each county. At this point, actual orders for equipment were placed, staff members were trained, and implementation began. INPHO tracked the progress of the LAN setup and the WAN connection.

Resources

The INPHO project was initiated through a grant from CDC ($1.8 million over three years) in 1994. The original estimates for the project were about $4 million for initial implementation and $1.6 million a year to maintain the WAN. WSDOH also estimated an additional $1.5 million a year for LAN support. The Washington State legislature, through Washington's Public Health Improvement Plan, awarded $2 million for LHJ technology capacity development.

This allocation left a very big question as to who would pay the $1.6 million annual maintenance. WSDOH approached the Office of Financial Management (OFM) with a proposal to include the annual maintenance cost as part of the Justice Information Network that OFM was coordinating the feasibility of developing. OFM requested that WSDOH coordinate the INPHO effort with the Washington State Department of Information Services (DIS). WSDOH and DIS broached the idea of building INPHO as a shared network with the counties. DIS agreed to partner with WSDOH in this effort, which became the beginning of the Washington IGN. DIS would eventually take responsibility for maintenance of the network. Today, the use and maintenance of the network costs WSDOH only $124,000 a year. Training of county and/or LHJ staff to maintain the LAN environments resulted in elimination of the $1.5 million per year that WSDOH would otherwise need to allocate to LAN support.

Network Ownership

Throughout the development and ongoing support of the network, the ownership has changed. The LHJs, with WSDOH approval, purchased the LAN equipment and software, while WSDOH reimbursed the LHJs for their expenditures. This arrangement gave ownership and responsibility for the LAN equipment and software to the LHJs. This approach was well received. It allowed the LHJs to expand or modify their networks as part of their own network infrastructures without permission from the state. WSDOH maintained ownership of the WAN and equipment, insuring that the WAN would remain a sharable resource.

Once the network was successfully implemented, WSDOH negotiated with the Washington State Department of Information Services to transfer ownership of the WAN components to DIS. In turn, DIS agreed to allow WSDOH to use the network free for a period of two years. At the end of the two years, the INPHO network officially became the Washington State IGN. The WAN components that became the IGN were only those used to connect the county's primary network to the state. Other WAN components that connected LHJ remote offices to the counties were not included in the IGN. Ownership of these WAN components was given to the counties, so that the components would become part of the county's own network infrastructure.

Maintenance

The IGN support is being provided by the DIS, which is charging costs back to the users of the network. The counties entered an agreement that if they would house the IGN equipment and provide very minimal level support for it, they would be provided two years of free service. This agreement expired in June 1999, and today the counties are paying for their own usage.

Informatics

With the implementation of INPHO, public health in Washington has begun to use technology in everyday life, with applications ranging from e-mail to securing basic information about current events to conducting research. Smaller LHJs that, in the past, were left out of public health discussions surrounding legislation, budgets, and public health planning are now brought to the table through electronic discussion groups. Web-based training is becoming very affordable and available for staff who cannot usually leave the local health offices because of staffing needs and financial concerns. Though the network in itself is not the answer to spreading the knowledge of informatics, it is certainly an enabling technology.

Project Organization

The INPHO steering committee directed the overall activities of the project. This committee was made up of the WSDOH Secretary, a state health officer, a representative from the OFM, a representative from the DIS, a WSDOH Health Liaison Manager, the WSDOH Information Technology Director, the WSDOH Management Services Assistant Secretary, and the INPHO Project Manager and a Project Technical Coordinator.

The INPHO Workgroup was made up of staff from UW, from several LHJs, and from the WSDOH program staff.

This group worked on training issues, the design of the Web pages, e-mail, and listserves.

The full time INPHO project team consisted of only three staff members: the project manager, the project technical coordinator, and the technical expert.

Technology Used

The WAN was made up of T-1 frame-relay circuits with a committed information rate of 384 KB. TCP/IP is the only protocol allowed natively on the network. There are certain applications in use that tunnel other protocols within TCP/IP, though such tunneling is discouraged. Each county has a Cisco router for connecting to the WAN. The Cisco router is initially configured to prevent all inbound traffic except e-mail from accessing a county's network.

Lessons Learned by the INPHO Team

During the experience of implementing INPHO, project team members learned many valuable lessons. Some of these lessons are listed and discussed below.

Always Stay Focused on the Vision

The INPHO vision is to provide all public health officials access to authoritative, timely, accurate information. There are many roads to achieving this destination, but there are also some dead ends. INPHO tried to be as flexible as possible when it came to accommodating the county's technical preferences. When dealing with different technologies and approaches to connecting the LHJs to the network, INPHO made it very clear that the only thing that was not negotiable was that the LHJs would have access to authoritative, timely, accurate information. This information may be residing at the CDC in Atlanta, at the state health department, at other LHJs in Washington, or out on the Internet. The vision became the guiding principle in all INPHO activities.

Use Proven Technology, but Not Old Technology

When INPHO began, frame-relay technology for high-speed WANs was just emerging. The technology was proven to work well, and in many cases it cost significantly less for the same throughput as the traditional dedicated T-1 circuits. INPHO chose to use frame-relay technology, and this decision was well accepted by the county's technical staff because it was a new but proven technology. At the LAN level, we recommended that the counties use either the latest version of Novell's Netware or Microsoft's NT Server as their network operating systems.

Use National Standards but Avoid the Holy Wars

INPHO chose to use the basic Internet standards for communicating throughout the network. The SMTP was used for all external e-mail. TCP/IP was selected as the only protocol that would be allowed on the WAN, though tunneling of other protocols within TCP/IP was permitted if there was an application that required other protocols. INPHO chose not to attempt to set platform standards at the county level, though from a support and training standpoint, it would be more efficient to pick a standard LAN operating system and a single e-mail package. One reason for INPHO's decision to avoid imposing an operating system on local users is that there are very strong opinions and biases, especially when it comes to views of predominant vendors. For example, many prospective users were true Microsoft believers and steadfast Novell advocates, but there were also Macintosh and IBM supporters. INPHO avoided these "holy wars," because project team members believed that local resistance to attempting to set standards in these areas might have prevented achievement of the INPHO vision.

Each LHJ and County Is Unique: Avoid
Stereotyping in the Assessment of Needs

Making assumptions about a county's technical capability, political makeup, and needs based on size, fiscal status, or geography is dangerous. After all, it is the people and priorities that determine the technical capabilities and needs of a county. Politics, in fact, played a major part in INPHO's technical designs for the county portions of the networks. In Washington State, all LHJs are at the county level. But in many cases, effectively providing for public health in the communities required LHJs to maintain strong ties to the cities and their political structures.

The INPHO team made it a point to try to go into each jurisdiction without a preconceived notion of what to expect in terms of politics, technical ability, or the jurisdiction's desires. This objective approach paid dividends. Confounding stereotypical conceptions, INPHO team members found that some small counties had highly qualified technical staff and very solid information technology infrastructures, whereas other, larger counties lagged far behind in technological capacity. In addition, the relationship between the LHJ and a county was a key factor in determining how to approach the design and implementation of the project. In the best cases, the LHJ and the county IT staff had very good relationships, and cooperation was easy. In other cases, the LHJ and county staff actually disliked one another. In yet another case involving a large city, the LHJ did not want to partner with the county for fear that the city might feel alienated. Avoiding preconceptions about an LHJ's needs allowed the INPHO staff to identify such political and relational factors, and these factors in turn became crucial to the design and support structure for a network.

Politics Count and Are to Be Ignored Only at a Project's Peril

Ignoring the politics associated with a network project is like driving at high speed with your eyes closed. A "driver" may get lucky and progress for a while without an accident, but the odds are that he or she will come to a very unpleasant stop. Thus, understanding the history of the relationship between the county and the state is important. Knowing what has happened between a county and a state in the past and being sure to address resultant concerns are ways to insure that a project will not be negatively impacted by history. INPHO ran into several situations in which state agencies had come into a county office, installed a PC for a specific job function, and left without making provisions for local staff training or for support. The result was massive confusion—of the person with the PC left on his or her desk, and, even more so, of the county IT staff members expected to furnish the support. In other cases, state staff had loaded software on a county PC, changed the configuration, and left without ever notifying the county IT staff of the purpose and nature of the change.

In light of this history, INPHO made a commitment to the county IT staff never to make any changes to a PC or to a network without notifying IT staff in advance and updating it when changes were accomplished.

The INPHO team also designed technical solutions to mitigate some of the political situations. For instance, INPHO always made sure that county officers understood the public health nature of the project and that the LHJ was funding this project. Permitting the LHJ to become a source of project funds through WSDOH reimbursement became important to political acceptance of the project. Typically, an LHJ accounts for 1–3% of the overall county budget, while the criminal justice system typically makes up over 70%. The needs of the criminal justice system obviously take priority over public health needs. INPHO's decision to allow the LHJ to provide the funds to the county for the project put the LHJ in control. This solution was especially effective in the situations in which the political relationship between the county and the LHJ was poor. In the cases involving a large county and large cities, housing the WAN equipment in the LHJ provided the LHJ with leverage. Although the WAN remained part of the county's infrastructure and a means of connecting to the county network, the fact that the WAN equipment was housed in the LHJ left no doubt about ownership of the equipment and who was in control. In King County (Seattle is in King County), it took nine separate meetings with different groups and individuals to design a network architecture that was acceptable to everyone involved.

A Legislature Can Make a Liar Out of You in a Hurry

Throughout the implementation of INPHO, funding was always a tenuous issue. It was a given that the federal funds would not continue. INPHO team members had approval for state funds to underwrite operational costs for two years after the network was completed. INPHO had been telling the LHJs and counties about the funding arrangements and emphasizing that after two years of operations, funding was uncertain; at the same time, the LHJs would always have the option of paying for INPHO costs or else disconnecting.

However, the Washington State legislature developed other ideas. The 1997 legislature decided that the state should not be paying for a network that supported the counties. Accordingly, the legislature pulled the funding two years early. INPHO was not given an opportunity to explain that the network was primarily for the use of the state and that the counties were using it to access state systems. With the support of the Department of Information Services and the State Department of Health, the portion of the network that connected to the state was sustained by the state for the additional two years. The portion of the network that was used only by the counties was left to the counties to support. The counties begrudgingly did pay for those parts of the network.

Build It to Last

During the project, INPHO team members learned that, when building a system, staff should use quality equipment and software. Wherever possible, the system should be built so as to avoid or minimize ongoing costs. For example, in many cases, using fiber optic cable for connections is expensive up front, but the added growth capacity and the minimization or elimination of recurring costs make use of fiber optic cable very attractive. INPHO also used microwave for connecting offices in cases in which fiber was too expensive and a line of sight existed. Microwave proved to be not quite as reliable and maintenance-free as fiber, but it was substantially less expensive than data circuits, and it provided LAN speed bandwidth.

The Major Lesson Learned for the Informatics Practitioner

For the practitioner of the discipline of informatics, there is a major lesson stemming from the INPHO project: *Stay focused on the public health problem to be addressed by a project.* It is easy for people to get caught up in cool technology and to lose focus on the actual public health problem to be solved. However, it is essential for a public health practitioner to recognize that technology is a means, not an end. One experience of the INPHO project team illustrates this important principle. The first INPHO Web site was designed with a really attractive graphic that was very public health-oriented and featured links to several public health sites. The group that designed it was quite proud of it. The first training session that was given to an LHJ was going really well. The trainers were using the new Web page to show the LHJ staff how to surf the Web, and the participants were excited. Then one of the LHJ staff commented, "This is really cool, but how do I address the real questions we get every day? Today, I'm being asked, can a person use Hartz 1-3 flea shampoo to get rid of head lice on their children?" This one comment made the Web design group eliminate the "cool" graphics and instead develop a Web page that was much more information-driven.

The Future of These Types of Systems

We believe that the market for large networking projects for public health will diminish over time. As networks are constructed by use of nonproprietary technology and in particular by use of TCP/IP, the need for more networks will diminish while the need for increased network speed will continually rise. With the availability of new high-speed Internet connections such as cable modems and with digital subscriber lines (DSLs) becoming available to more and more remote communities, the emphasis will switch from connecting people to networks to providing services in a secure manner over existing networks. Many of the challenges addressed in this chapter will continue to be challenges, however. We will still face the challenges of the lack of trust between government entities, of making the technology fit into the day-to-day business practices of public health, and of fear of abuse of the Internet and of data and information. A major challenge for the future will be gaining the trust of the citizenry that government can provide systems that are easy to use, efficient, and convenient while also protecting personal data. One technology that will be a major player in public health's addressing this challenge is the Public Key Infrastructure (see Chapter 10).

Advancing Technologies That Will Change the Way Public Health Systems Operate: Public Key Infrastructure

The use of Public Key Infrastructure (PKI), in particular the use of digital signatures for authenticating users, is going to play a huge role in how public health will conduct business over networks. By focusing on authenticating people and securing information over the network, PKI will reduce the need for dependency on secure WANs and instead focus security closer to the source of the data. Networks will need to focus on increasing bandwidth and reliability to address the increasing use of multi-media and other forms of information sharing.

Questions for Review

1. Explain how access to the Internet paved the way for LHJs to be receptive to the INPHO project. What were the primary concerns of the LHJs with regard to access to the Internet?
2. Why did counties develop such mistrust of state agencies and agency systems?
3. Explain how the ingenuity of WSDOH staff helped to overcome obstacles posed by the poor telecommunications infrastructure in rural areas.

4. To what extent did counties and LHJs actually pay for the networks made possible by the INPHO project?
5. Explain the development process used by INPHO in working with each LHJ and county individually. What were the components of this process?
6. Why was it important for the INPHO team to leave most decisions regarding LAN components and configuration to the LHJs? What were the only requirements imposed on LHJs by the INPHO project, and why were these requirements important to the success of the project?
7. How did the INPHO project solve the problem of securing resources to underwrite the estimated $1.6 million in annual maintenance?
8. Why was an arrangement set up whereby the LHJs purchased LAN equipment and software and WSDOH reimbursed the LHJs? Why didn't WSDOH merely purchase the equipment and software directly?
9. How was staying focused on the vision for INPHO translated into action by the INPHO project team?
10. In what way did the INPHO project use national standards and avoid the "holy wars"?
11. Why was it valuable, indeed crucial, for the INPHO team to approach each jurisdiction without a preconceived notion of jurisdictional politics, technical ability, or desires and needs?
12. In what sense did recognizing the political environment surrounding the LHJs become important to the INPHO project's success?

27
The Community Health Information Movement: Where It's Been, Where It's Going

RICHARD D. RUBIN

All my life's a circle, sunrise and sundown.

— *"Circle," Harry Chapin, 1972*

Learning Objectives

After studying this chapter, you should be able to:

- Explain the reasons that community health information activities have been the focal point of the personal healthcare industry.
- Describe the history of the community health information movement.
- Understand the problems that prevented the successful implementation of previous community health information systems and describe possible future successful implementation strategies.

Overview

The history and evolution of the community health information movement can be considered a case study. Beginning with the Community Health Management Information System, an initiative of the John A. Hartford Foundation, and continuing through failed efforts to form community health information networks (CHINs), the movement has essentially progressed in a circular fashion, returning to its original starting point. The lessons learned from the long history of failures provide a blueprint for those who would succeed in providing community health information services. These lessons include the requirement to focus on information needs rather than wants; the importance of establishing information services on a business basis; as the model for building CHIN collaboration must fit in a competitive framework, recognition of the importance of defining roles clearly; the need to narrow the scope of community health information initiatives; and the acknowledgement that the privacy of health information as a legitimate concern. Ultimately, the success of the community health information movement resides in forming partnerships among health enterprises, vendors, and community groups. A few organizations are already encountering success with this model. Public health organizations can benefit substantially from becoming partners in such community health information initiatives.

Introduction

Circuitous is a very appropriate term to describe the meanderings of the community health information movement over the last 10 years. The movement has undergone various transformations, from community utility to public sector panacea to commercial network to reviled failure to dot.com dream and back to a community tool. The community health information movement has experienced highs, lows, and everything in between.

Examining this movement in the context of public health is a somewhat problematic proposition. At first glance, the phrase *community health information* sounds tailor-made for public health. If you knew nothing more than the name, you might assume this movement had been created and driven by public health to serve community needs. In fact, the community health information activities, as defined below, have largely been outside the province of public health. Public health has been an occasional participant, but rarely a driving force. It is the personal healthcare industry that has been the focal point for most community health information initiatives.

If there is one word to account for the prominence of personal health over public health in community health information activities, that word is *money*. Monetary issues have driven much of the community health information movement over the last decade. Most efforts were concerned with profit making or else they were designed to reduce the cost of care and/or administration. In either case, the personal health services industry was a far more lucrative target than the public health sector. Despite this emphasis, the community health information movement is an important area of study for public health professionals. The lessons learned over the past decade in trying to make a collaborative community-based program work are directly applicable to public health, which so often works in a similar environment. Also, public health professionals will have to find creative ways to leverage the information technology investments of the personal health industry if they wish to meet their own needs. Along these lines, this chapter will review the history of the movement, profile selected community health information activities, discuss specific issues of interest to public health, and speculate on future directions for the movement.

Definitions

Before proceeding further, it is important to narrow the scope of this chapter by defining terminology. The place to begin is with *community*. *Community* is a very familiar term to public health practitioners. It is used both to describe a collection of people bound by geography and those bound by a shared characteristic (e.g., disease or ethnicity). For the purposes of this discussion, *community* refers to the collection of individuals and organizations that comprise the health services market in a given geographic area. This definition deliberately encompasses a broad range of possibilities. The geography can be statewide, regional, or local. The market participants can include some or all of the stakeholders.

Like community, *health information* covers a vast landscape. For the purposes of this discussion, health information includes any data related to population or personal health services. Although many of the efforts that will be examined focus on a relatively narrow scope of data, there is no per se requirement to exclude any specific information from consideration.

There are a variety of terms appended to *community health information*. The most common is *network*. A community health information network is often referred to as a CHIN. This acronym is sometimes used to characterize all community health information activity. As will be discussed below, *CHIN* has a more specific meaning.

Finally, the term *movement* will also be used in conjunction with community health information. Although there are a variety of organizations that sprang up to address community health information activities of many types, there is no formal, exclusive, organized national collective of those organizations involved in community health information activities. The movement, as defined in these pages, refers simply to those individuals and organizations that have a self-declared interest in community health information activities.

History

To understand the current state of the community health information movement, it is first necessary to review the history.

Community Health Management Information System

The community health information movement could be said to have begun in 1990. That was the year the John A. Hartford Foundation, a private philanthropy based in New York City, first debuted its Community Health Management Information System (CHMIS) initiative. Under the leadership of its Program Director, Richard Sharpe, the Hartford Foundation had invested heavily in a variety of efforts to better manage health cost and quality. These programs were generally targeted at measuring some dimension of performance, identifying a path to improvement, and then applying this knowledge to drive change. Researchers, consumers, providers, purchasers, and payers were all involved in these programs to varying degrees.

In assessing the challenges faced by grantees in the cost and quality management program, Sharpe identified a common concern—lack of data. Across all domains, for all users, it was very difficult to make significant progress because the data needed to measure some dimension of performance was not readily accessible. Assessing performance, of course, is a prerequisite for improving performance. Therefore, Sharpe believed that the healthcare system would be unable to significantly improve performance in the cost or quality domains unless and until data could be made readily available to users. Specifically, Sharpe envisioned a blended data set that included claims data, selected clinical information, and demographics. When aggregated across a given community, this database could be used to assess population health, provider performance, effectiveness of selected treatments, cost and utilization of services, and a variety of other key performance measures.

Sharpe believed there was only one way to collect and aggregate this complex data set in a cost-effective manner. That was to create a robust electronic transaction processing system for the health industry similar to the information infrastructure enjoyed by the banking and financial services industry. This system would be known as the Community Health Management Information System, or CHMIS. CHMIS was to be comprised of three key components:

1. *The organization.* CHMIS was assumed to cover a given geography, usually a state. The CHMIS organization was a collaborative body drawn from key stakeholders in the health community. While the organization was open to all, it was to be controlled by the demand side, consisting of purchasers and consumers. Demand-side control was seen as necessary to convince reluctant providers and payers to participate and share data. The organization was to govern and operate the system and establish rules for participation.
2. *The transaction system.* CHMIS envisioned an electronic network that carried transaction flows between health industry trading partners. The network would be built and operated by contractors hired by the organization and funded by fees on the transactions. As the transactions moved across the network, data elements would be extracted and shipped to the data repository.
3. *The data repository.* The heart of CHMIS was the data repository. This was a massive central database fed by the transaction system and governed by the organization. Subject to privacy and security limitations, the data repository would be accessible to all members of the community who wished to mine the information.

Although the details have changed over the years, the three basic components of CHMIS have endured and continue to this day to guide developers of community health information initiatives. These three basic components are now:

1. A community of stakeholders who agree to participate in a system and abide by rules in exchange for the benefits of connectivity.

2. An electronic network that links trading partners, facilitates information exchange, and enhances communication.
3. Aggregating and sharing information across enterprises to improve performance (these days, it is more likely to be virtual aggregation rather than physical).

In early 1991, the Hartford Foundation made a series of initial grants to community groups in Iowa, New York, Tennessee, and Washington State. Eventually, by the mid-1990s, the CHMIS grant program supported seven community sites directly (Minnesota, Ohio, and Vermont were added to the original group) and many other communities indirectly.

CHMIS was the first organized effort to advance the concept that health services stakeholders could be connected across enterprises (inter-enterprise.) Prior to CHMIS, the focus of health information networking had been either intra-enterprise or limited to a specific subset of the stakeholders. The Hartford Foundation and its grantees spent a great deal of time in the early 1990s promoting the CHMIS concept across the nation and within the health industry. In 1992, the CHMIS specifications were published jointly by the Foundation, by the sites, and by Benton International, a consulting firm retained by the Foundation. This detailed CHMIS design provoked a great deal of interest and opposition.

The key distinguishing aspect of CHMIS was the data repository. The transaction system was seen as a means to an end—populating the repository. This concept was very different from many following efforts that focused much more heavily on networking and administrative simplification. The data-centric focus was one of the major challenges the CHMIS initiative faced. Although many in the health services community were intrigued by the concept of linking the stakeholders electronically, they raised the following concerns:

Proprietary Data

For those on the supply side, the idea that their performance was going to be profiled based on data gathered by the repository was a significant problem. Concerns ranged from fears of being competitively disadvantaged to problems with methodology and fairness. The data-driven aspect of CHMIS, linked to a focus on performance, alienated many on the supply side.

Demand-Side Control

Supply-side concerns about performance profiling were exacerbated by the demand-side control over the governing organization. It felt to some industry participants as if CHMIS was being done to them rather than with them.

Privacy

Whereas the supply side was concerned with competitive issues, privacy advocates were worried about the confidentiality of personal health information. The potential threat to privacy posed by aggregating health information was profound. The CHMIS sites and the Hartford Foundation acknowledged this concern and worked aggressively with the privacy community to address concerns. Although the issue was mitigated over time, it never went away.

Feasibility

The CHMIS initiative arose prior to the Internet revolution. Many of the technology people in health services liked the concept, but they questioned whether it could ever be achieved. Technical, financial, and political constraints were all identified. In particular, the nonstandardized, heterogeneous hodgepodge of disparate information systems present in most healthcare communities seemed an insurmountable barrier to seamless connectivity. In some sense, the very grandeur of the CHMIS idea was its major failing. To many, CHMIS was seen as too big to be true.

The Public Sector: Health Care Reform

As CHMIS geared up in the early 1990s, it shared the stage with another more prominent movement, health care reform. At the national and the state level, reformers zealously attempted to solve the myriad problems afflicting the health system. Some reform initiatives were market-based; most, however, were more oriented to the public sector and the power of legislation and regulation. Cost and access were the focus of most reform initiatives. However, many of these efforts included health information on the reform agenda.

In many respects, the health care reform movement was stillborn. The action never matched the rhetoric, and the failures of the Clinton reform plan in 1993–1994 dissipated much of the movement's energy. However, a few states did enact comprehensive reform bills and included health information to some degree. Not coincidentally, three of the CHMIS states, Washington, Vermont, and Minnesota, were among the group that passed legislation.

The public sector community health information efforts varied considerably, as did the rest of reform packages. Minnesota created a public-private partnership, the Minnesota Health Data Institute (MHDI) that still exists today. Vermont addressed the health information issue at more of a conceptual level and had not really implemented much when the law was swept away in the health care reform backlash of the mid-1990s. The Washington State health information proposal was the most comprehensive and far-reaching, and it is the one that will be discussed here.

The 1993 Health Care Reform Act in Washington State was extraordinarily comprehensive. It totally reworked the state's health system. The law has been described as "Clintonesque," in that it was similar to the proposals advanced by the President. One component of the law, passed in April 1993, was the Health Services Information System (HSIS). Not surprisingly, HSIS was also very comprehensive in nature. A la CHMIS, the heart of the system was a comprehensive data repository that would be used by the state to assess and control the healthcare marketplace. Others would also be granted access to the data, as appropriate to meet their health information needs. A transaction system was assumed, and in place of the CHMIS organization, HSIS would be governed by the state.

Between 1993, when HSIS was created, and 1995, when it was repealed along with most of the rest of the reform law, the state Department of Health in concert with the state Health Services Commission engaged in extensive planning work. Everything from financing to data sets to privacy was assigned to committees for consideration and review. It is hard to assess HSIS in isolation. HSIS was part and parcel of the 1993 Act and therefore was subject to all the complex political currents that buffeted the short-lived bill. However, it is instructive to examine why HSIS struggled. Some of the concerns were similar to CHMIS:

Data Aggregation

Even though it was the state gathering the data rather than a private community group, many were horrified at the thought of a giant central repository. This was one issue about which the right wing and the left wing shared a common view. Both segments of the political spectrum were alarmed at the thought of the state's possessing a data resource of this magnitude. The privacy issue was perhaps the single biggest factor in the demise of HSIS.

Feasibility

HSIS was also too big to be true to most people. Furthermore, the technologists in the health industry were even more skeptical of the state's ability to pull it off than they were of CHMIS.

Funding

HSIS was essentially an unfunded mandate. The law required HSIS to come into existence, but there was very little state money budgeted to bring the system about. A specific funding source was not identified in the controlling legislation. It was presumed that the private sector would build the system. However, the private sector had little interest in spending money to achieve public sector data gathering objectives.

Going into the 1995 legislative session, HSIS was on life support. By the end of the 1995 session, the legislature mercifully put HSIS out of its misery. HSIS was the high-water mark for comprehensive community health information initiatives undertaken by the public sector. As will be described later in this chapter, other public sector efforts of more modest scope continued. However, the mid-1990s marked the beginning and the end of the states' efforts to implement CHMIS-like systems.

CHIN

There were members of the community health information movement who were quite taken by the network aspects of CHMIS but were alienated by its data-centric focus. This wing of the movement saw community health information initiatives as primarily a means to forge communication links among health industry stakeholders and to simplify administration. Members of this movement deliberately excluded any concept of a central database. In fact, it was an article of faith among this group that data owners must keep full control over their information if the community effort was to be successful. This wing of the community health information movement can be broadly characterized as CHINs.

CHINs were the natural heirs to the CHMIS vision. They had learned from the struggles of the CHMIS movement and the failures of the public sector. Although CHINs varied enormously across communities, they can still be said to have some common design elements, as shown in Table 27.1.

CHINs enjoyed quite a heyday from 1994 to 1996. There was even a CHIN trade association, the Comnet Society. Every conference on health information networking featured CHINs. Comnet estimated that over 500 CHIN-like entities existed across the country.[1] (Coment's numbers were never fully validated and should be viewed with caution.) Some saw CHINs as the salvation

TABLE 27.1. Common design elements of CHINs

Design Element	Characteristics
Ownership	CHINs were largely driven by the supply side. Hospitals, integrated delivery systems, health plans, and trade associations all sponsored CHINs in one geography or another. Consumers, government, and purchasers were largely absent from the CHIN movement.
Commercial involvement	CHINs were very much a commercial undertaking. Major health information technology companies actively pursued the CHIN business. Ameritech, IBM, several major banks, and others staked out the CHIN market as theirs. In some cases, the vendor sponsored the CHIN. In other cases, they worked for a community group sponsoring the initiative.
Network-centric	Consistent with the name, CHINs were oriented around networking solutions rather than databases. Linking trading partners and exchanging information was the key goal. Reduced costs of administration were the major selling point. Some saw the CHINs as *the* community network. Others saw them as a network-of-networks that would tie together rather than replace enterprise networks. The latter view was more common among CHIN proponents.

of the industry. However, like CHMIS, even during the high times, there were many doubters. The anti-CHIN faction made the following arguments:

Feasibility

The focus might be different, but CHINs had done little to solve the endemic networking problems of the health industry that had foiled CHMIS. The absence of standards, a proliferation of proprietary products, and old legacy systems made common connectivity horrendously expensive. Few were willing to pay such a price.

Politics

Taking the demand side away removed the onus of being pressured from above. However, constituting governing bodies with supply-side stakeholders effectively meant putting competitors together around the table. This created a complex set of political agendas.

Trust

To move forward with a CHIN, enterprises were effectively being asked to entrust mission-critical information systems to cumbersome cooperative groups. This left many chief information officers and chief executive officers feeling queasy. They were not confident the CHIN could execute.

The Inward Focus

One component of the CHIN debate was less about the "how" of the CHIN and more related to why. A number of the naysayers questioned the whole premise of inter-enterprise connectivity. They took the position that all they needed to do was wire up the stakeholders behind their four walls, and that would be that. They saw no business rationale for inter-enterprise connectivity.

By late 1995 and early 1996, the CHIN movement was in serious trouble. High-profile CHINs, Chicago being the best example, were flailing and failing. Comnet was struggling, and the organization eventually closed down. The major CHIN vendors reduced or terminated their involvement in the industry. As fast as the CHIN movement had risen, it now crashed. To this day, a CHIN is a metaphor to many for a big, expensive failure. It is not at all uncommon for a community health information initiative sponsor to start off describing his or her effort by insisting, "We're *not* a CHIN."

Enter the Internet

The community health information movement was in serious jeopardy. CHMIS, the public sector, and CHINs had all sounded great in their promises and then failed to deliver much of substance. The intra-enterprise advocates were saying, "I told you so." The movement was at best moribund. Most

community stakeholders did not see a need for a community health information infrastructure. Those that did see the need could not see a way to make it
happen. Then, a new trend emerged that changed everything—the Internet.

The Internet revolution has been thoroughly documented and chronicled.
This chapter will not revisit this subject. Suffice it to say that the importance
of the Internet revolution to the community health information movement
cannot be overstated. The rapid deployment and adoption of Internet technology rescued the movement from the brink and offered immediate benefits:

Taking the "Why" Question off the Table

Community health information advocates spent much of their time on "mis-
sionary" work. They needed to convince increasingly skeptical healthcare
communities that connectivity would and should happen. As long as the
debate raged around the why question, little concrete progress could be made
on implementation. By the end of 1997, the long-running debate of inter-
enterprise versus intra-enterprise had been decisively resolved in favor of
inter-enterprise. It was clear that simply connecting up within the four walls
of the enterprise would not cut it in a "wired" world. The Internet was demonstrating the benefits of the seamless network the "community" missionaries
had always described.

Providing the Means

Although the primary struggles of the movement to date were more political
than technological, the absence of a means to execute the vision, even for
those who were convinced of the need, was problematic. Internet technology
offered a relatively cheap, increasingly ubiquitous, standards-based means to
link community stakeholders. The Internet answered the most important aspect of the "how" question. It was clear that some form of Internet technology
was going to be the ultimate community health information network.

Leveraging Investment

For a community health information initiative to succeed, there had to be a
supporting infrastructure. Individual enterprises had to invest in automation,
move data from paper to electronic form, and train and provide incentives for
users. The lure and the promise of the Internet brought forth significant levels
of information infrastructure investment. Hospitals, health plans, physicians,
and government began to see health information technology as a key strategic investment. Similarly, on the commercial side, risk capital began to flow
to the healthcare information technology (IT) vendor community.

This convergence of the Internet and the community health information
movement spawned a new breed of initiatives. Tyler Chin, of Faulkner &
Gray, described them as "CHINInternets" (T. Chin, personal communication,

1997). These initiatives have seized on the promise of the Internet in many different ways to meet the shared health information needs of their communities. In many cases, the sponsors of these efforts explicitly acknowledged the problems of the past and sought to build their new models on a firm foundation of lessons learned. Before reviewing specific initiatives, it is helpful to consider the key lessons learned.

Lessons Learned in the Community Health Information Movement

As can be seen from the history described, there were many lessons to learn from the CHMIS, CHIN, and public sector experience. Although the learning experience varied across markets, it is possible to distill a set of the most salient lessons that seem to predominate in all settings:

- *The need to differentiate between needs and wants and to target needs.* A *want* is defined as something nice to have. A *need* is something that someone will pay for. Targeting needs is critical. Even in the not-for-profit environment, someone has to pay in order for progress to be made. Many of the community health information initiatives that failed never adequately appreciated the distinction between needs and wants. They generated considerable excitement by discussing all the functionality that frustrated health industry stakeholders had long wanted but were largely unwilling to invest in. Then, when the call came for funds, the sponsors heard the refrain, "I assumed someone else would pay for it." These initiatives ended up trying to fulfill big dreams with small budgets, a recipe for failure. Savvy community health information operators have learned to cut through the wants and to focus on the needs.
- *The need to build the business case for a concept.* Much of the early work in the community health information movement was related to sharing the vision. The need was so profound that it seemed more important to solve the systematic problems rather than quibble over how to fund the solutions. This ignored the day-to-day reality faced by the enterprises participating in the community endeavor. These enterprises faced demands for IT solutions well out of proportion to the budget dollars available to fund them. The enterprises tended to prioritize those solutions that addressed urgent needs and could be justified on a business basis. To secure community investment required a clear delineation of the benefits that will be generated. Long-term vision might inspire, but a good return on investment is more likely to engender support and participation.
- *The need to focus on more than a network.* Prior to the Internet revolution, most of the community health information initiatives focused most of their energies on developing a network capability. The emergence of Internet technology as a network solution allowed community organizers to expand their vision. Whereas some community groups leveraged Internet

technology to deploy private networks (Intranets or Extranets), many other groups focused their energies in other complementary areas—for example, development and implementation of standards, security and privacy practices, education and training, applications, etc. The presence of Internet technology has freed the community health information movement to go beyond CHINs and offer more than just a network.

- *The need to use the competitive versus the collaborative model.* Idealists in the community health information movement cherished the hope that much of the health information infrastructure would be built on a cooperative basis. The growth of the commercial IT sector has proven this belief false. In addition, many of the enterprises that comprise the local health services community have their own electronic strategy. These enterprises are not looking to either a community group or a commercial entity to meet their needs. Rather, they plan to do it themselves. In fact, many of these enterprises explicitly reject a collaborative strategy because they see their electronic-health (e-health) initiatives as a means to competitively distinguish themselves. This has forced community health information groups to acknowledge a fundamental truth: most of the health information infrastructure will be built under the competitive model. The challenge for community groups is to prioritize those limited collaborative components of the overall infrastructure that most effectively leverage and support the competitive investments being made.
- *The need to define roles.* The early community health information initiatives perceived the need to "do it all." They saw few ready partners at hand and assumed that if they did not address a key component of the community infrastructure, it would not get built. To some degree, this perception placed community groups into a competitive situation with others working to achieve similar objectives. As the movement matured, community groups recognized that they could not and should not attempt to build the entire health information infrastructure. There are roles for many different types of players. Linking and leveraging the amalgam of talent and resources devoted to improving the health information infrastructure makes far more sense then working at cross-purposes. The community groups need the enterprises, and vendors to be successful in their work. The vendors and enterprises can accelerate what they are trying to achieve with the help of the community groups. Clearly defining roles and constantly seeking to build and strengthen partnerships are now seen as crucial aspects of the work of a community health information group.
- *The need to narrow project scope and to avoid creeping incrementalism.* Trying to live down the claim of being "too big to be true" has dogged many of the more ambitious community health information efforts. Focus has become an important element of success. Most current community health information initiatives have narrowed the scope of their work considerably from the halcyon days of CHMIS. Taking slow, measured, clearly defined steps that address urgent business needs of key stakeholders

is widely seen as the most likely path to success for community health information initiatives.

* *The need to address privacy matters.* The concerns about health information privacy first encountered by CHMIS have continued to proliferate. The gradual automation of the health industry, coupled with highly publicized security failures, have sensitized many policy makers, media people, and ordinary consumers to the need to protect the privacy of personal health information. For many people, their health records are the most sensitive data they have. Although the community health information movement has always seen itself as a force for social good, privacy advocates see any aggregation of health information as a potential threat. Privacy and security concerns are here to stay, at least for the immediate future. Addressing these concerns is both an obligation and an opportunity for the movement.

The Community Health Information Movement in Action

The lessons described are best understood in the context of specific initiatives. Listed below are six leading community health information initiatives. Together, these six organizations illustrate the past, present, and future of the community health information movement.

Minnesota Health Data Institute

The Minnesota Health Data Institute (MHDI) is a unique public/private partnership in the state of Minnesota. MHDI operates as a private, not-for-profit organization; yet, it was created by the Minnesota legislature in 1993. The 21-member board, comprised of purchasers, providers, payers, the public sector, and consumers, works closely with the Minnesota Commissioner of Health to accomplish its mission:

> "To design and implement an integrated state wide health care data system to support the information needs of health care consumers, purchasers, providers, payers, policymakers, and researchers in measuring and improving the quality and efficiency of health care services in Minnesota."[2]

MHDI has programs in quality measurement, electronic commerce, and privacy. MHDI has lived through the evolution of the community health information movement. It was originally a CHMIS site, and it sought to execute its mission on the comprehensive scope of the CHMIS vision. However, early on, the community leaders recognized that the full-scale CHMIS approach would not work in Minnesota. They sought instead to create a CHIN-like approach. Their solution was a private Intranet called MedNet.[2]

MedNet sought to match the community governance of CHMIS with the "network-of-networks" CHIN concept.

MedNet was not designed to be the sole network in the community. It was envisioned as a means to link the existing networks of key health care enterprises. MedNet enjoyed early success as some of the major market participants connected to the network. However, usage was limited, and transaction volumes suffered. In an effort to boost network usage and diversify its electronic-commerce (e-commerce) offering, MHDI pioneered an eligibility application, the central query system (CQS). The CQS was designed as a common eligibility portal for public sector and private sector eligibility data. Minnesota Medicaid was the initial source of eligibility content. In addition to the CQS and MedNet, MHDI delivers educational services related to e-commerce and recently to issues related to the Health Insurance Portability and Accountability Act of 1996 (HIPAA).

MHDI has also grappled with the privacy issues. It played a key role in helping Minnesota draft its health privacy laws. Since then, MHDI has expanded its work in this area to include Public Key Infrastructure (PKI). Along with groups in four other states (Washington, North Carolina, Massachusetts, and Utah), MHDI participates in the national HealthKey program that is exploring approaches for deploying PKI in health care.[3]

Recently, MHDI evolved its e-commerce offering in a new direction. MHDI and the Pointshare Corporation entered into an agreement to outsource CQS and MedNet. MHDI decided it was better able to achieve its objectives by leveraging the capabilities of a private company. Pointshare saw MedNet and CQS as a cost-effective way to enter a market and deliver services. This type of partnership highlights the creative approaches community health information initiatives are taking to achieve their goals. MHDI is unique in structure, experienced in the gyrations of the community health information movement and innovative in its program design. Those interested in the progress and potential of the movement will closely watch MHDI as it moves into the future.

Utah Health Information Network

The Utah Health Information Network (UHIN) is the only statewide CHIN that really achieved success. Whereas the CHMIS sites struggled and most CHINs never got off the ground, community leaders in Utah had the vision and capability to organize and implement a statewide network. In 1993, UHIN was incorporated as a nonprofit company with a mission to provide the consumer of healthcare services with reduced costs and improved healthcare quality by creating and managing an electronic value-added network, standardizing healthcare transactions, and gathering and providing data to a statewide repository. A board that is selected by the membership governs UHIN. The UHIN membership capitalized the company and funds the operation of the network. In addition, UHIN has received support from the state of Utah.[4]

UHIN understood early on the "wants versus needs" dilemma and the requirement to make a business case. The organization focused tightly on a limited scope of work and required anyone who wanted to play to have a stake in the game. Although UHIN is a classic community health information network, it takes great pride in emphasizing that it runs the network as a business. UHIN leaders know that community participation is voluntary and predicated on the network's capability to meet its customers' needs.

Currently, UHIN offers an electronic data interchange (EDI) solution for healthcare claims and remittances that serves all interested payers and providers in Utah. As the organization looks toward the future, UHIN envisions expanding its suite of services to include:

* Eligibility
* Referrals
* Patient records
* Lab tests
* Digital images

In the conduct of its business and in its role as community educator, UHIN heavily emphasizes the importance of standards. UHIN has taken a leadership role within the sate of Utah to help the healthcare community get ready for HIPAA and the requirement to implement national standards for common healthcare transactions. In addition, UHIN has diversified its work in two other areas. First, like MHDI, UHIN is one of the five participating state organizations in the HealthKey program. UHIN sees the emerging importance of privacy and security and wants to explore ways to make it work on a cost-effective basis for all participants. Second, UHIN recently entered into an innovative arrangement with the Utah Department of Health to collect data that is legally required by statute. For those data sets mandated by law, members may use UHIN to submit to the state. This arrangement highlights a clever and efficient arrangement to meet public health information needs by leveraging a community asset. UHIN will continue to explore creative ways to keep pace with the changing face of e-commerce, serve its customers, and apply its most valuable commodity—the commitment of its members.

New England Healthcare EDI Network

The New England Healthcare EDI Network (NEHEN) is a fairly recent entrant to the community health information scene. It offers another interesting model for how community efforts can evolve through partnership. In the mid-1990s, the Massachusetts Health Data Consortium (another HealthKey participant) brought together key stakeholders to explore how best to address shared e-commerce needs. These enterprises were very clear that they did not want to create what they deemed a CHIN. To them, a CHIN was a single network solution for all. In contrast, they sought a means to keep their independence and engage in collaborative activities of limited scope. In this context, the Massachusetts Health Data Consortium created and operated the Affiliated Health Information Networks of New England.

Initially, the affiliated group focused primarily on information and education as it considered how best to work toward its vision of "non-CHIN" collaboration. In 1997, the group hit on an idea for a network-of-networks model that would meet the requirement to offer common benefits while preserving individual discretion. This idea was NEHEN. NEHEN was created with five key benefits in mind:

- A tool to achieve HIPAA compliance;
- Delivery of service efficiencies through EDI;
- Reduced time to implement EDI on a large scale;
- Maintenance of individual business flexibility; and
- Reduced cost of EDI implementation through coordination and standardization.

The founding members of NEHEN included major healthcare payers and providers in New England (Harvard Pilgrim Health Plan, Tufts Health Plan, CareGroup, and others). The founders sought a private partner to staff the effort, to bring it to fruition, and eventually to operate the network. They selected Computer Science Corporation (CSC) for this purpose.[5]

To get buy-in, CSC embarked on an extensive communications effort with key executives. CSC emphasized how NEHEN could address urgent business needs and provide a positive return on investment. Once the decision was made to proceed, CSC created the network infrastructure with a secure Extranet and a thin layer of software at each enterprise location. The network initiated operations with the eligibility transaction. As of 2001, NEHEN was generating 12,000 eligibility inquiries per day.[5] NEHEN intends to move forward with other HIPAA-compliant transactions, including claims, referrals, remittance, and others.[6]

NEHEN is a blend of the community model and the commercial IT world. Incubated in a community not-for-profit setting, NEHEN has now incorporated as a limited liability corporation. The network is governed by its member participants and is open to any enterprise that wishes to join and adhere to common practices. CSC operates the network at the behest of the members. NEHEN is now being seen by other e-commerce companies as a cost-effective platform to conduct their business. The possibility exists that NEHEN will become the common health information network for both health industry participants and the vendors that serve them.

Wisconsin Health Information Network

When knowledgeable people talk about CHINs and describe the failure of the concept, they may add, "except for WHIN." Just as UHIN is seen as the one statewide CHIN that succeeded, the Wisconsin Health Information Network (WHIN) is often seen as the one community-based CHIN that succeeded. WHIN began where others ended up: as a partnership between Ameritech, a large telecommunications company, and Aurora Health Care, a major integrated delivery system based in Milwaukee. The genesis for this partnership was the effort Aurora made in the 1980s to connect physician offices to Aurora's hospital information system (HIS). In working with the physician community and other stakeholders to connect and share information, Aurora began to sense both the need for inter-enterprise connectivity and the challenge of bringing it about. After surveying members of the community, Aurora and Ameritech concluded that a single hospital solution was not the right way to proceed. It made far more sense to develop an "all-community" solution.[7]

In 1992, Aurora and Ameritech responded to the community's concern by creating WHIN. Since that time, WHIN has enjoyed steady growth and a reputation as the most visible and successful CHIN in the country. WHIN offers a comprehensive list of services including:

- Network access
- Clinical information
- Eligibility data
- Referral processing
- On-line document retrieval
- E-mail
- Electronic forms

Because of its hospital roots, WHIN offers a deeper level of functionality to hospital and physician participants than most other community health information networks. The recipe seems to have worked. WHIN currently has over 1200 physicians and 3000 total subscribers generating over 100,000 transactions a month. It is also worth noting that as a for-profit company, WHIN is profitable.[7]

As the CHIN market deteriorated nationally, Ameritech got out of the business. WHIN is now owned and operated by Aurora. WHIN has worked hard to justify the benefits of a community health information network. In 1994, WHIN published an independent study conducted by the University of Wisconsin. The study was designed to assess the impact of the CHIN. Sample findings about the impact of WHIN include[8]:

- Savings of $5.10 for medical record requests handled by WHIN for the hospital
- Savings of $1.00 for referral requests and $2.50 for clinical information requests handled by WHIN for physician offices
- Benefits such as rapid response time, fewer lost charges, and decreased patient stays in hospital

WHIN now seeks to consolidate its gains and potentially expand its offering to neighboring markets. It endures as the role model for a successful CHIN.

Healtheon/WebMD

Many people would not consider Healtheon/WebMD as a community health information initiative. Instead, they would see the company as a vendor or a "dot.com." However, an examination of the objectives of the company in light of the evolution of the community health information movement makes it clear that Healtheon/WebMD may be the ultimate end-state of the movement.

Healtheon/WebMD (recently renamed WebMD) describes itself as follows:

> "WebMD provides connectivity and a full suite of services to the healthcare industry
> that improve administrative efficiencies and clinical effectiveness enabling high quality
> patient care. The Company's products and services facilitate information exchange,
> communication and transaction between the consumer, physician, and healthcare
> institutions."[9]

Change the names and this could easily be a statement from the early days
of CHMIS. Indeed, it could be argued that WebMD has an even more ambitious plan than CHMIS and the CHINs. WebMD seeks to wire up the healthcare
industry "end-to-end" on a national basis.

WebMD is really an aggregation of health information technology companies
that have been acquired over the years by Healtheon, the original organization.
This national conglomeration of companies includes physician practice management systems, consumer health information sites, claims processors, network
service providers, and others. Its breadth of offering, matched with strategic partnerships, has positioned WebMD as the dominant player in its market space.

This dominant position provided the company with enormous capital resources
after it went public. Even with current market fluctuations, the total market valu-
ation of WebMD is well into the billions. WebMD's list of corporate partners and
investors reads like a who's who of industry. The result is a war chest that most
community health information groups could only dream about. However, the
clout and scope of the company has also caused problems. Some have been
concerned by the potential for WebMD to overwhelm, dominate, and
disintermediate healthcare enterprises. The creation of a rival organization,
MedUnite, by major health plans was a direct response to WebMD. The company
has also struggled to seamlessly integrate the component companies into a single,
efficient, operating entity. As a consequence, WebMD's fortunes and the prospects of the e-health sector it leads have been depressed recently.

The question for the community health information movement is whether
WebMD and other e-health companies will displace the movement, push enterprises closer to community-based alternatives in a defensive reaction, or eventually emerge as a powerful partner and enabler. Many on Wall Street and on main
street will be watching with great interest to see how the story plays out.

Pointshare

Like WebMD, Pointshare is a commercial organization. However, it has a very
different strategy. Pointshare derives its strategy from the premise that health
care is a local service. The company believes that in order to deliver value, it
must operate at the community level. Pointshare positions itself as a national
leader in connecting healthcare communities with secure online business
services that enhance communications, improve the delivery of patient care,
and increase operating efficiency. To achieve this objective, Pointshare provides the following offering:

- Connectivity
- Eligibility
- Referrals
- Clinical messaging
- Access to medical content

Pointshare also carries other value-added services on its network, including access to an Internet-based immunization tracking system operated by public health and a private company.[10]

Pointshare is smaller and more regionalized than WebMD. It is interesting to note that Pointshare is based in Washington State and also operates in Minnesota. These are two of the states discussed as leaders of the community health information movement. This overlap is not coincidental. Pointshare has long supported and participated in community health information efforts. The company sees such community groups as blazing a trail for adoption and use of its services. Where communities have come together to address shared information needs, Pointshare believes it will find a more receptive market for what it sells.

Specifically, in Washington State, Pointshare is working with a community collaborative called the Network Advisory Group (NAG). NAG is a consortium of major payers and providers dedicated to coordinated implementation of HIPAA. Pointshare is the initial intermediary that links the payers and providers together. In Minnesota, as previously mentioned, Pointshare has partnered with MHDI to operate its network. Like WebMD and other e-health companies, the challenge for Pointshare will be to deliver on the promise of e-health in a less favorable investment climate. Pointshare is trying to demonstrate that community health information networks are not only a social good, but that they can also be good business

The Future

Using a circle as a metaphor for the community health information movement means we come back to our starting point or near to it as we examine the future and the implications for public health:

"Do it all together" is not going to work. The original vision whereby a small group of community leaders in a top-down model wired up the world and governed a unitary system is not palatable to the health industry or to community stakeholders. Furthermore, it is not consistent either with the nature of Internet technology or the nature of the commercial organizations seeking to harness it. The health information infrastructure must permit discretion at the individual enterprise level and perhaps even at the individual user level.

"Do it all alone" is not going to work either. Those most deeply opposed to the early vision of the community health information movement believed there was no need for inter-enterprise connectivity or collaboration. They expected to "own" on an exclusive basis all of their trading partners. These trading partners would be connected directly to a single enterprise, and that supposedly would solve the problem. The evolution of the healthcare market place with many-to-many relationships already made this a questionable strategy. The Internet revolution makes it a suicidal strategy. Like it or not, health enterprises will be sharing data, customers, and trading partners for the foreseeable future. The question is not if enterprises need to connect to others, but how.

"Just let somebody do it for you" does not appear that it will work as a concept. The commercial organizations moving into the community health information space had high hopes that they would assume a role similar to the one CHMIS identified 10 years ago. As the intermediary at the heart of the network, they would sign everyone up, route traffic, extract data, and get rich on the value they provided and the huge volumes of transactions they moved. It is too soon to be definitive about this concept; however, the early returns seem to indicate that this model won't fly. Major health enterprises fear the intermediary will either assume a monopoly role and mistreat them or assume their role and disintermediate them. Furthermore, enterprises increasingly see e-health as a means to competitively distinguish themselves. Therefore, they are reluctant to turn it all over to a third party.

"Do it in partnership" seems to be the direction the market is currently headed. The need for interoperability is a key driver of the partnership approach. Health services is a many-to-many market place. This means there is a tremendous cost to all participants if everyone does their work in isolation. Interoperability is a critical component of any robust health information infrastructure, just as it is in other industries. In this context, the enterprises, the vendors, and the community groups are finding common ground. The enterprise holds the data and sometimes the customers everyone wants access to. However, the enterprise generally lacks the necessary capital, IT talent, and field force to establish connectivity and get it used. The vendors have the capital, the resources, and the incentive to execute on infrastructure development. However, without the content and the customers, they have no way to make the connectivity and applications valuable. The community group usually lacks the capital, the content, and the resources. However, the community group is often in the best position to build trust, foster collaboration, and educate the stakeholders—all prerequisites for the successful pursuit of interoperability. As can be seen with the examples profiled, enterprises, vendors, and community groups are already finding exciting ways to partner.

What does this partnership approach mean for public health? It suggests that public health needs to move aggressively to join the partnership. With limited budgets and the requirement to assess populations, public health organizations have wonderful opportunities to leverage the investments of the personal health industry and the vendor community. Going it alone makes no more sense for public health than it does for the healthcare enterprises.

Specific partnership opportunities abound and are already under way in some communities. These include:

- *Immunization tracking.* In Washington State, public health, Pointshare, and a company called HealthRadius are partnering with health plans and providers to see if the same network used to transact the administrative and clinical business of health care can be leveraged to track immunizations.
- *Vital statistics.* UHIN and the Utah health department are piggybacking reportable information on the same network developed for handling administrative transactions.
- *Lab results.* Public health is attempting to extract and aggregate surveillance information from clinical laboratory findings. Many enterprises and the vendors that serve them have identified clinical results reporting as a priority for the messaging services they are building and deploying. This suggests a cost-effective partnership could be structured to accommodate all users.
- *Consumer information.* Vast sums are being spent to attract consumers to the Internet and particularly to medical content sites (WebMD, drkoop.com, etc.). These initiatives offer public health a vehicle to disseminate information on prevention.

As the community health information movement enters its second decade, a different sort of promise beckons than was glimmering 10 years before. At the beginning of the cycle, it was sharing grand visions and trying to make it all come true at once. Now, the vision is entrenched, and the field is crowded with those who want to help bring it about. The challenge for the community health information movement is to make the right "picks"—pick an area of focus, pick the right role, pick a good set of partners, and concentrate resources to execute successfully. Over the next 10 years, the goals of the movement's founders can finally be realized.

Questions for Review

1. Briefly explain why personal health care has been given priority over public health in community health information activities.
2. Explain why the Community Health Management Information System (CHMIS) initiative of the John Hartford Foundation failed.
3. Why did the public health care reform effort in the 1990s fail?
4. Explain why CHINs failed, in spite of the fact that they had learned from the struggles of the CHMIS movement and the failures of public health care reform.
5. In what ways did the emergence of the Internet rescue the community health information movement?
6. Why is building a business case important for any initiatives of the community health information movement?

7. In what sense did the collaborative model of the community health information movement prove false?
8. Explain why the Utah Health Information Network (UHIN) succeeded as a CHIN, when so many other CHINs failed. What differentiated UHIN from these failed efforts? Explain why the Minnesota Health Data Institute has been a successful initiative.
9. Explain the shortcomings of the following concepts of providing community health information:
   a. "Do it all together."
   b. "Do it all alone."
   c. "Just let somebody do it for you."
10. Explain what using the partnership approach means for public health in the community health information movement.

References

1. Furukawa M. Peake T. *Profiling America's Health Information Networks.* Atlanta, GA: COMNET Society; 1995.
2. Minnesota Health Data Institute Web site. Available at: http://www.mhdi.org/. Accessed April 4, 2002.
3. HealthKey Web site. The HealthKey Collaborative: A Shared Vision. Available at: http://www.healthkey.org/. Accessed April 4, 2002.
4. Utah Health Information Network Web site. Available at: http://www.uhin.com/. Accessed April 4, 2002.
5. Pizzo S. Healthcare's napkin network. *Baseline* magazine. February 4, 2002. Available at: www.baseline.com.
6. Computer Sciences Corporation Web site. Available at: http://www.csc.com/industries/healthservices/knowledgelibrary/762.shtml. and www.csc.com/industries/health.services/casestudies/1140shtml. Accessed April 4, 2002.
7. Brennan P, Schneider S, Tornquist E. The Wisconsin Health Information Network. In: *Information Networks for Community Health.* New York: Springer-Verlag; 1997:73–99.
8. Wisconsin Health Information Network Web site. Available at: http://www.whin.net/. Accessed April 4, 2002.
9. WebMD Web site. Available at: http://www.webmd.com/. Accessed April 4, 2002.
10. Pointshare Web site. Available at: http://www.pointshare.com/. Accessed April 4, 2002.

28
Developing the Missouri Integrated Public Health Information System

GARLAND LAND, NANCY HOFFMAN, AND REX PETERSON

Learning Objectives

After studying this chapter, you should be able to:

- Describe the requirements, the architectures, system development areas, and common processes of the Missouri Integrated Public Health Information System.
- Explain the challenges posed by the Missouri system and the approaches taken to mitigate those challenges.
- Discuss the keys to success and lessons identified by the implementers of the Missouri system.

Overview

The Missouri Health Strategic Architectures and Information Cooperative (MOHSAIC), an initiative of the Missouri Department of Health (MDOH), is one of the best-known successful undertakings to develop an integrated public health system to serve both state and local public health needs. MOHSAIC was to replace more than 60 different program-specific computer systems serving individual health programs. The challenges faced by system developers were daunting. They included locating sources of funding for a very expensive project, acquiring qualified staff and contractors, coordinating system development across programs that often preferred their own dedicated systems, dealing with conversion of data from legacy systems, and encountering entrenched resistance to business reengineering. The means by which MDOH addressed these challenges to build an integrated system are instructive. The keys to success included locating sources of funding, dealing with both internal and external politics, securing top-level promotion and support, developing a strategic plan to guide the project, and involving users at all levels in the design of the system. The keys also involved the system designers' developing a solid reputation by beginning construction in areas where support for MOHSAIC already existed, a tactic that helped overcome resistance in other program areas. The wisdom of the decision to design and implement MOHSAIC is already apparent at all levels of use of the integrated system. An integrated immunization register and a surveillance component are only two examples of the many benefits that the integrated system offers.

Introduction

In 1992, the Missouri Department of Health (MDOH) had over 60 different program-specific computer systems serving individual health programs. The systems ran on a variety of platforms, since there were no hardware or software standards. This situation had developed over the years in part because various federal agencies provided specific computer systems or funded the development of categorical systems. State-funded information systems were also developed as stovepipe systems that only met specific categorical needs.

Many programs developed their information systems with their own staff, and so there was no central inventory for the MDOH regarding what systems existed and what data were being collected. Client data were based upon categorical programs rather than being person-specific across programs. There was no easy way to share data among programs because there was no common identification number used by the various systems. This situation hindered the assessment and policy development capabilities of the MDOH.

The information systems did not support the ability to integrate services. At the local public health agency (LPHA) level, this affected delivery of services to the clients. Clients were viewed as program participants instead of individuals who could have multiple health needs. Because local agencies had to rely on numerous non-integrated computer systems for their information, they were unable to attend to the total health needs of their clients in a coordinated fashion.

Secondary to the problem of integrating services was the cost and difficulty of maintaining over 60 systems. Although all systems supported most of the same functions (registration, service tracking, report production, etc.) and contained many of the same clients and data elements, there was little coordinated maintenance of the various systems. The lack of standard hardware and software architectures made any central support difficult. This led to costly duplication of development and maintenance of the systems. Programs that did not have federal funding or strong state support could not afford to have an information system, which led to inefficiencies.

Approach

Development of MOHSAIC Plan

The MDOH's strategic plan, *Public Health Agenda for the '90s—Healthy Missourians 2000,* [1] contained eight strategic goals. One of these goals pertained to strengthening the information systems for public health in Missouri. This goal had several specific objectives that address the development of an electronic communications system to integrate services at the state and local levels. A comprehensive assessment of MDOH's organizational strengths and weaknesses revealed that in terms of overall strategic use of communications technology, MDOH's information systems development was spotty.

It became clear to the department director that to reach MDOH's year 2000 goals, an integrated system was needed. It also became clear that a new approach to systems development needed to be adopted. Other Missouri state agency information systems staff were beginning to adopt information engineering (IE), a methodology originated by Clive Finkelsten[2] to develop information systems. The decision was made that the MDOH would also use this methodology. It was decided that an outside consultant experienced in the methodology would be needed to guide the MDOH through the process.

In September 1992, the MDOH engaged a consultant experienced in IE methodology. An initial project to create an Information Strategy Plan (ISP) was implemented and called the Missouri Health Strategic Architectures and Information Cooperative (MOHSAIC) project. IE differs from traditional methods in the following ways:

- IE analyzes functions and data independent of the organizational structure of the agency.
- With IE, users are intimately involved in all stages of the process; the initial stages focus on high-level goals and involve the department's senior management. The later stages analyze more detailed information and involve lower level program staff.
- IE conveys conceptual ideas through the use of diagrams or pictures. Symbols, such as colored boxes and interconnecting lines, represent data, activities, and their interaction at various levels of abstraction.

Development of the ISP required the commitment of 80–90% of six senior managers' time for a period of 14 weeks. All divisions of the MDOH were represented on the team. The first step in the process was to assess all the information systems in the MDOH and identify all the functions performed by the department and the data needed to perform these functions. The team members captured this information in an electronic form. Team members defined each data element and process to ensure clear communication with future workgroups and program developers. As the software application was developed, additional design sessions with program level staff increased the level of detail. This team created a long-range plan for information systems development that transcended organizational boundaries or units.

A second team consisting of representatives from a rural area, a city, a large metropolitan health department, and one manager from the original team was formed. The same consultant facilitated a review of the functions performed by the local public health agencies and the data needed to perform these functions. The ISP developed by this group was identical to that of the first

ISP with the exception of expanding a few activity definitions. The definitions were expanded and the two plans were consolidated to create a single plan that addressed the information needs for public health in Missouri.[3]

As the ISP was being developed, it was tailored to the specific needs of the department. The strategic goals outlined in *Public Health Agenda for the '90's—Healthy Missourians 2000,* the Institute of Medicine report *The Future of Public Health,*[4] interviews with departmental management, and the extensive experience of the ISP MOHSAIC team members were used to ensure a good fit. This resulted in a plan that was based on the core functions of public health—i.e., assessment, policy development, and assurance. The plan integrated the critical success factors, strategic issues, and information and technical needs necessary for the department and local public health agencies to achieve their goals.[3]

Both groups identified a number of requirements for the integrated system. These included provisions that:

- The same standards would be used to capture all data.
- All data would be included in a single integrated system.
- One technical platform would be used.
- Records would be client-centered to allow a holistic view of client versus episodic or single service information.
- The system would support data sharing among public health agencies and staff.
- The system would support the capture of demographic and other client information one time to reduce the amount of redundant information that must be entered and stored.
- The system would be designed for the MDOH and the local public health agencies that are independent of the MDOH.

It was anticipated that all these requirements would eventually result in comprehensive, high-quality, compatible data and more efficient, cost-effective use of limited resources.

The ISP consisted of three architectures: (1) information, (2) business systems, and (3) technical. The information architecture showed the relationship between functions performed and data. The business systems architecture detailed this relationship into business areas and business systems from which information systems are developed. The technology architecture established the necessary hardware and software to support these systems. The ISP also provided the architectures for a statewide information network to link public and private healthcare providers electronically.

These architectures were broadly designed, and they formed the framework to guide systems development. The ISP enabled the MDOH to manage technical and coordination issues on an ongoing basis so that it could incorporate new technology and build new systems as needed. This arrangement allowed seamless access to data regardless of where those data resided based on current appropriate technology. Together, these provided architectures for creating and managing information from a public health functional perspective regardless of organizational structure. All the core public health functions of assessment, assurance, and policy development, including management functions, were addressed.

The ISP identified eight major areas for system development: (1) clients and services, (2) public health profiles, (3) policy and planning, (4) finance, (5) personnel, (6) property and materials, (7) constituent and public relations, and (8) legal affairs. Clients were broadly defined as "actual or potential recipients of public health services." They include a person, family or group of persons; things that are regulated, such as child care, hospitals, home health agencies, sewage, lead abatement, etc.; and environmental clients such as water systems, food manufacturers, land fills, toxic waste, etc.

The plan also identified similar processes that occur with all types of clients. This common functionality included dealing with inquiries and complaints, capturing common demographic information through registration, scheduling services, creating a baseline client profile, creating and managing an inventory of supplies, and service/care plan management. Development of these generic processes supported the grouping of similar programs by component and allowed the integration of client data.

Development Around Public Health Clients

The ISP made recommendations on priorities for application development. It was determined that the area that supported 80% of the functions performed by the department and by local public health agencies was related to clients and services. Developing an application that captured data on the client and the services they received would support the core function of assurance.

The information systems staff was divided into three teams. The initial team supported the "person" client, health management, component. The initial application development focused on the generic registration (demographic information), generic appointment scheduling, generic inventory, and program specific immunization/tuberculosis (TB) information. This health management application formed the basic infrastructure to support a statewide immunization register that was later expanded to include family planning and service coordination services. Plans are to include all public health services, including a Web-based birth certificate and newborn hearing and metabolic screening.

A second team developed and implemented the surveillance component that supports the mandated reports of communicable diseases, sexually transmitted diseases (STDs), HIV/AIDs, lead, and TB. A third team focused on regulatory "clients." This component supports the licensing/certification functions performed by the department. These include narcotics and dangerous drugs, hospitals, home health agencies, hospices, child care, lead abatement workers, and emergency medical services and food establishments.

Development and Implementation Steps

Plan the Technology Architecture

Before MOHSAIC, the MDOH had applications running on an MVS mainframe, a UNIX mid-range computer, and both Macintosh and IBM-compatible personal computers (PCs) written in a variety of languages and using six different relational database management systems. The department had three separate e-mail systems and multiple word processing systems, electronic spreadsheets, and graphics software. The ISP technology architecture included a plan to migrate this variety of disparate technologies into a single network that would serve the entire department and eventually the state's local public health agencies. The proposed architecture included a department-wide Novell network; IBM-compatible PCs for client workstations; GroupWise e-mail, scheduling and task tracking; the Microsoft Office products (MS Word, Excel, PowerPoint, and MS Access), and Internet access. UNIX servers and the state mainframe would continue to support large applications and could be accessed by all users on the Novell network.

Find Financial Support

The MDOH was quick to accept the proposed ISP technical architecture, but slow to implement it because of funding issues. Although the department was expending significant funds maintaining the existing disparate systems, these systems had to be maintained during the transition so money could not immediately be diverted. In 1994, the department agreed to a network allocation scheme that would charge each network user an annual network fee. The total annual cost of the network, including network software, network hardware (excluding the client PCs), network technicians, help desk staff, and trainers, would be divided by the total number of users for the annual user fee. With the exception of a small amount of maternal and child health block funds and some preventative health block funds that were used in the development of the ISP and general design, the network allocation fee provided MOHSAIC with its first source of funds. However, it addressed only the MDOH's local-area network (LAN). Significant funding was needed for other functions of MOHSAIC.

To keep initial costs under control, the department gathered all Microsoft licenses that existed throughout the department and applied them to upgrades. The MDOH's original agreement with Microsoft was a concurrent license agreement rather than named users, so very few new licenses were needed. The MDOH also allowed existing Macintosh users to connect their computers to the network with the understanding that they would have to replace them with IBM-compatible PCs when the computer's useful life was over. The annual network fee has remained in the range of $1,800–$2,300 per user since the inception of the network. Increased network functionality and cost of relocations (MDOH moved its entire central office and seven of its district and area offices) have offset the savings from paying off the start-up costs.

The MDOH completed installation of the network in its main office in less than six months; it then began installing routers and leasing dedicated lines to remote sites, including the state public health laboratory, an off-site division, six district offices, and three area offices by 1998. The MDOH has 1,300 employees on the network and 13 sites connected throughout the state.

During 1996–1997, the MDOH expanded the network to include 114 local public health agencies throughout the state. The local agencies were connected with frame relay lines varying in speeds from 56 kb to 384 kb. Initially, the LPHAs were given access only to MDOH's major applications (Women, Infants, and Children [WIC], vital records, MOHSAIC, and intranet), but in 2000 MDOH began providing the LPHAs e-mail, Internet access, and broadcast fax capabilities.

Funding for the installation of the wide-area network (WAN) that connects remote department sites and local public health agencies was provided by the Centers for Disease Control and Prevention's (CDC) initial Information Network for Public Health Officials (INPHO 1) grant and a $750,000 general revenue appropriation. To support the ongoing costs of the WAN, an allocation scheme was developed that allocates the cost to the programs using the WAN (WIC, vital records, immunizations, etc.) based on the amount of transactions generated by their applications.

A CDC Health Alert Network (HAN) grant provided funds for the MDOH to increase functionality to the LPHAs over the WAN. Office automation, e-mail, Internet access, desktop video streaming, broadcast fax, and some two-way video conferencing were provided to LPHAs at no cost to them.

Whereas finding funding for the network was challenging, it was a mild challenge compared with the challenge of finding funds for development of the integrated public health information system. Almost all the department's funding was program-specific, and the providers of the funding ranged from hesitant to strongly opposed to using their program-specific funds for developing a system that was not dedicated to serving their program. As a result, MOHSAIC is unusual in that the MDOH's information management unit, Center for Health Information Management and Evaluation (CHIME), rather than the programs receiving benefits from the system, acquired the majority of the development funds. For some programs, this was a disadvantage, because they saw the system as a CHIME project and never fully participated as equal partners. This resulted in an abnormal number of changes after implementation, because insufficient information was provided during analysis. However, other programs did see this as an excellent opportunity to obtain a system they needed but could not afford, and these programs eagerly participated in the development.

MOHSAIC has been built using 12 federal and state funding sources. Table 28.1 shows the funding sources and amounts for fiscal years 1996–2002, the development period for MOHSAIC. The funds were used for both development and maintenance costs during that time period. Because implementa-

TABLE **28.1.** MOHSAIC funding sources, 1993–2002

Medicaid	$6,107,000
General revenue	6,021,000
Immunization program	2,054,000
INPHO II	2,250,000
HAN	1,890,000
Assessment initiative grant	1,290,000
INPHO I	700,000
NEDSS	695,000
Child care development block	220,000
MCH block grant	300,000
Other	115,000
Total	$21,732,000

tion of MOHSAIC was by components, there is no clear point in time where development ended and operations began.

Early in the development, the MDOH negotiated an agreement with the state Medicaid program. The agreement provided matching funds for development of components of MOHSAIC that directly benefited the Medicaid program. The MDOH was also able to acquire an ongoing state general revenue appropriation for MOHSAIC development that was used for the Medicaid match. The MDOH then received a second Information Network for Public Health Officials (INPHO 2) grant that was used to develop additional components of MOHSAIC. Federal funds were used to support 72% of the costs to develop MOHSAIC.

Acquire Qualified Staff and Contractors

Obtaining funding was just one of many difficult tasks facing MDOH during the initial stages of MOHSAIC. Acquiring sufficient skilled staff to develop and implement MOHSAIC proved to be an even larger task. Prior to the ISP, the department had 16 information systems programmer analysts, none of whom had experience in developing client-server systems or Oracle databases. Most of these staff members were needed to support the existing systems until MOHSAIC was implemented. Thus, the MDOH's initial plan was to purchase a commercial off-the-shelf software package that met most of the requirements determined in the ISP. However, the department was not able to find an integrated public health package that met even a small portion of the

ISP requirements. Therefore, the MDOH decided to obtain the necessary staff and develop the system in-house.

The MDOH began retraining existing staff in the skills needed for MOHSAIC and recruiting new staff with the needed skills. However, the Missouri capital, Jefferson City, is a relatively small community, and the need for information technology (IT) professionals in state government far exceeds the available resources. The MDOH realized it would need to develop new IT professionals in addition to undertaking its recruitment and retraining efforts. Thus, the MDOH began providing IT training to selected public health staff within the agency who had an interest and had demonstrated some ability in IT. Some of the selected staff were not able to make the adjustment to the IT field successfully, but the ones that did make the adjustment proved to be a very valuable asset. Their knowledge of public health and their understanding of the users' needs created better and more user-friendly applications.

Initially, the MDOH experienced high turnover rates among its IT staff. The high turnover rate was primarily caused by the state's salaries' being far below the national average for IT staff, but some also left because they did not feel MDOH would be successful in implementing MOHSAIC with the limited resources that were available in the early stages of its development. The state's personnel rules limited the salaries and benefits the department could provide IT staff. The MDOH addressed this issue by providing non-monetary rewards, including:

- Giving the staff considerable input into the technology used by MOHSAIC
- Providing extensive training, often out-of-state, for staff in the new technology
- Providing recognition for staff achievements whenever possible
- Promoting from within in most cases
- Providing flexible work schedules

Although all of these rewards helped reduce turnover rates, the success of the initial components of MOHSAIC probably had the greatest impact. During the past three years of the project, the turnover rate was only 2–3% annually, considered excellent in the IT industry.

Within a couple of years, MDOH developed a staff of trained and experienced programmers and technicians to develop, implement, and maintain MOHSAIC. However, it was not practical to develop all the employees needed from in-house staff alone for three reasons. First, MDOH was unable to find or train sufficient employees to develop the system entirely in-house. Second, had MDOH employed all development staff, these hires would be facing a significant layoff once MOHSAIC was completed and in a maintenance-only mode. Third, some development tasks required very specific skills for a short period of time, and it was not cost-effective to hire or train existing staff in these skills that would not be required on an ongoing basis. As a result, MDOH supplemented its IT staff by establishing contracts that provided consultants with a variety of skills. These consultants worked alongside MDOH IT staff and under the direction of MDOH's project manager. MDOH benefited not only from the work of the consultants. but also from the transfer of learning that occurred between the consultants and MDOH staff. During the peak of development, MDOH had 19 consultants supplementing its 25 programmer-analysts in developing MOHSAIC.

Define System Requirements

One of the major challenges in developing a large integrated system is the large amount of information that must be gathered and analyzed before actual coding can begin. To address this issue, MDOH used Joint Application Design (JAD) sessions to determine the requirements for MOHSAIC. The end users were the main participants in the sessions. A facilitator ensured that a JAD session was carried out in a thorough and orderly manner. The sessions were highly structured and designed to lead users through a discussion of all aspects of the system. The information systems staff who attended JAD sessions included analysts and modelers who designed the system as the users presented it. The JAD included a prototype of the system, so that users knew what their portion of the system would look like at the completion of design.

Select Common Identification Number

A decision was made in an early JAD session to share a common identification numbering system with the Department of Social Services (DSS). The two departments serve many of the same clients. The DSS's identification number is also the state Medicaid number; it provides immediate access to Medicaid eligibility data. The decision to share a common identification number initially provided some technology challenges, because the DSS applications run on the state's mainframe computer whereas MOHSAIC runs on a department UNIX server. However, the MDOH was able to develop an interface that allowed users to assign new identification numbers on the mainframe without having to manually log onto the mainframe. One of the main benefits of using this number is that Medicaid billing data can be easily imported into MOHSAIC.

Select Software/Hardware Architecture

MOHSAIC is a multi-tier system that was developed using Borland's Delphi. A thin client or Web browser client resides on the end-user's Windows PC and contains the entry screen and basic field edits. The middle tiers. which reside on Windows NT servers, contain the application logic. The data are stored in an Oracle database running on an AIX (IBM's version of UNIX) server. The advantages to this approach include:

- The memory and storage requirements for the end users' computer are reduced.

- The multi-tier system is more responsive, because the majority of the data transfers and operations occur between the middle tiers and the database server, which are connected by 100 MB Ethernet. Only minimal screen data is transferred over the much slower WAN (56–384 KB).
- Support is easier because the majority of the application is located in the central office instead of in the field.

Users located in the MDOH facilities or in the main facility of city and county public health agencies use the thin client and access the MOHSAIC transaction system over the MDOH dedicated high-speed network. Private healthcare providers with rights to use MOHSAIC can access the system via the Internet, using a Web browser.

Establish a Data Warehouse

The MOHSAIC transaction system is used to gather data and to track services provided to individual clients. The system is tuned for quick entry and access, but not for data analysis and ad hoc reporting. All data from MOHSAIC's transaction system, as well as data obtained from other sources, are loaded into the data warehouse. The MDOH data warehouse consists of an operational data store, an atomic data repository, and various data marts. Data are first collected and integrated in the operational data store before being moved to the atomic data repository. The atomic data repository is a normalized Oracle database that is used only for complex data analysis by professional research analysts. For other users, the data in the atomic data repository are moved to subject-specific data marts that are designed for rapid report production by nontechnical users. The users can use any Open Database Connectivity (ODBC)-compliant reporting tool to develop reports. Currently, MDOH users use MyEureka, Microsoft Excel, Microsoft Access, Epi Info, and Crystal Reports to develop ad hoc reports. County and city public health departments can download their county's data to generate reports and do analysis locally.

The MDOH Data Warehouse serves more roles than do normal data warehouses. These roles include:

- Collecting data from disparate state and local systems and integrating it into the MOHSAIC transaction system
- Providing infrastructure for MOHSAIC operational reports
- Proactively alerting managers to significant public health events
- Providing support for Intranet, Internet, and Extranet projects
- Providing support for data mining projects
- Collecting, managing, and providing metadata on the data warehouse data (metadata is information the users need about the data to be able to analyze it accurately)
- Integrating information from different public health programs into a cohesive and descriptive decision support model of public healthcare delivery

- Integrating information about diseases and other conditions of public health interest in Missouri into a decision support model for scientific and management inquiries

Develop Training Strategies

A major consideration was how to train the MOHSAIC users who are located all over the state. Although it was agreed that initial formal classroom training would be required, the MDOH realized that extensive initial and ongoing training was not realistic, given the volume and locations of the users. Therefore, efforts were made to make the system as intuitive as possible so that minimum training would be required. The developers followed normal Windows standards for pull-down menus, scrolls, buttons, etc., so that experienced Windows users could use their existing knowledge for most operations. In addition, documentation that described all screens and the data elements on the screens was provided each user as a reference.

Formal classroom training is provided in the MDOH's six district offices whenever new major releases are made. Agencies using MOHSAIC are strongly encouraged to send at least two representatives to the formal training classes. These representatives are responsible for training any additional staff in their agency.

Provide User Support

A critical success factor for MOHSAIC is its toll-free help desk. No matter how effective the training is, there will be a need for ongoing end-user support. Initially, the MDOH staffed its help desk with existing information technology staff, but the staff were not happy with the job and had difficulty relating to end users possessing minimal technology skills. To solve this problem, MDOH recruited people with good interpersonal skills and an interest in information technology and then provided them IT training. A number of the new recruits came from within the MDOH, so they came with knowledge of the MDOH and an understanding of the users' problems. The MDOH help desk now constantly receives praise for the patient and understanding assistance provided by its staff.

Challenges

In undertaking this project, MDOH confronted numerous challenges. This section will list and discuss these challenges.

Large Systems Projects Typically Fail

A study by The Standish Group found that 31% of all development projects are canceled before completion.[5] The larger the system, the greater is the likelihood of failure. Because integrated systems are by necessity very large, there is a high risk involved in attempting to develop them. In addition, integrated systems present greater risk because of the

- effort required to coordinate across many programs;
- need to obtain support from many programs;
- difficulty of obtaining funding;
- magnitude and complexity of the task of converting numerous existing data systems with different formats and data definitions into a single database; and
- confidentiality rules that are unique to each program.

Coordination Across Programs Is Difficult

Integrated systems are often sold on the basis that they are less expensive to develop and maintain than multiple stovepipe systems. Although this is true, development and maintenance of integrated systems require far greater coordination than stovepipe systems. Without a well-defined methodology and good automated design tools, the coordination and the amount of data involved would soon become overwhelming.

The MDOH began MOHSAIC development using the information engineering (IE) methodology. Following this methodology, the MDOH began with a top-down approach to analysis. The high-level models developed in the ISP created the framework for the subsequent detailed JAD sessions with end users. The information obtained from the detailed JAD sessions adds detail to the ISP models but does not alter the original framework.

As more and better tools for object-oriented (OO) development methodology have become available, the MDOH has migrated to an OO approach but still maintains the top-down design that was initiated in the ISP.

Even after the system is implemented, coordination among the various programs is still a major consideration. Changes requested by one program need to be analyzed to determine impact on other programs. Because of this, good change management policies are necessary.

Categorical Programs Don't Necessarily Support Integrated Systems

Because an integrated system is typically mandated from the top, the individual categorical programs often will not initially support the project. There are several reasons for this support refusal, including:

- The programs may have pride of ownership in their existing stovepipe systems. Unless a system is very old, the existing program staff were probably active in the design of the system and may even have had their own information technology staff develop the system. They believe the system is meeting their needs, and they have no desire to replace it.

- The programs may fear that their requirements will not get the attention needed to ensure that their needs are met.
- The programs may believe they will have to compromise some of their specific requirements. This is a legitimate concern, inasmuch as the various programs will have to arrive at common data definitions and formats requiring compromise on their parts.

Large Health Agencies Already Have an Information System

Some of the larger metropolitan health agencies have invested time and resources to develop data systems to support their agencies. Often, these systems support financial and billings systems critical to the agency. However, these systems lack the statewide perspective of the client. Participation is dependent on meeting the billing needs of such large agencies and providing data access for ad hoc reporting. To elicit metropolitan support, the MDOH created an electronic exchange of information for vaccines and surveillance data.

Pooling of Funds Is Difficult

One of the main reasons that stovepipe information systems were developed and supported was the existence of categorical federal and state funding. Programs received funding with specific limitations to spend the money only to support the activities of the program. In the early development stages of MOHSAIC, there were many conversations, roadblocks, and frustrations over the concept of pooling categorical monies to support an integrated system. Program managers at the state level and federal levels had no policy framework that allowed for the pooling of categorical monies to build an integrated system.

These barriers started to break down when the CDC promoted the development of a state investment analysis to support using a portion of categorical funding for data integration. In 1998, the MDOH was one of the first states to develop an investment analysis that laid out our strategy for data integration. However, MDOH later learned there was no formal procedure for CDC's approving an investment analysis. The analysis was meant to assist a state in obtaining program support for using categorical funds for data integration. It did not mandate that funds be used for data integration. Because most programs already had limited funding, MDOH did not require them to support MOHSAIC with their core funds.

The exception to this practice was the immunization program. The program had been financially supporting two metropolitan registries and a different stand-alone application in 99 rural LPHAs. They stopped support of all these systems and provided their funds to MOHSAIC. They received in return a statewide immunization registry that interfaced with the MDOH birth/death system and the DSS's Medicaid system.

The main strategy that MDOH used in gaining program financial support for MOHSAIC was to use newly appropriated monies instead of trying to rebudget existing funds. During the project period, there were several new state laws and federal grants that involved the creation of data systems. It became the policy of the MDOH that any new information system would be developed as part of MOHSAIC. These funding sources became new funding opportunities for MOHSAIC. This approach prevented the wars that would have taken place if MDOH had tried to reallocate budgets. However, it also meant MDOH had to realign development priorities as new funding sources emerged. Because the system was being developed in a modular fashion, any new funding source ultimately benefited other programs that could use some of same source code that was developed for a specific program.

Enterprise-Level Systems Are Expensive to Develop

The total development costs for MOHSAIC are estimated to be nearly $24 million. Although this is a significant amount of money, it has to be evaluated in terms of the benefit derived in performing the core functions of public health. Although no firm figures are available, MDOH feels certain that the development costs for an integrated system are significantly less than development costs of comparable standalone systems.

The single, integrated system will provide even more savings in maintenance. Because of common modules and common code, MDOH estimates that it will take 50% fewer staff to maintain. The data warehouse, typically a very expensive maintenance application because of the constant requirements to link and cleanse records, will be relatively inexpensive to maintain. All internal data loaded into the data warehouse already have a common identification number and meet standards on definitions and quality that typically do not exist in developing an enterprise data warehouse.

Throughout the MOHSAIC development, funding was a major issue, and tight budget restraints were ever-present. However, there were costs incurred as a result of redevelopment of portions of the application because of changing technology that might not be as prevalent for new developments starting today. Certainly technology change will continue to occur at an increasing rate, but the basic architecture is likely to be more stable in the near future than it was in the early and middle 1990s. When the MDOH began the ISP, the standard application architecture for Missouri state government was the mainframe computer with dumb terminals. MOHSAIC was initially targeted for this environment but was implemented as a two-tier client server application. It has since been rewritten as a multi-tier client server application, and the thin client is now being converted to a Web browser client. Although it is impossible to project future technology with much accuracy, it appears that future technology will enhance the multi-tier, browser interface application rather than replace it.

Integrated Systems Compound Confidentiality Issues

Creating an integrated public health information system compounded confidentiality issues. To address confidentiality issues, the MDOH created a workgroup with representatives from all areas of the department. The group reviewed all federal and state laws that addressed the sharing of information for specific medical diagnoses, conditions, or funded services. Portions of the data with more strict requirements for access and sharing were identified. The group reviewed and revised MDOH administrative policies and contract language related to confidentiality to provide clear direction to staff. Each of the program staff had to agree and document which collected portions of the client information could be shared. The OIS staff was given direction on confidentiality requirements. This staff created a security application that limited the data a user could access by user role and function. The MDOH computer system access forms were modified to reflect these roles and functions. Each completed request was forwarded to staff responsible for the data for review and required signature. For physicians and other providers not formally contracted with the MDOH, a memorandum of agreement (MOA) was developed. This MOA defines responsibilities related to confidentiality of both parties and must be signed by both parties prior to the grant of access.

The implementation of the Health Insurance Portability and Accountability Act of 1996 (HIPAA) will change the legal and regulatory environment for managing client's medical information. The MDOH will review and revise its policies to meet these requirements.

Legacy Data Conversion Is Difficult

One of the tasks that MDOH underestimated was the effort required to convert data from legacy systems to MOHSAIC. Among the problems encountered in this process were:

- Different formats for data that were used in the many systems. Many of these were relatively easy to convert, but some such as systems that used a single "name" field instead of first, middle, and last name fields were difficult.
- Most of the legacy systems did not have standards for entering data such as street address and city into fields. As a result, these fields contained misspelled words and non-standard abbreviations.
- Often, the design of the legacy system failed to include critical data, and the users of the system worked around the design flaw by entering the critical data in unstructured memo or note fields.
- Many of the older systems did not have sufficient edits to ensure that only allowable codes were entered.
- Many of the legacy systems did not provide sufficient identification data to permit unique identification of the client.

Even though the MDOH purchased automated tools to assist with the conversion, the conversion was a highly labor-intensive process. For many of the smaller legacy systems, the MDOH found that it was less expensive to re-key the data into MOHSAIC rather than to convert the data.

Resistance to Business Reengineering

The integrated public health information system supports changes in how clients and data flow through an organization. It reduces the amount of redundant data that must be entered into a system. Not all system users or program staff embraced providing services to clients in a noncategorical manner. Some agencies had designed their facilities to support specific program functions, such as WIC or family planning. The ability to integrate services impacted how clients were scheduled for and received services. This impact often altered the traffic flow through the agency.

Historically computers were provided to support staff who were responsible for entering data. The most effective use of MOHSAIC is for professional staff to enter data on services at the time they are provided. Professional staff were not always supportive because they lacked expertise in using computers. Some stated that data entry was not their job, whereas others felt that entering the necessary data would increase the time spent documenting services and reduce their time with each client. Many LPHAs stated that they lacked the financial resources to purchase additional computers for professional staff.

Keys to Success: Lessons Learned

There are several lessons learned from the MDOH experience in developing MOHSAIC that can be considered keys for success in developing other integrated public health information systems.

Provide Sufficient Resources

As previously mentioned, MOHSAIC was a $24 million project. When the initial discussions began in 1992, the budget and funding sources were not identified. During the early stages of the project, it became obvious that considerable resources would be required. The project went through some significant delays initially because sufficient funds were not available.

Later in the life cycle of the project, funding was not a major issue because the project began to gain a positive reputation at the state and federal level and funding sources opened up based upon the early success of the project. A positive development was that as MOHSAIC was built, the funds started flowing. From a negative perspective, not having sufficient initial funding meant losing key staff members who did not want to be involved in an underfunded project. It also delayed the project, dampening the enthusiasm and creating uncertainty about support.

Developing an integrated system is very expensive. The extensive resources required for such a project must be acknowledged early on. A plan is needed on how to find those resources.

The Major Challenge to Building an Integrated System Is Politics

Because of the large amount of money required to develop an integrated system, one can be lured into thinking that the main issue is finding the money. hiring competent staff or contractors, and making the right technical design decisions. All of those are significant factors, but the real key to success is to remember that building an integrated system is as much a matter of politics. management, and interpersonal relationships as it is employing current technology.

A categorical stovepipe system can have a lot of appeal to a program manager. Stovepipe systems can be designed to support the straightforward critical needs of a program. Program managers feel they have control over a stovepipe system. The program can recognize how any money spent on such a system will benefit them. The program can define a stovepipe system to meet its needs without having any outside entity controlling standards and decisions. Available funds can be spent on a stovepipe system without consideration for other agency priorities. Although an integrated system has other obvious benefits listed previously, a program manager may see only what the program is losing. and not necessarily what the program is gaining in moving to an integrated system. To overcome these negative tendencies requires considerable managerial support and expertise.

Building an Integrated System Requires Top-Level Promotion and Support

MDOH tried to overcome potential program resistance in several ways. First, it was made clear that developing MOHSAIC was a MDOH activity that had the total support of the director and the deputy director of the MDOH. The deputy director of the MDOH took an active role in the early stages of the system and served as the official sponsor. He held several meetings with the top and middle managers of the MDOH to give progress reports on the direction the MDOH was taking. There was no question that MOHSAIC was coming from the director's office and had the full support of that office.

Because the development of MOHSAIC took much longer than anticipated. it was important to keep the MDOH staff informed about its progress. This was done through several communication media, including articles in newsletters, presentations at staff meetings, and e-mail updates.

The MDOH formed an information systems advisory committee that had representation from each major division in the MDOH. The advisory committee made recommendations to the department director. The department director made the final decisions on implementing new policies relating to network fees, confidentiality, standards, etc. This process kept all divisions involved, but the control was still in the director's office as opposed to CHIME's being the final authority.

For many reasons, MOHSAIC had a long gestational period. Not unlike any pregnancy, a successful birth outcome is not only dependent on the skill of the physician performing the delivery, but even more important, on the prenatal nurturing and caring during the pregnancy. MOHSAIC was dependent on the technical skills of the development staff, but even more important was the consistent nurturing of the process by department executive staff.

Most of MOHSAIC was developed under the terms of three directors of the MDOH. Each of these directors had a strong public health background and understood the importance of information. These directors also showed strong leadership in ensuring that the MDOH operated as a single agency, rather than as an umbrella agency housing separate categorical programs. There was a major emphasis placed upon interprogram cooperation and coordination. It is uncertain whether MOHSAIC could have been successfully developed if the departmental emphasis on cooperation had not existed at that time.

A Large-Scale Project to Build an Integrated System Requires a Strategic Plan

Critical to the success of MOHSAIC was the creation of a strategic plan. This plan continues to provide direction for the development of information systems in the MDOH. As new or enhanced data needs are identified, they are mapped back to the plan to determine just how they fit into the overall system. Information systems staff identify whether portions of the system have already been developed or are scheduled for development and determine what other units might have similar needs and the resources needed.

Without this critical "roadmap," staff would not understand how new data system requests relate to the MDOH. The plan has also been critical in developing grants to show just how funds would be expended to complete portions of an integrated system.

In the Development of an Integrated System, There Is a Need to Centralize Information Systems in the Department of Health

In any agency, the need to centralize infrastructure technicians should be obvious. There must be one network, one set of standards, one e-mail, etc. for an agency to be able to communicate and exchange data efficiently. However, the decision about whether to centralize or decentralize IT development staff has been debated for decades. There are clearly benefits and disadvantages to both approaches. However, if the agency is dedicated to development of an integrated system, the decision to centralize staff is crucial to the project's success. At MDOH, a decision was made shortly after starting MOHSAIC to centralize all information technology staff and the high-level data analysis staff into one unit, CHIME, with a director who reported directly to the department director. This has been one of the key factors to MOHSAIC's success.

Start Building an Integrated System in Areas Where Support Exists

The developmental stages of MOHSAIC were often based more on serendipity rather than on conformity to a plan. When a program manager showed interest and support and funding was available, then many times that confluence of events drove decisions about development priorities. Because MOHSAIC was so large, MDOH realized that it could not be swallowed in one gulp and that we had to nibble away at it. MDOH found it could start almost anywhere and develop modules that not only supported the immediate application but also built the foundation for later applications. By starting where program support was strong, MDOH built a track record that helped when it moved on to programs where support had not been immediately evident.

One of the benefits of building MOHSAIC in an incremental fashion was that the programs whose components were developed later in the cycle could see the functionality of the system that was already developed and could recognize its applicability to their program. An integrated system can create many new functionalities that a stand-alone system cannot support. However, program staff may not recognize that potential until they see it in operation.

One of the real challenges was what to do when a program needs an information system on a time schedule that did not conform to the MOHSAIC schedule. Several times, program managers found stand-alone software that they felt met their needs and wanted to purchase the software, instead of waiting for MOHSAIC. Approving or disapproving such a purchase is a difficult political decision, because if MDOH denied the request, it created a negative atmosphere for MOHSAIC. However, if it approved the request, MDOH conceded to nonintegration. To handle this situation, MOHSAIC staff met with the upper level management to determine how critical it was to use a software system that did not conform to MOHSAIC. Sometimes, legislation or other political issues forced the decision to allow the purchase of the software. But in these cases, it was understood that MOHSAIC would eventually replace the application. In other cases, MOHSAIC time frames were negotiated so that it was not necessary to purchase the software.

A Major Focus Should Be on Making Data More Accessible

Information system developers often focus on the data model, standards, business rules, screen flow, and system design. Users, on the other hand, focus on how the system will improve efficiencies and produce reports that they did not have access to previously. During the early stages of MOHSAIC, staff often focused on the important development issues and slighted the reports and what the end users really needed. Initially, MDOH did not have the data warehouse infrastructure in place to complete the normal life cycle of the system. This led to some user dissatisfaction, because users were given a fancy data entry system with few reporting capabilities.

As the data warehouse infrastructure was built, staff made a commitment to have a data warehouse module operational when a transaction module was completed. This commitment required converting historical data, building the operational data store, and creating the user-defined reports. Most important was giving the users the ability to create their own ad hoc reports or to download a file into Epi Info or another software package for additional analysis.

One of the new opportunities with current information system development is that the users do not have to be totally dependent on programmers to develop reports. Our data warehouse not only integrates data for statistical analysis, but users also have access to appropriate data marts so that they can create their own reports. This approach has wide appeal among the users. Most program managers want to control a data system so that they can gain better access to their data. Through an integrated system, programs lose some control of the transaction software, but they actually gain more access to the data.

Involve Users at All Levels in System Design

A successfully designed system is one in which the users, who have an in-depth knowledge of their program, actively design the system. The MDOH sought involvement at all levels of the program, including field staff, clerks entering the data, managers, and local health staff. Weekly JAD sessions were held with the users to define the system requirements. When one or more of the users at different levels did not actively participate, the CHIME staff often had to return and redo the system later. Top-level managers typically did not participate in the JAD sessions; however, monthly meetings were held with upper management to demonstrate the progress that had been made on the components of interest to them. At times, these monthly meetings uncovered system design issues that were important to management but that were not discovered in working with lower level staff.

Equally important to the development of a successful component was having the contribution of information systems and statistical staff who knew the potential of data systems and how the data could be used. Several of the CHIME staff that developed MOHSAIC were former staff of the programs. They had both technical and program expertise. They knew how information technology could be used to improve work processes. This added perspective allowed the development of a system that was not just a mirror image of the system that was being replaced.

Benefits of an Integrated System

There are many programmatic benefits of an integrated information system. The following discussion describes a couple of examples.

Immunization Register

The integrated immunization register has provided a number of benefits to clients and providers of vaccines. The register creates a single record that reflects for each client all doses of vaccine that have been documented in the system, no matter how many providers have administered those vaccines. The record is available to system users statewide. When children move from one area to another in Missouri, their record is available to MOHSAIC users in their new home. This reduces the delay caused when a new user must call or contact a previous provider to obtain a copy of the child's record.

MOHSAIC users can rapidly access the client's immunization information and determine which vaccines are due. MOHSAIC users have reported that having access to this information has reduced the number of duplicate doses of vaccine children have received.

A feature of the system creates a list or notice for each provider of the children who are either due or past due for vaccine doses. System users can notify parents and prompt them to seek the needed vaccines. MOHSAIC clients are grouped by households. This grouping method allows an address and telephone number to be entered into the system once for all members of the household. When a record for any member of the household is accessed, an indicator will appear when any member of that household is due or past due for a dose of vaccine.

The Advisory Committee on Immunization Practices' vaccine recommendations are complex. The schedule for existing vaccines changes as new vaccines are added. MOHSAIC has a complex algorithm that determines the vaccines needed for each child. This feature has benefited WIC service providers, as they no longer must memorize the complex schedule to determine whether the clients they see need vaccines.

Another benefit of this integrated immunization register is the ability to interface with the state's Medicaid system to determine the Medicaid status of a client. In addition, managed care plans have contacted the MDOH for assistance in creating their Health Plan Employee Data and Information Set (HEDIS) indicators for their enrollees.

Surveillance

The surveillance component of MOHSAIC is designed to assist in the rapid response to events that have the potential to expand into major public health risks. Examples of such events are incidents of infectious or communicable diseases, discovery of environmental contaminants, or bioterrorism attacks. Whenever a Missouri healthcare provider becomes aware of a reportable disease, the information is immediately entered into MOHSAIC. MOHSAIC then automatically notifies a public health official, who is responsible for taking appropriate action to protect others from contracting the disease.

Because MOHSAIC is a centralized system, public health officials are able to respond to outbreaks that expand beyond city and county lines. The data are entered in the county which first learns of the disease, but the notification is sent to the public health official in the county who needs to do case follow-up.

Prior to MOHSAIC, surveillance was done on a case basis, and data on co-morbidity and individuals with multiple occurrences of the same disease were not available. Because MOHSAIC enters an individual only once in the system, all occurrences of reportable disease as well as the individual's immunization history are included in the single record. Thus, the public health worker has all information about the individual immediately available to him or her.

Development of the Information Systems Model Around Public Health Core Functions

The Institute of Medicine report, *The Future of Public Health*,[4] defined three core functions of public health—assessment, policy development, and assurance. The MDOH adopted this rubric and developed its strategic plan around these core functions, recognizing that data are essential to fulfill each of them.

The assessment function requires data in order to permit performance of a community diagnosis on the leading health problems and the trends and factors that are impeding healthy communities. Assessments can use programmatic data to determine unmet needs in a community. But, by definition, assessment requires population-based data that define the health problems of the entire community. One of the main challenges for communities in performing assessments is the lack of timely, readily accessible data at the community level.

To address this issue, the MDOH developed a Web site (available at: http://www.dhss.state.mo.us/) that provides over 300 county-specific health indicators grouped into 20 profiles, such as deaths, hospitalizations, communicable diseases, chronic diseases, injuries, prenatal, infant, child, etc. The profiles provide the number of events for each indicator, the county rate, and the state rate; the profiles also indicate whether the county rate is statistically different from the state rate and the quintile ranking. In addition, for each indicator, there is a resource page that provides information on the statistical definition, risk factors, intervention strategies, indicator reports, pertinent Web links, and other information that may be useful in conducting an assessment.

The MDOH Web site has an additional tool, Missouri Information for Community Assessment (MICA), to support the assessment function. MICA is an interactive system that allows the user to custom-design a table based upon available variables of a specific data file. The user can select from 15 data files, including births, deaths, hospitalizations, injuries, pregnancies, etc. The system allows for the creation of a table, a map, or a graph. Data can be displayed at the state, county, or ZIP code level. MICA allows public health agencies and other community groups to ask detailed questions and receive the answers in a matter of seconds.

The policy development function of public health requires data to establish goals and develop policies or programs that will respond to the needs identified through the assessment process. Some of the same data that are used for the assessment function are also used for policy development. Therefore, the county profiles and MICA on the MDOH Web site are useful for those designing health policies.

The assessment and policy development functions also require programmatic data to evaluate and redirect programs. Just as population-based data need to be readily available and in a format conducive for easy retrieval and analysis, so do program data. An effective analysis often requires data that are not restricted to categorical data collection systems. For example, the immunization program may want to know the immunization rate of WIC children or of children of women participating in a family planning program. The AIDs program may need to know the TB and STD co-morbidities of its clients. This type of data comes from the integrated data design of MOHSAIC. The specific data elements needed for assessment or policy development analysis is stored in a data mart of the data warehouse. The end user has direct access to the data warehouse and is able to custom design an inquiry using a commercial data retrieval software package.

The assurance function of public health is supported by the client-based transaction data of MOHSAIC. The design of MOHSAIC as an integrated system facilitates client-centered, rather than program-centered, service delivery.

Conclusion

Public health can no longer continue to develop stovepipe information systems. At the same time, Congress and the state legislatures will continue to fund categorical programs because of the nature of the political process. However, the expectations for government performance are increasing. Politicians and the public expect government programs to work together across bureaucratic lines, to weed out duplicative efforts, to fill service gaps with existing resources, to create policies that are practical and science-based, and to eliminate programs that do not work.

An integrated public health information system is one of the most effective ways to meet these high expectations. Through such a system, programs can share data and find new ways to coordinate activities. Redundant activities can be easily identified, and the resources can be reprogrammed. Person-centered, integrated data allow for more effective policy analysis and program evaluation.

However, creating an integrated system can be fraught with problems. The challenge of such an undertaking should not be underestimated. The Missouri experience highlights that there are several factors essential to a successful project. These factors include having a plan, having technical competence, managing the political environment, having top-level support, centralizing information systems, providing sufficient resources, insuring active program involvement, creating new functionalities, and making data more accessible.

MOHSAIC is an enterprise system that supports state and local public health activities. Other states may want to consider more modest approaches if several of the success factors are not present. For example, an integrated system could be developed around just one of the key components, such as health management, surveillance, or regulation. Although the benefits of these components are expanded through their interrelationships with each other, the components also have strong functional independence.

Missouri chose to develop a system that would meet both the state and local public health information needs. Each state must make the critical decision regarding the scope of the service that a system is to provide. A system that is designed just for state use would be much simpler to develop and deploy, but it may not meet the public health objectives desired of an integrated system.

Another consideration is whether to focus on linking stovepipe data systems through a data warehouse, rather than on integrating data through a transaction system. Such a linkage can be challenging because of the lack of standards across various systems. There probably is not a public health need to link all data systems. Therefore, an analysis would have to be conducted to determine what analytical functions are expected from such a data warehouse. If the primary objective is to have better data for assessment and policy development, as opposed to service delivery, then linking files through a data warehouse may be a preferred option. Investment in data warehousing software for data retrieval, so that users have better access to data, is an important consideration for this option.

In many cases, the answers to key public health questions do not require complex, integrated information systems and data warehouses. Often, the problem is that there is no easy way to retrieve and analyze data. In this case, a Web-based interactive system such as MICA may be the answer.

Each public health agency must determine the desirable role that data are to play in the agency. A decision must be made whether to focus on the assurance or assessment data needs or both. The critical success factors documented from the Missouri experience are important, regardless of the scope of any information systems project. With the emergence of managed care and the rethinking of the assurance functions, the role of public health is rapidly changing. At the same time, the demand for data continues to increase for surveillance, monitoring, and assessment. Integrated information systems are essential if public health is to respond and provide leadership in such an ever-changing environment.

Questions for Review

1. List and describe the inefficiencies of the program-specific computer systems that the integrated system replaced, and explain how the new integrated system addressed these inefficiencies.
2. Explain how the use of information engineering methodology made development of a MOHSAIC plan possible. Why was a plan important to the success of the project?
3. In what way was the use of two teams to develop the Information Strategy Plan efficient?
4. Why did application development center on the area of clients and services?
5. Explain how the MDOH found financial support for the project.
6. In what way did the decision to develop existing public health staff as IT professionals pay dividends? Why was the decision to hire consultants to assist with the project beneficial?
7. Explain how the use of Joint Application Design (JAD) sessions contributed to the success of the project.
8. Explain how system designers minimized training costs and dislocations while also providing the training necessary for users of the new system. How did the establishment of a toll-free help desk complement the training?
9. List and explain the reasons that program staff members with their own stovepipe systems sometimes resist the development and implementation of integrated systems. Why are large health agencies with an existing information system likely to resist an integrated system?
10. Explain how federal and state funding practices have contributed to the development of stovepipe information systems and thus created barriers to development of integrated systems.
11. Why was the strategy to use newly appropriated monies, rather than to re-budget existing funds, an important strategy for the success of MOHSAIC?
12. In what sense can it be said that integrated systems compound confidentiality issues?
13. Explain why conversion of data from legacy systems was difficult. In particular, why was re-keying the data from legacy systems into the MOHSAIC system necessary?
14. Explain why MOHSAIC system developers encountered resistance to the business process reengineering that an integrated system required. How did the developers deal with the resistance?

15. Why was top-level promotion and support of the MOHSAIC project essential to its success?
16. Why was it important to centralize information systems in the MDOH important?
17. In what way was beginning the building of MOHSAIC in program areas where support already existed important to the acceptance of the integrated system by other areas?
18. Why was involving users at all levels in the design of the integrated system a key to the success of the project?

References

1. Missouri Department of Health. *Public Health Agenda for the '90's—Healthy Missourians 2000*. Jefferson City, MO: Missouri Department of Health; 1992.
2. Finkelstein C. *An Introduction to Information Engineering: From Strategic Planning to Information Systems*. Wokingham, England: Addison-Wesley; 1989.
3. Missouri Department of Health. *Health Information 2000—Clients and Services Business Area Analysis 1*. Jefferson City, MO: Missouri Department of Health; 1993.
4. Institute of Medicine. *The Future of Public Health*. Washington, DC: National Academy Press; 1988.
5. The Standish Group. *Charting the Seas of Information Technology*. West Yarmouth, MA: The Standish Group; 1994.

29

Using Information Systems to Build Capacity: A Public Health Improvement Tool Box

Jerry A. Schultz, Stephen B. Fawcett, Vincent T. Francisco, and Bobbie Berkowitz

Learning Objectives

After studying this chapter, you should be able to:

- Define *public health improvement* and describe the challenges for building capacity for public health improvement.
- Describe the utility of having an information system for supporting public health improvement.
- Understand the background and context of the National Turning Point Initiative.
- Describe how the Internet-based "Public Health Improvement Tool Box" is used to enhance capacity, document systems change, and promote dialogue among those doing the work.

Overview

The National Turning Point Initiative, jointly funded by the Robert Wood Johnson Foundation and the W. K. Kellogg Foundation, is a major project dedicated to improving population health through an investment in strengthening and transforming the public health infrastructure. In this chapter, the methodology of the project and the ways in which the project is helping states and communities to improve public health are outlined. Much of the chapter focuses on changing and improving systems needed to help state and community partners to undertake activities associated with public health improvement. Central to this effort is the Internet-based Public Health Improvement Tool Box, developed by the Work Group on Health Promotion and Community Development at the University of Kansas. The PHI Tool Box provides access to information for supporting, documenting, and learning from the work of public health improvement. Although the initiative is ongoing and the lessons about it will come only later, the initiative and the PHI

Tool Box are exciting developments in the field of public health at the state and local levels.

Introduction

Public health improvement involves changing health-related outcomes and the conditions that affect them for all the people who share a common place or experience.[1] This is complex work: Different community conditions, such as access to health services or availability of support from community members, may affect distinct outcomes, such as population-level rates of immunization, adolescent pregnancy, or elders living independently.[2] Multiple and interrelated interventions, such as expanded programs or revised policies, may be needed to affect the conditions necessary for population-health improvement. In this dynamic and adaptive work, community and systems changes unfold over time and may adjust to reflect new barriers and opportunities encountered in the work. The task of public health improvement is to create conditions in which local efforts to promote health and well being can be successful.[3,4]

There are some important challenges in building capacity for public health improvement. First, improvement in population-level health outcomes involves bringing about systems changes—new or modified programs, policies, and practices at the state and local levels.[5,6] How can we best support efforts of state and local health departments to create the multiple and interrelated changes needed to make a difference with health outcomes? A second challenge is that the work of public health improvement cuts across disciplinary domains—including health, education, human service, business, and faith communities—and kinds of expertise, from professionals with disciplinary knowledge to community members with experience with local issues and situations. How do we best engage the different actors and organizations that can contribute to the varied and interrelated goals for public health improvement? A third challenge is that there are many different competencies needed for this work—for example, the skills of assessment, leadership, advocacy, social marketing, evaluation, and sustaining the initiative. How can we enhance the skills of a diverse group of professionals and community members needed to create conditions for community health? A fourth challenge arises because the common work of building capacity for public health improvement engages people across distances and over time. How do we connect those engaged in this work within and between states (and countries) and over the months and years required to make a difference? Finally, there is a high turnover among those doing this work. How do we build capacity among the generations of community members and professionals engaged in efforts to improve health outcomes at the population level?

To be useful, an information system for supporting public health improvement should have several attributes.

- It must be *easily available* to the different professionals and community members engaged in providing, retrieving, and using information to effect public health outcomes.
- It should be sufficiently *accurate and secure* to guide decisions and inspire confidence in its use.
- The information and supports should be *compatible* with the variety of goals and problems related to public health improvement.
- The content should be sufficiently *comprehensive* to reflect the varied information and skill building needs (e.g., assessment, strategic planning, leadership, grant writing).
- Gateways into the information should permit its *timely* access for people facing different issues and working on early or later stages of initiatives for public health improvement.
- The information should be *clear and compelling* enough to prompt and support action for public health improvement.
- It should be *friendly and supportive* to people with diverse experiences—including community members and professionals with limited training and those who operate from different domains of practice (e.g., public health, business, faith communities).
- It should be able to *connect people* working across distances and over time.
- Information should be *integrated* in a seamless support system for addressing multiple and interrelated outcomes. Finally, it must help *reduce inequalities* in resources available to support the work of public health improvement.

Public health informatics holds promise for contributing to the work of public health improvement.[7] Dramatic improvements in information technology permit widespread access to the means for building capacity for the work, documenting and evaluating public health initiatives, and learning through exchanges with peers and experts. More specifically, Internet-based systems have the advantages of standardized formats for gathering and reporting information, simplified and efficient ways to update it, and nearly universal access. Additionally, Internet-based systems may enhance the systems-oriented, integrated, and collaborative work necessary for public health improvement. Data systems can help focus attention on systems changes, analyze contributions across a variety of categories of concerns, and enhance collaboration among agents in different sectors, such as business or education, related to public health improvement. Finally, the new information technologies provide capabilities for building capacity in the many and varied people required for this work. Internet-based systems can help people gain access to skill-building information needed for the complex and adaptive work of public health improvement.

The purpose of this chapter is to describe an information system for building capacity for public health improvement as part of the National Turning Point initiative. Funded by the Robert Wood Johnson Foundation and the W. K. Kellogg Foundation, the mission of the National Turning Point initiative is to work with state health departments to enhance the infrastructure for public health improvement. Using the capabilities of the Community Tool Box (http://ctb.ukans.edu/) and the University of Kansas' Work Group on Health Promotion and Community Development (KU Work Group), we developed an Internet-based support system for this initiative known as the "Public Health Improvement Tool Box" (PHI Tool Box). This chapter describes the context for this work and the information system's several components:

1. *Tools for building capacity for the work*—tailored links to how-to information for a variety of relevant skills (e.g., assessment, leadership, evaluation)
2. *An on-line documentation system*—for entering, retrieving, graphing, and making sense of data on systems changes (i.e., new or modified programs, policies, and practices facilitated by participating state efforts for public health improvement)
3. *An on-line learning community*—for exchanges among peers and experts to guide and support public health initiatives.

We conclude with a discussion of potential challenges, strengths, and future prospects of such information systems for contributing to the work of public health improvement.

Background and Context: The National Turning Point Initiative

The National Turning Point Initiative (Turning Point: Collaborating for a New Century in Public Health, available at: http://www.naccho.org/project30.cfm) was funded by the Robert Wood Johnson and W. K. Kellogg Foundations and supported by the University of Washington National Office and the National Association of County and City Health Officials (NACCHO). Its vision and mission is to improve population health through an investment in strengthening and transforming the public health infrastructure. The working hypothesis is that strategic changes in the public health system can enhance the success of state and local efforts to promote and protect health and prevent diseases and injury. From January 1998 to December 2000, the two foundations funded 21 states and 41 communities to plan for and carry out public health systems change.

Turning Point began in 1998 with a two-year strategic development process using three primary methods:

1. It created a planning environment at the state and local level where committed stakeholders would plan collaboratively, analyze health issues and challenges, and promote system changes for public health improvement.
2. It developed a strategic planning document in each of the 21 states and 41 communities. The documents included plans to:

    a. assess and address gaps in system capacity;
    b. evaluate the public health workforce;
    c. identify necessary information and communication systems;
    d. develop a framework for stable financing; and
    e. identify strategies for formulating health policy.
3. Turning Point participants established a network of partners who could contribute to a health agenda in each state and community. These partners would collaborate to work on a variety of public health issues including
    a. eliminating health disparities among populations;
    b. assuring access to quality care;
    c. aggressively preventing infectious diseases;
    d. reducing risks for chronic diseases; and
    e. protecting the population from hazards and toxins in the environment.

The partners focused on building the system and infrastructure that could help address these issues. The infrastructure required for population health improvement includes, but is not limited to. (a) a skilled and competent workforce; (b) stable financing; (c) information systems and technology; (d) research and citizen involvement to guide policy development and implementation; and (e) collaboration among and between states, communities, and the multiple public and private organizations and institutions that contribute to health.

Two cohorts of states and one cohort of communities were involved in the planning phase of Turning Point. At the end of the planning phase, states were funded by the Robert Wood Johnson Foundation to implement a specific strategy highlighted in their strategic plans. Over a four-year period (2000–2003), the two state cohorts will collaborate to carry out different planned change initiatives. The communities, with funding from W. K. Kellogg Foundation. have addressed priorities in their strategic plans.

During development of the implementation phase of Turning Point. it became clear that the states and communities faced several common issues in building capacity for public health improvement. Although each state and community is unique in its approach to public health. commonly held areas for improvement included (1) performance management; (2) collaborative leadership; (3) information technology; (4) social marketing; and (5) modernizing public health statutes. To help assure a coordinated approach to these five areas, a third phase of Turning Point was created, The National Excellence Collaboratives. Turning Point states were given the opportunity to join one or more collaboratives to work jointly with state and local Turning Point partners and with national organizations such as the US Centers for Disease Control and Prevention (CDC), the Health Resources Service Administration (HRSA), the National Association of County and City Health Officials (NACCHO). and the Association of State and Territorial Health Officers (ASTHO). Each of the National Excellence collaboratives has created a shared vision, a mission, and a work plan that will culminate at the end of four years in a set of recommendations. products, tools, and pilot demonstrations.

For example, the Information Technology Collaborative had as its mission to assess, evaluate, and recommend to national policy makers innovative ways to improve the nation's public health infrastructure by utilizing information technology. Information technology would be used to improve data access, community participation in making public health decisions, and performance of the public health system. The initial goals of the collaborative were to

1. monitor health status to identify community health problems;
2. diagnose and investigate health problems and health hazards in the community;
3. inform, educate, and empower people about health issues;
4. develop policies and plans that support individual and community health efforts;
5. enforce laws and regulations that protect health and ensure safety;
6. mobilize community partnerships to identify and solve health problems;
7. link people to needed personal health services and assure the provision of health care when otherwise unavailable;
8. assure a competent public health and personal healthcare work force;
9. evaluate effectiveness, accessibility, and quality of personal and population-based health services; and
10. research for new insights and innovative solutions to health problems.

Supporting such a large-scale, multi-site, and multi-method initiative has been a particular challenge of Turning Point. Each funding foundation has created a national program office to provide guidance and technical assistance to the states and communities involved in Turning Point. The National Program Office for the W. K. Kellogg Foundation has been located at NACCHO. The Robert Wood Johnson Foundation's National Program Office is located at The University of Washington School of Public Health and Community Medicine. Several support challenges emerged during early implementation. How do we build capacity among state and local initiatives for the different competencies needed for systems change for public health improvement? How do we document and make sense of the unfolding of systems changes facilitated by state initiatives? And, how do we support learning among the Turning Point communities and states about the work of systems change for public health improvement?

Emerging Theory of Practice for Public Health Improvement

The model (or framework) for public health improvement used by the National Turning Point initiative is dynamic and interactive. For example, it is assumed that understanding of state and community contexts should guide action and intervention, which, in turn, should affect community and systems change for public health improvement. Systems changes, such as new programs for workforce development or revised public health statutes, will ultimately affect the context for public health improvement. The work is also iterative or repeating: for example, as time passes and issues change. the new context may beget renewed cycles of planning and action, another generation of systems changes, and further public health improvement.

The parts of this model are: (1) understanding context and collaborative planning: (2) action and intervention: (3) systems change: (4) enhanced infrastructure: and (5) improvements in population-level outcomes. This model integrates public health and community development perspectives.[1,6,8,9]

Understanding Context and Collaborative Planning

Collaborative planning. and related situation analysis. sets the stage for taking action targeted at public health improvement. Studying the context in which public health improvement occurs helps public health leaders and local people see the problems that states and communities face and how they are currently addressing them. The context can be influenced by a variety of factors, such as local people's dreams for healthier communities and disparities in income and health status. By bringing together stakeholders and accountable entities, states and communities can develop a broad perspective on public health improvement and how related issues might be addressed. Partnerships prepare and analyze state and community health profiles. They make available information about the local community's health concerns and analyze that information to help support locally determined plans for health improvement. The resulting agenda of state and community health issues should reflect not only the public health department's interests, but also those of a broader spectrum of community stakeholders, including the general public.

Collaborative planning brings together people and organizations with different experiences and resources to clarify their vision, mission. objectives, strategies. and action plans for bringing about community and systems changes. Partnerships for public health improvement might analyze the critical health issues to determine general underlying causes and contributing factors, how they operate in each state or community. and what interventions are likely to be effective in meeting goals for public health improvement. Partnerships might also develop an inventory of resources available to them that can be applied to selected public health improvement issues. They also develop health improvement strategies, such as social marketing and community coalitions that reflect an assessment of how available resources can best be applied to address locally identified concerns.

Action and Intervention

The planning process is followed by action taken to bring about public health improvement. Implementing strategies and interventions for public health improvement requires action by many different segments of the community or state (e.g., public and private health organizations, faith communities, schools, government). The particular mix of activities and actors will depend on the health issue being addressed and the local participants and resources. Some courses of actions are commonplace, such as conducting statewide social marketing campaigns against tobacco use, but others, such as changing public health statutes to protect water quality, may receive opposition. Establishing accountability for partners is important to help ensure successful implementation.

Systems Change

The aim of planning and taking action is to bring about community and systems change (e.g., new or modified policies, programs, and practices) related to public health improvement. Illustrative community and systems changes to be sought by a state partnership with a goal of reducing health disparities might include expanded programs (e.g., establishing and supporting peer educator programs in youth organizations and middle schools to encourage healthy living skills), new policies (e.g., reducing delays and waiting time in obtaining health care and preventative services), and modified practices (e.g., establishing city/state policies to create "healthy opportunity" zones that allow a tax credit for establishing neighborhood-based primary health facilities).[10]

Enhanced Infrastructure

When systems changes occur, the environment in which people attempt to effect public health improvement is transformed. By making the work easier and more rewarding, an enhanced infrastructure can influence the behavior of those who can contribute to public health improvement. For example, a systems change, such as a new Internet-based program for enhancing skills for community health promotion, can affect implementation of such efforts in multiple communities. Taken together, locally determined community and systems changes can support relevant behaviors of the many and varied actors needed for public health improvement.

Improvement in Population-Level Outcomes

Improvement in population-level outcomes, such as improvement in the incidence and prevalence of asthma or HIV/AIDS in the state or county, is the ultimate result of public health improvement efforts. It is hypothesized that an enhanced public health infrastructure can contribute to widespread behavior change needed to improve outcomes. It is important to develop a set of public health indicators of goal attainment that are accurate, available, and sensitive to state and community-determined efforts. Improved data systems can help monitor process and outcome to provide useful, formative information to guide decisions in the work of public health improvement.

Developing a Public Health Improvement Tool Box

Supporting programs for public health improvement efforts at state and community levels, such as those launched by National Turning Point, can aid implementation of this theory of practice. In collaboration with the National Program Office of Turning Point, we built a prototype Internet-based support system using the infrastructure of the Community Tool Box and other capabilities of the KU Work Group. The Public Health Improvement Tool Box (PHI Tool Box) is designed to promote public health improvement by connecting people with support tools for the work, documenting systems changes, and promoting learning through on-line exchanges.

The PHI Tool Box guides the users in choosing useful tools and pertinent information related to their current work. It also connects users to peers and mentors who can provide guidance specific to local contexts. The objective of the PHI Tool Box is threefold:

1. To *enhance capacity* for public health improvement through "how-to" learning modules and other tools found in the Community Tool Box;
2. To *document* the process of *systems change* related to public health improvement through the KU Work Group's on-line documentation system; and
3. To *promote dialogue* among peers and experts involved in public health improvement through a learning community that communicates through on-line forums.

Supporting and documenting the work, and learning with others, are activities that can enhance the infrastructure for public health improvement.

Audiences, Core Partners, and Assets in Development

There are a variety of audiences that might use a "tool box" for public health improvement. Leaders and staff of state and local public health departments who are doing the work of public health improvement can use it to seek information, document their efforts, or connect with other public health professionals working on common issues. People involved in health improvement initiatives through other sectors, such as faith communities or business, may also find the PHI Tool Box supportive of their efforts.

Support organizations, such as university-based research and training centers or advocacy groups, are also a primary audience. This information system can amplify their capacity to support national, state, and local public health improvement efforts. The PHI Tool Box contributes to the infrastructure by providing a framework for guiding these efforts and support materials that can make the work of public health improvement easier and more rewarding.

Similarly, those organizations that provide funds and resources for the work, such as government agencies or private foundations, can also benefit from enhanced support for public health related initiatives. Such information systems can optimize investments by enhancing competencies and shared learning about the work of public health improvement.

The development of the PHI Tool Box is based on the empirical and experiential knowledge of several core partners. The KU Work Group and the National Turning Point Initiative have joined efforts to develop and test an information system that brings together Internet-based technology, research-based learning systems, and deep experience with public health improvement efforts.

The KU Work Group, a research, teaching, and public service organization, has worked extensively with community and health development initiatives since 1990. The KU Work Group has actively developed tools and on-line technology that builds capacity and promotes learning among those doing the work of community health and development.[11–14] The National Program Office of the National Turning Point initiative at the University of Washington has drawn together a broad community of scientists and practitioners involved in public health improvement. By joining the experiential knowledge of the National Program Office and the KU Work Group's support capabilities, we seek to develop a valuable resource for public health improvement.

The PHI Tool Box is undergirded by the Community Tool Box. Operating since 1995, the Community Tool Box is designed to promote community health and development by connecting people, ideas, and resources. With support from the Robert Wood Johnson Foundation and other sources, the Community Tool Box team has created on-line learning modules for the variety of competencies required for the work (e.g., community assessment, strategic planning, leadership development, evaluation). Currently, the Community Tool Box has over 200 how-to sections and over 6,000 pages of useful information. The site received over 1.5 million hits and over 110,000 user sessions during the year 2000. In addition, the KU Work Group has developed an on-line documentation system by which clients can enter data on community and systems change, analyze data according to a theory of change, and produce graphs and private reports of accomplishments.

Core Components and Information Features of the PHI Tool Box

The work of public health improvement could be enhanced by an integrated and Internet-based system that brings together capabilities for support, such as easy access to how-to information for community assessment or evaluation and systems for documenting changes related to public health improvement and for learning through exchanges with peers and experts. The PHI Tool Box has three components: (a) a support system; (b) a documentation system; and (c) a learning community.

Supporting the Work

Drawing on the breadth of content of the Community Tool Box, we aim to create more depth of support for core activities in the work of public health improvement. The PHI Tool Box helps build capacity by linking users to how-to information relevant to their work. Hundreds of how-to sections can be accessed as users work on one element or another (e.g., community assessment, collaborative planning, taking action) of their respective frameworks for public health improvement (e.g., the Institute of Medicine's Community Health Improvement Process). Users can access how-to information about core competencies for public health improvement such as community assessment, strategic planning, intervention, advocacy, evaluation of process and intermediate outcomes, and resource generation, celebration, and renewal. Another gateway to tools, the troubleshooting guide, helps focus on the problems public health initiatives may face (e.g., we can't come to agreement on which systems changes to work on). The guide uses clarifying questions to lead the user to understanding the meaning of the situation and to link to "how-to" sections that help users decide the best course of action.

The support feature provides tailored links to on-line support tools in the Community Tool Box related to public health improvement. For example, one gateway to the tools is organized around the core competencies related to the "10 essential health services"[15,16]; another provides links relevant to the tasks of the Institute of Medicine's Community Health Improvement Process.[1] By invoking the Community Tool Box's Workstation feature, users can get outlines, links to how-to information, and examples to help produce products such as a leadership development plan, a strategic plan, a social marketing plan, or an evaluation plan. It provides connections to the National Turning Point initiative's internal structure for personal support and technical assistance. Links to other resources are also available.

Documenting Systems Changes

The on-line documentation system enables leadership in the National Turning Point initiatives to document valued accomplishments such as community and systems change—new or modified programs, policies, or practices related to public health improvement. It can also collect information about other events, such as resources generated for public health improvement and media coverage of the work. In addition, users can document success stories and lessons learned that connect discrete state initiatives in a common community of learners and doers. The database also records information about collaborating partners involved in accomplishing systems changes. Information from the documentation system can be used by multiple audiences to help them understand the effort, make adjustments, and ensure accountability.

The documentation system also collects information that allows the analysis of the potential contribution of systems change to public health improvement. The database of systems changes can be displayed to show the distribution of changes in the following ways:

- Primary goal/objective (e.g., the 10 essential public health services, monitor health status to identify community health problems. diagnose and investigate health problems and health hazards in the community)
- Primary strategy used to change behavior (e.g., modify access/barriers and opportunities, change policy)
- Duration of the change (e.g., one-time, ongoing)
- Penetration or exposure
  - for primary population (e.g., all, adolescents, African-Americans
  - through primary sector or setting (e.g., health organizations and providers, faith communities)
  - in primary places (e.g., list of specific states, cities/towns)
  - at primary level (e.g., neighborhood, city/town, county, state/tribe)

The on-line documentation system makes data entry easy and information available in real time, instantaneously. Participating state initiatives and support organizations have direct access to their data on systems change. Data collection is done in real time. helping avoid the delays of traditional retrospective reporting. The National Turning Point Office and the funders can also have immediate access to graphs and reporting based on this information. Information is entered through any Web browser (e.g.. Internet Explorer, Netscape Navigator) using data entry screens. The information entered is stored on a server at the KU Work Group.

Information capabilities include those of (a) reading on-line and printing reports of selected measures (e.g., systems change) for participating Turning Point state initiatives; (b) FTP (File Transfer Protocol) access to data for the National Turning Point office and state grantees for purposes of data management: (c) preformatted examples for how to use data in reports (e.g., model text, graphs. lists of accomplishments): and (d) on-line "helpful tips" to support how to enter and retrieve data and provide answers to commonly asked questions about documentation.

Information provided by the documentation system helps initiatives and funders to meet their needs for accountability and continuous improvement. It provides for a developmental approach. rather than merely a summative evaluation. The documentation system serves as a foundation for communication between stakeholders and for co-learning within and among state initiatives. The reports generated on-line by the documentation system encourage celebration and renewal of effort. In addition, the data and information on accomplishments produced through the system may be used to help secure further funds and resources.

The documentation system provides the basis for sensemaking.[13,17-19] Information from the documentation system can be used to develop a better understanding of how the initiative is functioning and possible contributions of systems change (an intermediate outcome) to goals related to improving the public health infrastructure (a more distant outcome). Some of the questions that can be answered include:

- Is the initiative facilitating community and systems change related to the mission? (i.e., by examining rates of change over time);
- What factors are associated with increased rates of community and systems change? (i.e., by examining what is associated with discontinuities in rates of change);
- Do public health experts regard the changes as important? (e.g., by using ratings of public health significance by constituents to "weight" the changes); and
- What is the contribution of community and systems changes to goals for improving the infrastructure? (e.g., by examining the distribution of systems changes among the 10 essential services).

Learning Through Exchanges with Others

Using a customized version of the on-line forum capabilities of the Community Tool Box, we created a forum or learning community for participants in the National Turning Point Initiative. Peers and experts can engage each other in dialogue about common issues and options for public health improvement. The forums are structured by topics chosen by the partners (e.g., assessing community health, developing coalitions). The forums create a virtual space where public health leaders can guide and be guided in solving problems that emerge in the work. For example, fine points of developing coalitions or social marketing can be discussed or valued ideas and resources shared. Because exchanges are archived, the forum permits cumulative learning among those doing (and exchanging ideas about) the work. In addition, thematic "conference" or discussion themes can be developed to support focused dialogue about different aspects of the work.

Plans for Implementation and Ongoing Learning and Improvement

Several strategies will be used to support use of the PHI Tool Box. First, training sessions on how to use the PHI Tool Box are provided for representatives of state initiatives at the periodic conferences for the National Turning Point grantees. These training sessions will include guided tours, tips on navigation, and practice and troubleshooting on using each component of the on-line system. These sessions provide hands-on experience in accessing relevant support materials in the Community Tool Box and the use of customized gateways, troubleshooting guides, searches, and other useful tools. Training in the use of the documentation system that includes entering data, generating reports, and sensemaking based on the data will also be provided. This training will also offer an opportunity for users to learn about and practice use of the learning community or forums.

The National Turning Point Program office will provide follow-up technical support such as in entering and retrieving data. Consultations with National Turning Point staff will help users interpret the data and possible interrelationships among the data. Annual follow-up consultation and training will be provided at national meetings of Turning Point grantees to enhance use of this support, documentation, and learning system for public health improvement.

The biannual meeting will also be used to assess and improve the PHI Tool Box. Focus groups will be conducted during each of these meetings. In addition, the PHI Tool Box has several user feedback systems built into each of its components. Users can suggest improvements in content and procedures, discuss alternative materials and approaches, and describe what works or does not work for them.

As participating Turning Point partners document the process of community and systems change, there will be enormous opportunities to learn about what works and the conditions under which public health improvement occurs. Ongoing data on systems change across sites can be used to better understand, support, and re-direct efforts for public health improvement. Online exchanges among peers and experts may help adapt state-based programs and practices and make sense of these widely distributed public health improvement efforts.

Some Potential Challenges, Strengths, and Future Prospects

Any information system to build capacity, such as the PHI Tool Box, should meet several important needs. First, the system should help state and local public health systems do the work of systems changes. How will it reduce the effort and make more rewarding the work of bringing about change within public health systems? Second, the work of population-level health improvement is not restricted to public health workers. The PHI Tool Box must have utility for a variety of users, who have varying levels of expertise. Will an educator, a business person, or a member of a faith community be supported in efforts to change programs or policies related to health improvement?

Third, the system should help users enhance the broad array of skills and competencies related to public health improvement. Does the information system provide access to learning resources for the appropriate and needed competencies? Fourth, a public health information system should connect public health leaders and workers both within and between states so that the sharing of guidance and successes can take place. It should also connect young practitioners with and help them share the wisdom of more experienced public health leaders. Finally, a public health information system should be a repository of useful information to help with continuity during periods of reduced staffing or gaps in the work force.

The strengths of the PHI Tool Box in supporting the work are numerous. Users can access the vast store of information available easily through any Internet-connected computer. Although not yet ubiquitous, Internet access to such information systems is growing rapidly. The amount of information available through the Community Tool Box is vast: it reflects the broad set of competencies needed for the work of public health improvement (e.g., assessment, leadership, sustainability). Though vast, the information being sought can be accessed through customized gateways, such as logic models, troubleshooting guides, and support links for the 10 essential services. Examples will illustrate application of competencies to specific health goals and problems (e.g., reducing disparities, increasing physical activity). The support material is written in language that is welcoming and friendly, with a limited jargon. Links are provided to connect the user to others who can provide more specialized information.

Through the PHI Tool Box, users can connect with other peers in an on-line forum or learning community or with experts or mentors associated with a national program office that can also provide guidance and assistance. The entire system of support, learning, and documentation is integrated. Users can garner data from the documentation system to help make sense of their initiative's efforts. For example, the data may suggest that systems change is not occurring. Depending on the user's assessment of the situation, it might be determined that the most appropriate partners are not involved. Support information might be accessed to prompt ideas for enhancing collaboration. In applying this information to the local context or situation, the user may seek guidance from peers and experts through the on-line learning community or mentoring component.

Future research and development can help establish and optimize the contribution of such Internet-based information systems to state and local initiatives for public health improvement. With refinement, Internet-based systems can help provide support and guidance, connect participants committed to improving health to each other and to needed resources, and document (and make sense of) comprehensive efforts. By building capacity for public health improvement, information systems can make the work easier and more rewarding. In so doing, it can help assure that all of us experience environments that promote and protect health and well being.

Acknowledgments

This work was supported, in part, by a grant from the Robert Wood Johnson Foundation and the National Office of the Turning Point Initiative. We thank those who give guidance to this work, including the Community Tool Box team and, especially, state and local public health workers and community members doing the work of public health improvement. Reprints may be obtained from the first three authors, Work Group on Health Promotion and Community Development, 4082 Dole Center, University of Kansas, Lawrence, KS 66045 or the last author, Turning Point National Program Office, 6 Nickerson, Suite 300, Seattle, WA 98109-1618.

Questions for Review

1. Explain why we refer to community-based efforts for public health improvement as complex, dynamic, and adaptive.
2. List and explain the challenges associated with building capacity for public health improvement.
3. List the attributes that an information system for supporting public health improvement should have.
4. Explain how public health information systems can contribute to the work of public health improvement.
5. List the qualities of the infrastructure required for public health improvement.
6. According to the experience of the National Turning Point Initiative, what challenges do states and communities have in common in building capacity for public health improvement?
7. Describe the parts of the model or framework used for public health improvement by the National Turning Point Initiative.
8. Describe the objectives of the Public Health Improvement Tool Box. What are its core components and information features?
9. What needs or challenges should an information system, such as the Public Health Tool Box, address? What are the particular strengths of the Public Health Tool Box?

References

1. Durch JS, Bailey LS, Stoto MA, eds. *Improving Health in the Community: A Role for Performance Monitoring.* Washington, DC: National Academy Press; 1997.
2. Fawcett SB, Francisco VT, Hyra D, Paine-Andrews A, et al. Building healthy communities. In: Tarlov A, St. Peter R. eds. *Society and Population Health: A State Perspective.* New York: New Press; 2000.
3. Fawcett SB, Francisco VT, Paine-Andrews A, Schultz JA. Working together for healthier communities: A research-based memorandum of collaboration. *Public Health Rep* 2000;115:174–179.
4. Roussos ST, Fawcett SB. A review of collaborative partnerships as a strategy for improving community health. *Annu Rev Public Health* 2000;21:369–402.
5. Fawcett SB, Francisco VT, Paine-Andrews A. Promoting health through community

development. In: Glenwick DS, Jason LA, eds. *Promoting Health and Mental Health in Children, Youth and Families*. New York: Springer-Verlag; 1993:233–255.

6. Fawcett SB, Paine-Andrews AL, Francisco VT, Schultz JA, et al. Empowering community health initiatives through evaluation. In: Fetterman DM, Kafterian SJ, Wandersman A, eds. *Empowerment Evaluation: Knowledge and Tools for Self-Assessment and Accountability*. Thousand Oaks, CA: Sage; 1996:167–187.

7. Yasnoff WA, O'Carroll PW, Koo D, Linkins RW, et al. Public health informatics: Improving and transforming public health in the information age. *J Public Manage Pract* 2000;6(6):67–75.

8. Glenwick DS, Jason LA. *Promoting Health and Mental Health in Children, Youth and Families*. New York: Springer-Verlag; 1993.

9. Green LW, Kreuter MW. *Health Promotion and Planning: An Educational and Environmental Approach*. 2nd Ed. Mountain View, CA: Mayfield; 1991.

10. Fawcett SB, Carson V, Collie V, Bremby R, et al. *Promoting Health for All: An Action Planning Guide for Improving Access and Eliminating Disparities in Community Health*. Work Group on Health Promotion and Community Development: University of Kansas, Lawrence, KS; 2000.

11. Fawcett SB, Francisco VT, Schultz JA, Berkowitz B, et al. The Community Tool Box: An Internet-based resource for building healthier communities. *Public Health* 2000;115:274–278.

12. Francisco VT, Paine AL, Fawcett SB. A methodology for monitoring and evaluating community health coalitions. *Health Educ Res* 1993;8:403–406.

13. Fawcett SB, Paine-Andrews A, Francisco VT, Schultz J, et al. Evaluating community initiatives for health and development. In: Rootman I, McQueen D, eds. *Evaluation in Health Promotion; Principles and Perspectives*. Copenhagen, Denmark: World Health Organization–Europe; 2001;241–270.

14. Schultz JA, Fawcett SB, Francisco VT, Wolff T, et al. The Community Tool Box: Using the Internet to support the work of community health and development. *Journal of Technology and Human Services*. 2000;17:193-215.

15. Institute of Medicine. *The Future of Public Health*. Washington, DC: National Academy Press; 1988.

16. US Centers for Disease Control and Prevention. *Public Health Practices*. Public Health Practices Program Office; 1994.

17. Fawcett SB, Paine-Andrews A, Francisco VT, Schultz JA, et al. Using empowerment theory in collaborative partnership for community health and development. *Am J Community Psychol*. 1995;23:677–697.

18. Fawcett SB, Lewis RK, Paine-Andrews A, Francisco VT, et al. Evaluating community coalitions for prevention of substance abuse: The case of Project Freedom. *Health Educ Behav* 1997;24:812–828.

19. Fawcett SB, Sterling TD, Paine-Andrews A, Harris KJ, et al. *Evaluating Community Efforts to Prevent Cardiovascular Diseases*. Atlanta, GA: Centers for Disease Control and Prevention, National Center for Chronic Disease Prevention and Health Promotion; 1995.

30
Using Data to Meet a Policy Objective: Community Health Assessment Practice with the CATCH Data Warehouse

James Studnicki, Alan R. Hevner, and Donald J. Berndt

Learning Objectives

After studying this chapter, you should be able to:

* Understand the basic concepts of data warehousing as applied to community health assessment practice.
* Explain the value of community health assessments and, in particular, the Comprehensive Assessment for Tracking Community Health (CATCH) data warehouse, as a tool for use in community health assessment.
* Describe the different data dissemination capabilities associated with data warehousing technologies and explain how CATCH uses the Internet to deliver information to local health planners.
* Explain the value of healthcare data warehousing for the investigation of complex public health issues, such as racial disparities in infant mortality.

Overview

The CATCH data warehouse, sponsored by numerous organizations and developed at the University of South Florida, is a state-of-the-art community health assessment tool in both its assessment methodology and in its use of data warehousing technology. In this chapter, CATCH and its usefulness for community health planning are described. A case study that illustrates the capabilities of CATCH to support research concerning community health issues is provided. In many ways, the CATCH data warehouse is the gold standard for community health assessment. Although its current applications focus on Florida community health issues, CATCH as a concept has implications for community health decision-making support on a national scale.

Introduction

The measurement and assessment of health status in communities throughout the world is a massive information technology challenge. The Comprehensive Assessment for Tracking Community Health (CATCH) methodology provides a systematic framework for community-level assessment that can be a valuable tool for resource allocation and healthcare policy formulation. CATCH utilizes health status indicators from multiple data sources, using an innovative comparative framework and weighted evaluation process to produce a rank-ordered list of critical community healthcare challenges. The community-level focus is intended to empower local decision makers and provide a clear methodology for organizing and interpreting relevant healthcare data. The effectiveness of the CATCH methodology is based on a data warehousing approach. The data warehouse allows a core set of reports to be produced at a reasonable cost for community use. In addition, on-line analytic processing (OLAP) functionality can be used to gain a deeper understanding of the healthcare issues. This chapter demonstrates the use of the CATCH data warehouse to perform an initial investigation of a critical healthcare issue—racial disparity in infant mortality. Ongoing research directions in community healthcare decision making conclude the chapter.

Community Health Assessment Practice

It is well documented that considerable variation exists in the health status of defined populations. This variation is evident when we compare large population groups, such as separate nations, states, or regions within a single country. Surprisingly, variation often persists within smaller population groups, such as census tracts or ZIP codes inside United States counties. These variations exist not only for what would be considered epidemiological health status outcomes (i.e., morbidity and mortality rates), but also for indicators that could be considered other dimensions or domains of population health, such as socioeconomic and demographic characteristics, the availability of health resources, patterns of health behaviors, and many other factors. To improve the health status of populations, a continuous monitoring and improvement system must be implemented. Such a system would require a comprehensive, objective, and uniform methodology for defining and characterizing the many dimensions that comprise the health status of a community.

In the United States, the Institute of Medicine (IOM) of the National Academy of Sciences, in its influential 1988 report *The Future of Public Health*[1] emphasized that assessment was one of the core functions of public health and recommended that there should be a regular and systematic collection, assemblage, and analysis of information on the health status and needs of communities. In 1997, the IOM Committee on Using Performance Monitoring to Improve Community Health outlined a community health improvement process through which communities can assess health needs and priorities, formulate a health improvement strategy, and use performance indicators as part of a continuing and accountable process.[2] The report called for a *community health profile* made up of sociodemographic characteristics, health status indicators, quality of life indicators, health risk factors, health resource indicators, and other measures that can be used to support priority-setting, resource allocation decisions, and the evaluation of health program impacts.

As part of the ongoing clarification of the public health role at the community level and the transition from a disease to a health focus and from a treatment to a prevention strategy, there has been recognition that partnerships and collaboration are necessary to support effective action.[3,4] Health organizations, public sector agencies, medical care providers, businesses, the religious community, educational institutions, and other community organizations are interdependent components of a multi-sectoral community health organization. The overall community must be empowered to make the necessary, and sometimes difficult, resource allocation choices to improve health through information, education, behavior change, and social support.[5] Such collaborative action at the community level must be informed by unbiased data describing the community's health status, needs, and resources. The community also needs the ability to track progress over time in meeting the community's healthcare goals.

The gap between current practice in community healthcare spending and the goals of collaborative community healthcare decision making is vast. The availability and quality of data on health indicators are problematic. There is little empirical evidence on the use, sharing, or strategies to integrate health data into decision making to provide guidance to community health organizations. While most of the literature on collaborative leadership and community engagement focuses on the process,[6,7] little attention has been focused on the effect of the availability of a common set of data, such as the community health profile, on the quality and inclusiveness of decision making. There is also scant information about the use of data and information technology to support and monitor the process.

The goal of this chapter is to present an outline of the Comprehensive Assessment for Tracking Community Health (CATCH) methodology and its implementation in a data warehouse. We illustrate the use of the CATCH data warehouse by performing a preliminary investigation of an important healthcare issue—racial disparity in infant mortality. This brief example portends the power of the data warehouse for in-depth research on many critical public health issues.

The CATCH Methodology

The University of South Florida's Center for Health Outcomes Research has developed the CATCH methodology to provide comprehensive, objective health status data for community health planning purposes. CATCH collects, organizes, analyzes, prioritizes, and reports data on over 250 health and social indicators on a local community basis. The CATCH methodology has been tested, refined, and validated over the past ten years. Reports have been prepared for 24 US counties, both within and outside of Florida. The CATCH methodology can be briefly described as shown in Figure 30.1.

Community health indicator data are gathered from a variety of sources. Secondary data sources include healthcare data reported by hospitals; by local, state, and federal health agencies; and by national healthcare groups. Primary data sources would include door-to-door or mail-in surveys. All healthcare data are normalized into common formats and organized into a community healthcare report card listing values for each important community indicator.

Each indicator value is then compared against the state average, a peer group of communities' average, and other interesting values (e.g., a national goal for that indicator). The results of these comparisons are organized into an n-dimensional matrix based on favorable or unfavorable comparisons against each comparison dimension. For instance, Figure 30.1 illustrates the layout of a two-dimensional comparison matrix based on state averages and peer averages. Community indicators that demonstrate unfavorable comparisons on all dimensions are highlighted as community health challenges.

Passing each indicator through a set of ranking filters prioritizes this set of health challenges:

• *Number affected*—Number of persons in the community affected by the indicator.

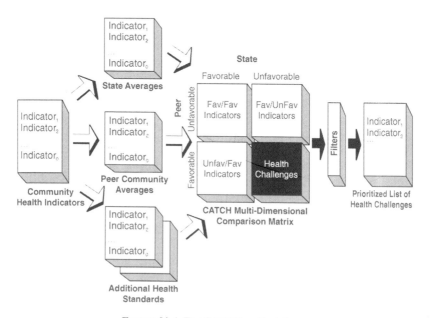

FIGURE 30.1. The CATCH methodology.

- *Economic impact*—An estimate of the direct cost per case for individuals affected by the indicator.
- *Availability of efficacious intervention*—An estimate of the relative degree to which treatment or prevention is likely to be effective.
- *Magnitude of difference*—The degree to which the community indicator is worse than the dimensional comparisons.
- *Trend analysis*—From a historical perspective, is the trend favorable or unfavorable, and what is the magnitude of change in the trend direction?

The community stakeholders are given an opportunity to weight the importance of each of these filters. The final product of the CATCH methodology is a comprehensive, prioritized listing of community healthcare challenges.[8] Up-to-date information on CATCH is available at the USF Center for Health Outcomes Research Web site at http://chor.hsc.usf.edu.

The CATCH Data Warehouse

The value of the CATCH methodology can be exploited most effectively through the use of data warehouse technologies. Here, we briefly describe the technology infrastructure of the CATCH data warehouse.

Limitations of Manual CATCH

Although the value of CATCH is incontrovertible, the ultimate deployment of CATCH throughout Florida and the nation has been constrained by several serious limitations:

- The handcrafted process is labor-intensive and slow. Hundreds of individual sources of data must be identified and contacted. Data are often provided in hard-copy formats that must be manually checked, validated, and then entered into spreadsheets. With manual methods, it takes three to four months to complete a CATCH report for a single county.
- Longitudinal trend analyses over many years are cost-prohibitive for most communities. Because each application is expensive and time-consuming, the capability to fund and produce annual assessments in a single community is limited.
- Most public health funding comes from state and federal governments. A statewide CATCH assessment would help to prioritize funding and serve to enable effective program evaluation based on quantifiable outcomes assessment. Because nearly all data elements available in Florida are available in most other states, there is reason to be confident that CATCH might be expanded nationally and even internationally. We are currently working on a national health assessment profile, using Florida as a case study.
- With the massive amount of healthcare data involved, many interesting

relationships and correlations of health status indicators can be found and investigated.

CATCH Data Warehouse Challenges

A CATCH data warehouse has been constructed to overcome these limitations, enabling both cost-effective report generation and ad hoc analyses of critical healthcare issues. The construction of a data warehouse for public healthcare data poses major challenges beyond those presented by the construction of a commercial data warehouse (e.g., retail sales). Such challenges include:

- Data come from a diverse set of sources. Healthcare data are published in a wide variety of formats with differing semantics. There are currently few standards in the healthcare field for data. The data integration task to build the data warehouse therefore requires significant effort.
- CATCH reports are disseminated to a diverse and geographically distributed set of stakeholders. The next section discusses the different dissemination modes that must be accommodated by the data warehouse.
- The data warehouse is required to support the activities of public policy formulation. The sociopolitical issues of healthcare policy impact design features such as security, availability, data quality, and performance.

Data Warehouse Design

Important missions of a data warehouse include the support of decision-making activities and the creation of an infrastructure for ad hoc exploration of very large collections of data. Decision makers should be able to pursue many of their investigations by using browsing tools, without relying on database programmers to construct queries. The emphasis on end-user data access places a premium on an understandable database design that provides an intuitive basis for navigating through the data. The star schema or dimensional model has been recognized as an effective structure for organizing many data warehouse components.[9] The star schema is characterized by a center fact table containing numeric information that can be used in summary reports. Radiating from the fact table are dimension tables that provide a rich query environment. This structure provides a logical data cube, with dimensions such as time and location identifying a set of numeric measurements within the cube.

The mission of the CATCH data warehouse is to support the automated and cost-effective application of the CATCH methodology as well as to enable more detailed analyses that were not possible through use of the coarse-grained data that typified past CATCH reports. The data warehouse design includes several levels of data granularity, from the coarse-grained data used in generic report production to actual event-level data, such as hospital discharges. The data warehouse includes major components at three levels of granularity, as illustrated in the data access pyramid found in Figure 30.2.

- *Report level*—Reporting tables with highly aggregated data are used to support the core CATCH reports, including comparisons between the target

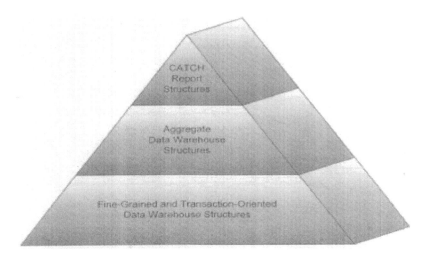

FIGURE 30.2. The CATCH data access pyramid.

county and peer counties. The aggregated data are derived from the underlying fine-grained data using stored procedures, which embody expertise and experience gained from performing CATCH assessments in the field. The aggregate tables provide fast interactive response for interactive access via data browsing tools and can provide the foundation for simple community-wide Internet access.

- *Aggregation level*—There are families of star schemas that provide true dimensional data warehouse capabilities, such as interactive roll-up and drill-down operations. These components have carefully designed dimensions that can be utilized by more sophisticated data browsing tools. The star schemas are populated by use of thorough data staging and quality procedures that usually involve processing detailed data sets extracted by various healthcare agencies and organizations. Typically, the data is aggregated and transformed for loading into a family of related star schemas that share important dimensions and support interactive OLAP techniques.
- *Raw data level*—For certain types of information, the design calls for retaining very fine-grained or even event-level data. An example is the hospital discharge data that includes each hospital discharge event for the more than 200 hospitals that are mandated to report such information in Florida. These data are retained at the transaction level because of the rich set of facts and dimensions available for analysis and the density of potential aggregations that result in negligible space savings.

These three levels of aggregation within the data warehouse combine to meet a wide range of reporting requirements and performance goals, thus providing a flexible basis for disseminating healthcare information to community decision makers.

Data Dissemination Modes

The human–computer interface is of paramount importance in the data warehouse environment and the primary determinant of success from the end-user perspective. To support analysis and reporting tasks, the data warehouse must have high-quality data and make those data accessible through intuitive interface technologies. The act of releasing data in a warehouse is in a very real sense the same as publishing those data in printed form: retractions in both media can be very painful. Once the data become accessible, they may be included in reports, forecasts, and analyses that form the basis of decision-making activities within an organization or a community. Therefore, data staging and quality procedures within the data warehouse are often among the most expensive and critical ingredients in providing a successful end-user experience.

The types of access in a data warehouse can be broadly categorized as *navigation* or *summarization* tasks. Navigation activities include data browsing, ad hoc queries, and traditional report generation. These tasks require human guidance and design to produce the appropriate queries, often presenting the results in tabular or graphical form. Though OLAP usually incorporates roll-up/drill-down features, the navigation style is highly interactive and driven by previous steps in data exploration.

Summarization tasks are algorithmic in nature. They apply techniques that summarize patterns in the data and usually produce models, often with some notion of reliability, which can be used to predict as well as to describe the underlying data. Traditional statistics and data mining techniques are often used as summarization tools. Thus, connectivity to statistical packages is an important interface component that allows analysts to use statistical techniques to confirm or more fully investigate interesting properties discovered through browsing in the CATCH data warehouse. The case study investigation in the next section illustrates our ability to explore data for interesting patterns. The following discussion focuses on the navigation tools and more traditional database access technologies being utilized in the project.

Data Browsing

Data warehouse browsing tools provide star query-like access through a flexible menu-based interface, with pull-down menus representing important data dimensions. These types of tools are easy to use, and they support some ad hoc exploration. However, they are usually controlled through some sort of administrative layer that determines the data available to end users. In the development of a flexible interface, there is a trade-off between the ability to express ad hoc queries and the ease-of-use that results from predefined constructs implemented by data warehouse designers and administrators.

As previously noted, the CATCH data warehouse consists of several levels of granularity from transaction-oriented data, such as hospital discharges, to summary data at the CATCH report level. Therefore, the interface requirements differ for each of the major components, especially with regard to the role of browsing tools. For instance, the browsing tools provide a convenient method for CATCH analysts to view the preliminary report results at a more detailed level than most community planners would want to sift through. Final report components may be generated by use of the browsing tools, or more likely they may be implemented as part of a reporting function that more fully automates the process.

A second and in some ways more important role for the browsing tools is to provide a flexible interface for more customized analysis. Healthcare issues highlighted by the CATCH methodology can be investigated more fully by using the finer levels of detail maintained in the data warehouse. These tasks might entail querying the true dimensional star schemas that include age, gender, race, and other dimensions, or even the event-oriented data, such as hospital discharges. Thus, the data warehouse allows the user to focus on issues such as differences in age or race with regard to specific health status indicators.

Report Generation

It is clear how the data tables and graphs from the browsing tools can be incorporated into comprehensive community health assessment reports. Reports allow quick and easy access to comprehensive summaries and more detailed collections of information from the data warehouse. This type of predefined and thorough reporting is critical for implementing a more automated CATCH methodology. For example, the comparison of target counties to peer counties, as well as to the state, are fundamental components of the original CATCH reports and important tools for community healthcare planners.

Ad Hoc Queries

Free-form queries formulated by use of Structured Query Language (SQL) provide a flexible ad hoc query capability for the more advanced user. This basic access mechanism is a standard relational database access path, but it requires some care in the data warehouse environment. Very large tables and ill-formed queries can conspire to produce some truly awful performance. Administrators and developers have been the most prevalent users of SQL in writing the procedures for constructing the data warehouse, as well as in providing queries and views for use by end-user tools.

Internet Access

Security issues, as well as a primary focus on research and development, have led to a conservative policy with regard to Internet access to the CATCH data warehouse. However, the use of the Internet to deliver information to local health planners is an important capability for the future. There are two ways to incorporate this capability within the data warehouse.

The first method for using the Internet is to save artifacts created by the research team in a format that allows delivery via the Internet. Many of the current tools have embedded support for this approach. The CATCH methodology has traditionally been centered on a large hard-copy report; much of this content could be recreated in Web-friendly form and easily disseminated to local health planners. The advantage of this approach is the continued role of a strong methodology, rather than a simple distribution of raw data with no guidance in how to apply analytic methods.

This method of Internet access was used effectively to distribute a CATCH assessment report throughout Miami-Dade County during the summer of 2000. The report was generated from the data warehouse in PDF formats. Figures 30.3 and 30.4 illustrate a sample Indicator Fact Sheet page and Indicator Comparison Chart page, respectively, from this report. The complete report of approximately 500 pages is available to the county policy makers and stakeholders via simple Web access.

A second approach is to provide dynamic access to the data warehouse via the Internet and allow direct queries by a larger community of end users. This approach will almost certainly have a role in the future, but the project will move cautiously in this direction. Most data warehouse vendors are moving to support Web-enabled data warehouses, so these types of tools will easily integrate into the current framework. Reliance on a Web-enabled tool set will minimize the need for customized Web development and will allow the focus of the project to remain on the content and evolution of a comprehensive community assessment methodology.

Case Study: Racial Disparity in Infant Mortality

Racial Differences in Health

Significant racial differences in health, disease, and mortality statistics concern researchers and policy makers across the nation and the world. Research frameworks for studying the role of race in health outcomes create confusion and active controversy as race becomes tangled with factors of ethnicity, culture, socioeconomic status, and demographics.[10] While the debate rages, health policy makers across the United States have made the elimination of racial disparities a top priority as a racial fairness issue. The first step to understanding racial health disparities must come from analyzing available health data and drawing conclusions based on what the data tell us.

We select *infant mortality* as a single health indicator to study for this data warehouse case study. Recent research on racial disparity in infant mortality illustrates the complexity of this health issue. Lillie-Blanton et al. perform a meta-analysis of the research literature on racial differences in four health measures—infant mortality, hypertension, substance abuse, and mortality from all causes.[11] Although socioeconomic conditions account for many observed racial differences in substance abuse and overall mortality, studies of infant mortality and hypertension show no clear relationships that help to explain the differences. Stockwell and Goza studied the impact of economic status on infant mortality in metropolitan Ohio communities.[12] They conclude that low-income whites and nonwhites at all income levels have significantly greater infant mortality rates

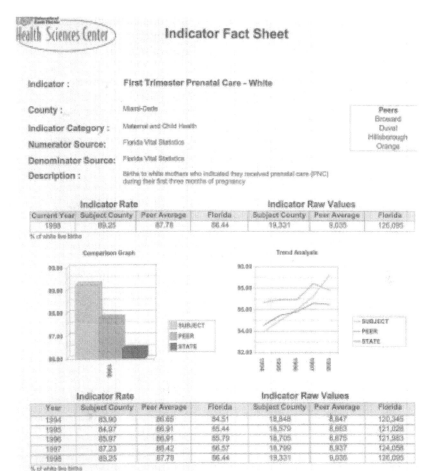

FIGURE 30.3. CATCH indicator fact sheet page. (*Source*: Center for Health Outcomes Research, University of South Florida.)

than the overall population. Din-Dzietham and Hertz-Picciotto show that higher levels of maternal education actually increase racial disparity in infant mortality.[13] Using data from North Carolina, they find that education beyond high school reduces the risk of infant mortality by 20% among whites but has little effect among nonwhites. Finally, even for extremely low risk (ELR) mothers, racial disparities are prominent. Alexander et al. report that ELR non-white mothers have 2.64 times greater risk for a small-for-gestational age (SGA) birth and 1.61 times greater risk of infant mortality.[14] These studies provide sobering evidence that racial disparity in infant mortality is a real and complex issue.

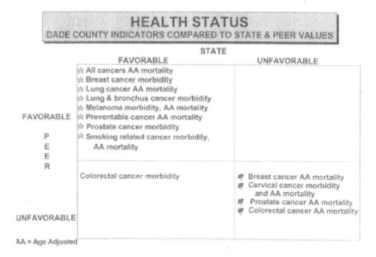

FIGURE 30.4. CATCH indicator comparison chart page. (*Source*: Center for Health Outcomes Research, University of South Florida.)

Racial Disparity in Infant Mortality Rates in Florida Counties

To study racial disparity in infant mortality rates (IMRs) in Florida counties, we begin by performing a cluster analysis of the counties based upon population. In this way, four groupings are defined:

- Group I—Small counties with less than 70,000 population (31 counties)
- Group II—Small medium counties with between 70,000 and 200,000 population (17 counties)
- Group III—Large medium counties with between 200,000 and 450,000 population (10 counties)
- Group IV—Large counties with over 450,000 population (9 counties)

To focus the analysis for the constraints of this chapter, we select the Group IV (large) counties, with 1990 census data and 1995 health indicator data for study. The goal of this study is to illustrate the ease with which the CATCH data warehouse can be used to support ad hoc investigations of interesting and timely health issues. The data warehouse is implemented using Oracle database software. The Oracle Discoverer interface provides efficient and easy-to-learn techniques for manipulating and viewing the desired data from the warehouse. Once initial observations and preliminary conclusions are made from the ad hoc investigation, then more rigorous data analysis can be performed to study the issue in more depth.

The first step of the analysis calculates the white and nonwhite IMRs for the nine largest Florida counties, as shown in Figure 30.5. The rates are based

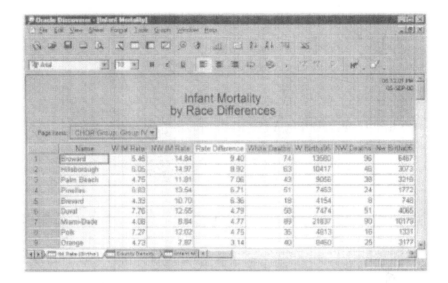

FIGURE 30.5. Rate differences.

on 10,000 live births. The greatest racial disparities are found in three counties—Broward, Hillsborough. and Palm Beach. Can we find characteristics among these three counties that might lead to an explanation of the higher racial IMR differences?

Population Density and Rurality

As seen in Figure 30.6, the 1990 data on county population and rurality shows little difference between the three counties and the other counties in Group IV. Broward is about 50% larger than the other two high-disparity counties. The three counties are largely urban. with Hillsborough, at 10.5%, the most rural. Observations on these data do not indicate that population or rurality plays a significant role in the racial IMR differences.

County Poverty and per Capita Income

In many research studies, socioeconomic indicators have been shown to play a significant role in racial health disparities.[11] Thus. we display county poverty rates and per capita income (1990 data) in Figure 30.7. Here, we find that Hillsborough has the second highest poverty rate among Group IV counties. With strong evidence from previous research, this fact may point to an explanation for the racial disparity in Hillsborough county. However. Broward and Palm Beach counties have relatively low poverty rates. Thus. we continue to search the data for other possible explanations for the disparities in these counties.

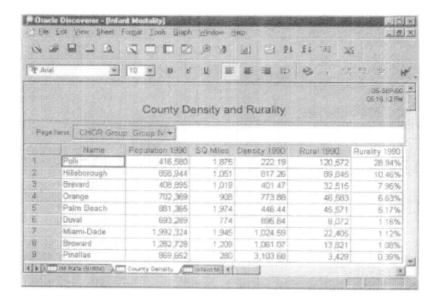

Figure 30.6. Density and rurality.

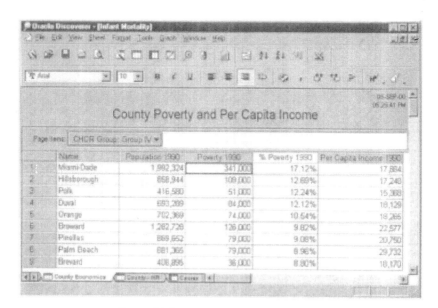

Figure 30.7. Poverty and per capita income.

County Population: Racial and Elderly Percentages

Next, we investigate the composition of the populations in the counties. Figure 30.8 shows the percentages of nonwhite and elderly (over 65) population in the Group IV counties. We note that Broward and Palm Beach counties have significantly greater elderly populations than most of the other counties. It is known that elderly populations tend to be conservative about the allocation of taxes to education and social programs. It is worth further investigation to see if this conservatism could be a contributing factor toward the racial IMR differences found in these two counties.

County Health Resources

The final data analysis studies the availability of health resources in the Group IV counties. Figure 30.9 illustrates the ratios of MDs, RNs, and LPNs in each county (number of resources/population). These data provide little indication that adequacy of health resources is a significant factor in racial IMR differences among counties.

Observations and Implications

The ability to rapidly design and execute ad hoc investigations is a compelling capability of the CATCH data warehouse. The availability of data at all three levels of the data access pyramid allows a researcher to move up and down the

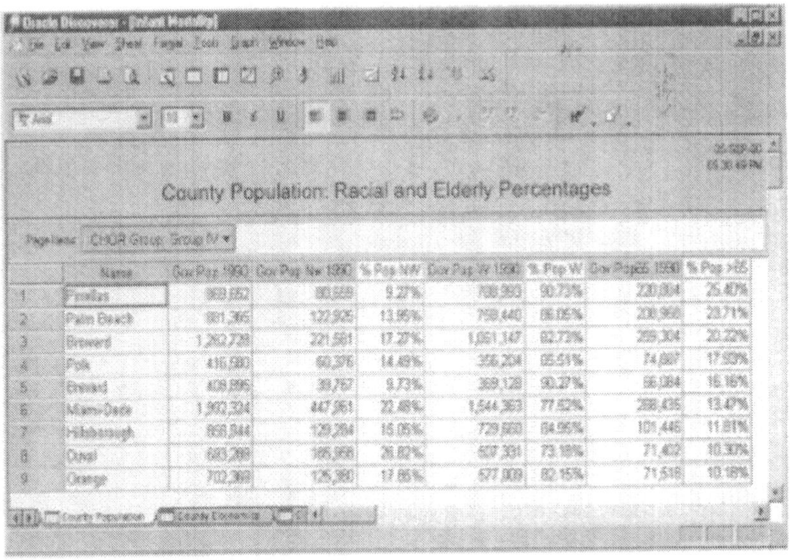

FIGURE 30.8. Population: Racial and elderly percentages.

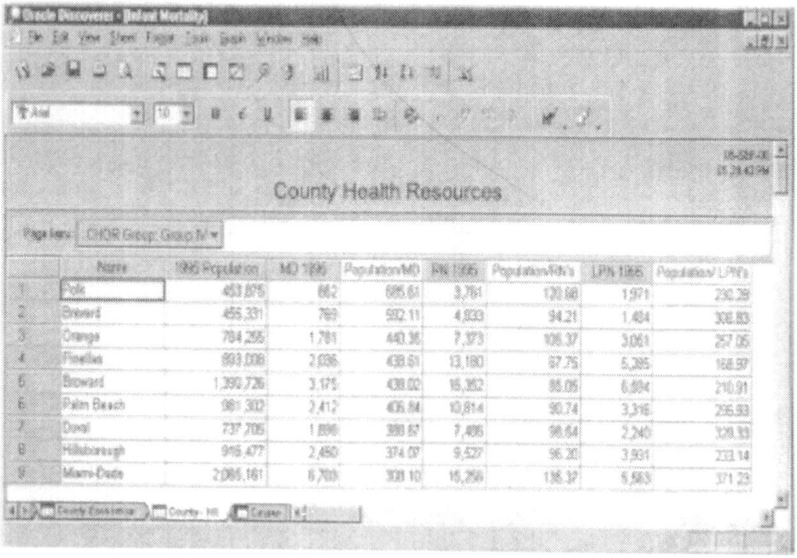

FIGURE 30.9. Health resources. (*Source*: Authors)

pyramid to group and order data in effective and revealing ways. The concise case study presented in this section aptly illustrates the use of the CATCH data warehouse for preliminary research investigations. Among the large Florida counties, we found three counties with above-average differences in white and nonwhite IMRs. A rapid analysis of potential explanations confirms the complexity of the racial health disparity issues found in the research literature.

Hillsborough County appears to confirm several previous studies that socioeconomic factors contribute to racial disparities. The high incidence of poverty seems to correlate with the high level of racial differences in IMRs. The implication is that the county should focus attention and resources on prenatal programs aimed at low-income nonwhite families. For example, a successful program to reduce the number of sudden infant death syndrome (SIDS) cases has been reported in the Chicago region.[15] Focused primarily in the African-American communities, the "Back to Sleep" program informs parents that infants should sleep on their backs for greatest safety.

On the other hand, racial disparities in Broward and Palm Beach counties seem to correlate with a high elderly population. Programs to bring greater awareness in the community of important health issues such as infant mortality may be called for. Counties with large retiree populations must achieve a balance of critical health programs that apply across the age spectrum.

These initial observations must be followed by more rigorous studies. We are performing ongoing research in Florida on racial disparities across many health indicators. Two examples of our in-depth data analyses on infant mortality are mentioned here.

Figure 30.10 shows a small portion of an extensive data table for infant mortality causes in Broward county from 1995 to 1997.

We find that white infant mortality causes differ from nonwhite causes in significant ways. For example, conditions of extreme immaturity and birth defects occur more frequently in nonwhite infant mortality. With the data warehouse as a repository of detailed birth and death certificate data, we can perform a more complete study of racial differences in causes of infant mortality.

The use of fine-grain data allows the application of detailed regression studies. A preliminary analysis finds that the county-specific racial disparity in infant mortality is not highly correlated with those factors that have high explanatory power for variation in total deaths and most major causes of death, such as heart disease, cancer, and stroke. We have conducted a preliminary multiple regression analysis utilizing the county infant mortality racial differential as the dependent variable (nonwhite infant death rate minus the white infant death rate). Explanatory variables were the percentage of the county population age 65 and over; the percentage nonwhite; the percentage living in poverty; a rurality factor; and the physician-to-population ratio, one important measure of health resource availability. The total amount of variation explained in the infant mortality racial disparity was less than 16%, ($R^2 = 0.157$). The same variables explain more than 60% of the variation in county-specific total age-adjusted mortality. The analysis suggests that there are a number of important research and measurement issues to be resolved in the study of the racial differences in infant mortality. Topics that require more study include:

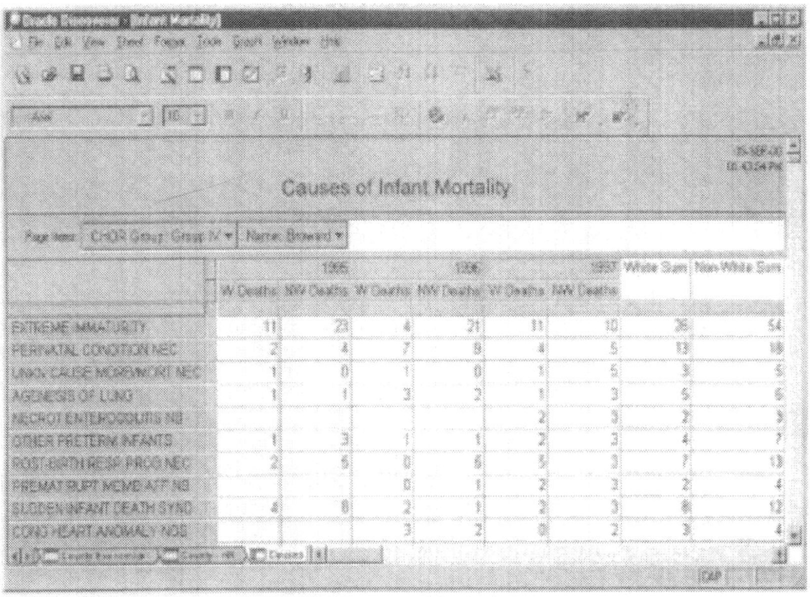

	1995		1996		1997		White Sum	Non-White Sum
	W Deaths	NW Deaths	W Deaths	NW Deaths	W Deaths	NW Deaths		
EXTREME IMMATURITY	11	23	4	21	11	10	26	54
PERINATAL CONDITION NEC	2	4	7	8	4	5	13	18
UNKN CAUSE MORB/MORT NEC	1	0	1	0	1	5	3	5
AGENESIS OF LUNG	1	1	3	2	1	3	5	6
NECROT ENTEROCOLITIS NB					2	3	2	3
OTHER PRETERM INFANTS	1	3	1	1	2	3	4	7
POST-BIRTH RESP PROB NEC	2	5	0	6	5	3	7	13
PREMAT RUPT MEMB AFF NB			0	1	2	3	2	4
SUDDEN INFANT DEATH SYND	4	8	2	1	2	3	8	12
CONG HEART ANOMALY NOS			3	2	0	2	3	4

FIGURE 30.10. Infant mortality causes 1995–1997.

- alternative measures to describe the racial disparity;
- the most appropriate form of analysis for grouped data (census tract, postal ZIP code, county);
- a conceptual framework that includes both individual and community variables combined in some way to maximize the amount of variation explained (requires matching individual to grouped data); and
- an enhanced understanding of the various causes of adverse birth outcomes.

Along with improvements in research design and methods, a data warehousing capability will greatly improve the effective use of population data in addressing these questions.

Conclusions and Effective Use of CATCH in the Communities

The CATCH data warehouse is the gold standard for community health assessment repositories in the nation. It is state-of-the-art in both assessment methodology and in data warehousing technology. We are just beginning to take advantage of the enormous potential of the data warehouse for research in critical healthcare issues. The sample case study on racial disparity in infant mortality that we have presented demonstrates how ad hoc investigations of health issues can be accomplished rapidly via the data warehouse interfaces, making effective use of the three levels of data access—reports, OLAP structures, and raw data at the base.

We are also planning a major research direction in the understanding of how individual communities can make best use of the reports and data from the data warehouse. The CATCH data warehouse will result in widespread distribution of data previously unavailable to most communities, as well as on-line access for specialized inquiry. Many issues arise as to how the communities will make most effective use of the CATCH data for healthcare decision making.

There is a rich literature on the decision-making process both with and without information technology. For example, Dennis et al. study the effects of minority influence on decision-making and find that the presence or absence of technology has very different effects.[16] Another important contributing area is the political process and its ramifications for decision making.[17] Certainly, policy making in health care is very much a political process.

The use of the CATCH methodology and the state-of-the-art data warehousing technology across many Florida communities will provide a rich research opportunity for studying many interesting issues concerning group decision making in community healthcare organizations. Some of the issues we plan to study include:

- The impact of the presence of a champion for specific actions
- The size and make-up of the decision-making group
- The speed of the decision-making process.

- The stakeholders in the process and their influence in the decision making
- Resource constraints faced by the community
- The political nature of the process
- The differential in access to data among the communities
- Information exchange patterns and practices
- The ease of access and usefulness of the data
- The presence of more thorough and structured data via the CATCH methodology
- The ability to produce customized analyses via the CATCH data warehouse

The complexities of each issue and the interrelationships among these issues make the design of research studies both a challenge and an opportunity. Research on healthcare decision making will focus on the communities' use of the CATCH information for healthcare planning.

Acknowledgments

Funding for the CATCH data warehouse project has come from the US Department of Commerce through the Technology Opportunities Program (TOP), Bear Stearns, the ORACLE Educational Program, and the many public and private corporations and agencies who have sponsored CATCH community assessments. The Florida Department of Health is a research partner. Research collaborators in the CATCH project include E. Gilbert, S. Hedge-Desai, S. Luther, R. Marsh, D. McCorkel, B. Myers, M. Nevrekar, M. Pearl, J. Slayton, and B. Steverson.

Questions for Review

1. Describe the community health assessment environment that makes a tool such as the CATCH data warehouse necessary for planners and decision makers.
2. Describe the methodology of CATCH in the gathering and processing of community health indicator data. How does CATCH compare indicator values to produce n-dimensional matrices? Explain how CATCH prioritizes indicators.
3. What have been the previous constraints in the widespread deployment of a manual CATCH system throughout Florida and the nation? In what ways does the CATCH data warehouse address these constraints?
4. List and describe the three levels of data granularity used in the CATCH data warehouse.
5. List and describe the data dissemination modes employed in the CATCH data warehouse. Explain the user capabilities provided by the data browsing tools offered by CATCH.
6. Explain the role of the Internet in the use of the CATCH data warehouse. What factors have led to adoption of a conservative policy with regard to Internet access?

7. Describe how the CATCH data warehouse supports the investigation of important public health issues.
8. Explain how the CATCH data warehouse will support community health decision making in Florida.

References

1. Institute of Medicine. Summary of Recommendations. In: Waterfall W, ed. *The Future of Public Health*. Washington DC, National Academy Press; 1988.
2. Institute of Medicine. Measurement Tools for a Community Health Improvement Process. In: Durch J, Bailey L, Stoto M, eds. *Improving Health in the Community, a Role for Performance Monitoring*. Washington, DC: National Academy Press; 1997.
3. Institute of Medicine. *Healthy Communities: New Partnerships for the Future of Public Health*. Washington, DC: National Academy Press; 1996.
4. Nakajima H. Editorial: New players for a new era. *World Health* 1997;50:3.
5. Cropper S. Collaborative working and the issue of sustainability. In: Huxham C, ed. *Creating Collaborative Advantage*. London: SAGE Pub; 1996.
6. Centers for Disease Control and Prevention. *Principles of Community Engagement*. Atlanta, GA: Centers for Disease Control and Prevention; 1997.
7. Chrislip D, Larson C. *Collaborative Leadership: How Citizens and Civic Leaders Can Make a Difference*. San Francisco: Jossey-Bass; 1994.
8. Studnicki J, Steverson B, Myers B, Hevner, A, Berndt, D. Comprehensive assessment for tracking community health (CATCH). *Best Practices and Benchmarking in Healthcare* 1997:196–207.
9. Gray P, Watson H. *Decision Support in the Data Warehouse*. Englewood Cliffs, NJ: Prentice-Hall; 1998.
10. Williams D. Race and health: Basic questions, emerging directions. *Ann Epidemiol* 1997;7:322–333.
11. Lillie-Blanton M. Parsons P. Gayle H, Dievler A. Racial differences in health: Not just black and white, but shades of gray. *Annu Rev Public Health* 1996;17:411–448.
12. Stockwell E. Goza F. Racial differences in the relationship between infant mortality and socioeconomic status. *J Biosoc Sci* 1996;28:73–84.
13. Din-Dzietham R. Hertz-Picciotto I. Infant mortality differences between whites and African Americans: The effect of maternal education. *Am J Public Health* 1998;88:651–656.
14. Alexander G. Kogan M. Himes J, Mor J. Goldenberg R. Racial differences in birthweight for gestational age and infant mortality in extremely-low-risk US populations. *Paediatr Perinat Epidemiol* 1999;13:205–217.
15. Chicago Department of Public Health. CDPH Announces Three-Point Plan to Address Infant Mortality and SIDS Rates in Chicago's African-American Community. Available at: http://w4.ci.chi.il.us/health/PressReleases/SIDS.html. Accessed April 4, 2002.
16. Dennis A. Hilmer K, Taylor N. Information exchange and use in GSS and verbal group decision making: effects of minority influence. *Journal of Management Information Systems* 1998;14:61–88.
17. Mintzberg H. *The Nature of Managerial Work*, New York: Harper and Row; 1973.

31
International Networking: Addressing the Challenge of Emerging Infections

Ann Marie Kimball and Tiffany Harris

Learning Objectives

After studying this chapter, you should be able to:

- Describe the Emerging Infections Network's current and future role in the prevention and control of emerging infections.
- Understand the application of an electronic disease surveillance system to an international trade organization's business needs.
- Describe the significant challenges to be addressed in implementing an information technology project that has as its user group representatives from multiple countries and professions that have varying approaches to political decision making and the acceptance and use of information technology.

Overview

The Emerging Infections Network (EINet) is a telecommunications network in the Asia Pacific geographic region. Developed and administered by the University of Washington with support from the Centers for Disease Control and Prevention and in partnership with public health officials of five Asia Pacific Economic Cooperation (APEC) economies. EINet focuses on providing education about and the prevention and detection of emerging infectious diseases that can have adverse impact on travel and trade relationships among nations. EINet provides a good example of the challenges inherent in developing and maintaining an international electronic network that connects nations with differing views and practices regarding data sharing. However, the working relationships fostered by networks such as EINet offer untold benefits for epidemic investigation and control of infections that cross international boundaries.

Introduction: The EINet (Emerging Infections Network)

EINet (Emerging Infections Network) is a telecommunications network in the Asia Pacific geographic region linking the 21 member economies of the Asia Pacific Economic Cooperation (APEC). It focuses on prevention and control of emerging infections that are of importance to trade and travel within the region. The University of Washington began the network with scientists from five Asia Pacific APEC economies in July 1996, as an international outreach effort, with support from the US Centers for Disease Control and Prevention (CDC). EINet was launched as an approved APEC project. It represents the first time such a trade community has prioritized emerging infections within an ongoing agenda of trade-related issues.

EINet dovetailed with a coincident initiative within APEC by the United States government to address the importance of emerging infections and their human, economic, and political costs to this trade community. The project is within the portfolio of the Industrial Science and Technology Working Group (ISTWG). Since EINet's inception, APEC also has approved several other projects in disease surveillance. Faculty and staff of the University of Washington School of Public Health and Community Medicine maintain the network.

EINet as an Informatics Project

International networking is a new approach to information sharing for disease control. Issues within such efforts include system design, technology incorporation, and content. Specifically, in designing such a system, who should be included? How should information flow? What type of information is most useful? Technological challenges include the diversity of hardware and software used by the potential network members and insuring compatibility in design so that access is not problematic. The adoption and continuing evolution of the Internet has solved many of these issues, and these Internet-based solutions were brought into the activities of this network. Content issues include insuring accuracy and timeliness; establishing and maintaining the balance between detailed surveillance data and more general disease alert information; and addressing confidentiality, data ownership, and security.

EINet is a telecommunications-based approach that has expanded and enhanced an existing trade-related telecommunications network (APEC EduNET). EINet carries a dialogue about the emergence of new disease to officials in trade and health ministries, to academics, and to other interested persons in APEC member countries. This dialogue is accomplished through the identification and inclusion of public health authorities in the network. As a result of this inclusiveness, EINet has a diverse user group that includes scientists, public health workers, and others with an interest in its content.

The goal of EINet is to create a utilitarian virtual public health community. EINet, which is free to its users, is moderated, and it provides information regularly. The network is also responsive to user input.

Existing resource materials and new didactic materials are directed to both scientists and policy makers. A rich Web site has been created for this network (http://apec.org/infectious/). Specific content on EINet includes reference material from existing library sources concerning the full range of emerging diseases of interest to the region. Initially, the CDC's "self-assessment instrument" was put forward as a means of describing the capacity of participating partners; however, this assessment work has been refined through two subsequent electronic surveys of the user group in 1997 and 2000.

The EINet Web site also includes distance learning materials for teaching about emerging infections. These materials are updated biannually. In addition, the EINet site links to other companion sites relevant to the Industrial Science and Technology Working Group (ISTWG) of APEC. The network's sources of information about regional outbreaks and other updates on the field are largely from outside its user group, although information from network users is increasing. APEC EINet is dedicated to providing timely information on issues of emerging infectious diseases (EIDs), enabling better collaboration by policy makers, health officials, and researchers throughout the Pacific Rim.

The Need for EINet

The combination of the emergence of new infectious diseases such as HIV/AIDS, the reemergence of old diseases, such as tuberculosis, and the growing resistance of diseases to available treatments, along with the worldwide increase in the speed and scope of travel and trade, has created a need for new and innovative surveillance strategies. In the world of trade, sudden trade embargoes or restrictions because of epidemic threats constitute a nontariff trade barrier that can be very costly to member states.

The emergence or resurgence and epidemic dissemination of infectious diseases such as dengue, tuberculosis, cholera, and others in the region is of particular concern. Dengue fever has expanded its traditional epidemiologic range; it now presents a major threat to Malaysia, Indonesia, Thailand, and other Southeast Asian countries. Cholera swept through Latin America in 1991 and 1992, involving three APEC economies: Peru, Mexico, and Chile. Tuberculosis is also a major concern throughout the region, and the HIV/AIDS pandemic has exploded definitively in Asia in the past six years.

While the increasing economic interdependence of the APEC member economies has created new wealth, the increased traffic of goods and people in the region poses new public health challenges. APEC is concerned about EIDs because they cause preventable illness and death, drain economies through the direct costs of treatment and hospitalization, generate indirect costs from time lost from work and reduced purchasing power, and lead to unfounded trade sanctions that hinder economic activity.

The emergence and re-emergence of infectious diseases has appropriately become an issue on the Science and Technology agenda of APEC. The US agricultural trade with other APEC economies exceeds $50 billion annually, according to 1999 figures.[1] However, outbreaks such as the Sakai (Japan) *Escherichia coli* 0157:H7 epidemic of 1996 threaten this trade and represent an unpredictable nontariff trade barrier to the United States. Transmission of multi-drug-resistant tuberculosis on extended airplane flights epitomizes a second, travel-related, type of EID that concerns APEC.[2]

Existing national and international public health disease reporting structures are not tailored to the needs of the new economic cooperation of the region. They do not permit the speed and the high level of interaction and flexibility essential to timely reactions to the EIDs that pose a particular threat to an interconnected economic cooperative. EIDs threaten the health of societies and therefore may provoke nontariff trade barriers as governments seek to protect vulnerable populations. They also impose direct and indirect economic costs. For example, India estimates a loss exceeding $1.2 billion due to trade and travel restrictions imposed during the putative outbreak of plague. Timely diagnosis and proactive public health cooperation with trading partner nations could have averted much of this economic damage.

Emerging infections require rapid, responsive collaboration among the scientific communities, governmental bodies, and commercial interests of member economies for effective prevention, surveillance, and control. Universities, as centers of scientific training and research, have an important role to play. However, university/government linkages will need to be strengthened to address this challenge.

The new paradigm of EIDs represents an entirely different educational framework for teaching about infectious diseases, microbiology, virology, epidemiology, and public health prevention and control. This framework sparked the creation of working groups and new curricula at universities across the United States. The University of Washington and Harvard University have had two of the most active working groups. New curricula were necessary to orient tomorrow's public health experts to the challenges posed by the "creation" of new pathogens through ecological pressure and through the potential for broad transmission of some pathogens by the routes of trade and travel. This same challenge faces the Asia Pacific. However, because bibliographic access is more limited, progress in building new curricula has been slower there.

EINet was created to address these issues for the 21 APEC economies. Originally known as the APEC Telecommunications Network for Emerging Infections, APEC EINet has focused on initiatives to:

- Help draw APEC's ISTWG into a policy initiative on EIDs. The "APEC Framework for Emerging Infectious Diseases" was approved at the ISTWG

meeting in Taiwan in March 1998; it now encompasses an action plan and
five projects on disease surveillance.

- Create a Web site offering data, reference material, and Web links to library
resources on EIDs.
- Produce a biweekly e-mail newsletter compiling disease alerts, APEC-
related news, and other relevant information from a number of sources,
including health professionals and the news media.
- Devise a distance learning curriculum, available on the Web site, that is
useful to health professors as well as to other scientists and policymakers.
- Visit sites and participate in international meetings to better assess and
promote the potential for increased use of information technology in
addressing emerging infections.

The Development of EINet

In 1993, the APEC Leaders Education Initiative called for "an investment in
our future generations by establishing an APEC Education Program to develop regional cooperation in higher education, study key regional economic
issues, improve workers' skills, facilitate cultural and intellectual exchanges,
enhance labor mobility, and foster understanding for the diversity of the region."[3] In response, representatives of APEC economies met in Seattle in May
1994 to establish new mechanisms, such as university-based "study centers,"
for sharing academic resources. Since then, the University of Washington has
been a leader among educational institutions collaborating on APEC projects.
In 1995, US Secretary of State Warren Christopher called for a telecommunications network initiative to link all APEC Study Centers to facilitate the
exchange of information and enhance collaboration. The University of Washington took the lead on this networking activity, and the product, the APEC
EduNet, provided the original backbone for the APEC EINet project.

Although health is not the focus of the APEC process, the issue of EIDs was
introduced by the United States in 1995 at a gathering of the APEC economies' cabinet-level science/technology officials (APEC 2nd Ministerial on
Science and Technology). Continued efforts by the United States and other
economies led to passage of a formalized policy framework on EIDs during
the meeting of the ISTWG in March 1998. "Self-funded" projects as well as
"projects proposed for funding" have been formally approved by the ISTWG.

Scientists from five APEC economies established EINet at the University of
Washington in 1996. EINet is funded through a cooperative agreement between
the University of Washington and the CDC. The University of Washington lever-
ages the budget by providing use of existing equipment, such as Internet servers.
The telecommunications technology that is used relies heavily on connectivity
over telephone lines and hubs of information processing at Internet servers. The
network includes an e-mail listserve and a Web site.

Originally, the EINet site included a password-protected site for viewing recent multi-drug-resistant tuberculosis surveillance data; however, the quality and timeliness of data from the member economies was not adequate to sustain this site.

An electronic survey was sent out early on to determine what users wanted. The results are presented in Table 31.1.

EINet's Web site and e-mail resources include biweekly bulletins that encapsulate recent news of disease outbreaks and public health from around the region. This newsletter was formatted according to a market survey. It may well be that our participants are ready for a more frequent, less formal use of e-mail communications. We have repeated our market survey in Year One (Spring–Summer 2000) of the new project. The CDC and other partners of the Committee on International Science, Engineering, and Technology Policy (CISET) interested in the Asia-Pacific networking collaborated with us in this survey effort. The survey was sent via e-mail and was carried out over our existing network, with additional e-mail addresses gathered from other sources. Respondents were asked to return the survey electronically via e-mail; however, a fax number and mail address were also provided. Nonrespondents were targeted with reminder e-mails.

A universe of 539 respondents with functioning e-mail addresses was initially identified and sent the survey. Ten percent of these addresses could not be reached. A total of 106 questionnaires were returned, representing 17 of the 21 APEC economies. No one from Chile, Russia, Papua New Guinea, and Brunei Darussalam responded. Enthusiasm for information-sharing remains

TABLE 31.1. EINet interest survey ($N = 29$)

Question	Response (%)
Found most useful (choose all that apply):	
Summary of surveillance reports of outbreaks in the Asia-Pacific region	52
Using the network to enhance collaboration through communication	24
Announcing new research developments	57
Announcing APEC EINet project activities and meetings	57
Summary of APEC conferences and summits	71
All of the above	33
Preferred frequency of communication:	
Once a week	48
Once a month	52

high, and support for usership appears to be increasing. However, security of information use and information transfer remains an unknown.

A problem with the use of an electronic survey in this setting is the creation of selection bias—those who respond to an electronic survey are likely the most computer literate with the highest computer usage. This makes close interpretation of the results of a given survey less useful. A longitudinal approach to detect trends may be a more appropriate application.

Political Issues

The APEC group exists largely through consensus building rather than through formal treaties among its partner economies. As a consequence, there is no treaty or legal basis for EINet to carry out disease surveillance, although it is a formal project of the APEC and a working ISTWG group. In addition, user access is variable due to "info politics" in the different economies.

Technical Issues

The technical issues encountered have been minimal, primarily because the strategy for implementation and maintenance relied on the capacity of the user group. In other words, the users themselves maintain their Internet access for their own use. The EINet network provides some additional incentive for maintaining electronic competence, but it does not by any means represent the only such incentive. By taking advantage of existing technology, the network has circumvented many technical concerns.

People Issues: Use of EINet

International networking is rife with "people issues" that figure strongly in the attempt to promote a timely, candid discussion across the Pacific about emerging infections. Although our network has been well subscribed and our bulletins extensively quoted in the region at all levels of national health systems, it has been less interactive than hoped. In fact, according to our most recent survey, only 23% of respondents could contribute information to the network on EID research updates. Whether the barriers are political, cultural, or technical has not been investigated.

Our initial effort within EINet was to compile surveillance information to describe drug resistance in tuberculosis; this effort was unsuccessful. The reasons were multiple. There were interprogrammatic jealousies within governments that prevented data sharing, concerns about the accuracy of testing that caused hesitation, and concerns about data ownership and control of information. Probably most important was the overall paucity of data collection. The rhetoric about surveillance for this serious threat overstated greatly the actual activity underway. The vision of prospective timely tracking of drug resistance in tuberculosis remains in the future for Asia Pacific.

The Impact of Advancing Technology on the Operation of the System

The advance of technology has pushed the development of the network ahead. Whereas initially our Web site development was constrained from the use of frames and images because of slow access in Asia, this constraint no longer exists. At the start of the project, many countries had little national coverage by the Internet, but now the majority has some coverage, and many have good coverage. The use of telephone calls and faxing to communicate has become much less necessary over the past four years.

What Was Learned in the Process of Thinking This System Through, Designing It, Implementing It, and Evaluating It?

The original vision for this effort was a surveillance and monitoring network. However, experience in the first three years of activity has resulted in the current network, which is actually a disease alert and information network, rather than a true surveillance network.

The future objectives are to:

- Create or enhance working relationships among organizations responsible for trade, travel, and public health on the Pacific Rim;
- Extend the capacity of APEC's developing economies to use information technology and the Internet for alerts and surveillance information locally, nationally, and internationally;
- Demonstrate, through evaluation, the value added when APEC and its member economies assign high priority to programs that seek to prevent and control trade- and travel-related infections; and
- Provide health professionals with technical content, direction, and Internet-based resources for learning about emerging infections in the Asia Pacific.

Implications for Informatics Practitioners and Lessons Learned

The experience of developing and implementing EINet provides several lessons for practitioners of public health informatics.

1. *It is important to be responsive to user needs.* The users are the key to the success of any network.
2. *Having incremental vision is crucial.* Not everything will work as planned, and implementers need to be willing to try and fail before finding the best solution.

3. *The network approach is broader than its technological base.* Electronic networking can only follow successful "human networking," and it is only as strong as the ongoing collaborative work that it provokes. It is our intention that this work be responsive to the concerns of the community within APEC and that our objectives accurately reflect the preoccupations of the region. We have been in contact with the Emerging Infections program of World Health Organization Geneva (WHO Geneva) and with the Western Pacific Regional Office of WHO in Manila regarding this new project, and we will continue to involve these and other interested parties as well.

Through the links created with this project, CDC and the University of Washington will initiate collaboration with an expanding number of APEC institutions focused on the areas of epidemiological and laboratory-based surveillance of emerging infections. Eventually, this collaboration will be institutionalized through ongoing long-term research work and other cooperative public health activities to facilitate the prevention and control of infectious diseases.

The Future for Systems Like EINet

EINet and such systems as ProMED and PACNET have demonstrated the potential power of international electronic networking in enhancing cooperation in disease surveillance and control. The future of the EINet will continue to be defined by the desires of its user group. Its current configuration will be expanded through outreach to lesser-developed countries in the region. Systems in Korea, Japan, Australia, Taiwan, and the United States have provided proof of the validity of the national concept of networking. EINet contributes the international proof. It is probable that as diagnostics improve and the timeliness of disease reporting is enhanced, electronic networks will be more, rather than less, important as "first alert" systems. The working relationships fostered by such networks carry untold benefits for epidemic investigation and control of infections that cross international boundaries.

Questions for Review

1. Explain why EINet was created. What problems did the network seek to address?
2. List and describe the services offered to public health officials by EINet.
3. Explain the process by which EINet was developed and the political/public health forces that were involved.
4. In what sense can it be said that international networking is rife with people issues?

5. What has been the contribution of advancing technology to the operation of the EINet system?
6. In what sense is a network approach broader than its technological base?

References

1. Office of Trade & Economic Analysis/Trade Development/International Trade Administration/U.S. Department of Commerce. US Foreign Trade Highlights, U.S. Trade by Commodity with APEC (20). Available at: http://www.ita.doc.gov/td/industry/otea/usfth/geoarea/rapec.txt. Accessed April 4, 2002.
2. Kenyon TA, Valway SE, Ihle WW, Onorato IM, Castro KG. Transmission of multidrug-resistant *Mycobacterium* tuberculosis during a long airplane flight. *N Engl J Med* 1996;334:933–938.
3. APEC Leaders Education Initiative at first annual summit of APEC leaders, Seattle, Washington. November 1993. http://www.apec.org/leaders_education_initiative.htm. Accessed April 4, 2002.

Suggested Reading

APEC Emerging Infections Network Web site. Available at: http://www.apec.org/infectious/. Accessed April 4, 2002.
EuroSurveillance Web site. Available at: http://www.ceses.org/eurosurveillance.htm. Accessed April 4, 2002.
International Society for Infectious Diseases. ProMED-mail. Available at: http://www.promedmail.org. Accessed April 4, 2002.
SEA-AIDS Web site. Available at: http://www.hivnet.ch:8000/asia/sea-aids/. Accessed April 4, 2002.
Kimball AM, Horwitch CA, O'Carroll PW, et al. The Asian Pacific Economic Cooperation Emerging Infections Network. *Am J Prev Med* 1999;17:156–158.
Kimball AM, Horwitch CA, O–Carroll PW, et al. The APEC Emerging Infections Network: Prospects for comprehensive information sharing on emerging infections within the Asia Pacific Economic Cooperation. *Emerg Infect Dis* 1998;4:472.

32
Case Study: An Immunization Data Collection System for Private Providers

WILLIAM A. YASNOFF

Learning Objectives

After studying this chapter, you should be able to:

- Describe the processes used by the Oregon Immunization case study to solicit provider compliance with reporting immunizations.
- List and describe the principles of informatics that were applied in developing a solution to the problem of securing immunization data from private providers.
- Examine the lessons learned from the Oregon case study and consider the implications of these lessons.

Overview

In this chapter, a first-person account is provided of an effort to design and build an immunization data collection system that would link private providers with an existing state registry. The system had to be efficient and also mesh well with existing provider work processes associated with administering immunizations in 1,500–2,000 private provider offices. The experience related here illustrates the application of many of the public health informatics principles that have been presented in numerous chapters of this book. It especially demonstrates the importance of involving prospective users in the development of solutions to problems and of recognizing that high-tech solutions are not always the most effective. Finally, the entire experience emphasizes that effective practice of public health informatics is more than a science; it is also an art requiring the exercise of imagination and human relations skills in meeting the needs of and dealing with the constraints posed by users.

Introduction

This case study illustrates a solution to one of the most common problems in public health informatics: data input. In building public health information systems, we are often in the position of needing input from users in the community outside our organizations. In such cases, it is a significant challenge to motivate users to cooperate. A significant part of eliciting that cooperation is the ability to provide a data input system that is compatible with existing procedures but does not impose substantial new burdens on the user.

As you review this case, try to stop at the end of each section and think about how you would approach the situation at that point. Then compare your ideas with those that were actually used. This suggestion is not meant to imply that the approach actually used in the case is ideal or even correct. Even the fact that the problem was solved does not necessarily validate the approach. After all, there are many ways to address system design problems.

As a means of focusing on key principles, some of the specific, but minor, problems that were solved in order to implement this solution have been omitted from this description. In particular, the many discussions that were needed to overcome skepticism about the both the possibility of solving the problem and the viability of the specific solution proposed are not described.

Background

When I began as director of Oregon's immunization registry in late 1994, my first priority was to determine what the biggest obstacles to full implementation of the registry would be. At that time, a public-sector immunization registry was already fully functional, serving every public clinic that provided childhood immunizations. However, this registry was part of a medical records system for public clinics, and it could not be used by private providers. In addition, over two-thirds of all the childhood immunizations at that time were administered in the private sector. Furthermore, the shift toward increased immunization delivery by private providers had already begun and was expected to accelerate in the next few years (currently, 82% of immunizations in Oregon are given by provide providers). The essence of my task, then, was to create an immunization registry for the private sector and then integrate it with the existing public sector registry.

Before becoming director of the registry, I had been involved with it for about six months as a consultant. During this time, a detailed business plan for developing the registry had been written. With this background, I did not experience much difficulty in identifying the three most difficult problems that I would need to solve in order to make the Oregon registry successful.

- First, and most important, an efficient mechanism for obtaining immunization information from private providers would need to be created.

In the public sector registry, computer terminals connected to a mainframe were available in each clinic. At the end of the day, clinic personnel entered all the immunizations that had been given. During the day, children's immunization records were immediately available through interaction with the terminal. However, this solution would clearly not be feasible for private providers; for them, it was expensive, time consuming, and inefficient.

- Second, an easily maintainable decision support system to produce immunization recommendations was needed. Although a simple decision support system already had been developed for the public sector registry, its lack of flexibility was already proving to be a major problem. A system that could easily accommodate all the existing and potential future ACIP recommendations was needed. This same algorithm would also be used to assess the immunization status of children and to determine the need for reminders and recall. (See Chapter 23 for more information about the system that was developed.)
- Third, a mechanism for financial sustainability of the registry would need to be established. Although there was federal funding available at that time for registry development, it was already clear that additional funds for continuing operations would not be forthcoming once the registry was completed. Without a solid plan for financial support, the entire project could be successful and yet be terminated because of a lack of funding. Indeed, the entire effort could be viewed as a futile exercise in the absence of a mechanism for continuing operational support.

This case study is focused on the first of these problems: developing an efficient mechanism for obtaining the immunization information from private providers. Solutions to the decision support and financial sustainability problems have been described elsewhere.[1,2]

Initial Analysis

In approaching the problem of private provider immunization input, my first task was to develop a possible solution—to conduct a requirements analysis. A key principle in this effort is that the users must be the final arbiters of any successful solution. However, users function best in this role when they are presented with one or more possibilities from which to choose. Naturally, users are not familiar with potential technical approaches to system design problems. It is the role of the system architect to first develop potential solutions that provide users with a framework for considering the problem.

My prior experience in pediatricians' offices as a medical student was extremely helpful to my analysis. I knew from this experience that the offices were extremely busy. Although the activities appeared somewhat chaotic, they followed well-defined procedures that would not be easy to change. My key assumption was that minimizing the time requirements imposed by any data collection system was the most important goal. Of course, had I not had experience with the target environment, my first step would have been to spend some time observing a private provider office or two so as to better understand the real user environment. Such direct experience is essential knowledge for the system developer.

In light of this previous experience, I generated my own list of the requirements that a private provider immunization input system would have:

1. Time requirements imposed on the users must be minimal;
2. The time delay between immunization and data submission should be short;
3. The process should fit into the existing paper work and activity flow;
4. The process should be interactive to permit delivery of immunization recommendations;
5. The security of any transmitted information must be guaranteed; and
6. The cost must be very low, especially for ongoing operation at an estimated 1,500 to 2,000 user sites and at registry headquarters.

I then used these requirements to exclude a number of possible solutions. For example, cost limitations clearly obviated installing any substantial equipment in the provider offices. Other available data indicated that only a very small percentage of private providers had computer systems, and even fewer used modems with those systems. In addition, the telecommunications infrastructure in rural Oregon at that time would limit effective modem speeds over ordinary telephone lines to 2400 baud in many areas, too slow for effective interaction.

I next focused on available communications tools in provider offices. Telephones and fax machines were the only such tools in widespread use. I was immediately attracted to the fax machine as an option because of its ability to transmit relatively large amounts of information quickly. I eliminated the telephone as a data input option, reasoning that a voice response system would at best be very time-intensive because of the need for manual transcription of transmitted information at registry headquarters. I was delighted to learn from a recently completed survey that over 90% of private providers already had fax machines in their offices.

Having selected fax machines as the communications tool, I regarded the rest of the solution as relatively straightforward. The providers would request a child's immunization record by telephone, using a voice response system. Each provider's fax number would be on file with the registry. The registry would immediately fax a history and the immunization recommendations. This fax transmission would include an identifying bar code. The provider would attach the history and recommendations to the patient's chart. The provider would merely blacken open circles next to the immunization recommendations to indicate which shots were given at that visit. This same sheet of paper would then be faxed back to the registry, where optical scanning would be used to read the blackened circles and bar code recognition would be used to identify the provider and the child.

This seemed to be a simple, elegant, and completely feasible solution that met all the requirements. The only remaining step was to get the endorsement of the users and then begin implementation. Little did I realize that my thinking to date would be only a tentative step in a very long march.

Meeting with the Users

Now that I had a solution to the input problem in hand, I was anxious to meet with the users to get their endorsement. In cooperation with the local medical societies, I arranged a dinner meeting of all the large pediatric practices. About a dozen pediatricians attended, and I began my presentation as they were eating dessert.

I started by reviewing the immunization problem in Oregon. At that time, Oregon had one of the lowest statewide immunization completion rates for two-year-olds in the nation, ranking 47th out of the 50 states. The pediatricians clearly shared our concerns about this low rate. I then discussed the progress that had been made in creating the existing public sector immunization registry. There was early evidence that the registry was already improving the immunization rates substantially in the population it served. I was very pleased to discover at the dinner that there was strong support in this group for establishment of a private sector immunization registry, including a clear appreciation of the benefits of the information it could provide.

I then reminded the providers that in order for a private sector immunization registry to work, they would need to supply information about every immunization given in their offices. It was apparent that most of them had not really considered the full implications of this requirement for their own practices. I described my proposal for sending immunization information to them via fax and collecting information by the same medium.

The reaction to my proposal was rapid and unanimous: the pediatricians told me, ever so politely, that such a system was completely and totally unworkable. In fact, they all seemed nearly incredulous that I had suggested such a ridiculous idea. A number of them pointed out that they administered so many immunizations in a day that handling two faxes for each one would totally overwhelm both their staff and the capacity of their fax machines. They made it very clear that they could not and would not participate in a registry that operated in this fashion.

This was not the feedback I had hoped for. Naturally, I was very disappointed that the pediatricians were so negative about what I thought was an elegant solution to the data collection problem. I was very concerned, because I knew that solving this problem was absolutely crucial to the success of the entire project. To make matters worse, it seemed that I had lost whatever credibility I had developed from the earlier part of the meeting.

My initial reaction was to try to engage them in a discussion of other possible solutions. As might be expected (and as I knew but had temporarily forgotten), my response to their objections was not productive at all. Typically, users cannot provide meaningful assistance in developing a technical solution to a system problem. The most productive interactions are usually based on the review of a proposed solution—which is what I had planned.

One clear mistake I had made in preparing for this meeting was failing to consider what I would do if my proposed solution was totally rejected. I was so convinced that my idea would at least form the basis for a workable system that I had not developed any backup plan.

As I listened to the pediatricians explain why various input methods could not work, I realized that the best I could do with this meeting was to understand the user requirements more clearly. I thought that if I could at least get a consensus about the requirements, I would have something to work with when I went "back to the drawing board" to develop a better option.

I therefore returned to the basic premise that they all supported the establishment of a private sector immunization registry. I was able to get these providers (with some grumbling, to be sure) to admit that they would need to enter data in some form in order for the registry to function. I next asked them to consider that this data entry process would require some of their time and that the amount of this time for each immunization would be greater than zero. Although all these points were obvious to me, it required some discussion before the pediatricians fully appreciated them.

I next turned to the issue of defining how much time they would be willing to devote to entering immunization data. I began with the question, "Would you be willing to spend one second to enter each immunization?" After some discussion, they agreed that this amount of time would be feasible. I then proceeded to ask if two seconds would be acceptable. For each increase in the amount of time, there was more and more discussion before they reached agreement. Three seconds generated substantial discussion before the group agreed that it was acceptable. Four seconds turned out to be too much—the consensus was that four seconds per immunization for data entry was simply not feasible. Later, after the meeting was over, one of the pediatricians approached me individually and shared his calculation showing that four seconds for each immunization would mean he would need to hire a new full-time staff person solely for this task.

With the three-second requirement clearly defined, I spent some time reinforcing it. I asked them to specifically agree that if I were (somehow) able to devise an input mechanism that met this criterion, they would support and use it. They unanimously agreed that they would. In retrospect, I believe their skepticism about the possibility that any solution could be developed to meet this requirement (a skepticism that I shared) may have encouraged them in reaching this agreement. Nevertheless, the meeting ended on a positive note, and I had clearly defined the key user requirement. I had no idea how a system could be developed to meet this requirement, but I was determined to return to the group with a solution.

Searching for the Solution

Now the really difficult work began. I consoled myself by looking back at my list of requirements. It turned out that these were all correct; I had simply not realized how crucial the time element for data entry would be to the providers. My original solution was obviously a dead issue, and I needed to develop a different one.

I began with a step-by-step list of the immunization process:

1. child arrives in the office;
2. check in at reception desk;
3. pull chart;
4. move child to exam room, put chart on door;
5. nurse reviews chart and talks to parent and child;
6. doctor reviews chart, talks to parent and child, examines child, writes orders;
7. nurse reviews orders, prepares immunizations;
8. nurse gives immunizations, records on chart;
9. chart, parent, and child to front desk to schedule next appointment.

In looking at this list, I focused very carefully on step 8. It seemed that this was the place in the process for collection of the registry data.

I decided to focus exclusively on data collection, ignoring for now the need to communicate the child's immunization history and recommendations to the provider. I clearly recognized that the 3-second input requirement was a very difficult one to meet, and therefore I wanted to look specifically at that part of the problem in isolation

I wish I could say that the idea that solved this problem occurred to me suddenly in a moment of inspiration. Such a moment would have been extremely exciting. But the reality was that the idea developed slowly over the next several months. In addition to spending time every day contemplating this problem, I read and explored input methodologies used in other time-critical situations. I had always thought that bar codes would be part of the solution because of the ease of both printing and scanning them. In fact, the previous registry director (Dr. Frank McCullar) had suggested issuing a set of bar code labels for every newborn and then peeling off a label in the provider's office each time an immunization was given. However, there were two serious problems with that approach: lost and forgotten bar code labels.

I arranged to visit several local companies that dealt with these types of problems. During these visits, I would describe the provider office environment and the stated 3-second requirement to see what suggestions might be forthcoming. While these visits did not directly result in a solution, they were helpful in elucidating and discussing possibilities as well as in familiarizing me with available input, scanning, and recognition technologies.

I kept returning to Dr. McCullar's idea for bar code labels. From the central registry's perspective, the idea of using such bar codes was very appealing as a data input mechanism because it would be fast, accurate, and inexpensive. Moreover, it occurred to me that the problems of lost and forgotten labels could be overcome by keeping these labels in the patient's chart in the provider's office. Peeling off a bar code label even seemed to meet the 3-second requirement. However, housing these bar codes at the provider's office introduced additional problems. For example, we knew that a very large fraction of children received their immunizations from two or more providers. How could such a set of bar codes be shared among two or more providers? A much bigger concern was how to insure that a bar code was submitted each time an immunization was given. Because data submission would be an extra step in the immunization process, it was inevitable that it would be missed in many cases, despite the best of intentions.

What could be done to design a system that would force the providers to submit the bar code reliably? I again considered step 8 in the process, the recording of the immunization information in the chart. It turns out that every pediatrician's chart has a special page for recording immunizations: the immunization record form. This form has been standardized, and copies of it are distributed by the American Academy of Pediatrics.

Each immunization uses one line on the form. The immunizations are grouped into the various series.

The presence of such a standard form in every child's chart made it a natural point to intervene to collect immunization data. I studied the immunization record form and considered the problem. I also thought about the key principle of accurate and complete data entry: it must be fully integrated into the business process. The central issue seemed to be integrating the bar codes with the immunization record form. I needed to find a method to force the nurse to peel off the bar code in order to record that the immunization had been given. Finally, it occurred to me to put the bar codes on top of the immunization record. Then, they would have to be removed in order for charting to occur.

But that idea would not work. Typically, when adhesive labels are peeled off, the underlying surface is a glossy plastic-like surface that does not accommodate writing. Nevertheless, I was encouraged at this point that I was close to a solution. The entire problem had come down to whether it was possible to stick a peel-off label to plain paper.

I began to pay close attention to every peel-off label I saw. All of them seemed to be stuck to a surface that did not accommodate writing. Then I got lucky. I happened to see a letter that the post office had forwarded because of a change of address. Affixed to the envelope was a yellow sticker from the post office. When

I peeled off the sticker, it came off easily, like a Post-it™ note. In fact, it was the same yellow color as the original Post-it™ notes and seemed to function in the same way, except that instead of featuring a single strip of adhesive at the top, this note's back was entirely coated with adhesive.

It now seemed that I had all the elements of a complete solution to the problem. I started to think about how bar codes on such a note could be placed on top of the immunization record form. But first, I had to address one more issue. Atlhough the standard immunization record form provided enough spaces to permit recording the immunizations in each series, there were many more options for possible immunizations than the number of spaces provided on the form. In order to have bar codes that were specific to every possible immunization, I would need many more spaces. Thankfully, this problem was relatively easy to solve. By rearranging the immunization record form into two columns, I was able to provide an option for every potential immunization while still allowing (just barely) enough space to record the appropriate information.

It seemed that I had found a potential solution to this difficult input problem. Now I had to figure out how to make it work.

Refining the Solution

The first step in pursuing this solution was to create a mockup so that people could understand exactly what this new form would look like. I arranged for the bar codes to be printed on label paper and attached to the Post-it™ notes, which were then affixed to a revised two-column immunization record form. Organizing all the needed information required several iterations. It was also clear that each form would need to be uniquely numbered and that a mechanism for associating a form with a particular child in a particular provider's office was needed. Also, forms suitable for receiving the peeled-off labels would be necessary.

The major issue at this point was to determine how these forms could be manufactured and, most importantly, whether their cost would be reasonable. To focus on this specific problem, I elected to hire consultants, since I was not familiar with the printing industry and wanted to get answers to these questions quickly. Such an assignment is a good example of a situation in which a consultant can be very helpful—there is a specific problem that requires specific expertise unavailable in-house.

Without much difficulty, I found a consultant, and he began his research. Within a few weeks, he had contacted several major printing firms, and the news was not good. First, it would be extremely difficult (translation: expensive) to affix the special adhesive notes to a form. Second, even if the notes could be affixed to the form, they would not be effective. It seemed that the adhesive used for such notes could not be expected to retain its properties for more than two years. Therefore, a form constructed as I envisioned it could not work: all the bar codes would fall off after two years. Since the childhood immunization record form must be utilized from birth until age six, using these notes was clearly unacceptable.

One printing firm, however, seemed particularly interested in this project, and I arranged a meeting with a representative of the firm. I described in detail the environment, the requirements, and the proposed solution. The company representative agreed to discuss the matter with her technical staff to see if a solution for manufacturing a suitable form could be found.

This time, the news was encouraging. Several weeks later, at a subsequent meeting, I was told that it might be possible to manufacture forms that would work in the way desired. This form would need to consist of three layers. The bottom layer would consist of plain paper; the middle layer would consist of label backing; and the top layer would consist of peel-off bar code labels. Cuts in the label-backing layer during manufacture and removal of each bar code label would also remove some label backing in the middle layer, creating a window to the plain paper below. The immunization information could then be written on the plain paper, which could be printed with any formatting information desired.

The problem was still not solved, however. The company was not sure that making cuts in the label backing would really work as intended. These cuts could not be complete, or else the label backing would fall apart during the manufacturing process. A workable design would require the use of small tabs to keep the label-backing layer together. These tabs would need to be strong enough to survive manufacturing, but easy enough to remove that the bar code labels could be used easily. Although the company had the technology to produce such a form, it had never done so before. Indeed, company representatives told me that such a form had never before been manufactured by anyone. The technical consultants within the company were reasonably sure it could be done, but a feasibility test would be required.

Another issue was that if the label came off with backing on it, this backing would need to be removed before the label could stick to anything, possibly a very cumbersome and time-consuming step. To address this contingency, the company proposed that the backing that was removed with a label be slightly smaller than the label itself. Hopefully, this arrangement would allow the label to be attached easily to plain paper without the necessity of removing the rest of the backing. Alternatively, the backing would be very easy to remove, since it would be smaller than the label itself. In any case, this design would clearly need to be tested as well.

Finally, there was the issue of cost. At this stage, the company really could not estimate what the final cost would be. However, company representatives understood that the cost of each form would need to be well under $1. Shortly after this discussion, we agreed to purchase a test batch of 1,000 of the forms at a cost of $4 each. We were hopeful that the final version could be manufactured at a considerably lower unit cost.

Before ordering the test batch of bar code forms, however, we needed to finalize the layout, decide how each child would be enrolled, and specify where the immunization bar codes would go when they were peeled off the form. We added a special bar code label with room for the name of the child and the provider at the top of the form. This label could then be attached to an enrollment form that would contain more detailed information. We designed small 3- by 5-inch forms for the immunization labels and had these printed in house. Each bar code form needed to be uniquely numbered. We wanted to use a number size that would accommodate any eventuality; therefore, we used a nine-digit number plus two alphabetic characters for the state abbreviation.

By this time, we had also addressed the issue of children who used multiple providers. Each bar code form would uniquely refer to a child-provider pair. In this way, a single child could have bar code forms in any number of provider offices. Wherever the immunization occurred, we would get a bar code indicating both the child and the provider. Thus, none of the bar code forms themselves would reflect a complete immunization record for the child; however, that was no different from the current immunization record forms.

Once the order was placed for the test batch of forms, we began to look for scanners that could read the forms at the central registry. We also began the process of designing our initial pilot test.

Pilot Testing

To make the pilot test most effective, we wanted to utilize provider offices that were representative of every type of practice. I also wanted to include providers that were very skeptical about the workability of this solution. We ended up dividing the providers into urban versus rural and large versus small. We recruited a total of nine practices to participate in the pilot testing during a one-month trial period. Each practice agreed to utilize the test forms in everyday work, enrolling children as they were seen.

We were very busy developing the complete system while we were waiting for the test forms to be produced. While the bar code forms were the central element in the system, we also needed enrollment forms, forms to receive the immunization and bar codes, a place to put the immunization bar code forms, and return envelopes. We also needed to develop training materials to explain the system to the pilot sites.

Figure 32.1 illustrates the enrollment portion of the system. When the child arrived in the office, a bar code form would be placed in the chart. The child's name would be entered on the label at the top of the form; that label would then be removed and affixed to the enrollment form. Additional information about the child would be entered on the enrollment form that would then be sent to the registry. The second identification label would be peeled off, placed on the parent immunization record form, and given to the parent. Removing the two name labels revealed two pre-punched holes in the top of the form that allowed it to be attached to the chart.

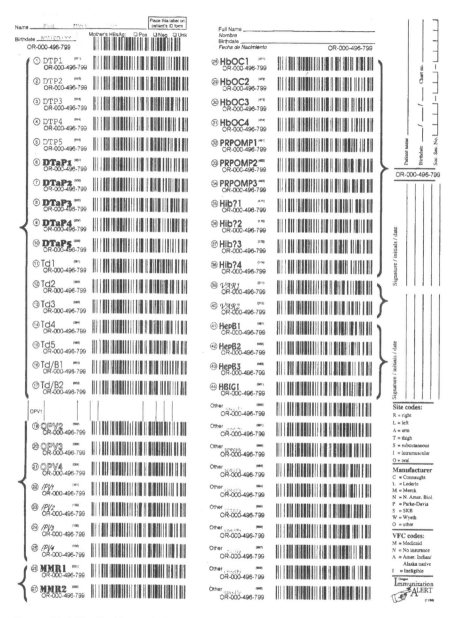

Figure 32.1. The final bar code form. At the top are two labels used for identification; holes beneath these labels are used to attach the form to the chart. Two columns of labels for the various immunization series constitute the majority of the form. Note that each type of immunization has a different font to aid users in distinguishing each series from the others. The right side of the form has, from top to bottom, identification information for the child (this information stays with the form), spaces for signature/initials/date of staff administering vaccines, and codes for use in filling out the form after the labels are removed. The OPV1 label has been removed to show the spaces for chart recording of immunizations: date, site, manufacturer, lot number, initials of provider, VFC code, and parental consent status.

Recording an immunization was a fast and simple process. A small paper form would be peeled off a pad of such forms affixed to the wall. For each immunization given, the bar code would be peeled off and transferred to the small form. After the date was written on the small form, it would be deposited in the receptacle also attached to the wall. On a weekly basis, all the forms in the receptacle would be collected, put in a postage-paid envelope, and mailed to the central registry. Figure 32.2 (right side) shows the process of recording an immunization.

Finally, the test forms arrived. We visited each of the nine practices and reviewed all the procedures for using the system. It was about a week before we started getting telephone calls from the test sites. Most of the calls were surprisingly positive—people really liked the system. However, they had many suggestions. We received numerous ideas for rearranging the form as well as suggestions related to the ancillary forms. For example, we originally had allowed room for only four immunizations on the small form—sometimes more were required (we ended up redesigning the form to accommodate up to six bar code labels).

The major concern expressed was that the bar code labels were difficult to peel off the form. Sometimes, peeling off one label would result in the entire form's coming apart. Our own extensive testing in our office confirmed that it was indeed necessary to be careful in peeling off the forms. We found from trial and error that it was necessary to hold on to the labels above and below the one that was being peeled off in order to avoid disintegration of the form. It also seemed that the small attachments of the backing of each label to the rest of the backing were too strong to allow smooth removal. We passed this information along to the manufacturer, which planned to correct this problem by making these attachments smaller next time. We also included an illustration of how to hold the forms above and below the one being removed in our updated training material.

After the test period was completed, we interviewed users of the system in each practice. We sorted and compiled all their suggestions and either incorporated them into the plans for the next version of the form or sent a written explanation to the practice detailing the reasons for not doing so. In this way, we not only collected extremely valuable information that helped improve the system, but we also reinforced our positive relationship with those practices who were willing to help us.

During this time, we also acquired and tested several scanners and developed the software needed to input information rapidly from the bar coded labels we were receiving. This work also required some thoughtful design. For example, the program to read the immunization bar code labels would make an audible " beep" every time it successfully read a new label, but it would not make such a noise whenever there was an effort to repeat a scan of a label that already had been read. In this way, the operator was able to perform the scanning process rapidly, with audible feedback so that no input was missed, while avoiding duplicate data entry from scanning a particular label more than once.

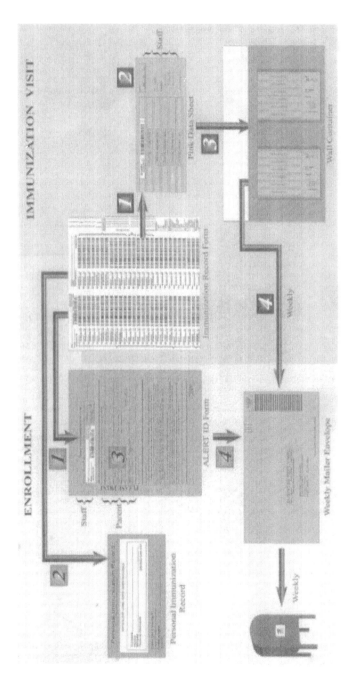

FIGURE 32.2. Illustration of the operation of the bar code system for immunization data collection. ENROLLMENT (left side): 1. Patient identification label filled out and placed on enrollment form ("ALERT ID Form"); 2. Second patient identification label filled out and placed on Personal Immunization Record (for family); 3. Parent/guardian completes demographic information on enrollment form; 4. Enrollment form placed in business reply envelope for weekly mailing to registry. IMMUNIZATION VISIT (right side): 1. Bar code label for immunization peeled off and affixed to pink data sheet; chart information entered on blank space left when bar code label removed: 2. Date and Vaccines for Children status entered on pink data sheet.: 3. Pink data sheet placed in wall container (note two pads of blank pink data sheets on front of container); 4. Accumulated pink data sheets transferred to business reply envelope and mailed to registry (weekly).

We also had defined a solution for communicating immunization information to providers. When the child arrived in the provider's office, the receptionist would make a call to a toll-free automated telephone system. Using telephone touch-tones, the receptionist would enter the bar code form number and receive acknowledgement of the information. That call would then be ended. The registry computer would then retrieve the immunization information for the child and generate a list of recommended immunizations for that visit. This information would then be sent via fax to the provider office—the fax numbers for all the offices would be on file. This fax, in turn, could then be included in the child's chart. The providers were comfortable with this mechanism because they could decide whether or not to request the immunization record. For those children who received all their immunizations in a single provider's office, the request would be unnecessary, thus resulting in fewer central registry faxes to the provider offices.

Statewide Rollout

As I led the planning effort to deploy this new system statewide, the key issues were production, distribution, marketing, and training. The order for a large quantity of bar code forms was just the beginning. We also needed enrollment forms, forms for attaching immunization bar codes, envelopes, wall-mounted pouches, and parent immunization record forms. We were very pleased that the bar code forms would cost only 21 cents each. (This cost was based on a very large quantity purchase. Although the large supply of forms reduced unit cost, it severely limited the ability to make any needed changes in the format for a long time.) However, we also needed to engage in careful management of the cost of all the ancillary materials. We ended up using an expandable file folder pouch as the wall receptacle for the peeled-off bar codes, and we devised a method to attach two pads of the forms to it, using clear plastic adhesive pouches. We calculated the quantity needed for each item and placed the orders.

Marketing the transition to the new system proved to be a huge task. We wanted to deploy the new system to about 1,500 providers over a one- to two-month time frame. We knew that we would need to visit each provider and that these visits would need to be either early in the morning before the practice opened or at lunchtime (to avoid interfering with patient visits). It was easy to see that handling this number of visits within such a short time frame would require the services of a large number of people. However, the immunization registry itself had a marketing staff consisting of only one person.

We had been, however, working closely with the Vaccines for Children program, which had a staff of four. We were able to arrange for these staff members to work with us to lead the bar code marketing efforts. In addition, we were very fortunate to have wonderful cooperation from the health plans that were supporting the registry. These health plans collectively agreed to detail 40 of their representatives to the registry for the rollout. These representatives routinely called on providers on behalf of the health plans and therefore were familiar with the issues involved in working with them. The marketing effort never could have been successful without the participation of the health plan representatives.

With this large marketing team in place, the challenge was then to organize and train them. We divided the state into four territories, and each of the Vaccines for Children staff members became a team leader for one territory. We arranged for a half-day training session for the entire marketing team to explain the bar code system itself as well as the plan for introducing this system to providers.

Developing the training materials proceeded in parallel with the planning efforts. We contracted with a video production firm to develop a 10-minute instructional video explaining how the bar code system operated in a provider office. We also developed a series of color overheads that explained the system step by step. Finally, we designed and produced a laminated wall poster that summarized the system's operation and that could serve as an ongoing reference for providers.

Distribution of materials was also a challenge. Each provider needed three to five boxes of forms of various types, the number depending on the size of the practice. Marketing representatives delivered most of this material to providers during their visits. However, we also shipped the materials when it was necessary to do so. This capability was especially helpful for serving provider locations that were distant from registry headquarters.

Initially, I decided to implement a voice response system to track the marketing process. The idea was that each marketing rep would call the system once a day and update the status of the provider offices. Although this was a technically workable solution, it turned out that the marketing reps would not use the voice response system. Rather, they wanted to be able to talk to a team leader to report progress, discuss problems, and share experiences. Therefore, we ended up managing the rollout process primarily through individual conversations and manual reporting.

Results

The rollout of the new system was very difficult, but it went reasonably well. Our training session for the temporary marketing reps enjoyed excellent attendance, and the questions that these marketing reps asked helped us to define important details of the process that had not been fully considered. In addition, these representatives were able to suggest very helpful revisions in the training materials.

At first, the rate of provider enrollment was very slow, a reflection of the time needed to schedule initial appointments. Once the marketing reps began visiting providers, however, we were able to sign providers up rapidly. More than half of the private providers were participating in the system by the end of the first month.

Of course, this sign-up rate was unsustainable. Those providers in easily accessible locations who readily agreed to participate had already been enrolled. To reach the rest of the providers, we needed a concerted effort, including (in some cases) direct calls I made to encourage providers to sign up.

As the quantity of enrollment and immunization bar codes increased at the central registry, we developed systems for handling the large flow of paper. It was also necessary to refine and streamline our data input process to be sure that our productivity could keep up with the workload. We were very pleased that the data collection system required the services of only two central registry staff members to enter all the data from the entire state.

At the end of two months, we had about 80% of the providers enrolled in the bar code system. At that time, almost all our 40 marketing reps returned to their regular positions. Through the additional hard work of the Vaccines for Children staff, we were able to sign up even more private providers over the next several months, bringing the final participation to over 90%. By this time, we were receiving data from well over 1,000 immunization visits every week.

The next challenge was to reinforce this enthusiastic response from the provider community by providing them with useful data in return. This challenge, however, turned out to be an insurmountable one for several reasons. First, the data we had on most children were incomplete. We had thought earlier in the process that we might be able to collect history information by using bar code forms, but the funds for the effort had not been forthcoming, and we had to abandon it. It would be a long time before our records were relatively complete. Therefore, any reports we produced would not be of immediate value.

In the end, our concerns about the lack of data completeness resulted in the decision not to provide any feedback to the providers. Since the providers had been expecting reports, albeit incomplete, many of them were disappointed, and there was some attrition in data reporting. However, for most of the providers, once they began using the bar code system, the process was simple and easy enough that they were willing to continue reporting even in the absence of any discernible short-term benefit to their practices.

I am pleased to report that as of this writing, 81% of the private providers of immunizations in Oregon continue to report data to the registry using the bar code system. This progress is in no small part due to the hard work and leadership of Barbara Canavan, who has been directing the immunization registry for the past several years. Among other changes in the program, providers now have the option to call registry staff to get immunization information in lieu of a feedback system.

Over time, there should be a transition from this reporting system to an electronic reporting system based on direct electronic transmission of immunization information. This transition is likely to occur either from billing records or directly from electronic medical records. However, in the meantime, the bar code system provides a useful and inexpensive method for obtaining this information from private providers.

The bar code immunization input system has also been applied in other environments. In New York City, it has been offered as an input option, and a small number of practices have elected to use it. In the state of Mississippi, the system is being used for private providers statewide.

Conclusion

This case study illustrates how a specific informatics problem related to data input was solved. It is important to note that the solution itself was not "high-tech" from the user's perspective. Indeed, its success may be attributed in large part to its conformity with the existing, paper-based data recording process.

This case illustrates both positive and negative lessons. On the positive side, the key success factors and the lessons learned include:

- the importance of securing user input in the design of a system;
- the need for system designers to develop a thorough understanding of user requirements; and
- the importance of being willing to respond effectively to user concerns.

There are also lessons to be learned from the early failures in this case. These lessons include:

- the importance of developing alternative solutions in the event that a preferred solution proves unacceptable to users;
- avoiding a bias in favor of highly technical approaches to problems that may lend themselves to simpler solutions; and
- the need for comprehensive planning for system design, development, and implementation, rather than using a plan-as-you-go approach.

In particular, I regret my lack of more complete preparation for the initial meeting with private providers. In approaching such a situation again, I would try to talk with individual users prior to such a meeting to develop a better appreciation of the feedback likely to be obtained from the entire group.

Finally, it is important to be open to a wide range of possibilities in solving informatics problems. Successful systems are not those that use the most sophisticated and complex technology. Rather, systems succeed when appropriate and cost-effective approaches are employed.

Questions for Review

1. In retrospect, how could the author have been better prepared for his initial meeting with the private providers? What specific steps could he have taken to anticipate provider needs and insure that he presented and refined an acceptable plan at this first meeting?

2. What was the guiding principle behind the author's identification of step 8 as the data collection point in the provider's work process? Why not step 9?
3. Explain why the use of bar codes was a more feasible solution than a telephone voice response system. What were the disadvantages of the latter? Why was the use of peel-off labels important? Why did the solution need to be integrated with the patient chart?
4. Why did the author make sure that private providers who were skeptical of the data collection system were included in the pilot testing? What are the advantages of including these providers?
5. In what way were the calls received by the central registry from providers participating in the pilot testing important to the success of the project? Interviews with providers after the pilot testing? Feedback from marketing representatives? What informatics principle does the handling of these calls, interviews, and conversations illustrate?
6. Explain how the author was able to stay within cost constraints in (a) avoiding the imposition of substantial costs on participants in the data collection system, (b) limiting additional costs to the central registry, and (c) marketing the data collection system and distributing the materials to providers.
7. What budgetary constraints limited fuller effectiveness of the system?
8. To what extent was the solution to the problem of adhesive backing of the note luck, and to what extent does it represent design creativity?

References

1. Miller PL, Frawley SJ, Sayward FG, Yasnoff WA, Duncan L, Fleming DW. Combining tabular, rule-based, and procedural knowledge in computer-based guidelines for childhood immunization. *Comput Biomed Res* 1997;30:211–231.
2. Canavan B. *Building and Sustaining an Immunization Registry*. Boston, MA: American Public Health Association; 2000.

33
Public Health Informatics in the National Health and Nutrition Examination Survey

Lewis E. Berman, Yechiam Ostchega, Debra S. Reed-Gillette, and Kathryn Porter

Learning Objectives

After studying this chapter, you should be able to:

- Explain the history and the goals and objectives of the National Health and Nutrition Examination Survey (NHANES).
- Provide examples of uses of the data provided by NHANES.
- Describe the quality assurance and quality control program for NHANES 99+.
- Describe the value provided by the development of the NHANES 99+ Integrated Survey Information System (ISIS).

Overview

The National Health and Nutrition Examination Survey (NHANES) provides an example of the use of technology and systems to collect data simultaneously in geographically distinct locations and make available crucial data related to public health. Through the development and use of the Integrated Survey Information System (ISIS), NHANES connects field personnel, mobile examination centers, contractors, and the Centers for Disease Control and Prevention (CDC)/National Center for Health Statistics (NCHS) headquarters for a continuous flow of data in near real time. It also makes those data available in a usable form to researchers and analysts. This chapter provides an overview of the NHANES methodology, objectives, and goals. It also describes an application of public health informatics that is both innovative and highly functional.

Introduction

The National Health and Nutrition Examination Survey (NHANES) is the cornerstone survey used for assessing the health of the US population. The program is an ongoing series of surveys that originated in 1960 as the National Health Examination Survey (NHES) or Cycle 1. Since the start of the program, there have been eight periodic surveys, as shown in Table 33.1.

The first three studies were conducted in the 1960s. Beginning in 1970, a nutrition component was added, and the name was changed to NHANES. Three of these surveys were conducted between 1970 and 1994. A special study of Hispanic populations (HHANES) in the United States was conducted from 1982 to 1984.

NHANES data have been used for numerous purposes, including:

- determining the prevalence of iron deficiency in the US population[1];
- estimating the prevalence of osteoporosis in the older US population[2];
- examining the prevalence of overweight among US preschool children[3]; and
- determining the correlation between US dietary fat intake and serum total cholesterol concentrations[4].

Perhaps one of the most significant uses of NHANES data is the development of the CDC growth charts.[5] These growth charts have been distributed

TABLE 33.1. Overview of NHES and NHANES

Survey	Years	Age Groups	Survey Emphasis
NHES I	1960–1962	18–79 years	Growth, development, and sensory defects
NHES II	1963–1965	6–11 years	Growth, development, and sensory defects
NHES III	1966–1970	12–17 years	Growth, developmental histories, school questionnaires, medical examination, including x-rays and laboratory tests
NHANES I	1971–1975	1–74 years	Selected chronic diseases
NHANES II	1976–1980	6 months to 74 years	Detailed personal interview, health examination, and nutrition interview
HHANES†	1982–1984	6 months to 74 years	Detailed personal interview, health examination, and nutrition interview focused on Hispanic population
NHANES III	1988–1994	2 months and older	Detailed personal interview, health examination, and nutrition interview
NHANES 99+	1999–Present	All ages	Detailed personal interview, health examination, and nutrition interview

worldwide and are used by nearly every US pediatrician. Their applicability extends to assistance program eligibility, growth hormone therapy, and international comparisons.

The primary objective of NHANES is to collect high-quality health and nutrition data and release it in a timely manner. In accordance with this objective, NHANES has the following goals:

- To estimate the number and percentage of persons in the US population and in designated subgroups with selected health conditions and risk factors
- To monitor trends in the prevalence, awareness, treatment, and control of selected diseases
- To monitor trends in risk behaviors and environmental exposures
- To analyze risk factors for selected diseases
- To study the relationship between diet, nutrition, and health
- To explore emerging public health issues and new technologies
- To establish a national probability sample of genetic material for future genetic research
- To establish and maintain a national probability sample of baseline information on health and nutritional status

This national operation uses three mobile examination centers (MEC), each of which consists of four interconnected tractor-trailers that move to sites around the country, as shown in Figure 33.1.

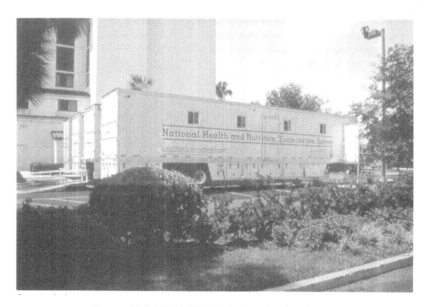

FIGURE 33.1. NHANES Mobile Examination Center.

Each year, NHANES visits 15 different sites, with operations lasting about eight weeks at each site. The timeline for advance arrangements, setup, testing, and examination is extremely tight, requiring planning that occurs many months before arrival at a geographic location or "stand." The logistics of operating such a study require telecommunications hook-up, power, sewage, water, and security.

The most recent survey, NHANES 99+, differs in several respects from previous surveys in this series in the following ways:

- NHANES 99+ is continuous, whereas previous surveys operated in a fixed timeframe. The sample design of the current NHANES is based on an annual survey of the noninstitutionalized, civilian US population. Each single year and any combination of consecutive years will comprise a nationally representative sample of the US population. Single-year prevalence estimates, however, are limited in terms of the stability of prevalence estimates due to the limited number of survey participants in a single year.
- NHANES 99+ can be linked to other federal government data collections from the noninstitutionalized, civilian US population.
- Survey content can be changed from year to year, depending on the complexity, reliability, and validity of the health measure. Emerging public health issues can be incorporated into the survey within one year, instead of having to wait for the next NHANES cycle. Scientific advances in testing, newly developed protocols, and new equipment can be added to the survey within one or two years instead of a decade. Note, however, that it still takes about two years of data collection to have stable national estimates.
- NHANES 99+ features incorporation and reliance on information technology (IT) to collect data and insure high quality. IT features include a private frame-relay wide-area network, commercial off-the-shelf (COTS) equipment, local-area networking, relational database technology, a data replication architecture, development environments such as Blaise[6] and PowerBuilder,[7] and integration of biomedical equipment. The technology innovations in NHANES 99+ result in real-time data access, rapid and accurate data collection, reduced back-end data cleanup, and faster data release and analysis.

In this chapter, we will address the conduct and field operations of NHANES 99+ and the systems and information technology that make it functional.

Field Operation

As with previous NHANES surveys, the design for NHANES 99+ is a stratified multistage probability sample of the civilian noninstitutionalized population of the United States. To determine the areas of the country and individual households/participants to visit in a particular year, information is garnered from the US Census Bureau, from new housing development listings, and from a household listing process. This selection process occurs in four stages: (1) selection of Primary Sampling Units or PSUs (counties or small groups of contiguous counties); (2) selection of segments within a PSU (a block or group of blocks containing a cluster of households); (3) selection of households within segments; and (4) selection of one or more participants within each household.

Each year of the survey, approximately 5,000 people are interviewed in the household and examined in the MEC. To get sufficient representative sampling, 15 different PSUs are visited per year, with the number of participants at each PSU ranging from 300 to 500. Although a representative sample of the population is examined every year, it is necessary to use several years' worth of data to permit in-depth and stable analysis. This is especially true when the prevalence of a condition is low or when researchers want to analyze the data by several co-variables or make estimates for different population subgroups. Reliable estimates for breakdowns by various age, gender, race/ethnicity, and income groups are possible only by aggregating data from several years.

There is approximately one year of lag time between the start of sample design and the beginning of field operations. Approximately six to eight months before interviews and exams begin at a PSU (stand), a team of people works on the logistics related to the household interview and MEC examinations. This work includes leasing office space for the field staff, finding hotel rooms, conducting publicity/outreach, establishing relationships with local health officials, and receiving endorsements from community leaders and groups. For the MEC, space is leased for setting up the trailers, telecommunications are ordered, and security, water, power and sewage requirements, and build-outs are planned and developed.

Two to three months before household interviews start, an advance letter is sent to each potential participant, informing him or her that an interviewer will visit his or her home. Once the stand officially opens, a team of approximately 20 interviewers arrives at the stand to start the screening and interviewing process. When the interviewer arrives at the home, he or she shows an official identification and briefly explains the purpose of the survey. The interviewer then administers the household screener questionnaire solely to determine if people in the home are eligible to participate in the survey based on predetermined demographic criteria. If the person is eligible, the interviewer explains the household questionnaire and informs the participant of his or her rights and the CDC/NCHS confidentiality policy. If the person agrees to participate, the household interview is administered. Upon completion of the interview, the interviewer schedules a time for the participant(s) to be examined at the MEC. This flow is shown in Figure 33.2.

Household Questionnaire

The household questionnaire consists of three parts: screening, family interview, and sample person interview. The questions asked of each participant

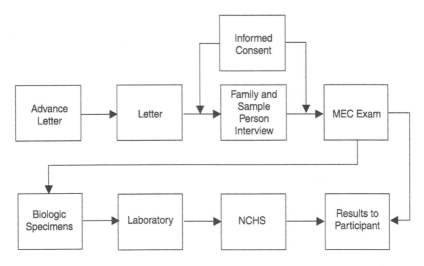

FIGURE **33.2.** NHANES 99+ operational flow.

depend on the participant's age and gender. These questions are related to health practices and experiences and in general are related to the medical components administered in the MEC. The family questionnaire portion is conducted with a designated family reference person; it includes information that applies to all members within the family. The queries elicit information concerning family structure, income, food security, and housing characteristics. Table 33.2 provides an overview of the content of each of the household administered questionnaires.

A set of exclusion criteria questions is incorporated into the household interview to determine an individual's eligibility for certain MEC components. For example, if an individual has indicated a prior heart attack in the medical conditions section of the questionnaire, that individual would be excluded from the cardiovascular fitness component within the MEC. These exclusionary data items are "shared" across the components within the MEC and are accessed by the MEC component subsystems at the time of the exam. Not only does this practice reduce respondent burden by eliminating the need to re-ask the same or similar questions, but it also insures data consistency across components.

The MEC and the Home Exam

Upon the arrival of a survey participant at the MEC, a coordinator greets the participant, verifies basic demographic information (age, gender, date of birth), and directs participants to the appropriate exam rooms. The coordinator is the last individual to verify and, if necessary, correct this basic demographic

TABLE **33.2**. Screener and household questionnaires

Component	Location of Interview	Information Collected
Screener	Household	Household composition, identification of families, family relationships, demographics, food security, and sample person identifications
Family questionnaire	Household	Demographics, dust collection, family income, food security, health insurance, housing characteristics, interview management, lead dust observation, pesticide exposure, and smoking
Sample person interview	Household	Acculturation, audiometry, blood pressure, cardiovascular disease, demographics, dermatology, diabetes, diet behavior and nutrition, dietary supplements and medicines, digital symbol substitution, early childhood, hospital utilization, immunization, kidney conditions, medical conditions, miscellaneous pain, occupation, oral health, osteoporosis, physical activity, physical functioning, respiratory health and disease, social support, smoking and tobacco use, tuberculosis, vision, weight history

information. In addition to a coordinator, each MEC team consists of a physician, a dentist, two dietary intake interviewers, three certified medical technologists, four health technicians, one phlebotomist, two interviewers, a home examiner, and one data manager. Because two MECs are open at any given time, with a third traveling to another location, two complete MECs teams are staffed. A description of each of the examination components is shown in Table 33.3.

The exam center typically has two examination sessions a day. These are held either in the morning, the afternoon, or the evening to allow for the flexibility required by survey participants. The examination centers are open five to six days each week, including Saturday and Sunday. Saturday is the most popular day for examinations. Figure 33.3 shows the distribution of exams by day of the week. Household screening and interviewing begin three weeks before the start of the examinations. This advance screening and interviewing allows sufficient time to schedule participants for exams. Typically, the schedule is loaded with more participants at the start of the exam period. In a typical four-hour exam session, there can be as many as 14 participants moving through the MEC. Although the majority of participants complete the examination, some do not.

TABLE 33.3. Examination components in NHANES 99+

Component	Location	Measurements
Anthropometry	MEC/Home exam (limited)	Height, weight, circumferences (calf, thigh, arm, abdomen), and skin folds (triceps and subscapular)
Audiometry	MEC	Otoscopy and tympanometry
Balance	MEC	A standardized Romberg test of standing balance on firm and compliant support surfaces
Bioelectrical impedance analysis (BIA)	MEC	Total body water, body cell mass, and fat-free body mass using a low-level electric charge
Cardiovascular fitness	MEC	The component uses a treadmill (walking only) to take a survey participant to approximately 80% of maximal heart rate to measure oxygen consumption
Dietary recall	MEC	Detailed information on all foods and beverages consumed during the previous 24-hour period (midnight to midnight)
Dual energy x-ray absorptiometry (DXA)	MEC	Bone mineral content, bone mineral density, total body fat, and lean muscle mass
Laboratory	MEC/Home exam (limited)	Sexually transmitted diseases, latex allergy, DNA, insulin/C-peptide, glycohemoglobin, glucose, lipids, albumin complete blood count, and many laboratory analytes
Lower extremity disease	MEC	Foot abnormalities, evaluation of touch pressure sensation, ankle brachial systolic pressure
MEC audio computer-aided self-interview (ACASI)	MEC	Alcohol use, drug use, mental health, sexual behavior, smoking and tobacco use
MEC computer-aided personal interview (CAPI)	MEC	Alcohol use, current health status, kidney function, physical activity, reproductive health, and tobacco use
Muscular strength	MEC/Home exam (timed walk only)	Timed 20-foot walk and measurement of the isokinetic strength of the right knee extensors
Oral health	MEC	Dental sealant, tooth count, coronal carries, orofacial traumatic injuries, dental fluorosis assessment, pain, gingival bleeding, loss of attachment, and root caries
Physicians' exam/ blood pressure	MEC/Home exam	Heart rate for participants 0–4 years of age; radial pulse for participants 5 years and over; and blood pressure for all participants 8 years and over
Tuberculosis skin testing	MEC/Home exam	Reactions to two different TB skin tests
Vision	MEC/Home exam (near card only)	Distance vision, refractive error, shape of the cornea, distance eyeglass prescription, and near vision

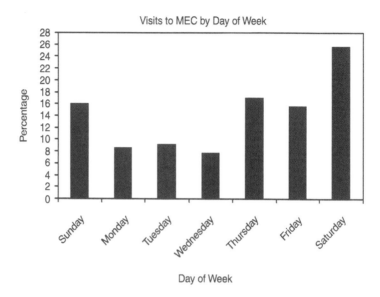

Figure 33.3. Percentage of MEC visits by day of week for the first year of NHANES 99+.

Reasons for incomplete exams include late arrival, early departure, refusal to do some exams, or physical limitations. To help insure that participants receive, at a minimum, several core components, a team relies on a prioritized list of components. For example, anthropometry, blood pressure, and venipuncture are higher priority than the cardiovascular fitness exam.

Although the MEC is outfitted with a hydraulic lift for wheel-chair accessibility, there are people who cannot endure travel to the MEC for an exam. For these people, a scaled-back home exam, consisting of only those measures that can be done reliably in the home, is administered.

Upon completion of the examination, each examinee is paid for his or her time and for travel. An examinee is also given a partial report of findings that contains information collected within the MEC. For example results of the vision, blood pressure, complete blood count, hearing, and dental exams are provided. Other results are mailed to participants later, as results are made available from the laboratories or data graders. The complete report of findings is typically sent out 12 to 16 weeks after the exam. Figure 33.4 shows a portion of the final report of findings.

Quality Assurance and Control

During NHANES III, postsurvey data verification and cleanup was an intensive operation, taking nearly three and a half years. Unlike NHANES III, however, the data from NHANES 99+ is immediately available on a server located at NCHS and at the home office of the data collection contractor. A comprehensive, continuous, and tightly integrated quality assurance (QA)/quality control (QC) program is in place for NHANES 99+, resulting in expedient data release. Because of careful planning, the first year of NHANES 99+ data was released only six months after the end of the first year of data collection to collaborators who help support and contribute to the program.

QA/QC is one of the most important aspects of this study, because the integrity of the conclusions drawn by the study is in large part determined by the quality of the data collected. There are two basic components of insuring data integrity: QA and QC. QA consists of those activities that take place before data collection or in improving and refining data collection; QC consists of those activities that take place during and after data collection.[8] Manual development, training/retraining before and during the survey, and certification of examiners and feedback are part of the QA process. Component completion rates, validation of household interviews, contractor and subcontractor debriefings, examiner performance, reliability, and validity, MEC examination flow, and equipment performance are part of the QC process.

The NHANES 99+ data sets need to be of the highest attainable accuracy and precision within the usual limitations dictated by acceptable procedures and reasonable cost. Two sources of error that may affect quality can occur during data collection activities. These error sources are:

- Sampling error that relates to survey sampling methodology
- Nonsampling error that relates to nonresponse bias and measurement inaccuracy

These errors can be either random or systematic. Systematic errors are a consistent deviation from true measurements, and they are of more concern. The overall goal for NHANES 99+ QA/QC is to reduce systematic error and objectively measure the extent to which this type of error exists. Data errors and biases are to be caught at the earliest possible stage of QA/QC. A major precept of this effort is to follow simple quality control measures before taking more difficult and costly steps.[9] In addition, software can be used to automatically provide QA/QC in standardized, appropriate, understandable, and useful summary tables and graphs.

Two sources of error may enter into the data collection activities. One source, sampling error, is the failure to identify all of the units comprising the population of interest.[10] The second source is nonsampling error that can result from many sources, including nonresponse error and measurement error. Nonresponse error results from the failure to collect data on all persons in the sample. For example, a participant may not have time, may be physically limited, or may refuse to participate in some or all components in the MEC.

Measurement error refers to inaccuracy in measurement. Such errors may be the result of numerous factors. For example, examiners may not take accurate measurements or may provide inaccurate instructions to the participant.

National Health and Nutrition Examination Survey

Final Report of Findings

> These measurements were obtained as part of a survey and do not represent a medical diagnosis. Interpretation of these measurements must be made by a physician.

Date of Examination: April 13, 1999
Participant Name: John Q. Public
Participant Age At Interview: 43 years
Participant Age At Exam: 43 years
Participant Gender: Male
SP ID: 123456

Body Measurements

Height/Length.   5 ft. 9 in.
Weight   179.0 lbs

For a person of your height, your weight is above the range of a healthy weight, and you may be overweight.

Blood Pressure and Heart Rate

		Optimal	Normal	Acceptable
Systolic Blood Pressure	126 mm Hg	< 120	< 130	< 140
Diastolic Blood Pressure	90 mm Hg	< 80	< 85	< 90
Resting Pulse Rate	64 bpm			

The participant's blood pressure is mildly high. Based on the Sixth Report of the Joint National Committee on Detection, Evaluation, and Treatment of High Blood Pressure. NIH Publication, 1997.

Dental

The dental examination of the National Health and Nutrition Examination Survey is not, and is not intended to be, a substitute for the examination usually given to persons seeking care from their own dentists. Neither a dental history nor x-rays are taken, and therefore the findings are solely the result of what can be seen at the time of the examination.

The examining dentist recommends that you continue your regular routine care.

• No findings

FIGURE 33.4. A portion of the final report of findings mailed to a participant 12 to 16 weeks after the MEC exam.

National Health and Nutrition Examination Survey

Final Report of Findings

Laboratory

Lab Test	Result	Units	Flag	Reference Range
Glucose	88.0	mg/dL		60.0 - 109.0
Glycohemoglobin	—	%		
ALT	37.0	U/L		0 - 40.0
AST	28.0	U/L		0 - 31.0
Alkaline Phosphatase	51.0	U/L		39.0 - 117.0
Albumin	5.1	g/dL		3.2 - 5.2
Bicarbonate	25.0	mmol/L		22.0 - 29.0
BUN	19.0	mg/dL		6.0 - 19.0
Calcium	9.9	mg/dL		8.4 - 10.2
Cholesterol	243.0	mg/dL	high	0 - 199.0
Triglycerides	918.0	mg/dL	high	0 - 199.0
HDL	—	mg/dL		
LDL	—	mg/dL		
Serum Creatinine	0.7	mg/dL		0.4 - 1.2
GGT	112.0	U/L	high	11.0 - 51.0
LDH	145.0	U/L		94.0 - 250.0
Phosphorus	4.2	mg/dL		2.6 - 4.5
Sodium	138.0	mmol/L		133.0 - 145.0
Potassium	4.7	mmol/L		3.3 - 5.1
Chloride	103.7	mmol/L		96.0 - 108.0
Total Protein	7.4	g/dL		5.9 - 8.4
Uric Acid	5.3	mg/dL		3.4 - 7.0
Bilirubin	1.7	mg/dL	high	0 - 1.0
Eryt. Protoporphyrin	—	ug/dL, RBC		
Serum Folate	—	ng/mL		
RBC Folate	—	ng/mL, RBC		
Iron	82.0	ug/dL		32.0 - 181.0
TIBC	—	ug/dL		
Serum Ferritin	—	ng/mL		
Transferrin Saturation	—	%		
Blood Lead	—	ug/dL		
T4	—	ug/dL		
TSH	—	uIU/mL		
Total PSA	—	ng/mL		
PSA Ratio	—	%		

*** Test not done on this age group
** Results Still Pending
— Test Not Done
<< Lower than Limit of Detection
>> Above the Limit of Calibration

nchs Kathryn Porter MD CDC

John Q. Public, 123456, April 13, 1999   Page 6 of 6
National Center For Health Statistics, 6525 Belcrest Road, Room 900, Hyattsville, Maryland 20782.

FIGURE 33.4. *(continued)* A portion of the final report of findings mailed to a participant 12 to 16 weeks after the MEC exam.

Measurement drift over time and change in personnel can be another cause for this error. Measurement error can also result from a participant's not understanding examination instructions or from diurnal variation in biomedical indicators. Finally, instruments that are poorly calibrated or equipment changes can also contribute to inaccurate measurements.

The specific objectives for NHANES 99+ QA include the following:

- Insuring proper examiner training as demonstrated by certification procedures and recertification procedures
- Identifying, evaluating, and selecting remedies to problems by using individual and group feedback and retraining
- Using gold standard examinations (GSE) to compare exam measurements between MEC technicians and recognized experts
- Calibrating equipment to help insure consistency

As part of NHANES 99+ QA, a comprehensive training program has been instituted. In large part, this program consists of appropriate examiner training that requires significant practice time for the health examiners (3 to 6 months) and less time for household interviewers and other staff. This program employs adult learning theory, which emphasizes practical hands-on learning for the adult learner.[11] The training provided is therefore hands-on in order to provide ample practice time in the MECs, with little class time. In addition, because staff turnover is expected in such a long-term survey, NHANES 99+ QA makes provisions for training new staff members. To insure that replacement staff members receive training that is consistent with that offered to previous examiners, the comprehensive training program uses a modular approach. The advantage of this approach is that it breaks down complex components to simple tasks that can be standardized and easily updated. For example, in the cardiovascular fitness component, one training session is dedicated to teaching the health technician how to use the blood pressure and heart rate monitor. Another session is dedicated to teaching the technician how to demonstrate walking on a treadmill to the participant. Trainees master individual modules before they practice an entire component in a training session. In essence, training can be conceptualized as a closed loop consisting of modular training, practical experience in the MEC and in the field, and feedback resulting in changes to the training modules.

NHANES 99+ has objective procedures in place for certifying health technicians soon after the start of the study. In addition, exam component project officers have developed objective skill lists for the majority of the components. The advantages of developing these skill lists are that (1) a skill list can be used to certify new examiners, (2) a skill list provides an objective way to assess examiners skills, (3) a skill list can be used to recertify examiners, and (4) a skill list provides feedback during annual retraining. Table 33.4 provides an example of a skill list in the assessment of blood pressure measurements.

GSEs are used to measure the agreement between a recognized expert and an examiner. This methodology functions by conducting examinations on the same

TABLE **33.4.** Example of a blood pressure skill list

Performance Items	Satisfactory	Unsatisfactory	Comments
Procedure explanation	✓		
Participant positioning before/ during exam	✓		
Examination environment is kept quiet		✓	Noise from other components inter-fered with hearing heartbeat
Radial pulse palpation	✓		
Adherence to resting intervals	✓		
Arm circumference measure-ment	✓		
Cuff size selection	✓		
Cuff fit test		✓	Physician forgot to do this
Inflation rate on all measures	✓		
Brachial pulse palpation	✓		
Stethoscope placement	✓		
Deflation rate on all measures	✓		
Tubing disconnect between measures	✓		

participant during a single exam session. It serves to identify potential problems and is didactic in nature. Components utilizing a GSE include audiometry, blood pressure, body measurements, oral health, and tuberculosis skin readings.

All biomedical equipment used in NHANES 99+ is subjected to stringent machine calibration. The frequency and complexity of equipment calibration varies from once per day to once per month and from very simple to detailed and time-consuming calibration. For example, in anthropometry, calibrated weights are placed on the digital scale, and the readout is captured to assess the state of the device. Alternatively, audiometry requires detailed assembly of calibration equipment and tedious testing to assure the reliability of the audiometer. Of note is that some of the equipment calibration exceeds manufacturer recommendations because of the need to use the devices extensively.

The specific objectives for NHANES 99+ QC are to:

* Determine the cause of component noncompletion; and
* Assess the nature and extent of measurement errors.

For each component, a completion rate consists of the ratio between the number of people examined and those eligible for the component, further segmented by age, gender, race/ethnicity, examiner, and cause. As noted earlier, participants may not complete an exam for a variety of reasons. Regardless of the reason, the impact of noncompletion manifests itself in the analytic utility of the data. For example, a low completion rate may create higher standard error in the estimates. Therefore, the component completion rate is continuously monitored.

In addition, each component is evaluated on the basis of several indicator variables. Typically, these values are the outcomes for a component. In anthropometry, one of the outcome variables is body mass index (BMI). Out-of-range BMI values may provide clues to problems associated with equipment, with technicians, with an outlier, or with a real change in the population. Another example of an indicator variable is systolic or diastolic blood pressure. Although the range of systolic blood pressure readings may be acceptable, it is plausible that other measurement problems can arise, such as an end-digit preference.[12] In such a case, the examiner prefers to record blood pressure with a preferred end digit (i.e., 140, 150, 160 rather than 142, 158, 164). The presence of such an end-digit preference is cause for retraining and recertification of the examiner.

Reporting Results to Survey Participants

The NHANES 99+ data collection system allows each person to get his or her initial examination findings immediately at the conclusion of the exam. Abnormal findings detected during the MEC exam are automatically flagged, and the MEC physician is electronically alerted to discuss these results with the participant before he or she leaves the exam center. In addition, when participants return for a tuberculosis (TB) skin test reading, a computer system allows the readings to be generated as a report that explains the TB skin test result. When indicated, the TB report contains a referral to a nearby clinic for further evaluation. As previously indicated, a final report of findings (ROF) is sent to participants approximately 12 to 16 weeks after the examination. This report contains all examination findings and requires time to compile, because laboratory measurements and data from the whole body scan (DXA) must be analyzed and transmitted electronically back into the ISIS database before results can be sent to the participant. Laboratory results requiring early reporting, such as abnormal glucose levels, are reported to participants as soon as possible. Laboratories notify the NHANES medical officer by fax or by uploading abnormal laboratory results to an FTP site.

The connectivity between the exam centers, laboratories, and headquarters allowed the NHANES survey to plan and implement an innovative protocol for reporting sensitive test results back to survey participants. Test results for sexually transmitted diseases (STDs) are not mailed out. Instead, individuals are instructed to call a toll-free phone number and provide a password for their results. A health educator uses a computer system to verify the password, give STD and human immunodeficiency virus (HIV) test results, and record the outcome of the post-test counseling. Persons tested for STDs such as *Chlamydia trachomatis, Neisseria gonorrhoeae,* herpes simplex type 2, and HIV receive pretest counseling by the MEC physician, along with instructions on how to get test results. As a privacy measure, results are provided only if the survey participant can correctly identify his or her password.

Information Management and Survey System Development

It is necessary to provide a brief description of past practices if the reader is to understand how information technology (IT) has revolutionized NHANES 99+. Previous NHANES (I and II), HHANES, and NHES surveys relied solely on paper and pencil data collection efforts. Questionnaires were in booklet form, and examination technicians recorded measurements on data entry forms that were designed for each component. After data collection, keypunch operators manually entered data onto a key-to-tape or key-to-disk operation. Because of keypunch limitations, all data collection relied on an 80-column record format. Each form included basic demographic data items such as gender and date of birth. Because demographics were collected in multiple places, this data was reconciled after keying to find a "best" value.

The NHANES III data system was automated, in that most of the medical components had electronic forms housed on workstations in each examination room. This arrangement precluded the need for manual key data entry operations for getting paper and pencil form data into a computer, as had been done on the surveys prior to NHANES III. Most data were entered into computers by the medical technicians in the MEC, rather than by automated capture from biomedical equipment. Some minimal data checking was performed on the electronic forms at the point of collection. However, the process of data reconciliation was still required. During the first phase of NHANES III, the household questionnaire was still in paper booklet form because of the lack of portable, rugged computers. Phase one questionnaires required keying operations; the keyed and electronic forms of the questionnaire then required reconciliation. The second phase of the survey implemented a computer-assisted personal interview (CAPI) system on personal computers.

System Requirements

The vision for NHANES 99+ was a system that verified data at the point of entry, contained shared common data elements, reduced the burden on the participant, and required minimal back-end data reconciliation and portability of data across surveys. This vision led to the development of a real-time data collection system. It was also envisioned that the use of COTS products and biomedical machines with electronic interfaces would enable the data to undergo a more timely QA/QC process, enabling staff to intervene earlier and correct problems in the survey. The basic requirements that were needed to support this vision are summarized in Table 33.5.

TABLE 33.5. NHANES 99+ information system requirements

Requirement	Description
Audit	Maintain an audit trail for data modification.
Configuration management	Version control for all applications.
COTS	Reliance, where possible, on commercial off-the-shelf equipment.
Documentation	All manuals, checklists, and training materials related to the information systems shall be available on-line from within any software application.
Editing	Point-of-entry data editing and validation. This shall include support for both hard and soft edits.
Flexibility	All systems shall be designed and implemented to be scalable, flexible, and expandable.
Graphical user interface	Development of a graphical user interface standard that applies to all systems developed.
Operating system	Development of systems to operate under Microsoft Windows 95, 98, and NT.
Operational support	Support survey planning and design, data collection, data receipt, quality assurance and control, communication of examination findings to survey respondents, data review, data editing, data analysis, generation, and documentation of public use data products and tracking of survey respondents.
Security/confidentiality	System security functions shall be built into all processes to ensure the integrity of the data and to protect the confidentiality of survey participants.
Timeliness	Delivery of data from the point of origin back to NCHS within 24 hours of entry.

The Integrated Survey Information System (ISIS)

All these information system requirements were incorporated in the design of the Integrated Survey Information System (ISIS) now in use. ISIS includes the entire software, hardware, database, and network architecture. Essentially, ISIS is a collection of customized subsystems linking the field office, the MEC, contractors, and NCHS during field operations. Figure 33.5 provides a schematic of the data flow that is accommodated by ISIS.

The flow of data is over a private WAN. The WAN connects the field offices to the contractor home office, and connects the contractor, in turn, to NCHS. This connectivity allows real-time data transmission from the field back to headquarters, allowing immediate operational feedback. Data transmitted between the MEC and the field office, the field office and contractor headquarters, and the contractor and NCHS are encrypted.

External laboratories are connected to the contractor via the Internet. The electronic data management system responsible for laboratory data interchange is not a real-time system, because laboratory processing occurs in batches. Consider, for example, a survey participant whose blood is drawn during the physical examination. Some of the simpler laboratory processing, such as a complete blood count, is done at the MEC, whereas the majority of analytes are processed at distant laboratories. This arrangement precludes immediate feedback; as a result of survey scheduling, it requires batch processing of the blood. Laboratories return blood results to the contractor and to NCHS headquarters in two to three months. Note, however, that abnormal results are delivered to NCHS as part of the early reporting system, so that these results are communicated to the participant as quickly as possible.

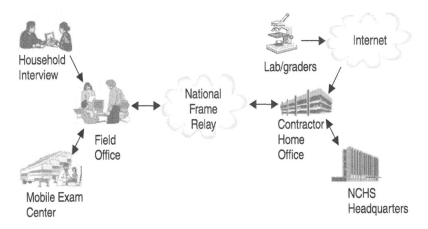

FIGURE 33.5. The NHANES 99+ data flow.

ISIS offers state of the art capabilities. Some of the technologies include a private WAN; an integrated electronic data dictionary and meta-data; client-server technology; data replication; and built-in disaster recovery. The ISIS infrastructure can support changes in the survey requirements to reflect changing public interest and priorities, if necessary. Most importantly, compared with previous surveys, ISIS allows NCHS to reduce significantly the time required to transfer, process, and publish the data. The impact of all of this technology was the production of edited data sets and documentation only six months after the end of the first year of the survey. By comparison, it took three and one half years to produce public use data sets from NHANES III.

ISIS has been designed to support all phases of the survey, using technologies robust enough to handle the demands of the distributed computing environment: survey planning and design; data collection; data receipt and control; quality assurance; communication of examination findings to sample persons; data review; editing; analysis; data archiving; and generation and documentation of public use data products. The technology in ISIS allows these activities to occur in parallel.

For the household interview and collection of self-reported information, ISIS is augmented with laptop-like computers called pentops. These CAPI instruments are programmed in Blaise, which allows for complex question routing, multiple language support (i.e., English and Spanish), modular design, form-like user interface design tools, and data manipulation tools. While the household interview is conducted independently of ISIS, the interviewer uploads the data to the field office server upon return to the field office. From there, the interview is replicated across the WAN back to the contractor and the NCHS servers. In addition to CAPI, ISIS also contains audio computer-assisted self-interviewing (ACASI) technology in the MEC for use in asking sensitive questions. For example, sample persons use ACASI, in privacy via touch screen and headphones, to respond to questions about illicit use of drugs and sexual behavior. The participant can hear the questions through the headphones or read them on a screen and then enter a response, using the keyboard or a touch screen.

Data Editing

As we have previously indicated, one of the most important aspects of ISIS is more efficient and timely data release. In part, this efficiency and timeliness is a product of reducing the data preparation work needed to release data sets. This reduction in preparation work, in turn, is a result of bringing data collection and editing together within the NHANES 99+ CAPI instruments and MEC component subsystems. Editing can occur either at the record level or at some level of aggregation of individual records. It can also occur at many stages of a survey, from the data collection stage through the data summarization stage. When editing occurs at the point of collection, where a participant is available for consultation, the result is fewer errors and less office editing.[13,14]

NHANES 99+ uses two types of automated CAPI and MEC component subsystem edits:

- Hard edits resulting from a user's attempt to enter a value that is inconsistent with the domain defined and approved by NCHS. For example, if, during the blood pressure exam, the examiner attempts to enter a diastolic value higher than the systolic value, the system automatically requires the examiner to correct the values.
- Soft edits stem from the ability of an interviewer to override a warning message and enter a value inconsistent with the domain or constraints defined and approved by NCHS. For example, skin fold measurements higher than the 99th percentile applicable to NHANES III data delineate the soft edit range. Values entered outside this range cause a soft edit warning message to be triggered; the examiner must either modify the value entered or else override the system to accept the value.

If there is a determination of an error after data collection is completed, there is a process for correcting the data directly in the database, outside the originating subsystem. For instance, suppose a participant recalls answering a question improperly in the MEC interview and wants to correct the response after the exam data have been submitted. In such a case, the field staff can document the change and forward a request to the data collection contractor. The data collection contractor provides a written description of the change and asks NCHS for approval to make the change in the database. In this manner, the edits are documented in the event that they must be deleted at a later date.

Meta-data and Item-Naming Conventions

Increases in the variety and uses of data create a need to formalize the manner of describing both the data and its uses. Business data is created, maintained, and accessed through business processes that are implemented through applications.[15(p52)] Simplistically, meta-data includes at least data about data (item meta-data) and data about processes (process meta-data). Process meta-data includes information automatically captured in computer-aided software engineering (CASE) tools.

Collected from many disparate sources, item meta-data are stored in the NHANES 99+ database. These meta-data serve a variety of functions. For instance, they allow for tracking of data changes over time, deriving new data from source data, maintaining detailed descriptions for each item, and automated generation of data documentation (e.g., data dictionaries or codebooks). Item meta-data for NHANES 99+ include the date at which the measurement or question is implemented, the database table the item resides in, the data type, a textual description of the item, historical information, applicable edits, the English and Spanish text of the question, instructions for asking the question, target age and gender group, response categories, skip patterns, and references to related data items. Figure 33.6 presents an example of the

Database Item Name	Version Info	Node Sequence	Target Population
DUQ060	1.3	89	Males/females 12- 19 years old

Database Table	SAS Label
ANL_DUQ	How old were you when you tried any form of cocaine, including crack or freebase for the first time?

Hard Edits	Soft Edits	Sybase Data Type	SAS Data Type
0 – 120	<None>	Numeric	Numeric

English Text:	How old were you when you tried any form of cocaine, including crack or freebase for the first time?
English Instructions:	VERBAL INSTRUCTIONS TO PARTICIPANT: Please enter an age. ENTER AGE IN YEARS.
Response Categories:	999 = Don't know 777 = Refused (skip to question DUQ160)

FIGURE 33.6. A Subset of the NHANES 99+ metadata for one data item and the corresponding format in a data dictionary.

NHANES 99+ metadata for one item, together with the corresponding format in a data dictionary.

Such meta-data require the use of consistent standards not only in the information itself, but also in the naming of items. Although the database system being used, Sybase, supports relatively long item and table names, there is a limitation on the naming conventions that can be used, because the data eventually must be integrated with statistical software packages such as SAS. (SAS version 6 and earlier impose an eight-character item name length. SAS version 8 allows for 32 character item-name lengths.) To accommodate in-house and external users who have not migrated to new versions of SAS or to comparable packages, NHANES 99+ uses an eight-character item name.

In addition, an important part of the conventions used for item naming is that the name itself must impart a basic description of the item to the user. For example, if an item were named "ITEM0001," little information is immediately transferred to the user. Conversely, items such as "GENDER," "RACE," and "AGE" provide immediate recognition of the underlying data values. NHANES 99+ uses the first two characters of the item name to identify the general topic of the item (e.g., MEC component or questionnaire section), the third character identifies the mode of data collection, and the remaining positions in the item name more fully describe the data item. Thus, an item name is represented as T T M D D D D D, where "T" represents topic, "M" represents mode of data collection, and "D" represents a brief description of the measurement or question. Example item names are:

- DUQ060: Drug use question 060 from the household questionnaire: "How old were you when you tried any form of cocaine, including crack or freebase for the first time?"
- BPXSYS: Blood Pressure measurement from the MEC exam—systolic
- BPXDIA: Blood Pressure measurement from the MEC exam—diastolic
- MCQ010: Medical Condition question 010 from the household questionnaire: "Has a doctor or other health professional ever told {you/SP} that {you have/s/he/SP has} asthma?"

Network and Database Replication Architecture

The NHANES network is composed of several LANs that are connected to enterprise networks at NCHS/CDC and at the data collection contractor. The NHANES 99+ WAN consists of the following interconnected LANs:

- NCHS/NHANES headquarters LAN
- Data collection contractor NHANES headquarters LAN
- A LAN at each of the three MECs
- A LAN at each field office (FO)

Because a primary requirement of ISIS is to move data from the field back to NCHS within 24 hours of collection, ISIS employs a WAN to provide real-time data collection for most data. Once the network connection is open and data are collected in an MEC or a FO, the data are transmitted to the data collection contractor and to NCHS instantaneously. An exception is the household interview; data from this source are delivered to NCHS as soon as the interviewer uploads the case to the field office server.

On a macro level, the WAN operates by connecting the MEC to the FO and the FO to the data collection contractor. The MEC-to-FO connection is typically an integrated services data network (ISDN) connection operating at 64 kilobits per second. In the event of failure on the MEC-to-FO ISDN line, ISIS rolls over onto a standard analog line that operates at 56 kilobytes per second. The FO is connected to the data collection contractor by an asymmetric bidirectional frame-relay connection. The bandwidth from the FO to the data collection contractor is 64 kilobits per second and 128 kilobits per second in the opposite direction. Should the bandwidth requirements of the survey change, the capacity in either direction can be incrementally modified. In addition, there are redundant ISDN and analog lines connecting the data collection contractor to the FO in the event of a failure of the frame-relay. These lines are also configured for automatic rollover. The data collection contractor is connected to NCHS by a dedicated T1 line operating at 1.5 megabits per second. Figure 33.7 provides an overview of the NHANES 99+ network architecture.

This network architecture supports the replication of data between the field sites and the contractor facilities and NCHS. The data moving from the field to NCHS and to the data collection contractor reside in highly normal-

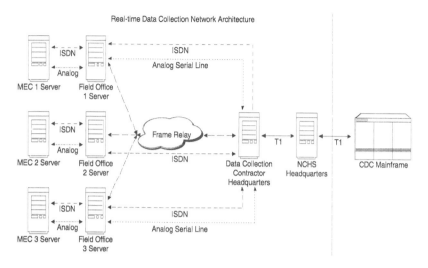

FIGURE 33.7. The NHANES 99+ network architecture.

ized relational databases that use the Sybase relational database management system (RDBMS). This database is called the "collection" database. Primarily computer specialists use the collection database due to the complexity of an RDBMS, the knowledge needed of the underlying database model, and the experience needed in the structured query language (SQL) used to query the database. Conversely, most analysts at NCHS are not familiar with an RDBMS, with database models, or with SQL, but are very experienced with analytic software tools such as SAS.

In the past, most analysts at NCHS have been using SAS housed on an IBM mainframe to perform processing. For the first year of the survey, all data sets were processed on a regular schedule and converted to SAS data sets that were migrated to the mainframe. Although this method satisfied the analysts, keeping up with the data processing requirements necessary for this data migration to occur, quickly became a heavy burden. Moreover, it is not reasonable to expect analysts to convert to the database environment for their work. In fact they would lose much of their capability if they relied on the structured query language (SQL), rather than on statistical packages such as SAS, to perform their analyses.

For this reason, NCHS designed a second or "analytic" database for use by analysts. This second database is essentially a denormalized and flattened version of the collection database. In essence, the tables have been restructured so that extensive joins are unnecessary. By using PC SAS (which is very similar to mainframe SAS) and SAS Access, analysts can connect directly to the analytic database to support micro and macro editing, research, QA/QC processing, and data release. This reliance on tools that are already familiar to the analysts significantly reduced the learning curve and transition time.

Data Systems Security and Protection

The recent wave of e-mail viruses and network attacks has forced IT programs to take a much more aggressive security stance. Protecting assets such as ISIS requires careful planning and the development of policies and procedures. The threats to ISIS can be both internal and external to the organization, and they can vary in impact. Table 33.6 provides a listing of some of the internal and external threats.[16]

These threats pose potential risks to NHANES 99+ network service, servers, desktop systems, physical office space, and to the MECs and laboratory

TABLE 33.6. NHANES 99+ internal and external security threats

Description	Internal or External
1. Inappropriate access to or disclosure of confidential data	Internal
2. Unauthorized modification or deletion of survey data	Internal
3. Disclosure of personal user accounts or passwords	Internal
4. Downloading of confidential data to unapproved media or machines	Internal
5. Failure to secure equipment or computer rooms	Internal
6. Workstations lacking appropriate security such as screensavers	Internal
7. Lack of a robust database and server backup and recovery program	Internal
8. Breaching of the network, firewalls, routers	Internal/External
9. Interception of sensitive data transmitted through e-mail	Internal/External
10. Introduction of virus infected e-mail into workstations and servers	Internal/External
11. Unauthorized entry into NHANES work areas	Internal/External
12. Network attack	Internal/External

equipment. To reduce risk, NHANES has defined and implemented security policies and procedures. These policies and procedures range from the mundane, such as the removal of modems and floppy disks on laptop and desktop computers, to more sophisticated methods of detecting intrusions and probing the network and systems for vulnerabilities. Following are some of the security risks and the associated preventative measures instituted in ISIS:

1. Threats to network service: NHANES 99+ maintains redundant connections to the field. Primary service consists of a frame-relay network with backup ISDN and analog communications. In the event of failure on the frame-relay network, there is an automatic rollover to ISDN or analog service. This system has proved to be extremely effective with little downtime.
2. Threats to databases and systems: to alleviate shutting operations down because of system failure, the system uses redundant servers and uninterruptible power supplies (UPS). The UPS have a three-hour charge to insure clean power; shutdown procedures; and a messaging system to alert staff in the event of a power failure. The servers on the MEC are configured so that a backup server automatically comes into operation in the event of a failure of the primary server. Each of the servers contains a redundant array of independent disks (RAID) configured with mirroring. This arrangement prevents loss of data in the event of a disk failure. Power failures have occurred and disks have failed, but the UPS and systems have worked as planned, without loss of data or downtime.
3. Threats to desktop systems: standard desktop PCs are deployed for examination components so that the survey is not dependent on proprietary solutions (with the exception of specialized biomedical equipment). In addition, software is developed within a standard software development environment to insure consistency across all systems. Each system is connected to a small UPS to insure clean power and a safe shutdown in the event of a major failure.
4. The threat of a physical break-in to the MECs: the MECs have a security system that automatically contacts local police and appropriate staff in the event of a break-in or fire. The MEC is also monitored for temperature and humidity changes. Certain locations use on-site security to protect resources.
5. The threat of laboratory equipment failure: because collected blood samples must be refrigerated on-site before shipment, freezers are connected to temperature monitors to help insure the equipment is operating properly. In the event of freezer failure, the system notifies appropriate staff so that the likelihood of sample loss is minimized.
6. The threat of viruses: to reduce the risk from viruses, several systems, policies, and procedures have been implemented. First, field systems do not have e-mail capability. In addition, desktop systems and servers are regularly scanned for viruses. The development environment at the data collection contractor does allow for e-mail service, but it uses an antivirus

package for protection. In addition, email and other services are not allowed over the dedicated T-1 connecting NCHS to the data collection contractor.

7. The threat of network attacks: ISIS utilizes a WAN that is connected to NCHS, contractor corporate offices, the MECs, and the FOs. In the event of an attack on corporate facilities, ISIS can be disconnected from these resources either physically or logically. The NCHS and the contractor corporate offices can disconnect themselves from the field in the event that the NHANES 99+ network experiences an attack. NCHS staff members routinely scan and probe the network to detect potential vulnerabilities. In addition, the routers and servers utilize several layers of protection to reduce the likelihood of an attack.

8. Threats to contractor and NCHS staff desktop computers: these systems are protected with virus scanning software at the desktop and server level, and they have screensaver password protection and LAN and e-mail passwords. The physical space is protected with keycard access systems and door locks. Passwords are routinely checked to insure that they cannot be easily cracked.

Principles Guiding the Integration of Components into the Health Examination

In the coming years of NHANES 99+, some examination components will be dropped, and other components will either modified or supplemented. The MEC and ISIS have been developed to allow for this flexibility. Integrating new components into the health examination requires considerable planning and analysis. Table 33.7 provides a set of guidelines constituting criteria to be used in determining whether to add components.

TABLE 33.7. NHANES 99+ guidelines for adding components

Guideline
1. Public health relevance
2. Reliable and validated instrument
3. Cost
4. Complexity and implementation of the protocol
5. Time to complete the examination
6. Adherence to IT standards for hardware interfacing and software development
7. Easily integrated into the information architecture

An example will demonstrate the complexity of modifying or introducing a new component to the exam. As is well documented, melanoma is on the rise in the United States.[17] In particular, dysplastic nevus (abnormal mole) is understood to be a precursor to melanoma,[18] and to date no national study has been conducted to establish the prevalence of this condition. Therefore, NHANES 99+ is a good vehicle to assess the magnitude of this public health issue. Because of the tight labor market for dermatologists, it is impractical to put a dermatologist in the MEC and keep him or her in the field for several years. Therefore, NCHS had to consider alternatives for an NHANES 99+ dermatology exam.

During the NHANES 99+ pretest in 1998, the use of existing computer technology and digital cameras for the dermatology component was evaluated. This study showed that the camera equipment had insufficient resolution and was extremely slow at capturing and delivering the data. Compounding the problem was that the image quality was deemed insufficient for diagnosis.[19] In light of these findings, the dermatology component was not included in the exam until reliable means for capturing the data were found. The NCHS staff, working in partnership with the National Cancer Institute and the National Institute of Arthritis, Musculoskeletal and Skin Diseases, recently conducted a formal validation study to evaluate the relevant issues. Results of this study are pending.

Superficially, it appears relatively simple to take several digital images of a participant. However, several constraints make the use of digital images a difficult protocol. First, the pictures are taken in an MEC exam room with limited space, because the room also accommodates the anthropometry component. This crowding limits the distance of the subject from the camera, the type of lighting that can be used, and the location of flash units. In addition, because a mole can be as small as five millimeters, a high-resolution digital camera must be used to retain sufficient information to review the image. This requirement translates to larger image files, more disk space, and longer data transmission time between the digital camera and the computer. However, even these considerations do not account for the difficulty of taking a "good" picture or for the challenge of doing so within a short time frame (several minutes). Moreover, the participant does not return to the trailer in the event that the data collected is of poor quality. Because there is only one visit to the MEC, it is imperative that the component be relatively easy to administer, repeatable, capable of producing high quality data, and capable of being standardized.

The dermatology component of the exam must also lend itself to standardization, because national prevalence estimates are established with this data. Another consideration is that this component must be completed quickly to avoid interference with the efficiency of MEC operations. After all, there are many exams in the MEC, and there is the possibility of substantial wait time if a session has many participants, because a person can be blocked from an exam while another participant is being examined. An overarching goal is to reduce the time burden on the participant by restricting the time of each exam. In the case of dermatology, eight minutes is allotted to snap, download, review, and, if necessary, re-shoot the pictures. Thus, the protocol must be straightforward and simple to administer without taking an inordinate amount of time.

The validation study for the procedure of adding dysplastic nevus as a condition to the NHANES 99+ included the use of a newer high-resolution digital camera with a faster connection between the camera and workstation. This innovation resulted in taking fewer pictures, because more skin area could be captured in one shot, and faster movement of the data to the PC. From a purely operational standpoint, the new equipment and procedures will make addition of the component possible. However, the images from the validation study must be read and compared to the in-person readings to determine whether using digital equipment is as reliable as in-person diagnosis. If the agreement is high, then this component will enter the exam.

Discussion and Conclusion

The diverse nature of NHANES data attracts a wide variety of users who evaluate health issues and prospectively influence policy and national health priorities. Some of the primary users of NHANES and NHES data have been researchers in public health. The richness of the NHANES data sets extends the usage beyond the public health community to include industry, other government agencies, policy makers, and students. While the NHANES data are particularly important for evaluating the nation's health, they are also being used for information technology research and development.

For example, during NHANES II and III, x-ray films were taken of the cervical spine, lumbar spine, hands, and knees, resulting in over 27,000 films. The logistics involved with using the x-ray films can be overwhelming. Shipping and receiving these films and film degradation resulting from environmental conditions all combine to discourage wide access to these data.[20] In fact, the films have been borrowed from the NCHS record center only nine times since 1974 (J. Findlay, National Center for Health Statistics, private communications, July 1994).

Yet, there was an obvious need for wider access to the film data. In response to this need, the cervical and lumbar spine films have been digitized and are now available on the Internet through the National Library of Medicine.[21] This unique data resource has spun off numerous avenues for research, including determining optimal scan resolution for digitizing hand x-ray films,[22] image compression,[23] and Internet image archives.[24] In short, NHANES has stimulated research in seemingly unrelated areas.

Integral to NHANES 99+ is the infusion of information technology to meet the objective of releasing high-quality data in a reasonable timeframe. To meet this objective, administrators have invested substantial resources in the creation of ISIS, including devoting significant time in early stands to identify and correct problems with the system and training staff in its use. One of the most important advantages of the technology is the reduction in data errors and in the time needed to prepare a data set for public release. The data edits built directly into the software permit data to be available almost immediately over the NHANES 99+ WAN. The real-time nature of NHANES 99+ makes intervention and feedback a real possibility, because QA/QC can be accomplished sooner.

These improvements come with a price, however, in the form of heavier reliance on higher skill levels of the employees who operate NHANES 99+. For example, the high reliance on technology and the complexity of ISIS require a higher degree of skill on the part of interviewers and examiners than was necessary for operation of the pen-and-paper methods that were used in previous surveys. In addition, the complexity of this system requires highly skilled computer programmers, database modelers, and system and network administrators. In this economy, these people are in high demand, a fact that makes it difficult to recruit and retain staff. It is our belief that the spirit of the project, the challenge of the work, and the visibility and importance of the work have resulted in relatively low staff turnover.

The up-front work in designing the ISIS database, network architecture, and meta-data has resulted in a framework with flexibility for future changes and technology transfer. We envision an innovative approach to future data collection, an approach that uses smaller, self-contained mobile examination units in defined population NHANES (Community-HANES) studies. This development, in turn, will allow for the assessment of public health issues in smaller and more specific communities. Many of the existing component subsystems, the network architecture, and the database design could be used with Community-HANES. Thus, the ideas, systems, and processes currently used will help drive the design of future health examination surveys.

Questions for Review

1. List the key differences between NHANES 99+ and previous surveys, and explain how these differences represent the value of the application of informatics to public health.
2. Describe the features of NHANES 99+ that provide for the privacy, confidentiality, and security of individual health information. How has the application of informatics contributed to the effectiveness of these features?
3. Explain how NHANES 99+ addresses sampling error and nonsampling error. How has automation of error detection contributed to the accuracy of NHANES 99+ data?
4. Explain why proper examiner training is important to NHANES 99+. Why is examiner skill level important, and what errors could result without inter- and intra-technician reliability?

5. Explain the difference between quality assurance (QA) and quality control (QC) in the NHANES 99+ survey. What issues do each address?
6. How do participants in NHANES 99+ receive the survey results related to them, and what provisions are made to safeguard access to sensitive information related to sexually transmitted diseases? How does NHANES 99+ address participant reluctance to divulge sensitive lifestyle information to interviewers?
7. Explain why data from external laboratories are not available in real time in NHANES 99+.
8. How does ISIS use an Intranet?
9. Describe the data editing features of ISIS. At what point can data be edited? To what extent does automation contribute to better editing practices?
10. Describe how NHANES incorporates consistent standards in the naming of items. Why are these item-naming standards necessary?
11. Describe the ways in which NHANES 99+ addresses (a) internal and (b) external security threats.

References

1. Looker A, Dallman P, Carroll M, Gunter E, Johnson C. Prevalence of iron deficiency in the United States. *JAMA* 1997;277:973–976.
2. Looker AC, Orwoll ES, Johnston CC, et al. Prevalence of low femoral bone density in older U.S. adults from NHANES III. *J Bone Mine Res* 1997;12:1761–1768.
3. Ogden C, Troiano R, Briefel R, Kuczmarski R, Flegal K, Johnson C. Prevalence of overweight among preschool children in the United States, 1971–1994. *Pediatrics.* 1997;99:E1.
4. Ernst N, Sempos C, Briefel R, Clark M. Consistency between US dietary fat intake and serum total cholesterol concentration: The NHANES Surveys. *Am J Clin Nutr* 1997;66(Suppl):956S–972S.
5. Centers for Disease Control and Prevention. National Center for Health Statistics. 2000 CDC Growth Charts: United States. Available at: http://www.cdc.gov/growthcharts/. Accessed April 4, 2002.
6. The Blaise System Homepage. Available at: http://neon.vb.cbs.nl/blaise/. Accessed April 4, 2002.
7. Sybase. Building International Applications with PowerBuilder 5 and 6. Available at: http://my.sybase.com/detail?id=47737. Accessed April 4, 2002.
8. Whitney C, Lind B, Wahl P. Quality assurance and quality control in longitudinal studies. *Epidemiol Rev* 1998;20:71–80.
9. Liepins G, Uppuluri V. *Data Quality Control: Theory and Pragmatics.* New York: Marcel Dekker; 1990.
10. Foreman, E. *Survey Sampling Principles.* New York: Marcel Dekker; 1991.
11. Knowles M, Holton E, Swanson R, eds. *The Adult Learner: The Definitive Classic in Adult Education and Human Resource Development.* 5th Edition. Houston, TX: Gulf Publishing Co.; 1998.
12. Perloff D, Grim C, Flack J, et al. Human blood pressure determination by sphygmomanometry. *Circulation* 1993;88:2460–2469.

13. Pierzchala M. Business survey methods. In: Cox BG, Binder DA, Chinnappa BN, eds. *Business Survey Methods*. New York: John Wiley & Sons; 1995:425–441.
14. Pierzchala M. A review of the state of the art in automated data editing and imputation. *Journal of Official Statistics* 1990;6:355–377.
15. Devlin B. *Data Warehouse from Architecture to Implementation*. Boston, MA: Addison-Wesley Longman; 1997:41–62.
16. Evans L. DHES/IMB Database Security Study. Internal Report to the Division of Health Examination Statistics/Information Management Branch. Centers for Disease Control and Prevention, Hyattsville, MD. August 2000.
17. Notice to readers: National Melanoma/Skin Cancer Detection and Prevention Month—May 2000. *MMWR Morb Mortal Wkly Rep* 2000;49:354.
18. Koh H, Geller A, Miller D, Lew R. Can screening for melanoma and skin cancer save lives. *Dermatol Clin* 1991;9:795–803.
19. Ostchega Y, Berman L. Preliminary Findings from the NHANES 99 Pilot Test Dermatology Component. Internal Report to the Division of Health Examination Statistics. Centers for Disease Control and Prevention, Hyattsville, MD. December 1998.
20. Berman L, Long L, Thoma G. Challenges in providing general access to digitzed xrays over the Internet. In: *Proceedings of the 23rd AIPR Workshop*, October 12–14, 1994, Washington, DC; 1994:2368–2422.
21. National Library of Medicine Web site. Available at: http://archive.nlm.nih.gov/. Accessed April 4, 2002.
22. Ostchega Y, Rodney L, Gin-Hua G, et al. Establishing the level of digitization for wrist and hand radiographs for the Third National Health and Nutrition Examination Survey (NHANES III). *J Digit Imaging* 1998;11:116–120.
23. Berman L, Long L, Pillemer S. Effects of quantization table manipulation on JPEG compression of cervical radiographs. Presented at the Society for Information Display, 1993 International Symposium, Seminar and Exhibition; Seattle, Washington; May 16–21, 1993.
24. Thoma G, Long L, Berman L. A client/server system for Internet access to biomedical text/image databanks. *Comput Med Imaging Graph* 1996;20:259–268.

34
Epilogue: The Future of Public Health Informatics

William A. Yasnoff, Patrick W. O'Carroll, Denise Koo, Robert W. Linkins, and Edwin M. Kilbourne

Learning Objectives

After studying this chapter, you should be able to:

- List and explain the three major challenges that public health informatics must address if the discipline is to be of maximum benefit to public health practice
- Explain why agreement on data and communications standards, along with policies to support data sharing and mechanisms and tools for accessing and disseminating data and information in a useful manner, are essential prerequisites to development of coherent, integrated national public health information systems
- List and define the steps that public health leaders must take in order to expand the practice and maximize the benefits of public health informatics

Overview

The future and the promise of public health informatics depends upon public health's ability to address three grand challenges. These challenges are developing coherent, integrated national public health information systems; developing closer integration between public health and clinical care; and addressing pervasive concerns about the impact of information technology on confidentiality and privacy. That future and promise also depend upon the ability of leaders in public health to promote recognition of the need for public health informatics at all levels and to provide the necessary training and the physical infrastructure/architecture to support effective practice of the discipline. The new and evolving discipline of public health informatics is the key to systematically and scientifically exploiting an opportunity to benefit the public's health.

The extent to which informatics will continue to improve, indeed transform, the practice of public health will be determined by the ability of public health professionals to address some major challenges to the discipline. It will also depend on the willingness of the leadership in public health to recognize the need for public health informatics and provide the necessary training and the physical infrastructure/architecture for its use.

Major Challenges for Public Health Informatics

Although there are numerous ways in which information science and technology can improve public health practice, there are three areas that represent grand challenges for public health informatics. These areas are (1) developing coherent, integrated national public health information systems; (2) developing closer integration between public health and clinical care; and (3) addressing pervasive concerns about the impact of information technology on confidentiality and privacy.

Developing Coherent, Integrated National Public Health Information Systems

One major goal of public health informatics is ensuring the capacity to assess community problems in a comprehensive manner through the development of integrated nationwide public health data systems. Developing such a capacity will require a clear definition of public health data needs and the sources for these data, consensus on data and communications standards—to facilitate data quality, comparability, and exchange—and establishment of policies to support data sharing, along with mechanisms and tools for accessing and disseminating data and information in a useful manner.

Because electronic reporting will increasingly form the basis for surveillance systems, developmental efforts must also address issues such as unambiguously defining the specific medical conditions that trigger various types of automated data transmissions, working with reporting organizations to ensure that they have appropriate software and electronic communications capabilities, and ensuring that there is adequate capacity for analysis of the tremendously increased volumes of public health data that are anticipated.

Agreement on standards is particularly challenging because of the diverse needs of the many groups who record and use health information, including providers, payers, administrators, researchers, and public health officials. As Daniel B. Jernigan, Jac Davies, and Alan Sim have pointed out in Chapter 11, most of the coding systems and standards currently in use have not previously taken into account public health data needs, and public health's interests are not uniformly regarded as consistent with the business needs of other organizations.[1]

However, the Health Insurance Portability and Accountability Act of 1996 (HIPAA) mandates that the Secretary of the Department of Health and Human

Services (HHS) adopt data standards for the electronic transmission of administrative and financial data related to health care (see http://aspe.os.dhhs.gov/admnsimp and Chapter 19). This legislation and the recent release of the final regulation by HHS have provided the impetus for various standards development organizations and terminology groups to work collaboratively to harmonize their separate systems. Recognizing the importance of standards, several programs at the Centers for Disease Control and Prevention (CDC) are actively involved with the established standards development organizations (SDOs), such as Health Level 7 (HL7). For example, the National Center for Injury Prevention and Control is coordinating a national effort to develop uniform specifications for data entered in emergency department patient records.[2] In addition, CDC has embarked on several agency-wide standards-related activities through its Health Information and Surveillance Systems Board (HISSB), including proposing HL7 standards for data elements important to public health and ensuring that the views of all our public health partners are represented at the SDOs.

Developing Closer Integration Between Public Health and Clinical Care

A second major challenge for public health informatics is facilitating the improved exchange of information between public health and clinical care. Much of the data in public health information systems still comes from forms filled out by hand, which are later computer-coded. Even where reporting is electronic, initial data entry is typically still manual. This results in serious underreporting of many reportable diseases and conditions.[3]

Data need to flow automatically to public health from clinical and laboratory information systems. When these data are appropriately compiled by public health information systems, they should allow more rapid and accurate assessments and disease control responses, as well as the formulation of improved clinical guidelines and interventions. Conversely, automated presentation to clinicians of prevention guidelines has been shown to improve clinical care,[4] and there are numerous other ways in which the skills and activities of the public health community (e.g., community outreach) could work to the benefit of clinical care. Electronic information sharing and data exchange provide the means by which we can better integrate public health and clinical care activities, but a great deal of creativity and hard work are needed to take full advantage of these opportunities.

Addressing Pervasive Concerns About the Impact of Information Technology on Confidentiality and Privacy

Finally, as numerous chapters in this book have pointed out, privacy, confidentiality, and security are pervasive and persistent challenges to progress in public health informatics. Information systems are correctly perceived by the public to be a double-edged sword—whatever is done to make integrated, comprehensive information more easily available for laudable and worthwhile purposes must of necessity create new opportunities for misuse. Public health often collects extremely sensitive personal medical information that has the potential for tremendous harm if improperly disclosed. Federal legislation that provides a fair and workable balance between individual privacy and the common good is needed to both reassure the public and establish legal guidelines for handling sensitive information. Although HIPAA will provide confidentiality standards for all health plans (including Medicare and Medicaid), clearinghouses, and providers who use electronic data, public health agencies need to adopt and enforce confidentiality policies that incorporate fair information practices,[5] and utilize state-of-the-art security measures to implement those policies.

Although public health has had an excellent record of information protection in the past, recent inappropriate releases of information and the lack of uniformly stringent policies across the nation are cause for concern.[6] To ensure successful information system development, public health informatics practitioners must therefore be fully cognizant of these issues and prepared with methodologies and technologies for addressing them effectively—for instance, through effective de-identification of data at the earliest possible opportunity in the aggregation process.

Maximizing the Contribution of Informatics to Public Health

Finally, if informatics is to deliver maximum benefit to the practice of public health, public health leaders must recognize the need for public health informatics and provide the necessary training and the physical infrastructure/architecture necessary for its effective use.

Recognition of the Need for Public Health Informatics

The field of informatics is still unfamiliar to most public health professionals. In consequence, public health leaders and others responsible for information systems and technology decisions are often not fully cognizant of the basic sciences of this discipline and the accumulated experience available. Without such awareness, the public health community has only recently begun to appreciate (for example) the need for both data standards and for a comprehensive information architecture for public health. This has contributed to the development of the current patchwork quilt of incompatible or nonintegrated surveillance and data systems found in public health agencies at every level.

The rapid evolution and widespread dissemination of general-purpose data management software and categorically focused public health surveillance and information systems has resulted in substantial exposure to the benefits of information technology without a complete appreciation of the underlying principles and practices required to successfully develop comprehensive integrated data systems that bridge programmatic boundaries. The ease of creating small, single-purpose systems tends to mask the inherent complexities of large-scale information system development, such as the need for well-informed planning and broad consensus. One of the main tasks of leaders in public health informatics is coordination and consensus building regarding the types of systems that should be developed and how they will interoperate.

Providing Training

Because information technology is now a critical part of the armamentarium of public health, some level of informatics training for both new and existing practitioners is essential. Just as every public health worker needs a basic knowledge of epidemiology, a basic understanding of public health informatics is now a necessity for effective practice in the information age. A deeper level of informatics training is needed by public health leaders and managers to successfully tackle their decision-making and management responsibilities with regard to information systems development projects. Hopefully, such understanding will improve reported systems development failure rates, currently in the 30% range.[7,8] Finally, a cadre of public health informaticians with comprehensive training and experience in both public health and informatics is needed to serve in leadership, research, and teaching roles, such as chief information officers for state public health agencies and informatics faculty at schools of public health.

The competencies and knowledge needed for a public health informatician include an understanding of the respective roles and domains of information technology (IT) and public health team members; the ability to develop and use an IT architecture; a working knowledge of information system development, networking, and database design; familiarity with data standards; a clear understanding of privacy and confidentiality issues, as well as security technologies; and skills in IT planning and procurement, IT leadership, managing change, communication, and systems evaluation research. Curricula are needed for developing these competencies at a basic level for the entire public health workforce, an intermediate level for public health managers and leaders, and an advanced level for public health informatics specialists and researchers. CDC has made some initial efforts to develop the needed educational programs through the public health informatics fellowship (see http://www.cdc.gov/epo/dphsi/informat.htm), the public health informatics course,[9] and a cooperative effort with the National Library of Medicine to help train public health workers in the effective use of the information resources available on the Internet. Eleven public health graduate programs in the United States already offer an informatics course, and an additional 13 are planning to do so within the next two years,[10] and cooperative efforts are underway to define informatics performance standards as part of the National Public Health Performance Standards program.[11] These and other efforts should continue and be expanded to address the public health informatics training needs of the current and future public health workforce.

Providing the Physical Infrastructure/Architecture

A prerequisite to the widespread use of powerful new information applications is the pervasive deployment throughout the public health system of modern computers that are interconnected through a standards-based network. In recent years, substantial progress has been made towards that goal. Beginning with the Information Network for Public Health Officials (INPHO)[12] and continuing with the Health Alert Network component of the bioterrorism preparedness initiative, CDC has made systematic efforts to improve the nation's public health telecommunications, information, and distance learning infrastructure by promoting Internet connectivity and other information infrastructure for state and local public health workers. Several other federal agencies (e.g., the National Library of Medicine) have also provided funds to promote Internet connectivity and use, and many state and local health departments have invested substantial resources of their own into computing and network technology.

In the private sector, the Robert Wood Johnson Foundation has awarded more than $20 million to develop immunization tracking systems, and others have joined this effort, including the Annie E. Casey, Wellness, Skillman, Flinn, and David and Lucile Packard Foundations.[13] Although less than half of all public health workers currently have modern, Internet-connected computers on their desks,[14] recent progress toward this goal has been remarkable. Just five years ago, for example, the computing and networking environment was such that most state and local public health professionals had never used e-mail. Today in many states, e-mail has become an indispensable communications tool used for every aspect of public health. We need to continue to expand our efforts until the entire public health system has a modern information, communications, and distance learning infrastructure supporting all critical public health data and information systems.

Conclusion

The confluence of improved information systems and technologies, new challenges to the public health system, and changes in the medical care system presents a unique opportunity not only to improve the efficiency and effectiveness of public health practice, but to transform fundamentally some aspects of public health practice itself. We believe the new and evolving discipline of public health informatics is the key to systematically and scientifically exploiting this opportunity to the benefit of the public's health.

Questions for Review

1. Explain why a consensus on data and communications standards is a prerequisite to development of integrated nationwide public health data systems.
2. Why is agreement on standards in public health data systems particularly challenging?
3. Explain the benefits to (a) public health and (b) clinical care of improving the exchange of information between public and clinical health care settings.
4. Why does maintaining privacy, confidentiality, and security remain a pervasive and persistent challenge to progress in public health informatics? What steps does public health need to take to address these issues?
5. To what extent have the rapid evolution and widespread dissemination of general-purpose management software and categorically focused public health surveillance and information systems resulted in the failure of public health professionals to develop a complete appreciation of the underlying principles and practices of public health informatics?
6. List at least five competencies and/or knowledge mastery fields required of a public health informatician.
7. Explain how the leadership in public health can contribute to the development of the physical infrastructure/architecture required for effective practice of public health informatics.

References

1. Harman J. Topics for our times: New health care data—new horizons for public health. *Am J Public Health* 1998;88:1019–1021.
2. National Center for Injury Prevention and Control. *Data Elements for Emergency Departments Systems (DEEDS), Release 1.0.* Atlanta, GA: Centers for Disease Control and Prevention; 1997.
3. Thacker SB, Berkelman RL. Public health surveillance in the United States. *Epidemiol Rev* 1988;10:164–190.
4. Elson RB, Connelly, DP. Computerized patient records in primary care: Their role in mediating guideline-driven physician behavior change. *Arch Fam Med* 1995;4:698–705.
5. Secretary's Advisory Committee on Automated Personal Data Systems. *Records, Computers, and the Rights of Citizens.* Washington DC: US Department of Health, Education, and Welfare; 1973.
6. O'Brien, DG, Yasnoff WA. Privacy, confidentiality, and security in information systems of state health agencies. *Am J Prev Med* 1999;16:351–358.
7. The Standish Group International, Inc. *Chaos: Charting the Seas of Information Technology.* Dennis, MA: Standish Group; 1994.
8. Southon FCG, Sauer C, Dampney CNG. Information technology in complex health services: Organizational impediments to successful technology transfer and diffusion. *J Am Med Inform Assoc* 1997;4:112–124.

9. O'Carroll PW, Yasnoff WA, Wilhoite W. Public health informatics: A CDC course for public health program managers *Proc AMIA Symp* 1998;472–476

10. Richards, J. *Informatics Training in Schools and Graduate Programs of Public Health.* MPH Thesis, Houston, TX: University of Texas-Houston Health Science Center; 1998.

11. Halverson PK, Nicola RM, Baker EL. Performance measurement and accreditation of public health organizations: A call to action. *J Public Health Manage Pract* 1998;4:5–7.

12. Baker EL, Friede A, Moulton AD, Ross DA. CDC's Information Network for Public Health Officials (INPHO): A framework for integrated public health information and practice. *J Public Health Manage Pract* 1995;1:43–47.

13. Watson B, Saarlas K, Hearn R, Russell R. The All Kids Count national program: A Robert Wood Johnson initiative to develop immunization registries. *Am J Prev Med* 1997;13(Suppl 1):3–6.

14. National Association of County and City Health Officials. Information technology capacity and local public health agencies. *Res Brief* 1999;4:1–2.

Index

Health Informatics Series
(formerly Computers in Health Care)

(continued from page ii)

Public Health Informatics and Information Systems
P.W. O'Carroll, W.A. Yasnoff, M.E. Ward, L.H. Ripp,
and E.L. Martin

Advancing Federal Sector Health Care
A Model for Technology Transfer
P. Ramsaroop, M.J. Ball, D. Beaulieu, and J.V. Douglas

Medical Informatics
Computer Applications in Health Care and Biomedicine, Second Edition
E.H. Shortliffe and L.E. Perreault

Filmless Radiology
E.L. Siegel and R.M. Kolodner

Cancer Informatics
Essential Technologies for Clinical Trials
J.S. Silva, M.J. Ball, C.G. Chute, J.V. Douglas, C.P. Langlotz, J.C. Niland,
and W.L. Scherlis

Clinical Information Systems
A Component-Based Approach
R. Van de Velde and P. Degoulet

Knowledge Coupling
New Premises and New Tools for Medical Care and Education
L.L. Weed

Healthcare Information Management Systems
Cases, Strategies, and Solutions, Third Edition
M.J. Ball, C.A. Weaver, and J.M. Kiel

Organizational Aspects of Health Informatics, Second Edition
Managing Technological Change
N.M. Lorenzi and R.T. Riley

Made in the USA
Lexington, KY
30 December 2012